# Immunology and Liver

FALK SYMPOSIUM 114

# Immunology and Liver


Edited by

**M.P. Manns**
Abt. Gastroenterologie/Hepatologie
Zentrum Innere Medizin
Medizinische Hochscule Hannover
Carl-Neuberg Str. 1
D-30625 Hannover
Germany

**G. Paumgartner**
Medizinische Klinik II
Klinikum Grosshadern der LMU München
Marchioninistr. 15
D-81377 München
Germany

**U. Leuschner**
Abt. Gastroenterologie
Zentrum der Innere Medizin
Klinikum der Johann-Wolfgang-Goethe-Universität Frankfurt
Theodor-Stern-Kai 7
D-60596 Frankfurt
Germany


*Proceedings of the Falk Symposium 114 held in Basel, Switzerland, 20–21 October, 1999 (Part I of the Basel Liver Week 1999)*


**KLUWER ACADEMIC PUBLISHERS**
DORDRECHT / BOSTON / LONDON

Library of Congress Cataloging-in-Publication Data is available.

ISBN 978-0-7923-8759-6

---

Published by Kluwer Academic Publishers, BV
P.O. Box 17, 3300 AA Dordrecht, The Netherlands.

Sold and distributed in North, Central and South America
by Kluwer Academic Publishers,
101 Philip Drive, Norwell, MA 02018, USA.

In all other countries, sold and distributed
by Kluwer Academic Publishers, Distribution Center,
P.O. Box 322, 3300 AH Dordrecht, The Netherlands

*Printed on acid-free paper*



Printed and bound in Great Britain by MPG Books.

# Contents

# List of Principal Authors

**F. Alvarez**
Gastroentérologie
University of Montreal
Saint-Justine Hospital
3175 Côte Sainte-Catherine
Montreal
Quebec, H3T 1C5
Canada

**B. Arnold**
Molekulare Immunologie
Deutsches Krebsforschungszentrum
Im Neuenheimer Feld 280
D-69120 Heidelberg
Germany

**U. Beuers**
Medizinische Klinik II
Klinikum Grosshadern der LMU
München
Marchioninistr. 15
D-81377 München
Germany

**F.B. Bianchi**
Dipartimento di Medicina Interna, Cardioangiologia, Epatologia
Università degli Studi di Bologna
Policlinico S. Orsola
Via Massarenti 9
I-40138 Bologna
Italy

**U. Broomé**
Department of Gastroenterology and Hepatology
Huddinge University Hospital
Hälsovägen
S-14186 Huddinge
Sweden

**E.L.R. Cancado**
Disciplina de Gastroenterologia
Hospital Das Clinicas da Faculdade de Medicina da USP
Rua Dr. Enéas de Carvalho Aguiar – 255 – 9°. Andar, sala 9159
CEP-05403/000
São Paulo, Brazil

**R.W. Chapman**
Department of Gastroenterology
John Radcliffe Hospital
Headington
Oxford OX3 9DU
UK

**A.J. Czaja**
Gastroenterology and Hepatology
Mayo Clinic
200 First Street SW
Rochester
MN 55905–0001
USA

**P. Donaldson**
Centre for Liver Research
The School of Clinical Medical Sciences
University of Newcastle
Framlington Place
Newcastle-upon-Tyne
NE2 4HH
UK

**M.E. Gershwin**
Division of Rheumatology, Allergy and Clinical Immunology
University of California at Davis
TB 192, School of Medicine
Davis, CA 95616–8660
USA

**E. Gleichmann**
Abteilung für Immunologie und Allergologie
Medizinisches Institut für Umwelthygiene
Auf'm Hennekamp 50
D-40225 Düsseldorf
Germany

**J. Heathcote**
The Toronto Hospital
University of Toronto
West Wing 4-828, Western Division
399 Bathurst Street
Toronto
ON M5T 2S8
Canada

**S.G. Hübscher**
Department of Pathology
The Medical School
University of Birmingham
Birmingham B15 2TT
UK

**E.F. Johnson**
The Scripps Clinic Research Institute
Department of Molecular and Experimental Medicine
Division of Biochemistry, MEM 255
10550 North Torrey Pines Road
La Jolla, CA 92037
USA

**R. Joplin**
Liver Research Laboratories
University Hospital
Birmingham B15 2TH
UK

**M.J. Lenardo**
Laboratory of Immunology
NIH-NIAID
9000 Rockville Pike
Bldg. 10, Room 11D09
Bethesda, MD 20892
USA

**U. Leuschner**
Medizinische Klinik II
Zentrum der Inneren Medizin
Klinikum der Johann-Wolfgang-Goethe-Universität Frankfurt
Theodor-Stern-Kai 7
D-60596 Frankfurt
Germany

**A.W. Lohse**
I. Department of Medicine
Johannes Gutenberg-University
Langenbeckstr. 1
D-55131 Mainz
Germany

**B. Ludewig**
Institut für Experimentelle Immunologie
Departement für Pathologie
Universitätsspital
Schmelzbergstr. 12
CH-8091 Zürich
Switzerland

**I.G. McFarlane**
Institute of Liver Studies
King's College Hospital
Denmark Hill
London SE5 9RS
UK

**J. Neuberger**
The Liver Unit
The Queen Elizabeth Hospital
Queen Elizabeth Medical Centre
Edgbaston
Birmingham, B15 2TH
UK

**M. Nishioka**
Third Department of Internal Medicine
Kagawa Medical University
1750-1 Ikenobe Miki-cho
Kita-gun
Kagawa 761-0793
Japan

**P. Obermayer-Straub**
Abteilung Gastroenterologie und Hepatologie
Zentrum Innere Medizin
Medizinische Hochschule Hannover
Carl-Neuberg-Str. 1
D-30625 Hannover
Germany

**G.R. Pape**
Medizinische Klinik II
Klinikum Großhadern der LMU München
Marchioninistr. 15
D-81377 München
Germany

**D. Pessayre**
INSERM U481
Hôpital Beaujon
F-92118 Clichy
France

**R. Poupon**
Service d'Hépato-gastroentérologie
Hôpital Saint-Antoine
184 rue du Faubourg Saint-Antoine
F-75571 Paris Cedex 12
France

**C.P. Strassburg**
Department of Gastroenterology and Hepatology
Hannover Medical School
Carl-Neuberg-Str. 1
D-30625 Hannover
Germany

**E.M. Tan**
WM Keck Autoimmune Disease Center
The Scripps Research Institute
10550 North Torrey Pines Road
La Jolla, CA 92037
USA

**B. Terjung**
Departments of Medicine and of Anatomy and Cell Biology
College of Physicians and Surgeons
Columbia University
630 W 168th Street
P&S 10-518
New York, NY 10032
USA

**V.K. Tuohy**
Department of Immunology, NB30
Lerner Research Institute
The Cleveland Clinic Foundation
9500 Euclid Avenue
Cleveland OH 44195
USA

**D. Vergani**
Royal Free and University College Medical School
University College London,
Department of Medicine
Gower Street Campus, Harold Samuel House
69–75 Chenies Mews
London
UK

**J. Węsierska-Gądek**
Institute of Cancer Research
University of Vienna
Borschkegasse 8a
A-1090 Vienna
Austria

**H.J. Worman**
Departments of Medicine and of Anatomy and Cell Biology
College of Physicians and Surgeons
Columbia University
630 West 168th Street,
10th Floor, Room 508
New York, NY 10032
USA

# Section I
# Basic mechanisms of autoimmunity

# 1
# Autoimmunity and autoaggression

B. ARNOLD

## INTRODUCTION

An understanding of the processes that ensure self-protection against the self-destructive capacity of the immune system is essential for antigen-specific tolerance induction in the treatment of autoimmune diseases and in clinical transplantation. It is therefore of crucial importance to define the molecular identity of the microenvironment leading mature lymphocytes either to tissue destruction or to tolerance after antigen recognition. Numerous animal models have been established, and various mechanisms resulting in tolerance or autoaggression have been reported. The enormous accumulation of data, however, has led to confusion rather than to a generally agreed view on how tolerance is induced and maintained under physiological conditions, and which changes permit the onset of autoimmune diseases. This chapter therefore summarizes changes in the view of self-protection in the past and then describes a model system of tolerance and autoreactivity to self-antigens on parenchymal cells.

## CHANGES IN THE VIEW OF SELF-PROTECTION IN THE PAST

Autoreactive T cells are involved in most organ-specific autoimmune processes leading to tissue destruction. Burnet's clonal selection postulated that self-reactive T cells must be eliminated to ensure self-protection. This view was experimentally supported by demonstrating reactivity to alloantigens either by *in-vivo* graft rejection or *in-vitro* induction of cytotoxic T lymphocytes (CTL) and the absence of responses to self-major histocompatibility complex (MHC) antigens in both assay systems. The term 'tolerance' described the consequence of this selection process preventing the immune system from reacting destructively against self. Autoaggression, on the other hand, was seen as a result of insufficient negative selection in the thymus, and activation of autoreactive T cells was considered the decisive step for the onset of an autoimmune disease.

This view changed when non-deletional mechanisms of tolerance were observed. Induction of unresponsiveness/anergy was firstly described as a consequence of stimulating $CD4^+$ helper T cell clones *in vitro* with antigen in the absence of co-stimulatory signals provided by antigen-presenting cells (APC)[1]. It was therefore proposed that T cell activation requires signalling through the T cell receptor (signal 1) as well as through co-stimulatory receptors (signal 2)[2]. In the meantime it has become clear that the term 'non-responsiveness' is inadequate because anergic T cells are still capable of producing lymphokines upon antigen stimulation[3]. This reactivity is, however, missed if only proliferation and interleukin 2 (IL-2) secretion is tested. As only bone-marrow-derived cells have been shown to express co-stimulatory molecules autoreactive T cells may be silenced by tissue cells by encountering the respective antigen, and thereby receiving only signal 1. Indeed, expression of an antigen only on thymic epithelium or only on peripheral tissue resulted in non-deletional tolerance *in vivo*[4,5]. However, in some animal models *in-vivo* tolerance to a 'foreign' alloantigen present during ontogeny judged by skin graft acceptance was accomplished by CTL responses *in vitro* against this alloantigen[4,6]. Thus, reactivity or non-reactivity to a given self-antigen was dependent upon the test system clearly showing that *in-vitro* proliferation and CTL assay might not be indicative of the *in-vivo* situation. Following studies on lymphocyte migration in the adult sheep[7], it is now widely assumed that in general naive T cells do not gain access to peripheral non-lymphoid tissues, in contrast to activated/memory T cells which can migrate into tissues. Consequently it has been argued that extrathymically expressed tissue antigens are ignored by naive T cells[8]. T lymphocytes with self-destructive capacity frequently found in healthy individuals could therefore represent either naive T cells with no access to the respective antigen, or tolerant T cells originating from a non-deletional tolerance mechanism. It was assumed that normal activation of the naive cells or reversal of tolerance has to be prevented in order to avoid autoaggression.

This picture, too, was revised when several groups reported that tolerance could be the result of T cell activation, expansion, and, consequently, activation-induced cell death[9]. Furthermore, it was recently shown that self-antigens which are sufficiently highly expressed in intact peripheral organs of adult mice could be presented to CD8 T cells in the draining lymph nodes by bone-marrow-derived cells via an exogenous class I-restricted pathway[10]. This cross-presentation could lead to tolerance based on deletion of the respective T cells in the absence of T cell help. The nature of the APC performing the cross-presentation is unknown, but dendritic cells seem to be good candidates because they can take up apoptotic cells and efficiently present their antigens via MHC class I. Finally, studies on transplantation tolerance claimed that the direct presentation of alloantigens by tissue parenchymal cells is a 'null event' resulting neither in T cell activation nor in tolerance[11]. Based on these results the concept has emerged that peripheral T cells ignore tissue-specific antigens unless they are presented by professional APC in the lymphoid compartments.

However, several objections to this view can be raised. First, if all self-reactive T cells found in healthy individuals represented naive T cells which have not been deleted either by negative selection in the thymus or by cross-presentation in the regional lymph nodes it would be difficult to understand the acceptance of autografts. As is known from the HY system, for example, the difference in one antigenic determinant is sufficient to cause skin graft rejection. Secondly, most of the studies mentioned above used adult animals either by confronting mature T cells with exogenous antigen or by transferring T cells specific for constitutively expressed endogenous antigen. In both cases events occurring during neonatal life may be missed.

## CONTROL OF NEONATAL TOLERANCE BY T CELL TRAFFICKING

The demonstration of large-scale trafficking of virgin T cells through extra-lymphoid tissues in fetal sheep[12] and newborn rats[13] opened the possibility of a direct contact between naive T cells with tissue-specific self-antigens on parenchymal cells resulting in tolerance induction. We recently confirmed these results by comparing the homing pattern of transferred lymphocytes in newborns and adults[14].

To test whether differential T cell migration through neonatal versus adult tissue would influence tolerance induction to tissue-specific self-antigens, we used a transgenic mouse model expressing the MHC class I antigen $K^b$ under control of the constitutively expressed keratin IV promoter on skin keratinocytes[14]. Since we are studying the effect of this extrathymic antigen on T cells with a corresponding TCR recognizing only the intact but not a processed form of the $K^b$ antigen (Des-TCR), we are dealing with a truly sessile antigenic determinant. These Des-TCR × 2.4KerIV-$K^b$ mice accept $K^b$-positive grafts and are therefore functionally tolerant despite the presence of $K^b$-specific T cells. 2.4KerIV-$K^b$ mice were crossed onto the Rag-2-deficient background and reconstituted as neonates or adults with bone marrow from Des-TCR transgenic mice. After efficient repopulation of the lymphoid compartments tolerance could be observed only in the neonatally reconstituted mice and was not detectable in the adult recipients. When skin autografts from tails were replaced onto the lateral thoracic wall of adult chimeras these mice showed chronic rejection accompanied by hair loss and scar formation. Apparently the adult environment of the Des-TCR × 2.4KerIV-$K^b$ mice, in contrast to the neonate, does not allow tolerance induction to sessile antigens expressed on keratinocytes. Blockage of T cell migration neonatally with antibodies directed against P- and E-selectin prevented tolerance induction. Thus, parenchymal cells such as keratinocytes and T cell migration in the neonate contribute to the control of autoreactive T cells.

## HARMLESS AUTOREACTIVITY VERSUS CHRONIC AUTOAGGRESSION

As mentioned above, the adult 2.4KerIV-$K^b$ chimeras rejected an autotransplant. Nevertheless, other parts of the skin also expressing the $K^b$ autoantigen were not affected, suggesting that the presence of activated self-reactive T cells is not sufficient to cause tissue damage in an intact organ.

Similarly, $K^b$-specific T cells were still present in the tolerant Des-TCR × Alb-$K^b$ mice, expressing $K^b$ only on hepatocytes[6]. We therefore asked whether the observed tolerance could be reversed *in vivo* and whether this would result in autoaggression. When these mice were challenged with syngeneic tumour cells expressing simultaneously the $K^b$ autoantigen and IL-2, reversal of tolerance was indeed achieved[15]. However, when in addition to breaking tolerance Des-TCR × Alb-$K^b$ mice were infected with a liver-specific pathogen or injected with bacterial CpG oligonucleotides, autoaggression occurred. These findings show that inflammatory stimuli as induced by CpG oligonucleotides are sufficient for autoaggression and exclude the need for molecular mimicry. Thus, in these systems at least two independent steps seem to be required for organ-specific autoimmunity: reversal of peripheral tolerance leading to activation of autoreactive T cells, and conditioning of the organ microenvironment by so far undefined inflammatory processes which enable the activated T cells to cause tissue damage.

## CONCLUSIONS

Some of the present confusion in the field is due to the changes in the definition of tolerance and in the view of how autoimmune destruction occurs. As long as absence of autoaggression was linked to lack of the respective T cell reactivity the assumption was supported that T cell activation is always the decisive step for induction of autoimmune diseases. Now, however, there are several examples such as the above-mentioned chimeras rejecting an autotransplant which demonstrate that the presence of activated T cells and the respective target structure in an intact organ do not necessarily lead to tissue damage. Following the present terminology we call this animal non-tolerant because we detect T cell reactivity *in vivo*. However, if we agree that tolerance represents a 'physiological state in which the immune system does not react destructively against the organism that harbours it'[16], this animal is clearly tolerant, as it does not suffer from an autoimmune disease. This is not just a semantic problem. So far most of the research in the field has focused on the prevention of T cell activation. Processes controlling autodestruction beyond T cell activation have mainly been neglected, although they might be of value for therapeutic intervention.

### References


1. Lamb JR, Skidmore BJ, Green N, Chiller JM, Feldmann M. Induction of tolerance in influenza virus-immune T lymphocyte clones with synthetic peptides of influenza hemagglutinin. J Exp Med. 1983;157:1434–47.
2. Mueller DL, Jenkins MK, Schwartz RH. Clonal expansion versus functional clonal inactivation: a costimulatory signalling pathway determines the outcome of T cell antigen receptor occupancy. Annu Rev Immunol. 1989;7:445–80.
3. Kruisbeck AM, Amsen D. Mechanisms underlying T cell tolerance. Curr Opin Immunol. 1996;8:233–44.
4. Corbel C, Martin C, Ohki H, Coltey M, Hlozanek I, Le Douarin NM. Evidence for peripheral mechanisms inducing tissue tolerance during ontogeny. Int Immunol. 1990;2:33–40.
5. Schönrich G, Kalinke U, Momburg F *et al.* Downregulation of T cell receptors on self-reactive T cells as a novel mechanism for extrathymic tolerance induction. Cell. 1991;65:293–304.
6. Schönrich G, Momburg F, Malissen M *et al.* Distinct mechanisms of extrathymic T cell tolerance due to differential expression of self antigen. Int Immunol. 1992;4,5:581–90.
7. Mackay CR. Homing of naive, memory and effector lymphocytes. Curr Opin Immunol. 1993;5:423–7.
8. Zinkernagel RM, Ehl S, Aichele P, Oehen S, Kündig T, Hengartner H. Antigen localisation regulates immune responses in a dose and time-dependent fashion: a geographical view of immune reactivity. Immunol Rev. 1997;156:199–209.

9. Rafaeli Y, Van-Parijs L, London CA, Tschopp J, Abbas AK. Biochemical mechanisms of IL-2-regulated Fas-mediated T cell apoptosis. Immunity. 1998;8:615–23.
10. Heath WR, Kurts C, Miller JFAP, Carbone FR. Cross-tolerance: a pathway for inducing tolerance to peripheral tissue antigens. J Exp Med. 1998;187:1549–53.
11. Gill RG, Coulombe M, Lafferty KJ. Pancreatic islet allograft immunity and tolerance: the two-signal hypothesis revisited. Immunol Rev. 196;149:75–96.
12. Kimpton WG, Washington RNP, Cahill RN. Virgin ab and gd T cells recirculate extensively through peripheral tissues and skin during normal development of the fetal immune system. Int Immunol. 1995;7:1567–77.
13. Halstead TE, Hall JG. The homing of lymph-borne immunoblasts to the small gut of neonatal rats. Transplantation 1972;14:339–46.
14. Alferink J, Tafuri A, Vestweber D, Hallmann R, Hämmerling GJ, Arnold B. Peripheral T cell trafficking controls neonatal tolerance to tissue-antigens. Science. 1998;282:1338–41.
15. Limmer A, Sacher T, Alferink J *et al.* Failure to induce organospecific autoimmunity by breaking of tolerance: importance of the microenvironment.Eur J Immunol. 1998;28:2395–406.
16. Schwartz RH. Immunological tolerance. In: Paul E, editor. Fundamental Immunology, 3rd edn. New York: Raven Press; 1993:677–731.

# 2
# Autoantibodies to insulin-like growth factor II mRNA-binding proteins in hepatocellular carcinoma

E. M. TAN, J.-Y. ZHANG and E. K. L. CHAN

## INTRODUCTION

Autoantibodies to intranuclear proteins which are located either in the nucleus or cytoplasm are being recognized with increasing frequency in many different diseases, including cancer[1–15]. Autoantibodies, especially antinuclear antibodies (ANA), have had a long history in the systemic autoimmune diseases such as systemic lupus erythematosus, scleroderma and Sjögren's syndrome[1,2]. Our interest in autoantibodies in cancer was stimulated by the observation that in hepatocellular carcinoma (HCC), there was a significantly increased prevalence of antinuclear antibodies compared with the precursor conditions, liver cirrhosis or chronic hepatitis (31% vs 13%)[11,12]. In countries where viral hepatitis is highly prevalent, patients with chronic hepatitis are being followed in hospital clinics at regular intervals, for treatment purposes as well as for early detection of transformation to liver malignancy. We have been able to observe that several patients show changes in their humoral antibody responses during transformation from the chronic liver disease phase to HCC[12]. This change in humoral immunity either takes the form of seroconversion from ANA-negative status to ANA-positive status or significant increases in titre and appearance of new antibodies during malignant transformation. An example is shown in Figure 1, in which a patient with liver cirrhosis had a progressive increase in ANA titre which preceded by more than 1 year the clinical detection of HCC (Figure 1A). Figure 1B shows Western blotting using the sera from this patient at the time-points indicated in Figure 1A. At time point iv, several new antigen–antibody systems were detected by Western blotting which were not present at time points i and ii. This change in the humoral antibody response could also be demonstrated by immunohistology (Figures 1C and 1D), where nuclear staining changed from nucleoplasmic (Figure 1C) to additional staining of nucleoli as shown in Figure 1D, corresponding to time point iv in Figure 1A. On the basis of previous studies in systemic autoimmune diseases, there is evidence that this

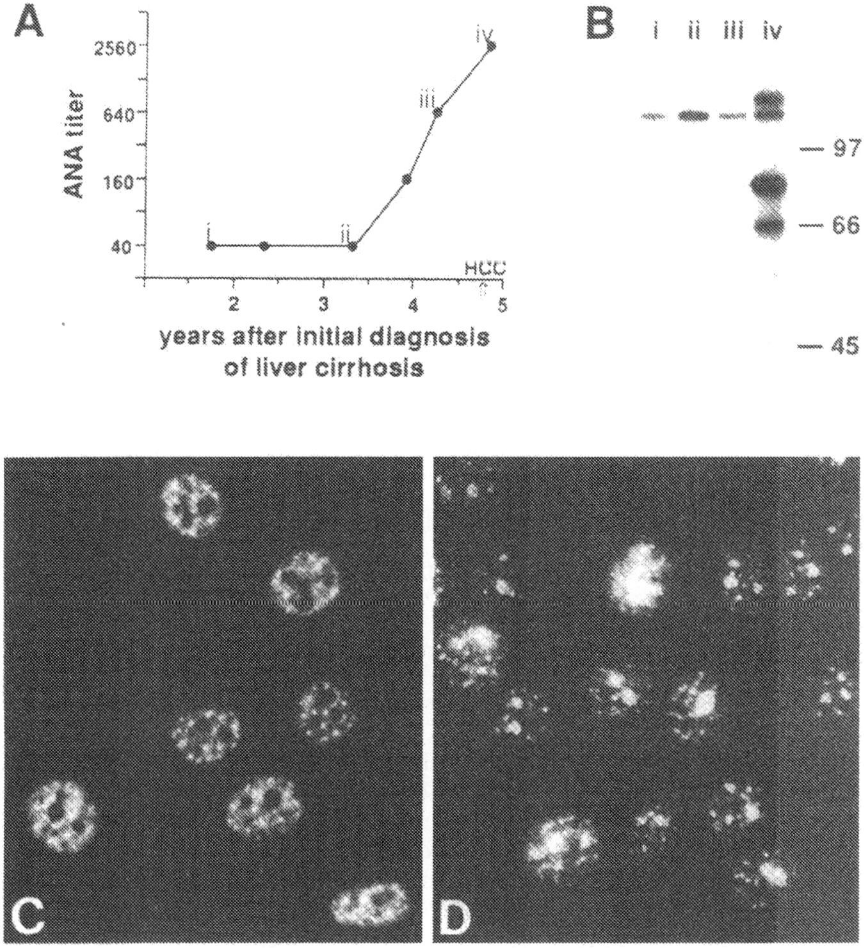


**Fig. 1** Increasing titres of ANA associated with new antibody specificities observed in patient N.K. who developed HCC. **A**: ANA patterns changed from nuclear speckles excluding nucleoli (*ii*, **C**) to nucleolar staining (*iv*, **D**). Arrow indicates the time-point when the diagnosis of HCC was made. **B**: Western blotting studies of nuclear extracts from HEp-2 cells were performed using sera collected at time points indicated by *i*, *ii*, *iii*, and *iv*. These studies confirmed the appearance of new antibody specificities in lanes *iii* and *iv* that were not present before the rise in ANA titre. Immunofluorescence on HeLa cells represented sera collected at time-points *ii* (**C**) and *iv* (**D**) (×500)

type of immune response is antigen-driven[16–18]. These novel antibody responses are therefore signals which point to intranuclear or intracytoplasmic molecules which might be playing some role in the malignant transformation process. Therefore, we have used antibodies in the sera of patients with HCC and other cancers as reagents to isolate, identify and characterize the target antigens. The serum from this patient at time point iv was used to isolate an intranuclear protein of 64 kDa which has structural motifs possessed in common by several other cellular proteins called the SR (serine arginine) family of proteins engaged

**Table 1** Antigen–antibody systems identified in HCC and other malignancies

| *Antigens* | *Properties/functions* | *Refs* |
|---|---|---|
| Fibrillarin | 34 kDa nucleolar protein | Imai *et al.*[11] |
| NOR-90 | 89, 93 kDa doublet proteins in nucleolus organizer region | Imai *et al.*[11] |
| B23 | 37 kDa nucleolar protein, also known as nucleophosmin, up-regulated in proliferation | Imai *et al.*[11] |
| HCC1* | 64 kDa nucleoplasmic protein, member of SR family of splicing factors | Imai *et al.*[13] |
| CENP-F* | 330 kDa doublet, nuclear matrix and centromere-associated | Casiano *et al.*[19,21], Landberg *et al.*[22], Rattner *et al.*[23] |
| $SG_2NA$* | 82 kDa WD-40 nucleoplasmic protein, highly expressed in S and $G_2$ phases of cell cycle | Muro *et al.*[14], Landberg and Tan[24] |
| DNA Topo II | DNA topoisomerase II | Imai *et al.*[25] |
| Cyclin B1 | Cell cycle nuclear protein | Covini *et al.*[26] |
| p62* | 62 kDa cytoplasmic protein, RRM-KH RNA-binding protein | Zhang *et al.*[20] |
| $\alpha$-enolase | Glycolytic enzyme (2-phospho-D-glycerate hydrolase) | Studies in progress |
| EF-1$\gamma$ | Elongation factor 1$\gamma$, 50 kDa protein of EF-1 complex engaged in 80S ribosome-mediated protein synthesis | Studies in progress |

* Four cellular proteins not previously reported in the literature.

in alternative splicing of precursor mRNA[13]. In the course of our studies we have now identified several antigens with this approach, and these are described in Table 1. Four previously unknown cellular proteins have been identified, including HCC1, the SR splicing factor mentioned above[13]; CENP-F, a 330 kDa duplex which is associated with the nuclear matrix and the centromere during mitosis[19]; $SG_2NA$, a 82 kDa nucleoplasmic protein highly expressed in the S and $G_2$ phases of the cell cycle[14] and, most recently, p62, a 62 kDa cytoplasmic protein which belongs to a family of insulin-like growth factor II mRNA-binding proteins[20].

Because we were using HCC as a model system in our studies where pre-cancer sera were available from the same patient, it became apparent that not all HCC sera containing antibodies were identifying antigens which were unique to the cancer phase of the patient's illness. As shown in Figure 1, a protein of high molecular weight was recognized as an autoantigen during the liver cirrhosis phase of this patient's illness and the antibody persisted at the time of conversion to malignancy. In a larger-scale analysis of serial samples of sera from certain patients, it was confirmed that many HCC patients already had circulating antibodies which had been present for many years during the chronic liver disease stage preceding cancer. As shown in Table 1, $\alpha$-enolase, a glycolytic enzyme (2-phospho-D-glycerate hydrolase), is an antigen identified by antibodies in HCC sera. Because of the concerns described above, we have performed a comprehensive study of the prevalence of anti-$\alpha$-enolase autoantibody in patients with other types of liver disease besides cancer, and the data are shown in Table 2. In two separate cohorts of HCC patients there was a prevalence of anti-$\alpha$-enolase in

**Table 2** Prevalence of $\alpha$-enolase autoantibody in human liver diseases

| *Liver diseases* | *No. tested* | *O.D.* in ELISA* 0.13–0.20 | *O.D.* in ELISA* >0.20 | *Total positive* |
|---|---|---|---|---|
| *Group 1 (from China)* | | | | |
| Acute hepatitis | 31 | 4 (12.9%) | 8 (25.8%) | 12 (38.7%) |
| Chronic hepatitis | 20 | 0 | 3 (15.0%) | 3 (15.0%) |
| HCC | 111 | 8 (7.2%) | 14 (12.6%) | 22 (19.8%) |
| *Group 2 (from Japan)* | | | | |
| PBC | 175 | 5 (2.9%) | 48 (27.4%) | 53 (30.3%) |
| HCC | 100 | 3 (3.0%) | 11 (11.0%) | 14 (14.0%) |

*Cut-off value 0.13. The arbitrary separation into two groups gives some indication of the proportion of high and low reactors.

22/111 (19.8%) HCC patients from China and in 14/100 (14.0%) HCC patients from Japan. However, in patients with acute and chronic hepatitis from both countries, it was observed that the prevalence of anti-$\alpha$-enolase was 38.7% in acute hepatitis and 30.3% in primary biliary cirrhosis. This study clearly shows that the $\alpha$-enolase antigen–antibody system is not unique to HCC, and suggests that its detection in HCC might be attributed to antibody already being present in precursor conditions. The results emphasize the importance of a comprehensive analysis of different types of patients for antibody prevalence before conclusions can be drawn regarding cancer relatedness.

## AUTOANTIBODIES TO p62, A RNA-BINDING PROTEIN OF THE RRM-KH FAMILY

While analysing a group of sera from HCC patients originating from Henan province in China, it was observed by Western blotting that a number of these sera were reactive with a protein which blotted in the region of 62kDa. This 62 kDa protein was expressed in high abundance in a T24 (bladder carcinoma cell line) and sera containing such antibodies were used to immunoscreen a T24 cDNA expression library. A full-length cDNA clone was isolated and the deduced amino acid sequence showed that it contained 556 amino acid residues with a calculated molecular size of 62 kDa[20]. The p62 contained two types of RNA-binding motifs, one consisting of two conserved RNP regions (RNP1 and RNP2) which comprised the RNA recognition motif (RRM). The other RNA binding region consisted of four repeats of the hnRNP-K homology (KH) domain[27] extending from approximately the first third of the protein to the C-terminus. Of great interest at this time was the finding that there were three other proteins in the gene sequence databases which showed very high homology to p62. Figure 2 shows the alignment of p62 with the other three proteins, KOC[28], ZBP-1[29] and B3[30]. In addition to the similar domain structure of all these four proteins, p62 had similarity/identity to KOC, ZBP-1 and B3 of 80.3/66.5%, 83.9/70.5% and 82.7/69.7%, respectively.

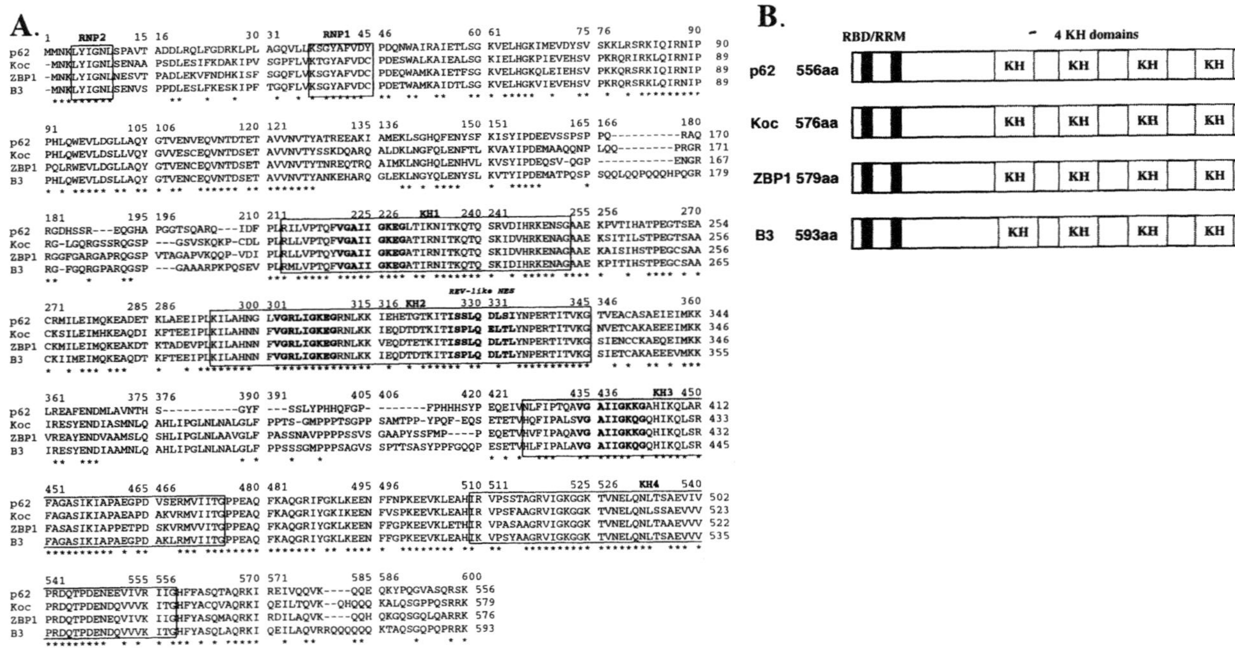


**Fig. 2** Similarity between p62 and three RNA-binding motif proteins Koc, ZBP1 and B3. **A**: The identities between p62 and the other three proteins are shown with an asterisk. **B**: The great similarity of the domain structures is shown. The RNA-binding domains with two conserved RNP regions, RNP1 and RNP2, and four KH domains are boxed. A nine-amino acid sequence (VGAIIGKE/KG) of unknown function in the first three KH domains is shown in bold, as is the REV-like nuclear export signal (NES) in the second KH domain

ZBP-1 was shown to bind to the 3′ UTR of beta-actin mRNA and the binding was mediated by a specific 54 nucleotide sequence[29]. ZBP-1 was highly concentrated in the lamellipodia or advancing edge of fibroblasts, and was suggested to be responsible for transport of beta-actin mRNA to these regions and therefore to be playing a role in regulating cell movement. KOC was isolated by differential selection of genes expressed in pancreatic cancer and was shown to be overexpressed in pancreatic cancer as well as in a number of other cancer tissues[28]. B3 was a protein which was shown to bind upstream of the *Xenopus* TFIIIA gene, and has been reported to be involved in developmental regulation of TFIIIA during oogenesis[30].

We developed an enzyme-based immunoassay to determine the prevalence of anti-p62 in HCC compared to chronic liver disease conditions and normal human sera, and the results are shown in Table 3. Anti-p62 was present in 21% of a cohort of HCC patients from Henan province in China, whereas it was not detected in several control groups of patients including 31 with acute hepatitis, 20 with chronic hepatitis, 26 who were asymptomatic HBsAg carriers and normal human sera. Thus, it appears that anti-p62 shows specificity for cancer and was not detected in the acute and chronic hepatitis patients examined. We have recently extended these studies to include 911 patients with diverse types of cancer and have observed that anti-p62 was present in a large variety of malignancies including oesophageal, breast, lung, colorectal, uterine, and ovarian cancers. Of the total of 911 cancer sera, 11.4% were shown to have antibodies to p62, indicating that the p62 antigen–antibody system is widely present among different malignancies. Of interest is a recent study describing the isolation and characterization of three genes encoding RRM-KH proteins[31]. The proteins were called insulin-like growth factor II mRNA-binding proteins (IMP). IMP-1 was the human homologue of ZBP-1 from the chicken and IMP-3 was identical to KOC. IMP-2 was identical to p62 except for an extra 43 amino acid residue insert between the KH-2 and KH-3 domains of p62. Thus, p62 and IMP-2 appear to be alternatively spliced products of the same gene. The investigators describing the IMP proteins were attempting to isolate cellular factors which bound to a specific IGF-II transcript called leader 3 IGF-II mRNA, and during the course of these experiments isolated the IMP-1, 2 and 3 genes. They also showed that the IMP bound to the 5′ UTR of leader 3 IGF-II mRNA and showed that IMP-1 and IMP-3 repressed translation of leader 3 mRNA transcript.

**Table 3** Prevalence of p62 autoantibody in human sera from Henan province by ELISA screening

| *Categories* | *Prevalence: patients with p62 antibody/ total patients with disease* |
|---|---|
| Hepatocellular carcinoma | 20/95 (21.1%) |
| Asymptomatic HBsAg carrier | 0/26 |
| Acute hepatitis | 0/31 |
| Chronic hepatitis | 0/20 |
| Normal human sera | 0/30 |
| Normal human sera* | 0/40 |

* This group of sera was obtained from the San Diego area.

Because of our finding that anti-p62 is found in HCC as well as other cancers, and of the report by Müller-Pillasch[28] that KOC mRNA is overexpressed in many human cancers, we are interested in pursuing the relationship of p62 with cancer. The observations of Nielsen *et al*[31] suggested a connection with IGF-II in that some members of the RRM-KH protein family were IGF-II mRNA binding proteins which were able to modulate translation. Further studies, such as those into the production of p62 and other RRM-KH transgenic mice, might provide insights into how this family of IGF-II mRNA-binding proteins could be involved in malignancy.

## References

1. Tan EM. Autoantibodies in pathology and cell biology. Cell. 1991;67:841–2.
2. Tan EM. Autoantibodies and autoimmunity: a three-decade perspective. A tribute to Henry G. Kunkel. Ann NY Acad Sci. 1997;815:1–14.
3. Burnham TK. Antinuclear antibodies in patients with malignancies. Lancet. 1972;2:2436–37.
4. Steiner M, Klein E, Klein G. Antinuclear reactivity of sera in patients with leukemia and other neoplastic diseases. Clin Immunol Immunopathol. 1975;4:374–81.
5. Thomas PJ, Kaur JS, Aitcheson CT, Robinson WA, Tan EM. Antinuclear, antinucleolar, and anticytoplasmic antibodies in patients with malignant melanoma. Cancer Res. 1983;43:1372–80.
6. Wasserman J, Glas U, Blomgren H. Autoantibodies in patients with carcinoma of the breast: correlation with prognosis. Clin Exp Immunol. 1975;19:417–22.
7. Pupa SM, Menard S, Andreola S, Colnaghi M. Antibody response against the c-erbB2 oncoprotein in breast carcinoma patients. Cancer Res. 1993;53:5864–6.
8. Dalmau J, Graus F, Rosenblum MK, Posner JB. Anti-Hu associated paraneoplasic encephalomyelitis/sensory neuropathy: a clinical study of 71 patients. Medicine. 1991;71:59–72.
9. Buckanovich RJ, Darnell RB. The neuronal RNA binding protein Nova-1 recognizes specific RNA targets in vitro and *in vivo*. Mol Cell Biol. 1997;17:3194–201.
10. Covini G, Muhlen CAV, Pacchetti S, Colombo M, Chan EKL, Tan EM. Diversity of antinuclear antibody responses in hepatocellular carcinoma. J Hepatol. 1997;26:1255–65.
11. Imai H, Ochs RL, Kiyosawa K, Furuta S, Nakamura RM, Tan EM. Nucleolar antigens and autoantibodies in hepatocellular carcinoma and other malignancies. Am J Pathol. 1992;140:859–70.
12. Imai H, Nakano Y, Kiyosawa K, Tan EM. Increasing titers and changing specificities of antinuclear antibodies in patients with chronic liver disease who develop hepatocellular carcinoma. Cancer. 1993;71:26–35.
13. Imai H, Chan EKL, Kiyosawa K, Fu XD, Tan EM. Novel nuclear autoantigen with splicing factor motifs identified with antibody from hepatocellular carcinoma. J Clin Invest. 1993;92:2419–26.
14. Muro Y, Chan EKL, Landberg G, Tan EM. A cell-cycle nuclear autoantigen containing WD-40 motifs expressed mainly in S and G2 phase cells. Biochem Biophys Res Commun. 1995;207:1029–37.
15. Winter SF, Minna JD, Johnson BE, Takahashi T, Gazdar AF, Carbone DP. Development of antibodies agaiinst p 53 in lung cancer patients appears to be dependent on the type of p53 mutation. Cancer Res. 1992;52:4168–74.
16. Tan EM, Chan EKL, Sullivan KF, Rubin RL. Antinuclear antibodies (ANAs): diagnostically specific immune markers and clues towards the understanding of systemic autoimmunity. Clin Immunol Immunopathol. 1988;47:121–41.
17. Tillman DM, Jou NT, Hill RJ, Marion TN. Both IgM and IgG anti-DNA antibodies are the products of clonally selective B cell stimulation in (NZB × NZW)F1 mice. J Exp Med. 1992;176:761–79.
18. Radic MZ, Weigert M. Genetic and structural evidence for antigen selection of anti-DNA antibodies. Annu Rev Immunol. 1994;12:487–520.
19. Casiano CA, Landberg G, Ochs RL, Tan EM. Autoantibodies to a novel cell cycle-related protein which accumulates in the nuclear matrix during S phase and localizes to kinetochores and spindle midzone during mitosis. J Cell Sci. 1993;35:73–85.

20. Zhang JY, Chan EKL, Peng XX, Tan EM. A novel cytoplasmic protein with RNA-binding motifs is an autoantigen in human hepatocellular carcinoma. J Exp Med. 1999;189:1101–10.
21. Casiano CA, Humbel R, Peebles CL, Tan EM. Autoimmunity to the cell-cycle dependent centromere protein p330[d]/CENP-F in disorders associated with cell proliferation. J Autoimmun. 1995;8:575–86.
22. Landberg G, Erlanson M, Roos G, Tan EM, Casiano CA. The nuclear autoantigen p330[d]/CENP-F – a marker for cell proliferation in human malignancies. Cytometry. 1996;190:143–5.
23. Rattner JB, Rees J, Whitehead CM, *et al.* High frequency of neoplasia in patients with autoantibodies to centromere protein CENP-F. Clin Invest Med. 1997;20:308–19.
24. Landberg G, Tan EM. Characterization of a DNA-binding nuclear autoantigen mainly associated with S phase and G2 cells. Exp Cell Res. 1994;212:255–61.
25. Imai H, Furuta K, Landberg G, Kiyosawa K, Liu LF, Tan EM. Autoantibody to DNA topoisomerase II in primary liver cancer. Clin Cancer Res. 1995;1:417–24.
26. Covini G, Chan EKL, Landberg G, Ochs RL, Tan EM. Immune response to cyclin B1 in hepatocellular carcinoma. Hepatology. 1997;25:75–80.
27. Burd CG, DFreyfuss G. Conserved structures and diversity of functions of RNA-binding proteins. Science. 1994;265:615–21.
28. Müller-Pillasch F, Lacher U, Wallrapp C *et al.* Cloning of a gene highly overexpressed in cancer coding for a novel KH-domain containing protein. Oncogene. 1997;14:2729–33.
29. Ross AF, Oleynikov Y, Kislauskis EH, Taneja KL, Singer RH. Characterization of a *gb-actin mRNA zipcode-binding protein. Mol Cell Biol. 1997;17:2158–65.
30. Pfaff SL, Taylor WL. Characterization of a *Xenopus* oocyte factor that binds to a developmentally regulated *cis*-element in the TFIIIA gene. Dev Biol. 1992;151:306–16.
31. Nielsen J, Christiansen J, Lykke-Andersen J,Johnsen AH, Wewer UM, Nielsen FC. A family of insulin-like growth factor II mRNA-binding proteins represses translation in late development. Mol Cell Biol. 1999;19:1262–70.

# 3
# Migration of microsomal autoantigens to the hepatocyte plasma membrane

**D. PESSAYRE, V. DESCATOIRE, P. DANSETTE, J. LOEPER, A. BERSON and M.-A. ROBIN**

## INTRODUCTION

Autoantibodies against microsomal autoantigens are present in some forms of drug-induced hepatitis, alcohol-induced liver injury, idiopathic autoimmune hepatitis, and viral hepatitis. For these autoantibodies to play a role in immune destruction the microsomal autoantigens would have to be inserted in, or transported to, the plasma membrane (PM) and would have to be exposed, at least in part, on the outer surface of the PM. The present review is mainly concerned with the immunogenicity, cellular transport, and PM expression of cytochromes P450 (CYP). Other microsomal autoantigens are briefly discussed.

## THE CYP SYSTEM

Animals have been subject to the relentless biological warfare of the plants that they ingest, as these plants defended themselves by developing new toxins[1]. Many of these vegetal toxins were liposoluble and could not be excreted in urine or bile. Clearly, animals that developed systems to transform liposoluble xenobiotics into water-soluble metabolites (that could be excreted in urine or bile), were more apt to survive. This evolutionary pressure probably explains the development of the CYP system[1]. By duplication of an ancestral CYP gene, divergent evolution of these genes, and so forth (new duplications followed by gene divergence), surviving animals were endowed with an entire range of CYP. Each CYP oxidizes different sets of xenobiotics (Figure 1). Due to the numerous CYP, most environmental liposoluble xenobiotics and most man-made drugs are metabolized by the CYP system. These CYP were strategically located in the liver (and small intestine) to partially metabolize ingested xenobiotics before they reach the systemic circulation.

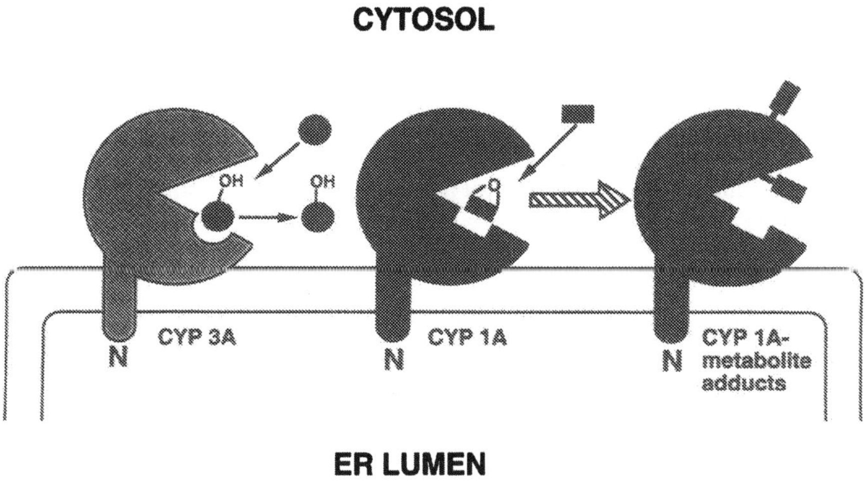


**Fig. 1** Diversity of CYP, main ER topology and formation of reactive metabolites. CYP have a similar general architecture. The N-terminal methionine and a few amino acids are in the ER lumen. A non-cleaved signal peptide/membrane anchor sequence crosses the ER membrane and the rest of the molecule protrudes into the cytosol, although part of it may be embedded in the outer moiety of the ER membrane. However, different CYP have different active sites and metabolize diverse sets of xenobiotics. Some drugs are transformed into chemically reactive metabolites that covalently bind to CYP (and other proteins)

Although the CYP system eliminates xenobiotics, it has the disadvantage of forming reactive metabolites that covalently bind to hepatic macromolecules, including CYP themselves (Figure 1). This covalent binding modifies hepatic proteins, which may interfere with the discrimination of self proteins from non-self proteins by the immune system.

## THE IMMUNE SYSTEM

The macrophagic and immune systems developed to fight bacterial, fungal or viral infections. The immune system is based *(a)* on the acquisition, during evolution, of different alleles of major histocompatibility complex (MHC) molecules that can each present different sets of peptides on the cell surface; *(b)* on the development, in each individual, by somatic mutation, of a whole range of helper T lymphocytes; *(c)* on the deletion or anergy of the helper T cells that recognize self peptides, leaving mainly those that recognize non-self peptides, and *(d)* on humoral and cell-mediated responses that cause the immunological destruction of cells presenting non-self proteins (humoral response) or non-self peptides (cell-mediated response)[2].

The superposition of the CYP and the immune systems creates a major problem for the distinction between self and foreign proteins. The covalent binding of a reactive metabolite to self proteins modifies these proteins (and peptides therefrom). These modified peptides may 'mislead' the immune system into mounting an immune attack against hepatocytes that harbour the modified proteins. This immune reaction is directed both against the Self (autoimmune targets) and against the modified Self (neoantigens).

## CYP AS AUTOANTIGENS IN DRUG-INDUCED HEPATITIS

Anti-CYP autoantibodies are present in the sera of patients with hepatitis due to some drugs.

### Tienilic acid

This uricosuric diuretic (also termed ticrynafen) was withdrawn from clinical use in the United States after more than 500 cases of hepatic injury and 25 fatalities were reported to the manufacturer[3]. Three-quarters of the cases exhibited cytolytic hepatitis, while the remainder had chronic hepatitis and/or cirrhosis[3]. The prompt recurrence of the disease in rechallenged patients suggested an immune mechanism[3]. Tienilic acid is transformed by CYP 2C (CYP 2C9 in humans, and CYP 2C11 in rats) into a reactive metabolite, presumably the thiophene sulfphoxide[4–6]. This metabolite has three alternatives. *(a)* It may react with an $H_2O$ molecule within the CYP 2C active site, and then lose $H_2O$, to form 5-hydroxy-tienilic acid. *(b)* It may covalently bind to nucleophilic residues at the active site of the CYP 2C protein. *(c)* It may leave the active site of CYP 2C and react elsewhere (possibly with nucleophilic sites on the surface of CYP 2C, with glutathione or with other proteins)[4–6]. However, when CYP 2C9-expressing yeast microsomes were incubated with tienilic acid and NADPH in the presence of glutathione (to trap the reactive metabolite that migrates away from CYP 2C9), the only protein that was alkylated was CYP 2C9[5].

In the sera of patients with tienilic acid-induced hepatitis there are anti-endoplasmic reticulum antibodies that show a specific immunofluorescent pattern on rat liver and kidney sections from untreated rats[7]. These autoantibodies have been termed 'type 2' anti-liver/kidney microsome (anti-LKM-2) autoantibodies to distinguish them from the 'type 1' autoantibodies (anti-LKM-1) found in some forms of viral or autoimmune hepatitis[8]. Anti-LKM-2 autoantibodies slowly decrease in titre after tienilic acid administration is stopped. They specifically recognize a conformational epitope of CYP 2C9 in humans[8–9], but recognize CYP 2C11 in rats (a major isoform in the adult male liver that exhibits 85% sequence identity with the human CYP 2C9)[10].

### Dihydralazine

This antihypertensive drug may cause acute cytolytic hepatitis, chronic hepatitis or cirrhosis in humans[11]. Subjects with dihydralazine-induced hepatitis have anti-CYP autoantibodies that slowly decrease in titre after dihydralazine administration is stopped[11]. These autoantibodies recognize rat liver but not rat kidney microsomes and are therefore termed anti-liver microsome (anti-LM) autoantibodies[11]. Anti-LM sera specifically recognize human *CYP 1A2* and rat *CYP 1A2*, two closely related isoforms that are mainly expressed in liver[11]. Dihydralazine is selectively transformed by rat and human CYP 1A2 into reactive radicals that covalently bind to rat and human CYP 1A2 proteins[12].

### Halothane

This anaesthetic agent leads to severe immunoallergic hepatitis in rare patients. Halothane is transformed by *CYP 2E1*[13] into a reactive trifluoroacetyl chloride intermediate that trifluoroacetylates diverse intraluminal microsomal proteins, as well as the *CYP 2E1* protein[14,15]. Halothane-induced hepatitis is associated with anti-CYP 2E1 autoantibodies[14,15].

### Ethanol

Alcohol is metabolized by both *CYP 2E1* and *CYP 3A4*[16], forming two reactive species: acetaldehyde[17] and the 1-hydroxyl ethyl radical[18] that covalently modify the *CYP 2E1* protein[19]. It is unknown whether *CYP 3A4* is also alkylated (although this would seem likely). Both anti-CYP 2E1 and anti-CYP 3A4 autoantibodies are found in alcoholic patients[20].

### Aromatic anticonvulsants

In hepatitis due to phenytoin, carbamazepine or phenobarbital, autoantibodies reacting with rat CYP 3A1[21], rat CYP 3A2[21,22], and a mouse CYP 3A isoform[22] have been detected. However, these human sera do not react with human CYP 3A4[22] and the nature of the human autoantigen remains speculative [23].

Thus, in the four cases in which the human autoantigen is known (i.e. in tienilic acid-, dihydralazine-, halothane- and ethanol-induced liver injury), the autoantibody is specifically directed against the particular CYP that transform(s) the drug into a reactive intermediate that covalently modifies the CYP protein[24].

## CYP–METABOLITE ADDUCTS AS NEOANTIGENS IN DRUG-INDUCED HEPATITIS

In patients with tienilic acid-, halothane-, or alcohol-induced liver injury there are not only anti-CYP autoantibodies, but also anti-CYP–metabolite adducts (Figure 2).

### Tienilic acid

Both immunoblot and flow cytometry have shown that the anti-LKM-2 sera of patients with tienilic acid hepatitis contain not only the previously described autoantibodies against unalkylated CYP 2C, but also antibodies directed against tienilic acid-alkylated CYP 2C[25]. After preadsorption on untreated rat liver microsomes (to eliminate autoantibodies against CYP 2C), these sera no longer recognized the PM of untreated rat hepatocytes on flow cytometry. However, these adsorbed sera recognized the PM of tienilic acid-treated rat hepatocytes. This PM labelling was markedly decreased when the sera were first reacted with tienilic acid (consuming the anti-adduct antibodies), or when an anti-tienilic acid antibody (which sterically masks the CYP–tienilic acid adducts) was first added. This PM labelling also decreased when an anti-CYP 2C11 antibody was first added, suggesting that steric

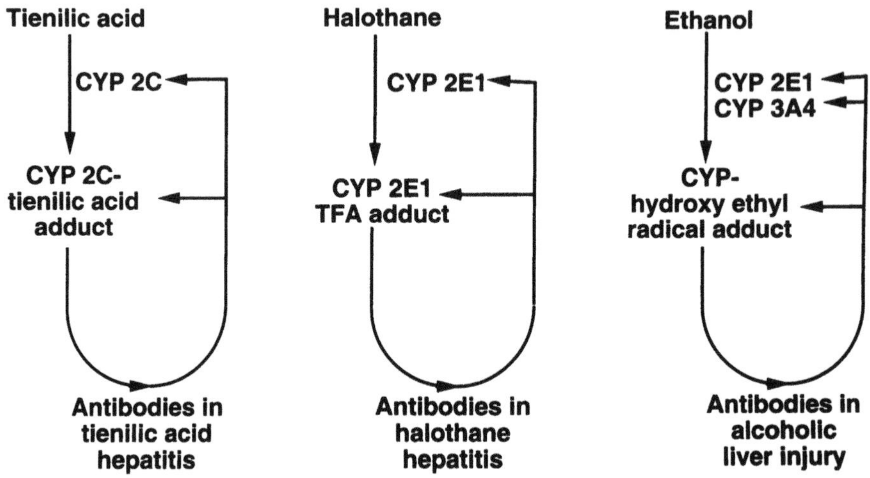


**Fig. 2** Drug-induced formation of anti-CYP autoantibodies and antibodies against CYP–metabolite adducts. TFA, trifluoroacetyl

hindrance caused by reaction of the anti-CYP 2C11 antibody prevented binding of the anti-tienilic acid–CYP 2C11 antibody[25]. These observations indicated that tienilic acid and CYP 2C11 were present on the same structure, i.e. tienilic acid-alkylated CYP 2C11[25]. Indeed, CYP 2C11 was the only protein alkylated by tienilic acid in PM immunoblots[25].

Interestingly, antibodies recognizing tienilic acid–protein adducts are also detected in the serum of patients who are treated with tienilic acid but do not develop hepatitis[26]. In these healthy recipients, antibody titres are lower than in patients with hepatitis[26]. This interesting observation suggests that the immune reaction is more frequent than previously imagined, although it is rarely severe enough to cause hepatitis.

## Halothane

In halothane hepatitis, although there are autoantibodies against CYP 2E1, there are also antibodies recognizing trifluoroacetylated (TFA) PM proteins[24]. Alkylated CYP 2E1 may be one of the PM target for these anti-TFA antibodies[24].

## Ethanol

Sera from alcoholic patients react with CYP 2E1-hydroxyethyl radical adducts present in microsomes[19] and PM[27] of ethanol-treated rats.

Thus in all three cases (tienilic acid, halothane, and ethanol), the alkylation of CYP proteins (modified Self) may lead to the appearance of both anti-CYP autoantibodies and antibodies against CYP–metabolite adducts (Figure 2).

## POSSIBLE MECHANISM FOR THE APPEARANCE OF ANTI-CYP AUTOANTIBODIES AND ANTI-CYP–METABOLITE ADDUCT ANTIBODIES IN DRUG-INDUCED HEPATITIS

Because hepatocytes do not normally express MHC class II molecules, initially they should not be able to present alkylated peptides to helper T cells (which recognize peptides presented by MHC class II molecules)[28]. Accordingly, alkylated hepatic proteins should first be released by hepatocytes for presentation by cells expressing MHC class II molecules, such as B lymphocytes or macrophages[28]. This release of alkylated proteins might occur during normal cell turnover of hepatocytes. However, any direct toxicity of the drug metabolite greatly increases the release of modified hepatic proteins and the likelihood of immunization[28]. Indeed, in halothane- or tienilic acid-induced hepatitis, the prevalence of infraclinical 'transaminitis' is much higher than that of severe immunoallergic hepatitis[29]. This suggests that direct toxicity may release neoantigens that cause immunization in a few patients[29].

The mechanism leading to the appearance of anti-CYP (auto)antibodies remains unknown. However, we suggest the following mechanism (Figure 3)[28].

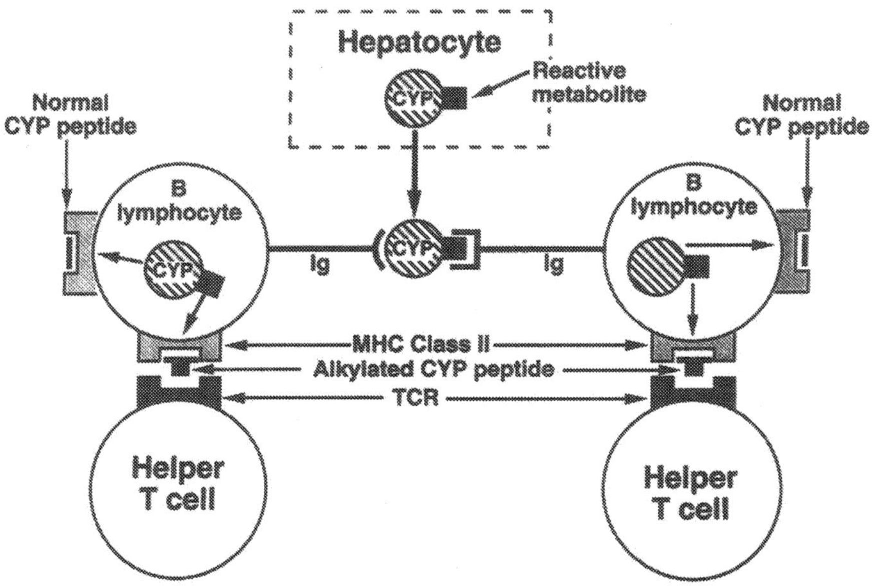


**Fig. 3** Hypothetical mechanism for the appearance of anti-CYP (auto)antibodies after CYP alkylation. Left part of the figure: after the death of a hepatocyte, the capture of an alkylated CYP by an autoreactive B lymphocyte (expressing a membrane immunoglobulin directed against a normal epitope of CYP) may lead to the presentation of alkylated CYP peptides and their recognition by helper T cells. This causes maturation of the B lymphocyte into a plasmocyte secreting an autoantibody against the normal epitope (see text for further explanations). Right part of the figure: if the immunoglobulin of the B cell recognizes the covalently bound reactive metabolite instead, the same mechanism will lead to an antibody recognizing the CYP–metabolite adduct. Normally the CYP protein is not alkylated and only unalkylated CYP peptides are presented. These normal peptides are not recognized by the T cell receptors (TCR) of helper T lymphocytes, and the B cells remain quiescent

Some B lymphocytes are autoreactive[30], but normally remain quiescent in the absence of stimulation by helper T cells[31]. Let us consider an autoreactive B cell expressing a membrane immunoglobulin that recognizes a normal, unalkylated CYP 2C epitope (Figure 3). After the death of a hepatocyte this autoreactive B cell may capture a CYP 2C molecule by its normal epitope (Figure 3). After internalization and processing of the protein, the autoreactive B cell may present peptides derived from the CYP molecule on its MHC class II molecules (Figure 3). Normally, the CYP is not alkylated, and the B lymphocyte only presents normal peptides. Since there are no helper T cells to recognize these normal peptides, the autoreactive B cell remains quiescent[28]. However, if the subject has taken tienilic acid the CYP protein is alkylated by the reactive metabolite (Figure 3). Thus, the B lymphocyte may present both normal and alkylated CYP peptides. T helper cells may recognize this 'modified Self' (Figure 3). This recognition may lead to bidirectional signalling, involving both the T cell, which is activated to proliferate, and the B cell, which undergoes clonal expansion and maturation[31,32]. The B cell will eventually secrete an autoantibody with the same specificity as the initial membrane immunoglobulin, that is, an autoantibody directed against a normal CYP-2C epitope (Figure 3). This hypothetical mechanism explains how CYP modification by covalent binding ('modified Self') could lead to the appearance of autoantibodies[28].

The same mechanism could also explain the formation of antibodies recognizing the reactive metabolite bound on the CYP molecule (Figure 3)[28]. Indeed, if the membrane immunoglobulin of a quiescent B cell can recognize the alkylated part of a CYP protein, this B cell could also internalize the CYP molecule, present alkylated peptides, and be stimulated by helper T cells (Figure 3). It would evolve into plasmocytes that would secrete an antibody with the same specificity, i.e. an antibody directed against the CYP–metabolite adduct (Figure 3). Other processes, involving multipartite interactions between Kupffer cells, helper T cells, B lymphocytes and hepatocytes, could also be involved in the generation of these anti-adduct antibodies[33].

Hepatocytes express MHC class I molecules, and this expression is greatly increased once the inflammatory reaction has started. Thus hepatocytes might express alkylated peptides on their surface[33]. These modified peptides could serve as targets for cytotoxic T cells, which could play a major role in the immune destruction of hepatocytes. In a previous review, multipartite interactions between Kupffer cells (as antigen-presenting cells), helper T cells (detecting the modified Self) and cytotoxic T lymphocytes (effector cells) recognizing modified peptides expressed by MHC class I molecules on the surface of hepatocytes (target cells) were suggested[33].

Whether the immune reaction is limited to CYP or also affects other proteins, may depend on the reactivity of the metabolite[28]. The reactive metabolite of tienilic acid is so highly unstable – it even reacts with water – that it has little chance to leave CYP 2C and react elsewhere. Only CYP 2C is alkylated, and the immune response only targets this CYP. In contrast, the reactive acyl chloride generated by halothane is stable enough to leave CYP 2E1 and to react with many other proteins. The immune response is directed not only against CYP 2E1, but also against a variety of different neoantigens and autoantigens[34].

Although all subjects produce the reactive metabolite and all subjects alkylate CYP (or other hepatic proteins), the immune reaction is only strong enough to cause immunoallergic hepatitis in a few subjects[28]. The reason for this individual susceptibility remains largely unknown. However, there is some evidence that two types of genetic factors may be involved. First, genetic metabolic factors may play a role[28]. Whereas alkylation of a few molecules of hepatic proteins could lead to uncommon (or infraclinical) immunization, more extensive alkylation of hepatic proteins could cause more frequent (or more severe) immunization. This could occur, for example, in subjects who are deficient in a metabolic pathway that normally diverts the drug away from the formation of reactive metabolites. Indeed, dihydralazine is either acetylated by the polymorphic N-acetyl transferase[2], or activated by CYP 1A into a reactive radical[12]. In slow acetylators a lower fraction of the dose is N-acetylated, leaving a higher fraction of the dose available for metabolic activation by CYP. The alkylation of hepatic proteins is more extensive and the incidence of hepatitis is higher in slow acetylators than in rapid acetylators [12]. However, about 50% of Caucasians are slow acetylators, whereas dihydralazine hepatitis is much less frequent, indicating that other susceptibility factors must also be involved.

A second type of genetic factor may be the polymorphism of MHC molecules[35]. Although the number of MHC molecules in an individual is small, each MHC molecule is extremely polymorphic in a given species. Each different allele of these MHC molecules presents largely different sets of peptides[2]. This diversity, although it does not protect the individual, protects the species by enabling some of its members to efficiently present a particular viral peptide and therefore survive viral pandemics. The diversity of MHC molecules may affect the likelihood of drug-induced immunoallergic hepatitis in a similar manner[35]. The presence or absence of a given MHC molecule may determine the efficient presentation of a peptide rendered immunogenic by the presence of a covalently bound metabolite. Indeed, one particular MHC molecule seems to favour hepatitis due to some drugs, while other MHC molecules seem to favour hepatitis due to other drugs[35].

## CYP AS AUTOANTIGENS IN IDIOPATHIC AUTOIMMUNE HEPATITIS, VIRAL HEPATITIS AND THE AUTOIMMUNE POLYGLANDULAR SYNDROME

### Idiopathic autoimmune hepatitis

Most patients with idiopathic autoimmune hepatitis exhibit antinuclear or anti-smooth muscle antibodies but do not exhibit anti-endoplasmic reticulum antibodies[36]. These patients are classified as having 'type 1' autoimmune hepatitis. A smaller group of patients (classified as having 'type 2' autoimmune hepatitis) rarely have antinuclear or antismooth muscle antibodies, but instead exhibit anti-endoplasmic reticulum autoantibodies in the absence of hepatitis C virus (HCV) infection[36]. These patients exhibit anti-liver/kidney microsome type 1 (anti-LKM-1) autoantibodies that recognize human CYP 2D6[37,38]. Both linear[39] and conformational epitopes[40] of CYP 2D6 are recognized by these anti-LKM-1 sera.

## HCV infection

A small percentage of the many patients infected with HCV (but none infected with HBV or HBV/HDV) exhibit anti-LKM-1 autoantibodies. These HCV-related anti-LKM-1 antibodies also recognize CYP 2D6[41,42], although some of them may also recognize CYP 2A6 (Georgios Dalekos and Michael Manns, personal communication).

## Autoimmune polyglandular syndrome type I (APS-1)

This genetic disease is mainly characterized by candidiasis, hypoparathyroidism and adrenal failure, but it also involves the liver in 10–15% of patients[43]. Both anti-CYP 1A2 and anti-CYP 2A6 autoantibodies are present in patients with APS-1[44].

## Mechanisms?

The mechanisms causing the appearance of anti-CYP autoantibodies in these diseases are unknown. Hypothetical mechanisms might be metabolic activation of endogenous substances, natural foodstuffs or food conservatives by CYP, molecular mimicry between CYP and yeast or viruses, and/or abnormal cutting of CYP by viral proteases or cell caspases (leading to *de-novo* presentation of otherwise cryptic CYP peptides).

# PRESENCE OF CYP IN THE PM

The presence of anti-CYP (auto)antibodies in several forms of hepatitis has generated renewed interest in the cellular biology, transmembrane topology and PM expression of CYPs. While some studies did not detect external expression of CYP 2D6[45–47], there is growing evidence that CYPs are indeed present in the PM of rat and human hepatocytes[14,25,27,48–54]. Loeper *et al.* reported the presence of several immunoreactive CYP in immunoblots of a PM fraction prepared from human hepatocytes and exhibiting low microsomal contamination[54]. These PM CYP co-migrated with purified CYP standards, without any detectable higher bands to suggest glycosylation[54]. PM CYP are complete (with the heme moiety) and are functional, exhibiting NADPH-supported monooxygenase activities[52,54]. Indeed, both NADPH–cytochrome *c* reductase activity[52,54] and the cytochrome P450 reductase (CPR) protein (Robin *et al.*, submitted manuscript) are present in the PM.

# VESICULAR TRANSPORT OF CYP TO THE PM

There is extensive flow of vesicles that migrate from the endoplasmic reticulum (ER) to the Golgi apparatus, and then to the PM (Figure 4)[25]. This migration is effected by molecular motors that associate with these vesicles and pull them along microtubules (Figure 4). Unless they are actively retained in the ER/Golgi compartments by specific retention or retrieval signal(s), ER proteins follow vesicular flow to the PM along microtubules, with a mean transit time of 15–30

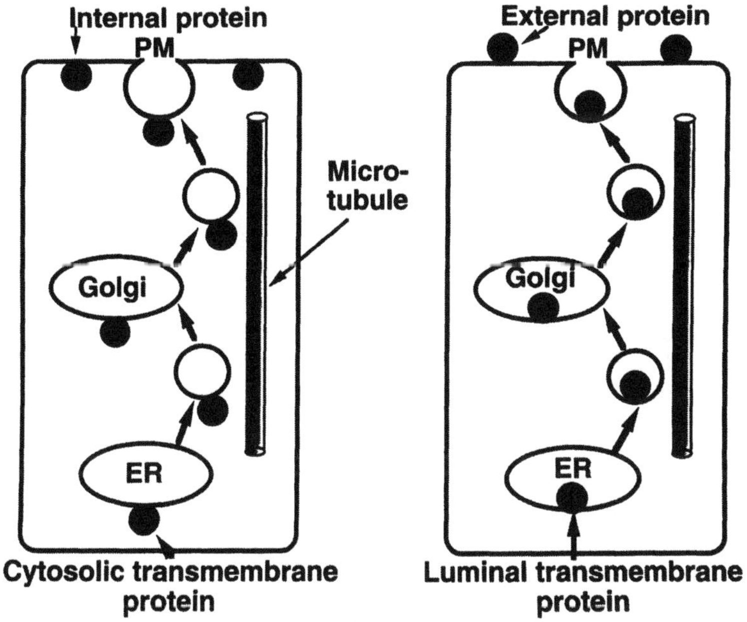


**Fig. 4** Vesicular transport of ER transmembrane proteins to the PM. Unless they are actively retained in the ER/Golgi compartments by specific retention or retrieval signal(s), ER proteins follow vesicular flow to the PM along microtubules. Proteins located on the cytosolic side of the ER membrane end up on the cytosolic side of the PM. Proteins located on the luminal side of the ER membrane finish on the outside of the PM

min. Proteins located on the cytosolic side of the ER membrane end up on the cytosolic side of the PM. Proteins located on the luminal side of the ER membrane finish on the outside of the PM (Figure 4).

CYP are synthesized by polyribosomes attached to the ER membrane and are cotranslationally inserted in the ER membrane where they remain anchored by a non-cleaved, N-terminal, signal peptide/membrane anchor sequence[55]. CYP are present in the Golgi[56] and CYP 2B[57], CYP 2C11 25, CYP 2C11–metabolite adducts[25], and CYP 1A1 and CYP 1A2 (Robin *et al.*, submitted manuscript) follow a vesicular route to reach the PM of rat hepatocytes. Cycloheximide, which interrupts protein synthesis; caffeine at 20°C, which decreases vesicular flow from the ER to the Golgi apparatus; brefeldin A, which redistributes Golgi structures back into the ER; and vinblastine or colchicine, which both inhibit the assembly of microtubules and the flow of vesicles along microtubules, all decrease the transport of these CYP to the PM[25,57]. Colchicine has similar effects *in vivo*, showing that the same vesicular transport is operating[25]. Thus, CYP follow a microtubule-dependent, vesicular route from the ER to the PM.

Pulse chase and immunoprecipitation experiments have indicated that only the recently synthesized CYP 1A2 molecules reach the PM (Robin *et al.*, submitted manuscript). Whereas ER CYP 1A2 was stably radiolabelled for several hours, radiolabelled CYP 1A2 reached the PM with a half-life of less than 30 min and then disappeared from the PM with a half-life of less than 30 min. Whether this short half-life in the PM is due to endocytosis[25] or some other mechanism remains to be investigated.

## PRESENCE OF CYP ON THE OUTSIDE OF THE PM

Incubation of non-permeabilized rat[52] or human[54] hepatocytes with diverse anti-CYP antibodies or affinity-purified human autoantibodies followed by peroxidase-conjugated secondary immunoglobulins resulted in peroxidase labelling of the PM on electron microscopy. With a flow cytometry analysis that excludes permeabilized cells (stained with propidium iodine), hepatocyte fluorescence was observed after exposure to anti-CYP 2B antibodies[54], anti-CYP 2C antibodies[25] or anti-CYP 1A antibodies (Robin *et al.*, submitted manuscript) and then FITC-labelled secondary immunoglobulins. These various observations suggested that CYP are oriented, at least in part, on the outside of the PM. This external orientation was confirmed by confocal scanning microscopy[25,57], which also showed the presence of CPR on the PM (Robin *et al.*, submitted manuscript). Finally, when hepatocytes were exposed to a membrane impermeant biotinylating agent, biotinylated CYP 1A and CPR were immunoprecipitated by anti-CYP 1A or anti-CPR antibodies (Robin *et al.*, submitted manuscript). All these techniques indicate that CYP (and CPR) are at least located, in part, on the outside of the PM.

## A MOSTLY EXTERNAL ORIENTATION OF CYP ON THE PM

To determine whether CYP are mostly or partly on the external surface, rat hepatocytes were exposed to immunoinhibitory anti-CYP 1A antibodies, extensively washed and then used to prepare PM. Ethoxyresorufin deethylation, an activity supported by CYP 1A, was totally inhibited, indicating that CYP are mostly located on the outside of the PM (Robin *et al.*, submitted manuscript). Similar observations were made in CYP 2D6-expressing yeast[58].

## A MOSTLY CYTOSOLIC ORIENTATION OF CYP IN MICROSOMES

CYP are mainly oriented as follows in the endoplasmic reticulum (Figure 1)[59–61]. The N-terminal methionine and a few amino acids are in the lumen, the signal/membrane anchor peptide across the membrane, and the rest of the molecule in the cytosol. ER CPR has a similar transmembrane topology[62]. External proteolysis experiments have confirmed this mostly cytosolic orientation of CYP 1A in microsomal vesicles (Robin *et al.*, submitted manuscript). However, some residual CYP 1A2 was observed and the percentage of this residual (intraluminal?) form was increased when vesicular transport was inhibited with colchicine (Robin *et al.*, submitted manuscript).

## SUGGESTED HYPOTHESIS FOR CYP TRANSPORT TO THE OUTSIDE OF THE PM

Vesicular migration, if any, of a cytosolic ER form to the PM should give a cytosolic PM form (Figure 4). To explain the external orientation of CYP on the PM, we suggest the following mechanism (Figure 5) (Robin *et al.*, submitted manuscript). Although ER CYP are mainly synthesized as cytosolic transmembrane proteins, these cytosolic forms might be retained in the ER/Golgi compartments by a cytosolic retention signal[63], and might not reach the PM. However, a fraction of newly synthesized CYP might achieve an endoluminal transmembrane topology (at some step of the vesicular transport system) and follow vesicular flow to the outside of the PM. This could explain why only newly synthesized CYP (i.e. the endoluminal form) reach the PM, while microsomes exhibit stable levels of [$^{35}$S]methionine for several hours (Robin *et al.,* submitted manuscript). With intraluminal CYP migrating to the PM with a half-life of less than 30 min and the cytosolic form being retained and slowly degraded with a half-life of 10 h, the steady state level of the intraluminal form of CYP is expected to be only a small percentage of total microsomal CYP, as indeed observed after external proteolysis (Robin *et al.*, submitted manuscript). Colchicine would increase the percentage of protease-resistant CYP in micro-

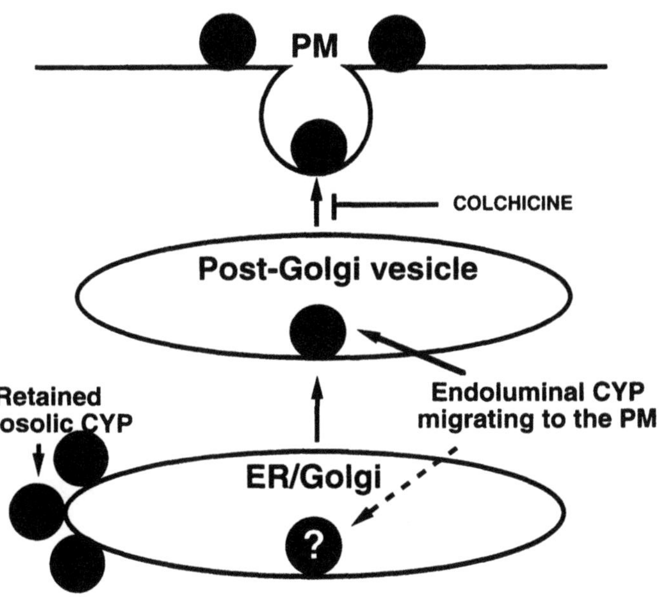


**Fig. 5** Suggested mechanism to explain the external orientation of CYP on the PM (Robin *et al.*, submitted manuscript). The major, cytosolic form of CYP could be retained in the ER/Golgi compartment(s) by a cytosolic retention signal. However, a fraction of newly synthesized CYP achieves an endoluminal topology (either in the ER itself or in a subsequent vesicular compartment) and follows vesicular flow to the outside of the PM. By interrupting vesicular flow along microtubules, colchicine increases the percentage of this intraluminal form in intracellular vesicles and decreases PM CYP

somes by interrupting transport of the intraluminal form (Robin *et al.*, submitted manuscript).

Thus, present data are consistent with three main hypotheses (Robin *et al.*, submitted manuscript). First, CYP may develop alternative transmembrane topologies during their synthesis in the ER. Dual topologies were demonstrated with a modified CYP 2D6 construct adding two positive charges to the N-terminal, pre-transmembrane peptide: 80% of this modified CYP 2D6 was on the cytosolic side of ER membranes, and 20% on the luminal side[64]. Natural CYP could also develop dual ER topologies, although with a much lower percentage of the intraluminal form.

Second, cytosolic ER CYP may migrate to post-Golgi vesicles and invert their topology in these post-Golgi vesicles and/or the PM[64]. Because microsomes contain vesicles derived from the entire vesicular transport system – and not just ER vesicles – the endoluminal form detected in microsomes is not necessarily located in the ER. Furthermore, CYP 2D6 was partly glycosylated when its intraluminal form was increased from not detectable to 20% by adding two positive charges to its N-terminal, pre-membrane sequence[64]. In contrast, wild-type CYP 2D6 was not detectably glycosylated[64]. With at most a few per cent of expected intraluminal natural forms of CYP, glycosylated forms may not be detected in microsomes. However, if an intraluminal CYP form did actually exist in the ER/Golgi compartments, if it were totally glycosylated and were selectively transported to the PM, then PM CYP would be expected to be mostly glycosylated. This expected enrichment of glycosylated forms in the PM is not observed, however, and wild-type PM CYP 2D6 is not detectably glycosylated[64]. This makes a strong case for the suggestion that CYP may achieve an endoluminal topology only after the ER/Golgi compartments[64].

Finally, this could occur post-translationally. About 30% of CYP 1A1 nascent chains escape control by the signal recognition particle and are synthesized as membrane-free polypeptides[65]. These polypeptides might post-translationally insert into diverse membranes[65]. Hypothetically, CYP might insert with the opposite topology in exocytic vesicles, perhaps due to the phospholipid asymmetry between the two membrane leaflets of these vesicles[66].

## POSSIBLE PATHOGENIC ROLE OF ANTI-CYP (AUTO)ANTIBODIES

### Tienilic acid

When tienilic acid hepatitis sera (exhibiting both anti-CYP 2C and anti-CYP 2C–tienilic acid adduct antibodies) were incubated with *(a)* human blood mononuclear cells from control subjects, and *(b)* hepatocytes from rabbits pretreated with both $\alpha$-naphthoflavone and tienilic acid, antibody-dependent cell-mediated cytotoxicity (ADCC) was observed[67], indicating that human anti-CYP 2C autoantibodies and/or anti-CYP 2C-tienilic acid adduct antibodies can be cytotoxic to hepatocytes.

### Halothane

Similarly, sera from patients with halothane-induced hepatitis (exhibiting both anti-CYP 2E1 and anti-TFA-CYP 2E1 antibodies) caused ADCC when hepatocytes from rabbits treated with halothane were incubated with blood mononuclear cells from human controls[68].

### Alcohol

Finally, sera from alcoholic patients (exhibiting anti-CYP 2E1 autoantibodies and anti-CYP 2E1-hydroxyethyl radical adduct antibodies) caused ADCC in ethanol-treated rat hepatocytes. This effect was blocked by preabsorbing the sera with human albumin complexed with the hydroxyethyl radical, which also eliminated the antibody reaction with the PM[27].

These observations suggest that the reaction of anti-CYP autoantibodies and/or anti-CYP-metabolite adduct antibodies with PM CYP and/or PM CYP–metabolite adducts may play a role in the immune destruction of hepatocytes in these diseases.

## URIDINE DIPHOSPHATE GLUCURONOSYL TRANSFERASE (UDPGT), EPOXIDE HYDROLASE, GLUTATHIONE TRANSFERASE AND ASIALOGLYCOPROTEIN RECEPTOR

### UDPGT

Certain patients infected with the hepatitis B virus develop coinfection or secondary infection with the hepatitis D virus, a deficient virus which can infect only HBV patients. In these HBV/HDV patients, anti-LKM-3 antibodies are directed against microsomal UDPGT[69]. UDPGT has a luminal ER topology[70]. The N-terminus of UDPGT and most of the protein, including the active site, is in the lumen; a transmembrane fragment then crosses the ER membrane, and a short tail of 19–26 amino acids, including the carboxyl terminus, protrudes into the cytosol[70]. A cytosolic di-lysine motif mediates retrieval of the protein from the Golgi apparatus and retrograde transport to the ER[71]. Thus the protein is not expected to be transported to the PM, unless it can partly escape this retrieval system. In that case the protein should end up on the external surface of the PM.

### Epoxide hydrolase

Antimicrosomal epoxide hydrolase autoantibodies are observed in patients with germander-induced hepatitis, and these autoantibodies recognize epoxide hydrolase on the surface of human hepatocytes (Loeper *et al.*, manuscript in preparation). Although ER microsomal epoxide hydrolase is mostly cytosolic, it has been suggested that a minor intraluminal form of epoxide hydrolase may be synthesized in the ER and could migrate to the outside of the PM[72].

### Glutathione S-transferases

Antibodies against *soluble* glutathione *S*-transferases are found in some patients with idiopathic autoimmune hepatitis[73]. It is possible (but to our knowledge still unproven) that some sera may cross-react with *microsomal* glutathione *S*-transferase[73], although the latter is a genetically distinct enzyme. The N-terminus of *microsomal* glutathione *S*-transferase is in the ER lumen while the active site is in the cytosol[74]. *Microsomal* glutathione *S*-transferase migrates to the Golgi apparatus[75] and the PM[76].

### Asialoglycoprotein receptor

Autoantibodies against the asialoglycoprotein receptor are found in some patients with idiopathic autoimmune hepatitis or with HBV or HCV hepatitis[77]. This receptor is expressed in hepatocyte PM[78].

## CONCLUSIONS

CYP and CYP–metabolite adducts follow vesicular flow to the PM. While ER CYP are mainly cytosolic, PM CYP are mainly external. We suggest that a fraction of newly synthesized CYP may enter the transport system in an endoluminal topology. It is not known whether this entry occurs in the ER or, more probably, at a subsequent step. The endoluminal CYP then follows bulk vesicular flow to the outside of the PM. Although cytotoxic T lymphocytes are probably involved in the immune destruction of hepatocytes, a possible pathogenic role of anti-CYP (auto)antibodies is suggested by ADCC experiments. Several other autoantigens are also transported to the PM.

### Acknowledgements

Some of the original studies cited in this review were supported by the European Union BIOMED 2 programme (BMH4-CT96-0658), the Programme Hospitalier de Recherche Clinique 95–96 and the Réseau Hépatox.

### References

1. Gonzales FJ, Nebert DW. Evolution of the cytochrome P-450 gene superfamily: animal–plant ‘warfare’, molecular drive and human genetic differences in drug oxidation. Trends Genet. 1990;6:182–6.
2. Germain RN. MHC-dependent antigen processing and peptide presentation: providing ligands for T lymphocyte activation. Cell. 1994;76:287–99.
3. Zimmerman HJ, Lewis JH, Ishak KG, Maddrey W. Ticrynafen-associated hepatic injury: analysis of 340 cases. Hepatology. 1984;4:315–23.
4. Lopez Garcia MP, Dansette PM, Valadon P *et al.* Human-liver cytochromes P-450 expressed in yeast as tools for reactive-metabolite formation studies. Oxidative activation of tienilic acid by cytochromes P-450 2C9 and 2C10. Eur J Biochem. 1993;213:223–32.
5. Lecoeur S, Bonierbale E, Challin D *et al.* Specificity of *in vitro* covalent binding of tienilic acid metabolites to human liver microsomes in relationship with the type of hepatotoxicity: comparison with two directly hepatotoxic drugs. Chem Res Toxicol. 1994;7:434–42.
6. Lopez-Garcia MP, Dansette P, Mansuy D. Thiophene derivatives as new mechanism-based inhibitors of cytochrome P450: inactivation of yeast-expressed human liver P450 2C9 by tienilic acid. Biochemistry. 1994;33:166–75.
7. Homberg JC, André C, Abuaf N. A new anti-liver–kidney–microsome antibody (anti-$LKM_2$) in tienilic acid-induced hepatitis. Clin Exp Immunol. 1984;55:561–70.
8. Beaune PH, Dansette PM, Mansuy D *et al.* Human anti-endoplasmic reticulum auto-antibodies appearing in a drug induced hepatitis are directed against a human liver cytochrome P-450 that hydroxylates the drug. Proc Natl Acad Sci USA. 1987;84:551–5.

9. Lecoeur S, André C, Beaune PH. Tienilic acid-induced autoimmune hepatitis: anti-liver and –kidney microsomal type 2 autoantibodies recognize a three-site conformational epitope on cytochrome P4502C9. Mol Pharmacol. 1996;50:326–33.
10. Pons C, Dansette PM, Amar C *et al.* Detection of human hepatitis anti-liver kidney microsomes (LKM2) autoantibodies on rat liver sections is predominantly due to reactivity with rat liver P-450 IIC11. J Pharmacol Exp Ther. 1991;259:1328–34.
11. Bourdi M, Larrey D, Nataf J *et al.* Anti-liver endoplasmic reticulum autoantibodies are directed against human cytochrome P-450 IA2: a specific marker of dihydralazine-induced hepatitis. J Clin Invest. 1990;85:1967–73.
12. Bourdi M, Tinel M, Beaune P, Pessayre D. Interactions of dihydralazine with cytochromes P4501A: a possible explanation for the appearance of anti-P4501A2 autoantibodies. Mol Pharmacol. 1994;45:1287–95.
13. Spracklin DK, Hankins DC, Fisher JM, Thummel KE, Kharasch ED. Cytochrome P4502E1 is the principal catalyst of human oxidative halothane metabolism *in vitro*. J Pharmacol Exp Ther. 1997;281:400–11.
14. Eliasson E, Kenna JG. Cytochrome P4502E1 is a cell surface autoantigen in halothane hepatitis. Mol Pharmacol 1996;50:573–82.
15. Bourdi M, Chen W, Peter RM *et al.* Human cytochrome P4502E1 is a major autoantigen associated with halothane hepatitis. Chem Res Toxicol. 1996; 9:1159–66.
16. Salmela KS, Kessova IG, Tsyrlov IB, Lieber CS. Respective roles of human cytochrome P-4502E1, 1A2, and 3A4 in the hepatic microsomal ethanol oxidizing system. Alcohol: Clin Exp Res. 1998;22:2125–32.
17. Behrens UJ, Hoerner M, Lasker JM, Lieber CS. Formation of acetaldehyde adducts with ethanol-inducible P450IIE1 *in vivo*. Biochem Biophys Res Commun. 1988;154:584–90.
18. Albano E, Tomasi A, Goria-Gatti L, Dianzani MU. Spin trapping of free radical species produced during the microsomal metabolism of ethanol. Chem Biol Interact. 1988;65:233–4.
19. Clot P, Albano E, Eliasson E *et al.* Cytochrome P4502E1 hydroxyethyl radical adducts as the major antigen in autoantibody formation among alcoholics. Gastroenterology. 1996;111:206–16.
20. Lytton SD, Helander A, Zhang-Gouillon ZQ *et al.* Autoantibodies against cytochromes P-4502E1 and P-4503A in alcoholics. Mol Pharmacol. 1999;55:223–33.
21. Leeder JS, Riley RJ, Cook VA, Spielberg SP. Human anti-cytochrome P450 antibodies in aromatic anticonvulsant-induced hypersensitivity reactions. J Pharmacol Exp Ther. 1992; 263:360–67.
22. Riley RJ, Smith G, Wolf CR, Cook VA, Leeder JS. Human anti-endoplasmic reticulum autoantibodies produced in aromatic anticonvulsant hypersensitivity reactions recognize rodent CYP3A proteins and a similarly regulated human P450 enzyme(s). Biochem Biophys Res Commun. 1993;191:32–40.
23. Leeder JS, Lu X, Timsit Y, Gaedigk A. Non-monooxygenase cytochromes P450 as potential human autoantigens in anticonvulsant hypersensitivity reactions. Pharmacogenetics. 1998;8:211–25.
24. Beaune PH, Pessayre D, Dansette PM, Mansuy D, Manns M. Autoantibodies against cytochromes P450: role in human diseases. Adv Pharmacol. 1994;30:199–245.
25. Robin MA, Maratrat M *et al.* Antigenic targets in tienilic acid hepatitis. Both cytochrome P450 2C11 and 2C11-tienilic acid adducts are transported to the plasma membrane of rat hepatocytes and recognized by human sera. J Clin Invest 1996;98:1471–80.
26. Bonierbale E. Mécanisme des hépatites immunoallergiques induites par l'acide tiénilique: activation métabolique de ce médicament et fixation covalente sur les cytochromes P4502C chez l'homme et le rat. Thèse de doctorat de l'Université Paris V, 1996.
27. Clot P, Parola M, Bellomo G *et al.* Plasma membrane hydroxyethyl radical adducts cause antibody-dependent cytotoxicity in rat hepatocytes exposed to alcohol. Gastroenterology. 1997;113:265–76.
28. Robin MA, Le Roy M, Descatoire V, Pessayre D. Plasma membrane cytochromes P450 as neoantigens and autoimmune targets in drug-induced hepatitis. J Hepatol. 1997;26(suppl.1):23–30.
29. Pessayre D, Larrey D, Biour M. Drug-induced liver injury. In: Bircher J, Benhamon JP, McIntyre N, Rizalto M, Rodes J, editors. Oxford Textbook of Clinical Hepatology 2nd edn. Oxford: Oxford University Press; 1999:1260–315.

30. Guilbert B, Dighiero G, Avrameas S. Naturally occurring antibodies against nine common antigens in normal humans. I. Detection, isolation and characterization. J Immunol. 1982; 28:2779–83.
31. Parker DC. T-cell dependent B-cell activation. Annu Rev Immunol. 1993;11:331–60.
32. Cambier JC, Morrisson DC, Chien MM, Lehmann KR. Modeling of T-cell contact-dependent B cell activation. IL-4 and antigen receptor ligation primes quiescent B cells to mobilize calcium in response to Ia cross-linking. J Immunol. 1991;146:2075–82.
33. Pessayre D. Role of reactive metabolites in drug-induced hepatitis. J Hepatol. 1995; 23(suppl. 1):16–24.
34. Gut J, Christen U, Huwyler J. Mechanism of halothane toxicity: novel insights. Pharmacol Ther. 1993; 58:133–55.
35. Berson A, Fréneaux D, Larrey D *et al.* Possible role of HLA in hepatotoxicity. An exploratory study with drug-induced idiosyncratic hepatitis. J Hepatol. 1994;20:336–42.
36. Homberg JC, Abuaf N, Bernard O *et al.* Chronic active hepatitis associated with anti-liver/kidney microsome antibody type 1: a second type of 'autoimmune' hepatitis. Hepatology. 1987;7:1333–9.
37. Zanger UM, Hauri HP, Loeper J, Homberg JC, Meyer UA. Antibodies against human cytochrome P-450db1 in autoimmune hepatitis type II. Proc Natl Acad Sci USA. 1988;85:8256–60.
38. Manns MP, Johnson EF, Griffin KJ, Tan EM, Sullivan KF. Major antigen of liver kidney microsomal autoantibodies in idiopathic autoimmune hepatitis is cytochrome P450db1. J Clin Invest. 1989;83:1066–72.
39. Manns MP, Griffin KJ, Sullivan KF, Johnson EF. LKM-1 autoantibodies recognize a short linear sequence in P450IID6, a cytochrome P450 monooxygenase. J Clin Invest. 1991;88:1370–8.
40. Duclos-Vallée JC, Hajoui O, Yamamoto AM, Jacqz-Aigrain E, Alvarez F. Conformational epitopes on CYP2D6 are recognized by liver/kidney microsomal antibodies. Gastroenterology. 1995;108:470–6.
41. Seeling R, Renz M, Bünger G, Schröter H, Seeling HP. Anti-LKM-1 antibodies determined by use of recombinant P4502D6 in ELISA and Western blot and their association with anti-HCV and HCV-RNA. Clin Exp Immunol. 1993;92:373–80.
42. Dalekos GN, Wedemeyer H, Obermayer-Sraub P *et al.* Epitope mapping of cytochrome P450 2D6 autoantigen in patients with chronic hepatitis C under interferon-$\alpha$ treatment. J Hepatol. 1999 (In press).
43. Ahonen P, Myllärmiemi S, Sipilä I, Perheentupa J. Clinical variation of autoimmune polyendocrinopathy–candidiasis–ectodermal dystrophy (APECED) in a series of 68 patients. N Engl J Med. 1990;322:1829–36.
44. Clemente MG, Meloni A, Obermayer-Straub P, Frau F, Manns MP, De Virgiliis S. Two cytochromes P450 are major hepatocellular autoantigens in autoimmune polyglandular syndrome type 1. Gastroenterology. 1998;114:324–8.
45. De Lemos-Chiarandini C, Alvarez F, Bernard O, Homberg JC, Kreibich G. Anti-liver microsome antibody is a marker for the rat hepatocyte endoplasmic reticulum. Hepatology. 1987;7:468–75.
46. Trautwein C, Gerken G, Löhr H, Meyer Zum Büschenfelde KH, Manns M. Lack of surface expression for the B-cell autoepitope of cytochrome P450IID6 evidenced by flow cytometry. Z Gastroenterol. 1993;31:225–30.
47. Yamamoto AM, Mura C, De Lemos-Chiarandini C, Krishnamoorthy R, Alvarez F. Cytochrome P-450IID6 recognized by LKM1 antibody is not exposed on the surface of hepatocytes. Clin Exp Immunol. 1993;92:381–90.
48. Jarasch ED, Kartenberg J, Bruder G, Fink A, Morré DJ, Franke WW. B-type cytochromes in plasma membranes isolated from rat liver, in comparison with those of endomembranes. J Cell Biol. 1979;80:37–52.
49. Stasiecki P, Oesch F. Distribution of enzymes involved in metabolic activation of polycyclic aromatic hydrocarbons among rat liver endomembranes and plasma membranes. Eur J Cell Biol. 1980;21:79–92.
50. Lenzi M, Bianchi FB, Cassani F, Pisi E. Liver cell surface expression of the antigen reacting with liver–kidney microsomal antibody (LKM). Clin Exp Immunol. 1984;55:36–40.
51. Satoh H, Davies HW, Takemura T, Gillette JR, Maeda K, Pohl LR. An immunochemical approach to investigate the mechanism of halothane-induced hepatitis. Progr Drug Metab. 1987;10:187–205.

52. Loeper J, Descatoire V, Maurice M *et al.* Presence of functional cytochrome P-450 on isolated rat hepatocyte plasma membrane. Hepatology. 1990;11:850–8.
53. Wu D, Cederbaum AI. Presence of functionally active cytochrome P-450 IIE1 in the plasma membrane of rat hepatocytes. Hepatology. 1992;15:515–24.
54. Loeper J, Descatoire V, Maurice M *et al.* Cytochromes P-450 in human hepatocyte plasma membrane: recognition by several autoantibodies. Gastroenterology. 1993;104:203–16.
55. Sakaguchi M, Mihara K, Sato R. A short amino-terminal segment of microsomal cytochrome P-450 functions both as an insertion signal and a stop-transfer sequence. EMBO J. 1987;6:2425–31.
56. Neve EPA, Eliasson E, Pronzato MA, Albano E, Marinari U, Ingelman-Sundberg M. Enzyme-specific transport of rat liver cytochrome P450 to the Golgi apparatus. Arch Biochem Biophys. 1996;333:459–65.
57. Robin MA, Maratrat M, Loeper J *et al.* Cytochrome P4502B follows a vesicular route to the plasma membrane in cultured rat hepatocytes. Gastroenterology. 1995;108:1110–23.
58. Loeper J, Louérat-Oriou B, Duport C, Pompon D. Yeast expressed cytochrome P450 2D6 (CYP2D6) exposed on the external face of plasma membrane is functionally competent. Mol Pharmacol. 1998;54:8–13.
59. De Lemos-Chiarandini C, Frey AB, Sabatini DD, Kreibich G. Determination of the membrane topology of the phenobarbital-inducible rat liver cytochrome P-450 isoenzyme PB-4 using site-specific antibodies. J Cell Biol. 1987;104:209–19.
60. Vergères G, Winterhalter KH, Richter C. Localization of the N-terminal methionine of rat liver cytochrome P-450 in the lumen of the endoplasmic reticulum. Biochim Biophys Acta. 1991;1063:235–41.
61. Black SD, Martin ST, Smith CA. Membrane topology of liver microsomal cytochrome P450 2B4 determined via monoclonal antibodies directed to the halt transfer signal. Biochemistry. 1994;33:6945–51.
62. Kida Y, Ohgiya S, Mihara K, Sakaguchi M. Membrane topology of NADPH-cytochrome P450 reductase on the endoplasmic reticulum. Arch Biochem Biophys. 1998;351:175–9.
63. Szczesna-Skorupa E, Ahn K, Chen CD, Doray B, Kemper B. The cytoplasmic and N-terminal transmembrane domains of cytochrome P450 contain independent signals for retention in the endoplasmic reticulum. J Biol Chem. 1995;41:24327–32.
64. Loeper J, Le Berre A, Pompon D. Topology inversion of CYP2D6 in the endoplasmic reticulum is not required for plasma membrane transport. Mol Pharmacol. 1998;53:408–14.
65. Addya S, Anandatheerthavarada HK, Biswas G, Bhagwat SV, Mullick J, Avadhani NG. Targeting of $NH_2$-terminal-processed microsomal protein to mitochondria: a novel pathway for the biogenesis of hepatic mitochondrial P450MT2. J Cell Biol. 1997;139:589–99.
66. Zachowski A, Henry JP, Devaux PF. Control of transmembrane lipid asymmetry in chromaffin granules by an ATP-dependent protein. Nature. 1989;340:75–6.
67. Neuberger J, Williams R. Immune mechanisms in tienilic acid associated hepatotoxicity. Gut. 1989;30:515–19.
68. Vergani D, Mieli-Vergani G, Alberti A *et al.* Antibodies to the surface of halothane-altered rabbit hepatocytes in patients with severe halothane-associated hepatitis. N Engl J Med. 1980;303:66–71.
69. Philipp T, Durazzo M, Trautwein C *et al.* Recognition of uridine diphosphate glucuronosyl transferases by LKM-3 antibodies in chronic hepatitis D. Lancet. 1994;344:578–81.
70. Yokota H, Yuasa A, Sata R. Topological disposition of UDP glucuronosyltransferase in rat liver microsomes. J Biochem. 1992;112:192–6.
71. Meech R, Mackenzie PI. Determinants of UDP glucuronosyltransferase membrane association and residency in the endoplasmic reticulum. Arch Biochem Biophys. 1998;356:77–85.
72. Alves C, von Dippe P, Amoui M, Levy D. Bile acid transport into hepatocyte smooth endoplasmic reticulum vesicles is mediated by microsomal epoxide hydrolase, a membrane protein exhibiting two distinct topological orientations. J Biol Chem. 1993;268:20148–55.
73. Wesierska-Gadek J, Grimm R, Hitchman E, Penner E. Members of the glutathione *S*-transferase gene family are antigens in autoimmune hepatitis. Gastroenterology. 1998;114:329–335.
74. Andersson C, Weinander R, Lundqvist G, DePierre JW, Morgenstern R. Functional and structural membrane topology of rat liver microsomal glutathione transferase. Biochim Biophys Acta. 1994;1204:298–304.

75. Luzio JP, Brake B, Banting G, Howell KE, Braghetta P, Stanley KK. Identification, sequencing and expression of an integral membrane protein of the trans-Golgi network. Biochem J. 1990;270:97–102.
76. Horbach ME, Sies H, Akerboom TPM. Purification of rat liver plasma membrane glutathione transferase. Eur J Biochem. 1994;222:91–6.
77. Treichel U, Gerken G, Rossol S, Rotthauwe HW, Meyer zum Büschenfelde KH, Poralla T. Autoantibodies against the human asialoglycoprotein receptor: effects of therapy in autoimmune and virus-induced chronic active hepatitis. J Hepatol. 1993;19:55–63.
78. Spiess M. The asialoglycoprotein receptor: a model for endocytic transport receptors. Biochemistry. 1990;29:10009–18.

# 4
# Caspase-10 mutations in the autoimmune lymphoproliferative syndrome type II

**J. WANG and M. J. LENARDO**

## INTRODUCTION

Apoptosis plays an essential role in maintaining homeostasis in lymphocytes. Antigen-provoked apoptosis of lymphocytes, or propricidal regulation, can be mediated by Fas (CD95/APO-1), tumour necrosis factor receptor (TNFR) and related molecules[1–5]. Other death ligands such as TRAIL and its corresponding death receptors DR4 and DR5 are expressed in immune cells, but their physiological functions are not well understood[6–11]. Recent experiments suggest that the fate of specialized antigen-presenting cells is also regulated during immune responses. Ingulli *et al.* (1997) have shown that antigen-bearing dendritic cells directly interact with antigen-specific T cells resulting in T cell activation and disappearance of the dendritic cells[12]. Because dendritic cells are potent stimulators of B cells and T cells, their turnover may be essential for regulating immune responses[13]. However, currently little is known about how this process is regulated.

We and others have identified the autoimmune lymphoproliferative syndrome (ALPS) as an inherited disease of lymphocyte homeostasis and defective apoptosis[14–19]. In ALPS type Ia this phenotype is associated with inherited mutations in Fas[20]. In ALPS type Ib systemic lupus erythematosus and lymphadenopathy are associated with inherited mutations in the FasL gene[21]. The *lpr* and *gld* alleles cause similar diseases in mice due to homozygous recessive mutations in the Fas and Fas ligand (FasL) genes, respectively[22–24]. ALPS type II is manifested by a related clinical phenotype and apoptosis defects in the absence of either Fas or FasL mutations[5,19]. The molecular basis for ALPS type II has not been previously identified.

Caspases are the effector molecules in the apoptosis pathways mediated by death receptors. Caspase-8 (casp-8) occupies a proximal position in Fas and TNFR signalling because it contains two death effector domains (DED) in its N-terminal prodomain. The DED allow casp-8 to interact with the DED of Fas-associated protein with a death domain (FADD)/MORT1. Homotypic interaction of the death domains in FADD and death receptors thus allow casp-8 to be recruited into the death-inducing signaling complex[5,25–27]. Deficiency in casp-8 causes prenatal mortality and a loss of TNF- and Fas-induced apoptosis in mice[28]. Caspase-10/Mch4/FLICE2 (casp-10) is a novel caspase homologous to casp-8 and linked to the casp-8 gene at the human chromosome locus 2q23[29,30]. Casp-10 induces apoptosis after transfection into MCF-7 cells[30], but its physiological role is unknown. Moreover, the participation of individual caspases in abnormalities of lymphocyte homeostasis and autoimmunity has not been defined.

Most ALPS patients we have examined prove to be ALPS type 1a. Recently we described two ALPS type II families with autoimmunity and pleiotropic apoptosis defects in multiple pathways, but no molecular abnormalities in Fas or FasL[31]. Rather, we found distinct inherited amino acid substitutions in casp-10 in each family that resulted in decreased apoptosis activity. In contrast to Fas mutations leading to ALPS type I, these casp-10 defects underlie a unique disorder of dendritic cell and lymphocyte homeostasis.

## RESULTS

### Clinical features and lymphocyte apoptosis defects

Patient 11 is an 11-year-old female who developed prominent non-malignant adenopathy and hepatosplenomegaly from 1 year of age. She had multiple autoantibodies and massive accumulation of T cells and B cells and an increase in $CD4^{-}CD8^{-}\alpha\beta T$ cells. Patient 11's mother also exhibited high levels of autoantibodies to nuclear antigens. In contrast, Patient 11's father and siblings are healthy. Patient 36 is a 10-year-old male who developed adenopathy, splenomegaly and non-infectious lymphocytic meningitis followed by optic neuritis, indicating a pattern of disparate inflammatory conditions. Lymphocyte phenotyping showed a dramatic T and B lymphocytosis and a significant increase in $\gamma\delta$ $CD4^{-}/CD8^{-}T$ cells. Both parents were clinically normal. Thus, despite normal Fas and FasL, both families manifested a loss of lymphoid homeostasis accompanied by autoimmune and inflammatory conditions.

In ALPS type I, T cell apoptosis induced by Fas or TCR cross-linking is abnormal[16]. We therefore also examined apoptosis in activated peripheral blood T lymphocytes (PBL) in kindreds 11 and 36. In Patient 11 and, to a lesser extent, her mother, apoptosis induced by T cell receptor (TCR) cross-linking and Fas cross-linking was decreased (Figure 1). We also examined apoptosis responses to a trimeric form of the TRAIL[32], and found defects in Patient 11 and her mother's lymphocytes, but not in ALPS type I patients (Figure 1 and data not shown). No apoptosis defects were found in the father and sisters of Patient 11 (Figure 1). Patient 36 also exhibited abnormal apoptosis responses to TCR, Fas, or TRAIL stimulation, while his parents exhibited modest but significant defects. Flow cytometry showed that Fas expression as well as apoptosis in response to staurosporine or lymphokine withdrawal were normal in Patients 11 and 36 (data not shown).

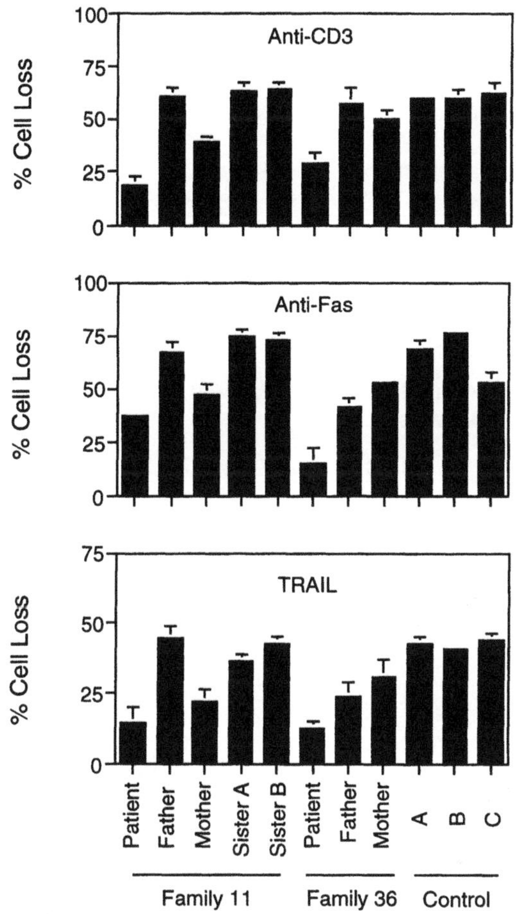


**Fig. 1** Lymphocyte apoptosis assays. Apoptosis of PBL were induced by 1 μg/ml plate-bound 64.1 (anti-CD3), 1 μg/ml CH11 (anti-Fas) or 1 μg/ml TRAIL at 37°C for 24 h and percentage cell loss was analysed as described[31]

## Identification of casp-10 mutations

We hypothesized that a molecule downstream of the death receptors might be deficient in these patients. Candidate gene approach revealed a casp-10 mutation in Patient 11; it was a C to T transition predicted to replace a leucine by phenylalanine in the p17 subunit of the protease (Figure 2A). In addition to the previously described casp-10 cDNA[29], we also detected a longer cDNA isoform (casp-$10_L$). Casp-$10_L$ encodes an insertion of 43 amino acids at the end of the prodomain identical to the prodomain of FLICE2, but its C-terminus was the same as the short casp-10 isoform[30]. The two isoforms were expressed equally. Approximately 50% of casp-10 cDNA (of either isoform) were mutant, implying heterozygosity. This was confirmed by direct sequencing of genomic DNA

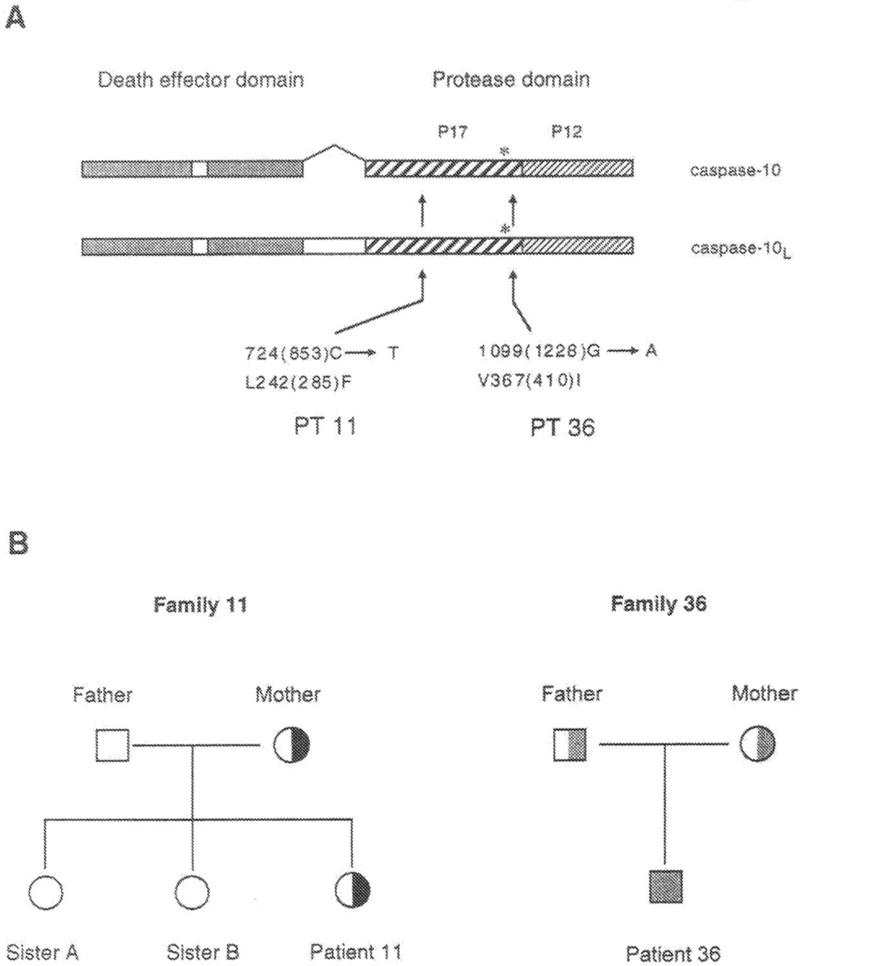


**Fig. 2** Casp-10 mutations. **A:** Diagram showing the location of casp-10 mutations in Patient 11 and Patient 36. The asterisk indicates the 'QACQG' active site. **B:** Pedigrees of families 11 and 36. Affected heterozygous individuals in family 11 are shown as partially filled symbols (dark). Affected heterozygous parents in family 36 are shown as partially filled symbols (grey), and Patient 36 who is homozygous is shown as a completely filled symbol (grey)

which revealed the wild-type C and mutant T nucleotides at the same position[31]. Genomic DNA sequencing in the parents revealed that the father of Patient 11 and two sisters carried only wild-type alleles, but her mother harboured both mutant and wild-type alleles[31]. Thus, the mutant casp-10 allele in Patient 11 was inherited from her mother (Figure 2B).

In Patient 36, sequencing of cDNA clones revealed a G to A transition predicted to cause a valine to isoleucine change 7 amino acids downstream of the QACQG active site in the p17 subunit of the casp-10 gene (Figure 2A). This mutation occurred in cDNA of both isoforms of casp-10. In contrast to Patient 11, no wild-type allele was detected in Patient 36, suggesting that the mutant allele is homozygous[31]. This was confirmed by genomic DNA sequencing[31]. Examination of the genomic DNA of both parents revealed that each was heterozygous for the mutant allele, indicating that the child had indeed inherited a mutant casp-10 allele from each parent (Figure 2B). Screening of DNA samples of normal unrelated donors from the general population and normal unrelated donors of the same ethnic groups as the patients revealed no casp-10 mutations of either Patient 11 or Patient 36 (data not shown). Therefore the casp-10 mutations in families 11 and 36 are not common genetic polymorphisms.

## Abrogation of apoptosis activities by casp-10 mutations

We next determined whether the altered forms of casp-10 were functionally defective. Expression constructs of both the long and short isoforms of the wild-type or the casp-10 mutants were transfected into HeLa cells together with a $\beta$-gal reporter construct. The cells were stained with X-gal and cell death was assessed in the blue transfected cells[31]. Either isoform of wild-type casp-10 induced significant cell death, but neither isoform of Patient 11 had detectable apoptotic activity in this assay (Figure 3A). Similar analyses of the Patient 36 casp-10 revealed a significant, albeit less severe, defect in apoptosis function (Figure 3B). Further quantitative analysis was performed with the bacterially-expressed casp-10 protease domain of Patient 11 fused to glutathione-*S*-transferase. The wild-type casp-10 fusion protein efficiently cleaved two different caspase substrates, DEVD-AMC and YVAD-MCA, but the Patient 11 mutant protein failed to do so. This suggests that the Patient 11 casp-10 is significantly defective in protease activity.

To explore how the heterozygous allele in Patient 11 and her mother could impair apoptosis, we co-expressed Fas with either the long or short isoform of the Patient 11 mutant casp-10 in 293 cells and found that apoptosis was sup-

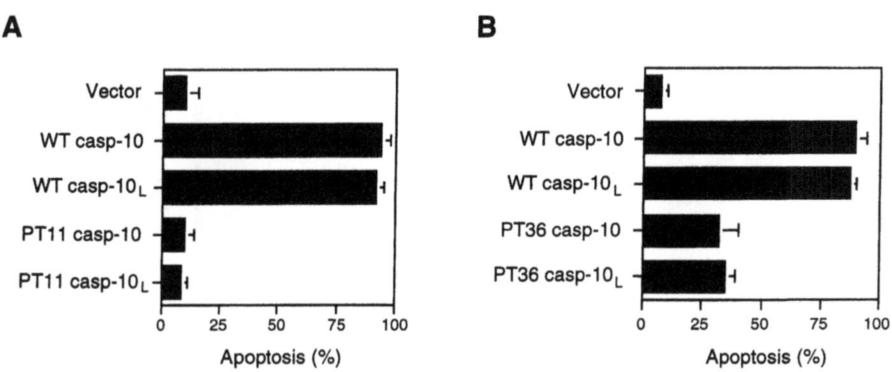


**Fig. 3** Defective apoptotic activities of mutant casp-10. HeLa cells were transfected with 2 $\mu$g vector control, wild-type casp-10, Patient 11 casp-10 (A) or Patient 36 casp-10 plasmid (**B**) in the presence of 0.6 $\mu$g $\beta$-gal construct DNA. Cells were fixed and stained for blue colour with X-gal 24 h after transfection. Percentages of apoptotic cells among the blue-transfected cells were quantitated under a microscope

pressed[31]. We also co-expressed the casp-10 mutants with the TNFR1, DR3, DR4 (TRAIL-R1) and DR5 (TRAIL-R2) receptors, and in each case the mutant caspase interfered with death induction[31]. The p35 inhibitor blocked apoptosis in all cases, indicating that the death observed was caspase-dependent[31]. By contrast, the mutant casp-10 did not interfere with apoptosis of transfected cells treated with ultravidet irradiation or staurosporine (data not shown). Hence, the abnormal casp-10 protein specifically interfered with multiple death receptor pathways, and not other apoptosis pathways. Transfection studies show that Patient 11 casp-10 is recruited into the DISC together with casp-8, and could thereby block caspase activation in a dominant fashion[31].

## Resistance of dendritic cells to TRAIL-mediated apoptosis

To explain the multiple autoimmune and inflammatory disorders in ALPS type II, we also examined how the Patient 11 and Patient 36 casp-10 mutations affect death receptor-associated apoptosis in antigen-presenting cells. We carried out direct ligand-dependent cell killing assays. We found that TRAIL induced significant dendritic cell death, whereas FasL and TNF-$\alpha$ had no measurable effects (Figure 4A and data not shown). Moreover, dendritic cells from Patient 11 and Patient 36 underwent significantly less apoptosis in response to TRAIL compared to ALPS type I patients and healthy controls (Figure 4A). Apoptosis defects were also observed in the mother of Patient 11 and to a minor degree in the parents of Patient 36 (Figure 4A). These data suggest that the casp-10 mutations in Patient 11 and Patient 36 affect TRAIL-induced death of dendritic cells.

To directly demonstrate that the defective casp-10 suppresses TRAIL-mediated apoptosis in dendritic cells, we used a retrovirus infection system to introduce the Patient 11 casp-10 mutant into dendritic cells[31]. Patient 11 casp-10 gene was inserted upstream of an internal ribosome entry site (IRES) and the

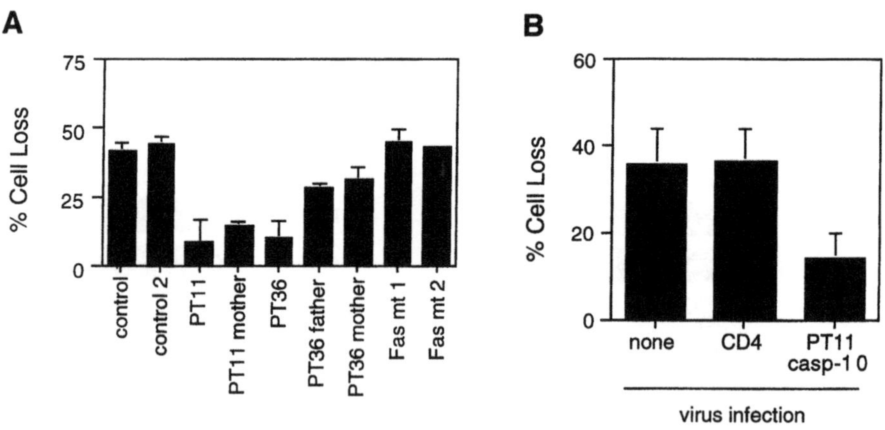


**Fig. 4** TRAIL-mediated killing of dendritic cells. **A:** Dendritic cells from Patient 11 and Patient 36, family members, normal controls and patients carrying Fas mutations were cultured with or without 1 $\mu$g/ml TRAIL at 37°C for 24 h. Percent cell loss was measured as described previously. **B:** Dendritic cells infected with retrovirus expressing CD4 or Patient 11 casp-10 and uninfected dendritic cells were cultured with or without 1 $\mu$g/ml TRAIL at 37°C for 24 h. Percentage cell loss was measured as described previously

GFP gene in a retroviral vector, allowing us to monitor the efficiency of viral transduction and viral gene expression by flow cytometry. Seventy per cent of the cells could be infected with either the retroviral construct carrying the CD4 gene (the control) or the vector encoding the Patient 11 mutant casp-10[31]. When we compared the virally transduced dendritic cells to non-infected dendritic cells, we found that TRAIL-dependent killing was significantly reduced in cells bearing the Patient 11 casp-10-expressing virus (Figure 4B). By contrast, dendritic cells infected with CD4-expressing virus were killed as efficiently as uninfected cells by TRAIL (Figure 4B). These data provide direct evidence that the Patient 11 mutant casp-10 dominantly interferes with TRAIL-mediated apoptosis in dendritic cells.

To determine the physiological significance of the dendritic cell apoptosis defect, we examined frozen sections of lymph node from Patient 11. We found that lymph node from Patient 11 exhibited unique large accumulations of CD83-bearing dendritic cells that were confined to the T cell areas of the lymph node[31]. This is not observed in normal controls or ALPS type I patients[31]. Thus, abnormal dendritic cell apoptosis is associated with overaccumulation of dendritic cells in the lymph node in ALPS type II which is not observed in ALPS type I.

## DISCUSSION

To our knowledge the mutations of Patient 11 and Patient 36 are the first reported inherited gene defects of a caspase associated with a human disease[31]. In Patient 11 the allele is heterozygous but the casp-10 protein encoded by its mutant allele is severely defective in autoprocessing and enzymatic function. Patient 36 has a different mode of inheritance. The deficiency of this mutant casp-10 is less severe but homozygosity of this mutation results in a significant impairment of apoptosis. We found certain similarities to mice and humans with Fas defects such as the overaccumulation of lymphocytes, especially $CD4^-CD8^-$T cells and autoimmune and inflammatory disorders. However, we also found an unprecedented defect in dendritic cell apoptosis in response to TRAIL and the overaccumulation of dendritic cells in the lymphoid tissue from Patient 11. The combined defect in lymphocyte and antigen-presenting cell apoptosis may have fundamental relevance to the pathogenesis of autoimmune disease in ALPS type II.

### Casp-10 connects to important apoptosis pathways

Casp-10 was originally identified in the expressed sequence tag database and transfection assays verified its function as a death-inducing caspase and indicated that it was recruited into apoptosis pathways especially involving DR4 and DR5[7,30,33,34]. Its function was poorly defined. We found that the casp-10 mutations in Patient 11 and Patient 36 impaired Fas-mediated apoptosis in lymphocytes and TRAIL-induced killing in both lymphocytes and dendritic cells. Moreover, transfection of the severely defective Patient 11 casp-10 curtailed apoptosis induction by Fas, TNFR1, DR3, DR4, and DR5. This suggests that casp-10 affects a signal integration point for apoptosis receptors. The downstream position of its effect at a point common to multiple cell death pathways could account for the severe pleiotropic autoimmunity and inflammatory disorders and abnormal cellular homeostasis in these two patients with ALPS type II.

The signalling role of casp-10 *vis-à-vis* its close homologue casp-8 is not understood. The casp-8 and casp-10 genes appear to be part of a gene duplication event in the human casp-8/10/c-FLIP locus (2q33, interval 204.7–205.4). It is now evident that casp-10 in its mutant form impairs apoptosis in the presence of a normal casp-8 gene. Genetic deficiencies of casp-8 have been shown to block Fas and TNF-induced apoptosis[26,28]. Thus casp-10 is unlikely to be a redundant form of casp-8. The third homologue in the locus, c-FLIP, contains multiple amino acid substitutions that abrogate its enzymatic function and can either impair or enhance apoptosis by associating with apoptosis signalling proteins in transfected cells[35–38]. In a manner similar to c-FLIP, the mutant casp-10 could interfere with casp-8 activation. Our data show that casp-8 and Patient 11 casp-10 can be co-recruited by FADD to Fas, but the relative contribution of either caspase to death induction by each of the death receptors is not defined. In family[36] the milder form of mutant casp-10 did not alone cause a strong dominant-interfering effect, as evidenced by the minor apoptosis defect in each parent who was heterozygous and clinically normal. This could imply that the severity of apoptosis defect may be correlated with clinical phenotype independent of any other genetic or environmental influences. Dominant negative as well as homozygous recessive mutants for casp-10 may be important tools to dissect these pathways in various immune cell types. A prime example may be dendritic cells, for which little is known about the pathways that govern their fate during and after immune responses.

## Dendritic cell homeostasis by apoptosis may be crucial for immune tolerance

Previous investigations of autoimmunity and apoptosis have focused almost exclusively on lymphocytes. It is now evident that the turnover of antigen-presenting cells is an important factor in the maintenance of tolerance. The differentiation and growth of dendritic cells has been well studied, but little is known about their fate after migration to the lymphoid organs [13]. The TNF family molecules CD40 ligand and TRANCE produced by T cells can promote the survival of dendritic cells in lymphoid tissue[39,40]. However, Jenkins and co-workers have observed that dendritic cells are directly eliminated in an antigen- and T-cell-dependent manner soon after an immune reaction[12]. We now show that activated T cells directly induced the death of dendritic cells. Moreover, of the three death-inducing cytokines produced by antigen-stimulated T cells that were tested, TRAIL, but not FasL or TNF, had the strongest apoptosis-inducing effect on dendritic cells. Moreover, casp-10 mutations impaired TRAIL-induced dendritic cell apoptosis. Corresponding to this apoptosis defect, we found a marked accumulation of dendritic cells in the T cell areas of the lymph nodes in Patient 11. Taken together with the findings of Ingulli *et al.*[12], and the fact that TRAIL is produced by T cells (as well as B cells, and monocytes)[11,41,42], the physiological disappearance of dendritic cells could be mediated by TRAIL. Similar lines of evidence indicate that this regulatory pathway is unimpaired by Fas mutations in ALPS type I.

Dendritic cell persistence could cause prolonged stimulation of T cells and B cells[13]. Usually, repeated antigen stimulation of activated T cells leads to apoptosis by the propriocidal mechanism[4]. Our data suggest that there is a cross-regulation in which TRAIL produced by T cells can induce dendritic cell apoptosis. However, in ALPS type II, both T cells and dendritic cells have impaired apoptosis responses and accumulate in T zones where the lingering dendritic cells could induce responses that do not normally take place. The combined apoptosis defects in two interacting cell types, i.e. dendritic cells and T cells, may be responsible for the disease phenotype in ALPS type II.

## Acknowledgements

We thank our colleagues L. Zheng, A. Lobito, F. Chan, S. Straus, J. Puck and J. Dale for their contributions to this work. J. Wang is a fellow of the Arthritis Foundation.

## References

1. Chinnaiyan AM, Dixit VM. Portrait of an executioner: the molecular mechanism of FAS/APO-1-induced apoptosis. Semin Immunol. 1997;9:69–76.
2. Russell JH, Rush B, Weaver C, Wang R. Mature T cells of autoimmune lpr/lpr mice have a defect in antigen-stimulated suicide. Proc Natl Acad Sci USA. 1993;90:4409–13.
3. Zheng L, Fisher G, Miller RE, Peschon J, Lynch DH, Lenardo MJ. Induction of apoptosis in mature T cells by tumour necrosis factor. Nature. 1995;377:348–51.
4. MJ. Lenardo. Fas and the art of lymphocyte maintenance. J Exp Med. 1996;183:721–4.
5. Wang, J., M. J. Lenardo. Molecules involved in cell death and peripheral tolerance. Curr Opin Immunol. 1997;9: 818–25.
6. Wiley SR, Schooley K, Smolak PJ *et al.* Identification and characterization of a new member of the TNF family that induces apoptosis. Immunity. 1995;3:673–82.
7. Pan G, O'Rourke K, Chinnaiyan AM *et al.* The receptor for the cytotoxic ligand TRAIL. Science. 1997;276:111–13.
8. Sheridan JP, Marsters SA, Pitti RM *et al.* Control of TRAIL-induced apoptosis by a family of signaling and decoy receptors. Science. 1997;277:818–21.
9. MacFarlane M, Ahmad M, Srinivasula SM *et al.* Identification and molecular cloning of two novel receptors for the cytotoxic ligand TRAIL. J Biol Chem. 1997;272:25417–20.
10. Marsters SA, Sheridan JP, Pitti RM *et al.* A novel receptor for Apo2L/TRAIL contains a truncated death domain. Curr Biol. 1997;7:1003–6.
11. Thomas WD, Hersey P. TNF-related apoptosis-inducing ligand (TRAIL) induces apoptosis in Fas ligand-resistant melanoma cells and mediates CD4 T cell killing of target cells. J Immunol. 1998;161:2195–200.
12. Ingulli E, Mondino A, Khoruts A, Jenkins MK. *In vivo* detection of dendritic cell antigen presentation to CD4(+) T cells. J Exp Med. 1997;185:2133–41.
13. Banchereau J, Steinman RM. Dendritic cells and the control of immunity. Nature. 1998;392:245–52.
14. Bettinardi A, Brugnoni D, E. Quiros-Roldan *et al.* Missense mutations in the Fas gene resulting in autoimmune lymphoproliferative syndrome: a molecular and immunological analysis. Blood. 1997;89:902–9.
15. Drappa J, Vaishnaw AK, Sullivan KE, Chu JL, Elkon KB. Fas gene mutations in the Canale–Smith syndrome, an inherited lymphoproliferative disorder associated with autoimmunity. N Engl J Med. 1996;335:1643–9.
16. Fisher GH, Rosenberg FJ, Straus SE *et al.* Dominant interfering Fas gene mutations impair apoptosis in a human autoimmune lymphoproliferative syndrome. Cell. 1995;81:935–46.

17. Kasahara Y, Wada T, Niida Y *et al.* Novel Fas (CD95/APO-1) mutations in infants with a lymphoproliferative disorder. Int Immunol. 1998;10:195–202.
18. Rieux-Laucat F, Diest FL, Roberts IA, Debatin KM, Fisher A, Villartay JP. Mutations in Fas associated with human lymphoproliferative syndrome and autoimmunity. Science. 1995;268:1347–1351.
19. Sneller MC, Wang J, Dale JK *et al.* Clincial, immunologic, and genetic features of an autoimmune lymphoproliferative syndrome associated with abnormal lymphocyte apoptosis. Blood. 1997;89:1341–8.
20. Straus SE, Lenardo MJ, Puck JM, Strober W, Sneller MC. Autoimmune lymphoproliferative syndrome: an inherited disorder of lymphocyte apoptosis. Ann Intern Med. 1999 (In press).
21. Wu J, Wilson J, He J, Xiang L, Schur PH, Mountz JD. Fas ligand mutation in a patient with systemic lupus erythematosus and lymphoproliferative disease. J Clin Invest. 1996;98:1107–13.
22. Watanabe-Fukunaga R, Brannan CI, Copeland NG, Jenkins NA, Nagata S. Lymphoproliferation disorder in mice explained by defects in Fas antigen that mediates apoptosis. Nature. 1992;356:314–17.
23. Takahashi T, Tanaka M, Brannan CI *et al.* Generalized lymphoproliferative disease in mice, caused by a point mutation in the Fas ligand. Cell. 1994;76:969–76.
24. Lynch DH, Watson ML, Alderson MR *et al.* The mouse Fas-ligand gene is mutated in gld mice and is part of a TNF family gene cluster. Immunity. 1994;1:131–6.
25. Boldin MP, Goncharov TM, Goltsev YV, Wallach D. Involvement of MACH, a novel MORT1/FADD-interacting protease, in Fas/APO-1- and TNF receptor-induced cell death. Cell. 1996;85:803–15
26. Juo P, Kuo CJ, Yuan J, Blenis J. Essential requirement for caspase-8/FLICE in the initiation of the Fas-induced apoptotic cascade. Curr Biol. 1998;8:1001–8.
27. Muzio M, Chinnaiyan AM, Kischkel FC *et al.* FLICE, a novel FADD-homologous ICE/CED-3-like protease, is recruited to the CD95 (Fas/APO-1) death-inducing signaling complex. Cell. 1996:85:817–27.
28. Varfolomeev EE, Schuchmann M, Luria V *et al.* Targeted disruption of the mouse Caspase 8 gene ablates cell death induction by the TNF receptors, Fas/Apo1, and DR3 and is lethal prenatally. Immunity. 1998;9:267–76.
29. Fernandes-Alnemri T, Armstrong RC, Krebs J *et al. In-vitro* activation of CPP32 and Mch3 by Mch4, a novel human apoptotic cysteine protease containing two FADD-like domains. Proc Nate Acad Sci USA. 1996;93:7464–9.
30. Vincenz C, Dixit VM. Fas-associated death domain protein interleukin-1beta-converting enzyme 2 (FLICE2), an ICE/Ced-3 homologue, is proximally involved in CD95- and p55-mediated death signaling. J Biol Chem. 1997;272:6578–83.
31. Wang J, Zheng L, Lobito A *et al.* Inherited human CASPASE10 mutations underlie defective lymphocyte and dendritic cell apoptosis in autoimmune lymphoproliferative syndrome type II. Cell. 1999;96 (In press).
32. Walczak H, Miller RE, Ariail K *et al.* Tumoricidal activity of tumor necrosis factor-related apoptosis-inducing ligand in vivo [See comments]. Nat Med. 1999;5:157–63.
33. Chaudhary PM, Eby M, Jasmin A, Bookwalter A, Murray J, Hood L. Death receptor 5, a new member of the TNFR family, and DR4 induce FADD-dependent apoptosis and activate the NF-kappaB pathway. Immunity. 1997;7:821–30.
34. Schneider P, Thome M, Burns K *et al.* TRAIL receptors 1 (DR4) and 2 (DR5) signal FADD-dependent apoptosis and activate NF-kappaB. Immunity. 1997;7:831–6.
35. Irmler M, Thome M, Hahne M *et al.* Inhibition of death receptor signals by cellular FLIP. Nature. 1997;388:190–5.
36. Rasper DM, Vaillancourt JP, Hadano S *et al.* Cell death attenuation by 'Usurpin', a mammallian DED-caspase homologue that precludes caspase-8 recruitment and activation by the CD-95 (Fas, APO-1) receptor complex. Cell Death Different. 1998;5:271–288.
37. Shu HB, Halpin DR, Goeddel DV. Casper is a FADD- and caspase-related inducer of apoptosis. Immunity. 1997;6:751–63.
38. Srinivasula SM, Ahmad M, Ottilie S *et al.* FLAME-1, a novel FADD-like anti-apoptotic molecule that regulates Fas/TNFR1-induced apoptosis. J Biol Chem. 1997;272:18542–5.

39. Anderson DM, Maraskovsky E, Billingsley WL *et al.* A homologue of the TNF receptor and its ligand enhance T-cell growth and dendritic-cell function. Nature. 1997;390:175–9.
40. Wong BR, Josien R, Lee SY *et al.* TRANCE (tumor necrosis factor [TNF]-related activation-induced cytokine), a new TNF family member predominantly expressed in T cells, is a dendritic cell-specific survival factor. J Exp Med. 1997;186:2075–80.
41. Marsters SA, Pitti RM, Donahue CJ, Ruppert S, Bauer KD, Ashkenazi A. Activation of apoptosis by Apo-2 ligand is independent of FADD but blocked by CrmA. Curr Biol. 1996;6:750–2.
42. Griffith TS, Wiley SR, Kubin MZ, Sedger LM, Maliszewski CR, Fanger NA. Monocyte-mediated tumoricidal activity via the tumor necrosis factor-related cytokine, TRAIL J Exp Med. 1999;189:1343–54.

# 5
# Mechanisms of virus-induced autoimmune disease

**B. LUDEWIG, P. AICHELE, R. M. ZINKERNAGEL and H. HENGARTNER**

## INTRODUCTION

Autoimmune disorders are diseases in which a vigorous immune reaction against certain self-antigens is induced, leading to pathological damage either in one organ or generalized in various tissues in the body. Generally, the immune system maintains a status of unresponsivenes towards self-antigens, while being able to mount an immune response against pathogen-derived antigens. Tolerance, at least on the level of T cells, is established and maintained by elimination of self-reactive cells in the thymus or, alternatively, when antigens are immunologically ignored because they are expressed at immunologically sequestered sites[1–3] or when antigens do not reach a certain concentration level in lymphoid organs[4,5]. Thus, the decision whether an autoimmune reaction is initiated is probably made when a previously ignored antigen is presented in sufficient amounts and over a certain time in secondary lymphoid tissues. It is likely that antigen presentation by professional antigen presenting cells, i.e. dendritic cells and macrophages, in lymphoid tissues is the key step in the initiation of an anti-self response and to break the status of ignorance. Accordingly, the central questions for the initiation of T cell-mediated autoimmune diseases are 'Which are the antigens that induce the primary immune response against the target organ?' and 'Which mechanisms lead to release of tissue antigen and subsequent presentation of these antigens in secondary lymphoid organs?'.

The mechanisms postulated to be involved in primary release of tissue antigens and/or initiation of a primary anti-self response include the following. (1) Autoimmunity due to responses against viral or other microbial structures that cross-react with one or more self-antigens has been termed 'molecular mimicry'[6,7]. (2) Mechanisms involving non-specific activation of T cells have been shown recently, including stimulation via cytokines secreted by 'bystander cells'[8]. Local virus infection and tissue destruction may create an inflammatory milieu for activation of self-reactive T cells[9]. (3) T cell-mediated protective immunity against viruses may directly contribute to immunopathologies[10]. An immune response initiated against a non-cytopathic virus, such as LCMV, may damage tissues infected with the virus via $CD8^+$ T cell-mediated and perforin-dependent cytotoxicity[11–14]. Furthermore, virus-induced damage of host tissues may trigger release of self-antigens leading particularly to spreading of Th cell responses from the original anti-viral specificity to an anti-self response[15].

Taken together it appears that the initial trigger of an autoimmune response in the majority of cases is an infection of the target organ with a virus or other pathogens. The immune response may then be directed against pathogen-derived antigens, pathogen antigens mimicking self-antigens or self-antigens that had been previously ignored. Clearly, a pathological autoimmune response develops only when these antigens are presented to the immune system in a minimal concentration for a sufficient amount of time to initiate and maintain the response.

Dendritic cells (DC) are the prime candidates to facilitate and regulate such transport of viral and self-antigens. Immature DC residing in the periphery, e.g. Langerhans cells in the epidermis or mucous membranes of the respiratory tract, form a network of sentinel cells to take up and process antigen for subsequent presentation to T cells[16,17]. It appears that for pathogens, such as Leishmania major or HIV, specific routing to lymphoid tissues by DC plays a major role for the initiation of the immune response[18–20]. Such transport is probably highly efficient as DC migrate rapidly from the periphery to local lymph nodes, and their turnover may be further enhanced by local production of pre-inflammatory mediators, e.g. by tumour necrosis factor (TNF) and lipopolysaccharide (LPS)[21–23]. In the context of virus-induced immunopathologies, DC-mediated transport of live viruses and/or viral proteins is probably the initiating event for the induction of the immunopathological sequelae.

## TRANSGENIC MODELS REVEAL MECHANISMS OF VIRUS-INDUCED AUTOIMMUNE DISEASE

Studies on the initiating events of organ-specific autoimmune diseases are often difficult because first, the triggering (probably viral) infectious agent is not yet known and, secondly, a long, usually asymptomatic phase precedes the clinical manifestation of the disease. In controlled transgenic approaches a transgene, e.g. a viral antigen, can be expressed in specific cells using tissue-specific promoters. Induction of an immune response against such defined neo-self antigens, for example by infection of the virus from which the transgene was originally derived, allows thorough evaluation of the early events of virus-induced immunopathological reactions.

A model that facilitates investigation of the development of virus-induced autoimmune diabetes comprises the transgenic RIP-GP mice which express the lymphocytic choriomeningitis virus glycoprotein (LCMV-GP) under the control of the rat insulin promoter (RIP) leading to expression of the neoself-antigen exclusively in the $\beta$ islet cells of the pancreas[2,3]. T cells ignore the peripherally expressed antigen and mice do not spontaneously develop autoimmune diabetes, defined as insulitis, destructive infiltration of pancreatic islets and hyperglycaemia. However, after activation of GP-specific T cells, e.g. by infection with

LCMV, an autoimmune response is induced leading to destruction of ß islet cells and diabetes between days 8 and 14 after infection[2].

## Dose and timing of antigen transport by dendritic cells to secondary lymphoid organs critically determines the outcome of an autoimmune disease

In order to investigate the involvement of antigen transport by DC for the initiation and maintenance of autoimmune diabetes in RIP-GP mice, DC constitutively expressing the immunodominant epitope GP33 of LCMV-GP (H8 mice)[24] were used to induce primary anti-ß islet cell responses. Single immunization of RIP-GP mice with an intermediate dose of H8-DC ($1–2 \times 10^5$) led to transient cytotoxic T lymphocyte (CTL) activation and insulitis; however, progression to diabetes could not be observed. Increasing the dose of H8-DC to $10^6$ led to an enhanced and slightly prolonged CTL activity accompanied by manifest, but mainly transient, diabetes in less than 50% of the immunized RIP-GP mice. Prolonging the CTL activity by repetitive immunization with H8-DC shifted the balance towards a more severe disease with an incidence of diabetes of > 90%[25] (Table 1). These findings are surprising, as H8-DC induce CTL activity and an elevation of CTLp frequencies that is approximately 10–100 times lower compared with LCMV infection[26]. This suggests that the CTL stimulation by repetitive DC immunization is an important factor contributing to the transition of the disease from insulitis to overt diabetes. Importantly, after induction of transient diabetes, mice remain normoglycaemic unless antigen is reintroduced by dendritic cells (B. Ludewig, unpublished data). Thus, this autoimmune response is self-limiting if antigen ceases to reach organized lymphoid tissues, it can be maintained if sufficient amounts of antigen are transported to secondary lymphoid tissues by DC.

It has been suggested that DC may pick up self-antigens released during tissue injuries and process these proteins via a not-yet-characterized class I pathway for presentation to $CD8^+$ T cells[27]. However, presentation of these antigens is probably limited by the turnover of MHC class I-restricted peptides on DC[28]. Comparison of constitutively GP33 expressing H8-DC and GP33-pulsed DC derived from non-transgenic C57BL/6 mice (B6-DC/GP33) allowed evaluation of the half-life of MHC class I-associated peptides on DC *in vivo* and the contribution of peptide turnover on the development of DC-induced autoimmunity. Constitutively GP33-presenting H8-DC and C57BL/6-DC exogenously pulsed with GP33 (B6-DC/33) and adoptively transferred into naive recipients induce a similar initial activation of the GP33-specific CTL pool (B. Ludewig, unpublished data) or secondary *in-vitro* cytotoxicity after restimulation[26]. However, even in an immunization protocol where the incidence of diabetes in RIP-GP mice was 100% after priming with H8-DC, B6-DC/GP33 did not induce diabetes (Table 1). In contrast to the strong and destructive infiltration after repetitive H8-DC priming[25], repetitive priming with B6-DC/GP33 resulted in a non-destructive insulitis with mainly peri-insular infiltration of T cells ($CD8^+$ and $CD4^+$) and only few B cells and CD11c-positive DC (B. Ludewig, unpublished results). Preliminary results indicate that the limited capacity of peptide-pulsed DC to induce autoimmunity is due to the relatively short half-life of

**Table 1** Role of CTLp frequencies and duration of the antigenic stimulus for the induction of autoimmune diabetes in the RIP-GP transgenic mice

| *Antigenic stimulus*[a] | *CTLp frequency*[b] | *CTL activity* | *Severity of insulitis*[c] | *Onset of diabetes* | *Incidence of diabetes(%)*[d] |
|---|---|---|---|---|---|
| 200 p.f.u. LCMV intravenously (i.v.) | Low | +++ | +++ | Days 8–14 | 100 |
| 200 p.f.u. LCMV i.v. | High | +++ | +++ | Day 4 | 100 |
| $2 \times 10^6$ p.f.u. Vacc-G2 i.v. | Low | ++ | + | – | 0 |
| $2 \times 10^6$ p.f.u. Vacc-G2 i.v. | High | +++ | +++ | Days 6–9 | 100 |
| $10^6$ H8-DC, single injection | Low | ++ | + to ++ | Days 9–13 | <50 |
| $10^5$ H8-DC, single injection | Low | + | + | – | 0 |
| $10^5$ H8-DC, repetitive injection | Low | + | +++ | Days 10–15 | >90 |
| $10^5$ B6-DC/GP33, repetitive injection | Low | + | + | – | 0 |

[a] Recipient mice were infected i.v. with 200 p.f.u. LCMV or $2 \times 10^6$ p.f.u. LCMV–GP recombinant *Vaccinia* virus (Vacc-G2) on day 0. Alternatively, mice were immunized i.v. either once with $10^6$ or $10^5$ H8-DC on day 0 or repetitively with $10^5$ H8-DC or peptide-pulsed B6-DC on days 0, 2, 8, and 12.
[b] Either RIP-GP or RIP-GP × TCR double-transgenic mice with low or high LCMV-specific CTLp precursor frequencies, respectively, were used as recipients.
[c] Insulitis was classified on day 14 or 21 by immunohistochemistry.
[d] Mice were scored diabetic with blood glucose >14 mmol/L on two consecutive measurements.
Adapted from refs 2, 26, 30 and Ludewig, unpublished results.

MHC class I peptides *in vivo*. The time-limited stimulatory capacity of peptide-pulsed DC did not significantly influence expansion of peptide-specific CTL, but strongly impaired their differentiation towards effectors (B. Ludewig, unpublished results). Thus, direct induction of CTL by DC with prolonged expression of the respective self-peptides is apparently a key step for the induction of destructive autoimmunity. Cross-priming or cross-presentation of self-peptides via DC27 for induction of autoimmunity is therefore probably highly demanding in terms of the quantities of the antigen needed. It remains an open question how and to what extent cross-presentation of both cellular and viral antigens via MHC class I by DC5[29] contributes to the development of autoimmunity in human disease.

Thus, together with previous results, important observations on quantitative aspects of autoimmunity have been made in RIP-GP mice. Infection of naive RIP-GP mice with LCMV generates a strong but time-limited CTL response that leads to destruction of ß islet cells in 8–14 days (Table 1). Elevation of CTLp frequencies in double transgenic mice expressing the LCMV-GP in the pancreas and a GP33-specific TCR on their CTL (RIP-GP × TCR) strongly accelerates disease (Table 1)[2]. Elevated CTLp frequencies also compensate for weak CTL induction by the less immunogenic LCMV-GP recombinant *Vaccinia* virus[30] (Table 1). The above-discussed experiments using DC for CTL induction against self-antigens, added a further dimension in the complex regulation of autoimmunity, that is the duration of antigenic stimulation by professional APC. Only when an antigen is presented on professional APC in a minimal dose, and for sufficient time, is a destructive autoimmune response achieved (Table 1). This is best achieved when the relevant antigen is produced by the DC in a directly presented manner. Presentation of exogenously added peptides, and probably also of whole proteinaceous antigens, is considerably more demanding due to the short half-life of MHC class I-restricted peptides on DC (Table 1). Therefore, these results clearly show that the integral of CTL activity, that is the CTL activity over time, is a critical parameter for the outcome of an autoimmune disease.

## Role of the local inflammatory milieu for development of autoimmune diseases

Local inflammatory responses with secretion of cytokines such as TNF-$\alpha$ or IL-2 may enhance virus-induced autoimmune responses. However, is such a chronic local inflammatory reaction alone sufficient to elicit a manifest autoimmune disease? Expression of TNF in pancreatic $\beta$ islet cells under the control of the RIP results in insulitis without diabetes both in RIP-TNF and in RIP-TNF × RIP-GP mice[30,31]. Importantly, the susceptibility for virus-induced diabetes is dramatically increased under such chronic inflammatory conditions, since RIP-TNF × RIP-GP mice develop diabetes after infection with LCMV-GP recombinant *Vaccinia* virus[30] (Table 2). Similarly, pancreatic expression of IL-2 results in enhanced lymphocyte traffic through pancreatic islets and up-regulation of MHC class I antigens. Manifest diabetes develops in RIP-IL-2 × RIP-GP mice only when an appropriate immunity against insulin-producing cells is initiated by infection with LCMV[32]. A more severe virus-induced immunopathology might also result from aberrant expression of co-stimulatory molecules in

**Table 2** Influence of local inflammatory and costimulatory stimuli on the development of diabetes in RIP-GP mice

| *Mice* | *Infection*[a] | *Insulitis*[b] | *Diabetes*[c] |
|---|---|---|---|
| RIP-GP | $2 \times 10^6$ p.f.u. Vacc-G2 i.v. | + | – |
| RIP-TNF | – | + | – |
| RIP-TNF × RIP-GP | – | + | – |
| RIP-TNF × RIP-GP | $2 \times 10^6$ p.f.u. Vacc-G2 i.v. | + | + |
| RIP-B7 | $2 \times 10^6$ p.f.u. Vacc-G2 i.v. | – | – |
| RIP-B7 × RIP-GP | – | – | – |
| RIP-B7 × RIP-GP | $2 \times 10^6$ p.f.u. Vacc-G2 i.v. | + | + |

[a] RIP-GP, RIP-TNF, RIP-TNF × RIP-GP, RIP-B7, RIP-B7 × RIP-GP mice were infected with $2 \times 10^6$ p.f.u. LCMV-GP recombinant *Vaccinia* virus (Vacc-G2) i.v. or were left untreated.
[b] Insulitis was classified by immunohistochemistry.
[c] Mice were scored diabetic with blood glucose < 14 mmol/L on two consecutive measurements.
Adapted from refs 2, 30, 31 and 33.

peripheral organs. Co-expression of LCMV-GP and the co-stimulatory molecule B7.1 on pancreatic $\beta$ islet cells does not lead to spontaneous diabetes or insulitis[33] (Table 2). However, infection of double-transgenic RIP-B7 × RIP-GP mice with LCMV-GP recombinant *Vaccinia* virus elicits insulitis and diabetes[33] (Table 2). Collectively these data show that a chronic local inflammatory environment strongly influences the susceptibility to virus-induced immunopathology.

Extensive infiltration of the target tissue with lymphoid cells is a prime hallmark of many autoimmune diseases. Interestingly, these focal accumulations of inflammatory cells often form an architecture similar to that seen in secondary lymphoid organs. Prominent examples of these morphological changes are found in Hashimoto's thyroiditis and in rheumatoid arthritis, where DC in the T cell areas of the synovi infiltrates locally and may present microbial antigens locally to T cells[34]. Similar organized infiltrates have been detected in human sporadic goitres[35] and in the pancreas of a diabetic patient[36].

The cellular composition of pancreatic infiltrates in the course of DC-induced autoimmune diabetes in RIP-GP mice showed the tendency to form organized lymphoid structures[25]. After DC priming early infiltrates consisted mainly of $CD8^+$ T cells that clearly outnumbered $CD4^+$ T cells. B cells were absent, whereas CD11c-positive DC were found also in these early peri-insular inflammatory lesions. Due to the continued stimulation of islet-specific CTL via DC, a more destructive insulitis developed with intra-islet infiltrations of $CD8^+$ and $CD4^+$ T cells, B cells and DC, accompanied by a severe loss of insulin-producing cells[25]. Later, formation of periductal lymphoid structures was found in the proximity of remaining insulin-positive islets. These newly formed lymphoid tissues showed a distinct compartmentalization into T and B cell zones, development of germinal centre-like structures, peripheral node adressin-positive high endothelial venules, and a strong infiltration with CD11c-positive DC25. Thus, autoimmunity induced by DC is strongly associated with the development of lymphoid neogenesis in the target organ.

However, as mentioned above, strong lymphoid infiltrates, e.g. induced by local production of TNF or lymphotoxin-$\alpha$[31,37,38] alone are not sufficient to mediate a manifest diabetes. Therefore, critical conditions for the induction and maintenance of destructive autoimmunity are: (1) activation of tissue-specific CTL in sufficient numbers and for a certain time, and (2) development of lymphoid tissue-like structures in the target organ helping to maintain the chronic inflammatory process. Antigen transport by DC is likely to be crucial for the initiation and maintenance of a specific CTL response and probably a key factor in the development of local organized lymphoid tissues.

## CONCLUSIONS

Based on the evidence obtained in the transgenic models, the likely scenario for the events leading to autoimmune manifestations after viral infections involves first the initial triggering event with acquisition of pathogen-derived antigens or self-antigen by DC. Secondly, these antigens have to be presented in local secondary lymphoid tissues by DC in a minimal concentration and for a certain time in order to overcome immunological ignorance. However, such an autoimmune response is self-limiting when the antigen is no longer transported to secondary lympoid tissues. Thus, in order to maintain an autoimmune response for development of a manifest autoimmune disease, DC have to activate self-reactive T cells in lymphoid tissues and/or transport pathogens persisting from the target organ to local lymphoid organs for a prolonged period of time. Alternatively, due to the chronic inflammatory process, lymphoid tissues might develop locally in the target organs, where DC locally may present antigen and thereby contribute to the maintenance of the autoimmune disease. Thus, it might be beneficial for the treatment of autoimmune diseases to specifically and locally manipulate antigen transport or antigen presentation by DC to avoid or reduce activation of self-reactive T cells.

### References


1. Barker CF, Billingham RE. Immunologically privileged sites. Adv. Immunol. 1972.25:1.
2. Ohashi PS, Oehen S, Buerki K *et al.* Ablation of 'tolerance' and induction of diabetes by virus infection in viral antigen transgenic mice. Cell.1991;65:305–17.
3. Oldstone MB, Nerenberg M, Southern P, Price J, Lewicki H. Virus infection triggers insulin-dependent diabetes mellitus in a transgenic model: role of anti-self (virus) immune response. Cell.1991;65:319–31.
4. Ferber I, Schonrich G, Schenkel J, Mellor AL, Arnold B, Hammerling GJ. Levels of peripheral T cell tolerance induced by different doses of tolerogen. Science. 1994;263:674–6.
5. Kurts C, Heath WR, Kosaka H, Miller JF, Carbone FR. The peripheral deletion of autoreactive CD8+ T cells induced by cross-presentation of self-antigens involves signaling through CD95 (Fas, Apo-1). J Exp Med. 1998;188:415–20.
6. Oldstone MB. Molecular mimicry and autoimmune disease. Cell 1987;50:819–20.
7. Oldstone MB. Molecular mimicry as a mechanism for the cause and a probe uncovering etiologic agent(s) of autoimmune disease. Curr Top Microbiol Immunol. 1989;145:127–35.
8. Tough DF, Borrow P, Sprent J. Induction of bystander T cell proliferation by viruses and type I interferon *in vivo*. Science. 1996;272:1947–50.
9. Horwitz MS, Bradley LM, Harbertson J, Krahl T, Lee J, Sarvetnick N. Diabetes induced by Coxsackie virus: initiation by bystander damage and not molecular mimicry. Nat Med. 1998;4:781–5.
10. Zinkernagel RM. Immunology taught by viruses. Science. 1996;271:173–8.
11. Cole GA, Nathanson N, Prendergast RA. Requirement for theta-bearing cells in lymphocytic choriomeningitis virus-induced central nervous system disease. Nature. 1972;238:335–7.

12. Zinkernagel RM, Haenseler E, Leist T, Cerny A, Hengartner H, Althage A. T cell-mediated hepatitis in mice infected with lymphocytic choriomeningitis virus. Liver cell destruction by H-2 class 1-restricted virus-specific cytotoxic T cells as a physiological correlate of the 51Cr-release assay? J Exp Med. 1986;164:1075–92.
13. Odermatt B, Eppler M, Leist TP, Hengartner H, Zinkernagel RM. Virus-triggered acquired immunodeficiency by cytotoxic T-cell-dependent destruction of antigen-presenting cells and lymph follicle structure. Proc Natl Acad Sci USA. 1991;88:8252–6.
14. Kagi D, Seiler P, Pavlovic J et al. The roles of perforin- and Fas-dependent cytotoxicity in protection against cytopathic and noncytopathic viruses. Eur J Immunol. 1995;25:3256–62.
15. Miller SD, Vanderlugt CL, Begolka WS et al. Persistent infection with Theiler's virus leads to CNS autoimmunity via epitope spreading. Nat Med. 1997;3:1133–6.
16. Steinman RM. The dendritic cell system and its role in immunogenicity. Annu Rev Immunol. 1991;9:271–96.
17. Banchereau J, Steinman RM. Dendritic cells and the control of immunity. Nature. 1998;392:245–52.
18. Moll H. Epidermal Langerhans cells are critical for immunoregulation of cutaneous leishmaniasis. Immunol Today 1993;14:383–7.
19. Spira AI, Marx PA, Patterson BK et al. Cellular targets of infection and route of viral dissemination after an intravaginal inoculation of simian immunodeficiency virus into rhesus macaques. J Exp Med. 1996;183:215–25.
20. Masurier C, Salomon B, Guettari N et al. Dendritic cells route human immunodeficiency virus to lymph nodes after vaginal or intravenous administration to mice. J Virol. 1998;72:7822–9.
21. Kimber I, Cumberbatch M. Stimulation of Langerhans cell migration by tumor necrosis factor alpha (TNF-alpha). J Invest Dermatol. 1992;99:48–50S.
22. Roake JA, Rao AS, Morris PJ, Larsen CP, Hankins DF, Austyn JM. Systemic lipopolysaccharide recruits dendritic cell progenitors to nonlymphoid tissues. Transplantation, 1995;59:1319–24.
23. DeSmedt T, Pajak B, Muraille E et al. Regulation of dendritic cell numbers and maturation by lipopolysaccharide *in vivo*. J Exp Med. 1996;184:1413–24.
24. Ehl S, Hombach J, Aichele P et al. Viral and bacterial infections interfere with peripheral tolerance induction and activate CD8+ T cells to cause immunopathology. J Exp Med. 1998;187:763–74.
25. Ludewig B, Odermatt B, Landmann S, Hengartner H, Zinkernagel RM. Dendritic cells induce autoimmune diabetes and maintain disease via *de novo* formation of local lymphoid tissue. J Exp Med. 1998;188:1493–501.
26. Ludewig B, Ehl S, Karrer U, Odermatt B, Hengartner H, Zinkernagel RM. Dendritic cells efficiently induce protective antiviral immunity. J Virol. 1998;72:3812–18.
27. Carbone FR, Kurts C, Bennett SR, Miller JF, Heath WR. Cross-presentation: a general mechanism for CTL immunity and tolerance. Immunol Today. 1998;19:368–73.
28. Cella M, Engering A, Pinet V, Pieters J, Lanzavecchia A. Inflammatory stimuli induce accumulation of MHC class II complexes on dendritic cells. Nature. 1997;388:782–7.
29. Albert ML, Sauter B, Bhardwaj N. Dendritic cells acquire antigen from apoptotic cells and induce class I-restricted CTLs. Nature. 1998;392:86–9.
30. Ohashi PS, Oehen S, Aichele P et al. Induction of diabetes is influenced by the infectious virus and local expression of MHC class I and tumor necrosis factor-$\alpha$. J. Immunol. 1993;150:5185–94.
31. Higuchi Y, Herrera P, Muniesa P et al. Expression of a tumor necrosis factor alpha transgene in murine pancreatic beta cells results in severe and permanent insulitis without evolution towards diabetes. J Exp Med. 1992;176:1719–31.
32. von Herrath MG, Allison J, Miller JF, Oldstone MB. Focal expression of interleukin-2 does not break unresponsiveness to 'self' (viral) antigen expressed in beta cells but enhances development of autoimmune disease (diabetes) after initiation of an anti-self immune response. J Clin Invest. 1995;95:477–85.
33. Harlan DM, Hengartner H, Huang ML *et al.* Mice expressing both B7-1 and viral glycoprotein on pancreatic beta cells along with glycoprotein-specific transgenic T cells develop diabetes due to a breakdown of T-lymphocyte unresponsiveness. Proc Natl Acad Sci USA. 1994;91:3137–41.
34. Melief MJ, Hoijer MA, Van Paassen HC, Hazenberg MP. Presence of bacterial flora-derived antigen in synovial tissue macrophages and dendritic cells. Br J Rheumatol. 1995;34:1112–16.
35. Kabel PJ, Voorbij HA, de Haan-Meulman M, Pals ST, Drexhage HA. High endothelial venules present in lymphoid cell accumulations in thyroids affected by autoimmune disease: a study in

men and BB rats of functional activity and development. J Clin Endocrinol Metab. 1989;68:744–51.

36. Jansen A, Voorbij HA, Jeucken PH, Bruining GJ, Hooijkaas H, Drexhage HA. An immunohistochemical study on organized lymphoid cell infiltrates in fetal and neonatal pancreases. A comparison with similar infiltrates found in the pancreas of a diabetic infant. Autoimmunity. 1993;15:31–8.
37. Picarella DE, Kratz A, Li CB, Ruddle NH, Flavell RA. Insulitis in transgenic mice expressing tumor necrosis factor beta (lymphotoxin) in the pancreas. Proc Natl Acad Sci USA. 1992;89:10036–40.
38. Picarella DE, Kratz A, Li CB, Ruddle NH, Flavell RA. Transgenic tumor necrosis factor (TNF)-alpha production in pancreatic islets leads to insulitis, not diabetes. Distinct patterns of inflammation in TNF-alpha and TNF-beta transgenic mice. J Immunol. 1993;150:4136–50.

# Section II
# Definition and spectrum of autoimmune hepatitis

# 6

# Definition and classification of autoimmune hepatitis 1999 (on behalf of the International Autoimmune Hepatitis Group)

I.G. McFARLANE

## INTRODUCTION

At the beginning of the 1990s there was considerable uncertainty about the diagnostic criteria for the condition which was then known as 'lupoid' or 'autoimmune chronic active' hepatitis (AICAH). It was recognized that the disease, which had been increasingly diagnosed during the 1970s and 1980s, was markedly heterogeneous with respect to its clinical and laboratory manifestations and possibly also its pathogenesis[1]. The hepatitis C virus (HCV) had been very recently identified[2,3] and early reports suggested that a high proportion of patients with presumed AICAH had HCV infections and, conversely, that many patients with chronic hepatitis C had features (notably mild to moderate hypergammaglobulinaemia and circulating autoantibodies) associated with AICAH[4–6]. Additionally, it was recognized that these features, as well as the histological changes of chronic active hepatitis, can often be seen at various stages in other liver disorders including primary biliary cirrhosis (PBC), primary sclerosing cholangitis (PSC), Wilson's disease and some forms of drug- and alcohol-induced liver disease. The advent of interferon (IFN) therapy for chronic viral hepatitis was also presenting a problem for clinical management because it was becoming apparent that IFN can provoke (or unmask pre-existing) autoimmune conditions and that accuracy of diagnosis was crucial[7].

Against this background in 1992 an international panel met in Brighton, UK, to review the diagnostic criteria for this condition. The panel comprised the nucleus of what shortly thereafter became the International Autoimmune Hepatitis Group, with 40 members from 17 countries. In the report of the panel's initial meeting[8], which became known as the 'Brighton Report'[9], it was acknowledged that the term 'chronic active hepatitis' (CAH) was beginning to outlive its usefulness and was no longer appropriate, since AICAH could become inactive during periods of treatment-induced or spontaneous remission without complete resolution, and use of the adjective 'chronic' was unnecessary for describing a disease that is *a-priori* chronic[10]. It was therefore recommended that the condition should be designated 'autoimmune hepatitis' (AIH).

## THE 'BRIGHTON REPORT'

This report recommended that AIH should be considered in any patient who presents with an unexplained acute or chronic hepatitic illness or biochemical liver test abnormalities in the absence of symptoms or signs of liver disease. It included a set of descriptive criteria and a proposed diagnostic scoring system which it was suggested could be used to classify patients as having either *definite* or *probable* AIH according to how closely their presenting features conformed to those of classic 'lupoid' hepatitis. This approach allowed for account to be taken of the features associated with the wider spectrum of the disease that was being seen in clinical practices, as summarized below.

### General features

The panel noted that there are no clinical, laboratory or histological features that are specific for AIH and that diagnosis depends on a combination of suggestive features together with careful exclusion of other causes of chronic liver disease. The salient points were the following:

1. The disease predominates among women but also affects men and can present at any age.
2. Onset is typically insidious, with fatigue, fluctuating jaundice and arthralgia as prominent features, but the disease can also present as an acute hepatitis or as an elevation of serum aminotransferase activity (revealed during routine clinical investigation) in the absence of obvious signs or symptoms of liver disease.
3. A family history of autoimmune or allergic disorders is common.
4. The serum biochemical profile shows a predominantly hepatitic pattern but the abnormalities do not reliably reflect severity of disease.
5. Hyperglobulinaemia with selective elevation of serum IgG is characteristic.
6. The large majority of patients are seropositive for anti-nuclear (ANA) and/or anti-smooth muscle (SMA), or type 1 anti-liver–kidney microsomal (LKM-1) autoantibodies.
7. In northern European caucasoids the disease is associated with inheritance of the truncated HLA B8-DR3 haplotype or the DR3 or DR4 allotypes while in Japanese patients the primary association is with DR4.
8. There are no morphological features that are pathognomonic of AIH but the characteristic histological picture is that of (what was formerly known as) CAH, i.e. periportal or periseptal piecemeal necrosis (interface hepatitis) with a predominantly lymphoplasmacytic infiltrate and often formation of liver cell rosettes, with or without lobular (or intra-acinar) inflammation and/or bridging necrosis.

9. Histological changes that mitigate against a diagnosis of AIH include prominent bile duct damage, granulomas, and other features such as siderosis or cuprinosis that are more suggestive of a different aetiology. The presence of lymphoid aggregates was considered to lack sufficient specificity to exclude AIH.

## Definite AIH

Classification as *definite* AIH required: (a) serum globulin, $\gamma$-globulin or IgG concentrations greater than 1.5 times the upper normal limit and serum $\alpha_1$-antitrypsin, copper and caeruloplasmin concentrations within the normal range; (b) seronegativity for markers of current infection with all known hepatotropic viruses; (c) absence of a history of parenteral exposure to blood or blood products, or excessive alcohol consumption, or recent exposure to potentially hepatotoxic drugs; and (d) seropositivity for ANA and/or SMA, or anti-LKM-1, at titres of greater than 1:80 in adults or 1:20 in children, as determined by immunofluorescence on rodent tissue sections.

## Probable AIH

This category allowed for a diagnosis of AIH to be made in patients who generally conform with the above criteria but who have: (a) less marked hyperglobulinaemia; or (b) abnormal serum copper and/or caeruloplasmin concentrations without evidence of Wilson's disease; or (c) lower titres ($\geq$ 1:40 in adults, $\geq$ 1:10 or 1:20 in children) of ANA, SMA or anti-LKM-1; or (d) a history of moderate alcohol consumption or exposure to hepatotoxic drugs with evidence of continuing liver damage after abstinence from alcohol or withdrawal of the drug. It also allowed for inclusion of the 10–20% of patients who present without ANA, SMA or anti-LKM-1 but have one or more of a range of other autoantibodies against 'defined' liver antigens. Additionally, patients who were anti-HCV antibody seropositive but otherwise fulfilled the above criteria could be provisionally included until their HCV infection status could be clarified.

## Subtypes of AIH

The panel noted a developing practice of subclassifying AIH according to serum autoantibody profiles, with ANA/SMA-positive cases being defined as type 1 AIH and those with anti-LKM-1 as type 2, and that further subdivisions were being proposed to take account of patients without these antibodies but who often had autoantibodies against liver-derived antigens, as well as patients with suspected AIH who had evidence of HCV infection. But the panel felt that it could not endorse these subdivisions (for other than research purposes) because they did not define distinct therapeutic groups and tests for most of the antibodies against liver-derived antigens were not widely available. It was acknowledged that there is a small proportion of patients who present with many of the features of AIH but also have histological, cholangiographic or other evidence of PBC or PSC. However, it was considered that there was insufficient information to classify these cases and it was recommended that they should not be included within the spectrum of AIH.

### Diagnostic scoring system

The diagnostic scoring system was originally designed as an adjunct to the descriptive criteria to provide an objective method for selecting relatively homogeneous groups of patients for research purposes. Points were allocated for each of the suggestive features described above, or deducted for features that were considered to mitigate against the diagnosis, to achieve an aggregate score that could be used to classify patients as having *definite* or *probable* AIH. In order to bias the scoring against cholestatic diseases the system included negative weighting for ratios of the elevations of serum alkaline phosphatase (ALP) to aspartate (AST) or alanine (ALT) aminotransferase activities that exceeded 3.0. The panel recommended that a diagnosis of *definite* AIH should not be made without histological assessment of a liver biopsy but, by defining minimum required parameters, the scoring system provided for a diagnosis of *probable* AIH to be made when histological assessment was not possible or available. Scoring for histology was delineated under 'additional parameters' and included negative weighting for evidence of bile duct damage and features suggestive of other causes of liver disease, as well as points accruable for autoantibodies against liver-derived antigens (in ANA/SMA/anti-LKM-1 negative patients) and HLA markers. Additionally, it was considered that a good response to immunosuppressive therapy is so characteristic of AIH that it should be used to reaffirm the diagnosis subsequently when the outcome of therapy became assessable, and various categories of response to which scores could be assigned were defined as: 'complete', 'partial', 'no response', 'treatment failure', and 'relapse'.

## REVIEW OF DIAGNOSTIC CRITERIA

The descriptive criteria and diagnostic scoring system proposed by the International AIH Group have subsequently been widely used by many investigators. During 1998 and 1999 the Group undertook a comprehensive review of the published data and of its members' own experiences in relation to the many new developments in diagnostic modalities for liver disease in general that have taken place since publication of the 'Brighton Report'. Two areas of development that have had particular impact on the diagnostic criteria for AIH are: (1) very marked improvements in the reliability, specificity and availability of tests for HCV, and significant advances in knowledge about infections with this and other hepatotropic viruses; and (2) increased understanding and awareness of the morphological changes associated with various liver disorders.

The review has revealed that the descriptive criteria appear to be robust and require only minor modifications to bring them into line with the above developments. It has reaffirmed that AIH predominates in women (although it is being increasingly recognized in men) and that it can present at any age. However, it was noted that the previous impression of a bimodal distribution in age at presentation (with peaks around puberty and between the 4th and 6th decades of life)[11] was probably an artefact due to patterns of patient referrals to specialist centres, and that in clinical practices elsewhere the large majority of patients present between the ages of 50 and 70 years[12,13] (Figure 1). The review has also reaffirmed that the presenting clinical, biochemical, immunological and histo-

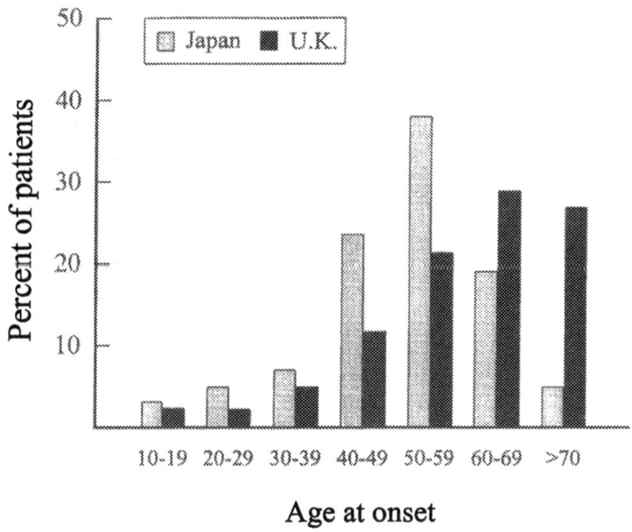


**Fig. 1** Distribution of age at onset in adults with autoimmune hepatitis presenting at gastroenterology clinics in Japan and the UK. Adapted from refs 12 and 13

logical features described in the 'Brighton Report' are appropriate, but it identified a requirement for a few changes to the specifications for exclusion of viral hepatitis and biliary diseases (see below).

There have been six major studies in which the scoring system has been applied to sufficient numbers of patients to allow for meaningful evaluation[12,14–18]. Review of the data obtained for the total of 983 patients in these six studies revealed that the overall diagnostic accuracy of the system (i.e. the number of patients correctly diagnosed as having or not having definite or probable AIH as a percentage of the total) was 89.8% (Table 1). Three of the studies included a total of 598 patients with AIH diagnosed according to previous Mayo Clinic criteria[14], or the 'Brighton Report' descriptive criteria[15], or the Japanese Ministry of Health criteria (which specify seropositivity for ANA)[12]. The overall sensitivity for confirming the diagnosis in these cases was 98.0%. In five studies the system was applied to 242 patients with chronic hepatitis C who were seropositive for ANA, SMA or anti-LKM-1 antibodies and/or had other features suggestive of AIH (hyperglobulinaemia and/or some degree of interface hepatitis on liver biopsy). None of these patients scored as having *definite* AIH but between 8.0% and 33.9% achieved scores within the range specified for *probable* AIH, giving an overall specificity of 80% for excluding AIH in patients with HCV infection and autoimmune markers. Two of the studies applied the system to a total of 143 patients with PSC, PBC or so-called 'autoimmune cholangitis' (AMA-negative patients with autoimmune features and cholestatic biochemical profiles and/or histological or cholangiographic evidence of biliary damage)[14,16]. Although only three (2.1%) of these patients scored as *definite* AIH, 53 (37.1%) achieved scores within the *probable* AIH range, giving an overall specificity of only 60.8% for exclusion of AIH in biliary diseases. In the majority of the patients with HCV infection or biliary diseases who scored as *probable* AIH the

**Table 1** Analysis of data from six studies of the sensitivity (for diagnosis of AIH) and specificity (for excluding AIH) of the International AIH Group scoring system

| Patient Group[a] | *n* | Mean (range) diagnostic Sensitivity | Mean (range) diagnostic Specificity[b] | Reference |
|---|---|---|---|---|
| AIH | 598 | 98.0% (97.3–100.0) | — | [12, 14, 15] |
| HCV | 242 | — | 80.0% (66.1–92.0) | [12–14, 17, 18] |
| Biliary diseases | 143 | — | 60.8% (44.8–64.9) | [14, 16] |
| Total | 983 | Overall diagnostic accuracy[c] = 89.8% | | |

[a]AIH = autoimmune hepatitis diagnosed by previous Mayo Clinic criteria [5], IAIH Group descriptive criteria [6] or Japanese Ministry of Health criteria [7];
HCV = patients with chronic hepatitis C with serum autoantibodies and other features suggestive of AIH; Biliary diseases = PBC, PSC and 'autoimmune cholangitis' (as defined in text).
[b]Note that none of the patients in the HCV group and only 5.2% of those with biliary diseases scored as *definite* AIH.
[c]Overall diagnostic accuracy = percent of total patients correctly diagnosed as having or not having AIH.

scores were borderline, i.e. only one or two points above the lower limit specified for a diagnosis of AIH. Indices which mainly contributed to this inappropriate scoring included the presence of ANA and/or SMA, mild to moderate elevations in serum immunoglobulins, low ALP:AST (or ALT) ratios, and inadequate weighting against histological evidence of bile duct damage.

Other relevant points revealed by the review of these and other published data are the following.

## Autoantibodies

The clinical utility of classifying patients according to autoantibody profiles, i.e. type 1 (ANA/SMA positive) and type 2 (anti-LKM-1 positive) AIH, remains uncertain because this classification is not exclusive[11]. Additionally, long-term follow-up of patients with type 1 and type 2 AIH has shown that, although there are some clinical, biochemical and histological differences, these two groups are similar with respect to severity of disease, prevalence of other autoimmune disorders in the patients and their families, and the eventual outcome[19]. Experience has also shown that seropositivity for antibodies against a soluble liver antigen (SLA) in the absence of ANA, SMA and anti-LKM-1, which it had been proposed classified a third type (type 3) of AIH, does not define a distinct subgroup[20].

The review noted that high titres of perinuclear staining antineutrophil cytoplasmic antibodies (pANCA, detected by immunofluorescence on ethanol-fixed neutrophils), which were previously thought to be a marker of PSC, reportedly also occur in up to 90% of patients with AIH[21-24]. The various autoantibodies against liver-derived antigens that were mentioned in the 'Brighton Report' continue to be of interest but tests for these are still not widely available. Subspecificities of ANA appear to have limited clinical implications in AIH[25,26] and reliance on anti-actin specificity of SMA can lead to missed diagnoses[27].

## Viral markers

The 'Brighton Report' criteria adequately discriminate between AIH and chronic viral hepatitis in patients with hyperglobulinaemia and serum autoantibodies, although minor adjustments to the scoring system are required to improve its specificity. However, in view of the advances in hepatitis virology that have been made since publication of that report, and because the hepatitis G virus (GBV-C/HGV) seems not to be an aetiological factor in AIH[28,29] and other agents (such as cytomegalovirus and Epstein–Barr virus) only very occasionally cause hepatitis, the previous requirement for exclusion of all known hepatotropic virus infections is considered expensive and unnecessary in most cases[14].

## Histology

Experience has shown that interface hepatitis as described in the 'Brighton Report' remains the characteristic histological picture in AIH, but that other features such as lymphoid aggregates, steatosis, siderosis, cuprinosis and bile ductule proliferation (which may occur to some degree in AIH even in the absence of cirrhosis) lack sufficient specificity to exclude AIH. Additionally, since the biochemical and immunological features of AIH can be seen in other disorders such as systemic lupus erythematosus in the absence of any significant liver involvement[30], the previous recommendation that *definite* AIH should not be diagnosed without histological assessment is reaffirmed.

## Genetic factors

The review has confirmed that AIH is particularly associated with inheritance of the HLA DR3 and DR4 allotypes in northern European caucasoids and with DR4 in Japanese patients, and that DR4 tends to occur more frequently in older patients whose disease is generally easier to control with immunosuppressive therapy[12,31,32]. Other HLA associations have been reported in caucasoids and other populations[33-36], and genetic differences in complement and cytokine metabolism and function may also be important[37-39].

## Overlapping syndromes

The diagnosis of acute and chronic viral hepatitis, drug (including alcohol)-induced liver disease and Wilson's disease, in patients with features of AIH (hyperglobulinaemia, autoantibodies and histological evidence of interface hepatitis) can now usually be made by other criteria, but the review has noted that there is insufficient negative weighting in the scoring system to exclude

AIH in patients with some forms of drug-induced hepatitis, of which the antibiotic minocycline is a typical recent example[40–43]. Patients with cholestatic disorders with features of AIH comprise a relatively small proportion of the total caseload in most clinical practices, but they continue to present difficult problems for diagnosis and clinical management. They have been variously described as 'autoimmune cholangitis', 'autoimmune cholangiopathy', or 'autoimmune sclerosing cholangitis'[44–48]. Given that AIH is frequently associated with various extrahepatic autoimmune disorders (e.g. thyroiditis, rheumatoid arthritis), the possibility that some patients with overlapping syndromes may have concurrent liver diseases (i.e. AIH and PBC or PSC) cannot be discounted. The present review has noted that there is still no universally agreed classification of these syndromes or of their nomenclature, and has highlighted a need for an international working party to clarify this. Overlaps with PBC (both AMA-positive and AMA-negative) are the most commonly reported, and the consensus now appears to be that such cases should be regarded as part of the spectrum of PBC and not as variants of AIH[49-54]. PSC overlapping with AIH is well recognized in children[48,44–57] and features of AIH can also be seen frequently in adults with PSC, although very few of the latter have combinations of these features with sufficient severity to satisfy the criteria for *definite* AIH[16]. Patients who qualify for a diagnosis of *definite* AIH, but who present with a cholestatic biochemical profile without any other evidence of biliary disease, do not appear to be a clinically distinct subgroup of AIH[58].

### Therapy

Although there have been recent reports attesting to the efficacy of other immunosuppressive agents[59–65], treatment with corticosteroids (± azathioprine) remains the standard therapy. The review reaffirms that a good response to corticosteroids is characteristic of AIH. However, it is noted that assessment of response to therapy can be problematic because: (a) it is heavily dependent on patient compliance (which can be difficult to monitor), and (b) occasionally patients with classic AIH who present with severe acute disease may not respond well to standard therapy. Thus, whereas a rapid and sustained response may be considered to reinforce the diagnosis, a poor response should not necessarily exclude AIH[14].

## DIAGNOSTIC CRITERIA FOR AIH IN 1999

The above review has revealed that the previous recommendations made by the International AIH Group appear to have generally stood the test of time. Thus, the diagnostic criteria for AIH in 1999 are essentially those which were specified in the 'Brighton Report'[8], with a few modifications to bring them up to date with current information and to improve the specificity of the scoring system for discriminating AIH from overlapping syndromes (particularly overlaps with PBC and PSC) and to simplify its use. These adjustments have been undertaken by the Group[67]. The important points are the following:

1. In view of the improvements in the reliability and availability of tests for hepatitis virus infections, exclusion of current infection with the hepatitis A, B or C viruses is considered adequate in most cases. Obligatory exclusion of *definite* AIH in patients with a history of parenteral exposure to blood or blood products who are seronegative for markers of infection with these viruses is no longer considered appropriate.
2. Patients with clinical, biochemical, histological or immunological features normally associated with AIH, but who also have histological or cholangiographic evidence of PBC or PSC, should be considered to have variants of these biliary diseases and not variants of AIH. The morphological features that should specifically exclude AIH are: (a) well-defined granulomas, and (b) bile duct changes typical of PBC or PSC (i.e. granulomatous cholangitis, or severe concentric periductal fibrosis, with ductopenia, established in an adequate biopsy specimen) and/or a substantial periportal ductular reaction (so-called marginal bile duct proliferation with a cholangiolitis) with copper/copper-associated protein accumulation. Other features such as lymphoid aggregates, steatosis, cuprinosis, siderosis, and bile ductule proliferation are considered to lack the necessary specificity to exclude AIH except when these changes (and particularly combinations thereof) are sufficiently prominent to raise doubts about the diagnosis.
3. Since testing for most of the more specialized autoantibodies against liver-derived antigens and for subspecificities of ANA and SMA is not yet widely available, and some subspecificities seem to have limited clinical implications while the use of others may lead to missed diagnoses, diagnosis of AIH in routine clinical practice will continue to rely on detection of ANA, SMA and anti-LKM-1 by conventional techniques for the time being. Although there has been a case report of AMA occurring in a child with *definite* AIH[66], patients with AMA should not normally be considered to have AIH. pANCA (detected by immunofluorescence on ethanol-fixed neutrophils) may be a useful addition to the diagnostic repertoire, especially for patients who present without ANA, SMA or anti-LKM-1. Diagnoses in the latter group may still be made on the basis of the combination of other features that are suggestive of AIH. It is recognized that subdivision of AIH into type 1 and type 2 is still in common usage and will probably continue to be used despite the limited clinical utility of this classification, but other subdivisions of AIH are not recommended at this time.
4. Adjustments to the scoring system relate mainly to increasing the weighting against overlapping cholestatic and AIH-like drug-induced syndromes. Scoring for 'partial response', 'no response' and 'treatment failure' in relation to immunosuppressive therapy is considered inappropriate, and cholangiography is recommended for all patients with an initial diagnosis of *definite* or *probable* AIH who do not respond to corticosteroids.

## References

1. Johnson PJ, McFarlane IG, Eddleston ALWF. The natural course and heterogeneity of autoimmune-type chronic active hepatitis. Semin Liver Dis. 1991;11:187–96.
2. Choo QL, Kuo G, Weiner AJ *et al.* Isolation of a cDNA clone derived from a blood-borne non-A, non-B viral hepatitis genome. Science. 1989;244:359–62.

3. Kuo G, Choo QL, Alter HJ *et al.* An assay for circulating antibodies to a major etiologic virus of human non-A, non-B hepatitis. Science. 1989;244:362–4.
4. McFarlane IG. Autoimmunity and hepatotropic viruses. Semin Liver Dis. 1991;11:223–33.
5. Magrin S, Craxi A, Fiorentino G *et al.* Is autoimmune hepatitis a HCV-related disease? J Hepatol. 1991;13:56–60.
6. Lenzi M, Johnson PJ, McFarlane IG *et al.* Antibodies to hepatitis C virus in autoimmune liver disease: evidence for geographical heterogeneity. Lancet. 1991;338:277–80.
7. Black M, Peters M. Alpha-interferon treatment of chronic hepatitis C: need for accurate diagnosis in selecting patients. Ann Intern Med. 1992;116:86–8.
8. Johnson PJ, McFarlane IG. Meeting report: International autoimmune hepatitis group. Hepatology. 1993;18:998–1005.
9. Mackay IR. Toward diagnostic criteria for autoimmune hepatitis. Hepatology. 1993;18:1006–8.
10. Ludwig J, McFarlane IG, Rakela J (Chairs). International working party report: Terminology of chronic hepatitis. Am J Gastroenterol. 1995;90:181–9.
11. McFarlane IG. The relationship between autoimmune markers and different clinical syndromes in autoimmune hepatitis. Gut. 1998;42:599–602.
12. Toda G, Zeniya M, Watanabe R *et al.* Present status of autoimmune hepatitis in Japan – correlating the characteristics with international criteria in an area with a high rate of HCV infection. J Hepatol. 1997;26:1207–12.
13. Parker DR, Kingham JGC. Type 1 autoimmune hepatitis is primarily a disease of later life. Q J Med. 1997;90:289–96.
14. Czaja AJ, Carpenter HA. Validation of scoring system for diagnosis of autoimmune hepatitis. Dig Dis. Sci. 1996;41:305–14.
15. Bianchi FB, Cassani F, Lenzi M *et al.* Impact of International Autoimmune Hepatitis Group scoring system in definition of autoimmune hepatitis. An Italian experience. Dig Dis Sci. 1996;41:166–71.
16. Boberg KM, Fausa O, Haaland T *et al.* Features of autoimmune hepatitis in primary sclerosing cholangitis: an evaluation of 114 primary sclerosing cholangitis patients according to a scoring system for the diagnosis of autoimmune hepatitis. Hepatology. 1996;23:1369–76.
17. Miyakawa R, Kitazawa E, Abe K *et al.* Chronic hepatitis C associated with anti-liver/kidney microsome-1 antibody is not a subgroup of autoimmune hepatitis. J Gastroenterol. 1997;32:769–76.
18. Dickson RC, Gaffey MJ, Ishitani MB, Roarty TP, Driscoll CJ, Caldwell SH. The international autoimmune hepatitis score in chronic hepatitis C. J Viral Hepatol. 1997;4:121–8.
19. Gregorio GV, Portmann B, Reid F *et al.* Autoimmune hepatitis in childhood: a 20-year experience. Hepatology. 1997;25:541–7.
20. Czaja AJ, Carpenter RA, Manns MP. Antibodies to soluble liver antigen, P450IID6, and mitochondrial complexes in chronic hepatitis. Gastroenterology. 1993;105:1522–8.
21. Hardarson S, La Brecque DR, Mitros FA, Neil GA, Goeken JA. Antineutrophil cytoplasmic antibody in inflammatory bowel and hepatobiliary diseases: high prevalence in ulcerative colitis, primary sclerosing cholangitis, and autoimmune hepatitis. Clin Microbiol Immunol. 1993;99:277–81.
22. Mulder AHL, Rorst G, Haagsma EB, Limburg PC, Kleibeuker JH, Kallenberg CGM. Prevalence and characterization of neutrophil cytoplasmic antibodies in autoimmune liver disease. Hepatology. 1993;17:411–17.
23. Targan SR, Landers C, Vidrich A, Czaja AJ. High-titer antineutrophil cytoplasmic antibodies in type-1 autoimmune hepatitis. Gastroenterology. 1995;108:1159–66.
24. Zauli D, Ghetti S, Grassi A *et al.* Anti-neutrophil cytoplasmic antibodies in type 1 and 2 autoimmune hepatitis. Hepatology. 1997;25:1105–7.
25. Czaja Al, Cassani F, Cataleta M, Valentini P, Bianchi FB. Antinuclear antibodies and patterns of nuclear immunofluorescence in type 1 autoimmune hepatitis. Dig Dis Sci. 1997;42:1688–96.
26. Chen M, Shirai M, Czaja AJ *et al.* Characterization of anti-histone antibodies in patients with type 1 autoimmune hepatitis. J Gastroenterol Hepatol. 1998;199:483–9.
27. Czaja AJ, Cassani F, Cataleta M, Valentini P, Bianchi FB. Frequency and significance of antibodies to actin in type 1 autoimmune hepatitis. Hepatology. 1996;24:1068–73.
28. Heringlake S, Tillman HL, Cordes-Temme P, Trautwein C, Hunsmann G, Manns MP. GBV-C/HGV is not the major cause of autoimmune hepatitis. J Hepatol. 1996;25:980–4.
29. Jongerius JM, Boland GJ, Van der Poel CL *et al.* GB virus type C viremia and envelope antibodies among population subsets in The Netherlands. Vox Sang. 1999;76:81–4.

30. Kooy A, de Heide LJM, Engelkens HJH, Mulder AH, van Hagen M, Schalm SW. How to diagnose autoimmune hepatitis in systemic lupus erythematosus? Hepatology. 1996;23:937–8.
31. Czaja AJ, Carpenter HA, Santrach PJ, Moore SB. Significance of HLA DR4 in type 1 autoimmune hepatitis. Gastroenterology. 1993;105:1502–7.
32. Czaja AJ, Strettel MDJ, Thomson LJ *et al.* Associations between alleles of the major histocompatibility complex and type 1 autoimmune hepatitis. Hepatology. 1997;25:317–23.
33. Manns MP, Kruger M. Immunogenetics of chronic liver diseases. Gastroenterology. 1994;8:243–9.
34. Marcos Y, Fainboim HA, Capucchio M *et al.* Two-locus involvement in the association of human leukocyte antigen with the extrahepatic manifestations of autoimmune chronic hepatitis. Hepatology. 1994;19:1371–4.
35. Vazquez-Garcia MN, Alaez C, Olivo A *et al.* MHC class II sequences of susceptibility and protection in Mexicans with autoimmune hepatitis. J Hepatol. 1998;28:985–90.
36. Bittencourt PL, Goldberg AC, Cancado ELR, Porta G, Laudanna AA, Kalil J. Different HLA profiles confer susceptibility to autoimmune hepatitis type 1 and 2. Am J Gastroenterol. 1998;93:1394–5.
37. Scully LJ, Toze C, Sengar DPS, Goldstein R. Early-onset autoimmune hepatitis is associated with a C4 gene deletion. Gastroenterology. 1993;104:1478–84.
38. Doherty DG, Underhill JA, Donaldson PT *et al.* Polymorphism in the human complement C4 genes and susceptibility to autoimmune hepatitis. Autoimmunity. 1994;18:243–9.
39. Cookson S, Constantini PK, Clare M, Underhill JA, Czaja Al, Donaldson PT. Multiple cytokine gene polymorphisms in type 1 autoimmune hepatitis. Hepatology. 1998;28:392A (abstract).
40. Gough A, Chapman S, Wagstaff K, Emery P, Elias E. Minocylcine induced autoimmune hepatitis and systemic lupus erythematosus-like syndrome. Br Med J. 1996;312:169–72.
41. Malcolm A, Heap TR, Eckstein RP, Lunzer MR. Minocycline induced liver injury. Am J Gastroenterol. 1996;91:1641–3.
42. Goldstein PE, Devier J, Cremer M. Acute hepatitis and drug-related lupus induced by minocycline treatment. Am J Gastroenterol. 1997;91:143–6.
43. Angulo JM, Sigal LH, Espinoza LR. Coexistent minocycline-induced systemic lupus erythematosus and autoimmune hepatitis. Semin Arthritis Rheum. 1998;28:187–92.
44. Ben-Ari Z, Dhillon AP, Sherlock S. Autoimmune cholangiopathy: part of the spectrum of autoimmune chronic active hepatitis. Hepatology. 1993;18:10–15.
45. Taylor SL, Dean PJ, Riely CA. Primary autoimmune cholangitis: an alternative to antimitochondrial antibody-negative primary biliary cirrhosis. Am J Surg Pathol. 1994;18:91–9.
46. Colombato LA, Alvarez F, Côté J, Huet MP. Autoimmune cholangiopathy: the result of consecutive primary biliary cirrhosis and autoimmune hepatitis? Gastroenterology. 1994;107:1839–43.
47. Michieletti P, Wanless IR, Katz A *et al.* Antimitochondrial antibody negative primary biliary cirrhosis: a distinct clinical syndrome of autoimmune cholangitis. Gut. 1994;35:260–5.
48. Mieli-Vergani G, Vergani D. Autoimmune hepatitis in children. In: Krawitt EL, Wiesner RH, Nishioka M, editors. Autoimmune Liver Diseases, 2nd edn. Amsterdam: Elsevier; 1998;425–32.
49. Goodman ZD, McNally PR, Davis DR, Ishak KG. Autoimmune cholangitis. A variant of primary biliary cirrhosis: clinicopathological and serologic correlations in 200 cases. Dig Dis Sci. 1995;40:1232–42.
50. Inverizzi P, Crosignani A, Battezzati PM *et al.* Comparison of the clinical features and clinical course of antimitochondrial antibody-positive and -negative primary biliary cirrhosis. Hepatology. 1997;25:1090–5.
51. Kim WR, Poterucha JJ, Jorgensen RA *et al.* Does antimitochondrial antibody status affect response to treatment in patients with primary biliary cirrhosis? Outcomes of ursodeoxycholic acid therapy and liver transplantation. Hepatology. 1997;26:22–6.
52. Heathcote J. Overlap syndromes of autoimmune hepatitis, primary biliary cirrhosis and primary sclerosing cholangitis. In: Krawitt EL, Wiesner RH, Nishioka M, editors. Autoimmune Liver Disease, 2nd edn. Amsterdam: Elsevier; 1998:449–56.
53. Kinoshita H, Omagari K, Whittingham S *et al.* Autoimmune cholangitis and primary biliary cirrhosis – an autoimmune enigma. Liver. 1999;19:122–8.
54. Neuberger J, Thomson R. PBC and AMA – what is the connection? Hepatology. 1999;29:271–6.
55. Wilschanski M, Chait P, Wade JA *et al.* Primary sclerosing cholangitis in 32 children: clinical, laboratory, and radiographic features, with survival analysis. Hepatology. 1995;22:1415–22.

56. Protzer U, Dienes HP, Bianchi L *et al.* Post infantile giant cell hepatitis in patients with primary sclerosing cholangitis and autoimmune hepatitis. Liver. 1996;16:274–82.
57. Roberts EA. Primary sclerosing cholangitis in children. In: Krawitt EL, Wiesner RH, Nishioka M, editors. Autoimmune Liver Diseases, 2nd edn. Amsterdam: Elsevier; 1998:433–47.
58. McNair ANB, Moloney M, Portmann BC, Williams R, McFarlane IG. Autoimmune hepatitis overlapping with primary sclerosing cholangitis in five cases. Am J Gastroenterol. 1998;93:777–84.
59. Danielsson A, Prytz H. Oral budesonide for treatment of autoimmune chronic active hepatitis. Aliment Pharmacol Ther. 1994;8:585–90.
60. Van Thiel DH, Wright H, Carroll P *et al.* Tacrolimus: a potential new treatment for autoimmune chronic active hepatitis: results of an open-label preliminary trial. Am J Gastroenterol. 1995;90:771–6.
61. Kanzler C, Gerken G, Dienes HP, Meyer zum Buschenfelde KH, Lohse AW. Cyclophosphamide as alternative immunosuppressive therapy for autoimmune hepatitis – report of three cases. Z Gastroenterol. 1997;35:571–8.
62. Nakamura K, Yoneda M, Yokohama S *et al.* Efficacy of ursodeoxycholic acid in Japanese patients with type 1 autoimmune hepatitis. J Gastroenterol Hepatol. 1998;13:490–5.
63. Heathcote J. Efficacy of ursodeoxycholic acid in Japanese patients with type 1 autoimmune hepatitis. J Gastroenterol Hepatol. 1998;5:457–9.
64. Schuppan D, Herold C, Strobel D, Schneider HT, Hahn EG. Successful treatment of therapy-refractory autoimmune hepatitis with mycophenolate mofetil. Hepatology. 1998;28:625A (abstract).
65. Alvarez F, Ciocca M, Canero-Velasco C *et al.* Short-term cyclosporine induces remission of autoimmune hepatitis in children. J Hepatol. 1999;30:222–7.
66. Gregorio GV, Portmann B, Mowat AP, Vergani D, Mieli-Vergani G. A 12-year-old girl with antimitochondrial antibody-positive autoimmune hepatitis. J Hepatol. 1997;27:751–4.
67. International Autoimmune Hepatitis Group report: review of criteria for diagnosis of autoimmune hepatitis. J Hepatol. 1999;31:929–38.

# 7
# Autoimmune hepatitis in Asia

**M. NISHIOKA**

## INTRODUCTION

Autoimmune hepatitis (AIH) appears to develop in patients when a genetically predisposed host is exposed to an environmental agent[1]. There are close associations with HLA DR3 and DR4 in patients with AIH. Interestingly, the prevalences of chronic viral infections are associated with the frequency of AIH, as indicated earlier by Mackay[2].

In Asian countries where there are major problems with regard to viral hepatitis, and there is a low prevalence of HLA B8 and DR3 phenotypes, the frequency of AIH may be low and AIH patients may have different characteristics and clinical outcomes compared to Europe and America.

Indeed, AIH in Japan is infrequent compared to other countries[3], and there are differences in characteristics and prognosis. However, the status of AIH in Asia has not been well studied. We tried to perform a mini-international survey which was designed to determine the incidence of AIH and other autoimmune liver diseases and their characteristics in Asian countries. The present status of AIH in Asia is reviewed.

## AUTOIMMUNE LIVER DISEASES IN ASIA

A mini-international survey was performed by sending questionnaires to well-known hepatologists of Asian Pacific associations for the study of the liver disease in 13 countries in Asia. Autoimmune liver disease (AILD) seems to be rare in Asia, although it was difficult to gather information. Almost all patients with chronic hepatitis were diagnosed as viral hepatitis in several countries. In addition, physicians do not provide care for many AILD patients. However, we were able to analyse the data returned from Taiwan and Thailand as well as those from Japan.

The results of a retrospective analysis of AILD patients in three different liver clinics are shown in Tables 1 and 2. AIH type I was present in those countries and predominantly in females. The age at onset of AIH seems to be younger in Thailand; the mean age was 41 years. AIH type II and PSC were not present in

**Table 1** Characteristics of autoimmune liver diseases in Asia – mean age at presentation and sex ratio

| | *Japan (Nishioka)*[a] | | | *Taiwan (Liaw)*[b] | | | *Thailand (Anuchit)*[c] | | |
|---|---|---|---|---|---|---|---|---|---|
| | *No. of patients* | *Age (years)*[d] | *Sex (F:M)*[d] | *No. of patients* | *Age (years)* | *Sex (F:M)* | *No. of patients* | *Age (years)* | *Sex (F:M)* |
| AIH type I | 27 | 53 (8–78) | 10:1 | 2 | 60–65 | 2:0 | 16 | 41.3 (24–79) | 15:1 |
| AIH type II | 1 | < 20 | 0:1 | 0 | | | 0 | – | – |
| PBC | 59 | 58 (25–79) | 9:1 | 46 | 54 (29–74) | 10:1.5 | 9 | 59.7 (47–85) | 9:0 |
| PSC | 4 | 54 (21–64) | 1:2.3 | 0 | | | 0 | – | – |
| AIC | 5 | 58 (32–76) | 1:1 | 14 | 54 (35–76) | 6:1 | 0 | – | – |

AIH: autoimmune hepatitis, PBC: primary biliary cirrhosis, PSC: primary sclerosing cholangitis, AIC: autoimmune cholangitis.
[a]Analysis of patients from 1988 to 1997, diagnosed in Department of Internal Medicine (Gastroenterology), Kagawa Medical University, Kagawa, Japan.
[b]Analysis of patients file of chronic liver disease documented from 1977 to 1998 in Liver Research Unit, Chang Gung Memorial Hospital, Taiwan.
[c]Retrospective analysis of the patients from 1988 to 1997, attending the liver clinic in the section of Digestive and Liver Diseases, Department of Medicine, Pramongkutklao Hospital, Bangkok, Thailand.
[d]Age: mean (range), F:M = female:male.

**Table 2** Clinical and histological findings of AILD in Asia

| | *Japan (Nishioka)* | | | | *Thailand (Anuchit)* | | | |
|---|---|---|---|---|---|---|---|---|
| | *Clinical feature* | *(%)* | *Histology* | *(%)* | *Clinical feature* | *(%)* | *Histology* | *(%)* |
| AIH type 1 | Asymptomatic | 28 | AH | 6 | Asymptomatic | 13 | AH | 13 |
| | General fatigue | 32 | CPH | 6 | Jaundice | 63 | CPH | 33 |
| | Hypochondralgia | 16 | CAH-2A | 22 | Gastrointestinal bleeding | 6 | CAH | 40 |
| | Jaundice | 11 | CAH-2B | 50 | Abdominal pain | 6 | Cirrhosis | 13 |
| | Fever | 6 | Cirrhosis | 16 | Oedema | 6 | | |
| | Arthralgia | 6 | | | Weight loss | 6 | | |
| PBC | Asymptomatic | 74 | Stage* I | 35 | Asymptomatic | 67 | Stage I | 14 |
| | Pruritus | 14 | II | 25 | Jaundice | 22 | II | 14 |
| | Jaundice | 12 | III | 28 | Postoperative jaundice | 11 | III | 28 |
| | | | IV | 11 | | | IV | 42 |

AH: acute hepatitis, CPH: chronic persistent hepatitis, CAH: chronic active hepatitis.
*Scheuer stage.

Taiwan and Thailand. Interestingly, AIH in Taiwan was extremely infrequent because only two cases were found in the past 20 years, while 46 patients with PBC could be found, as shown by Dr Liaw[4]. In Taiwan the carrier rate of HBs antigen is very high and 76% of patients with chronic hepatitis are positive for HBs antigen[4]. On the other hand, the frequencies of HCV and non-B, non-C virus are 21% and 3%, respectively. The high prevalence of HBV infection may be associated with the low incidence of AIH.

Clinical and histological findings are summarized in Table 2. The frequency of patients with severe AIH type I was high in Thailand. Sixty-three per cent of AIH patients had jaundice, while cirrhosis was less frequent, indicating that the frequency of AIH patients with acute severe onset is high in Thailand. There were no differences between Japan and Thailand in clinical or histological findings of PBC patients. However, advanced PBC patients such as Scheuer stage IV were often found in Thailand. Concurrent immunological disorders in AILD are shown in Table 3. Chronic thyroiditis is commonly seen in AILD in Asia.

## AUTOIMMUNE HEPATITIS IN JAPAN

### Prevalence

In Japan AIH was considered to be a rare disease 30 years ago. With the advent of diagnostic techniques such as detection of autoantibodies the number of AIH patients has increased[5]. The AIH Study Group, a subgroup of the Intractable Hepatitis Study Group, which has been sponsored by the Ministry of Health and Welfare of Japan, carried out a nationwide survey of AIH patients by sending

**Table 3** Concurrent immunological disorders in autoimmune liver disease in Asia

| | *Japan (Nishioka)* | *Taiwan (Liaw)* | *Thailand (Anuchit)* |
|---|---|---|---|
| AIH type 1 | RA: 9.8%<br>SJS: 9.8%<br>Thyroiditis: 9.8%<br>PBC: 2% | No | Thyroiditis: 19%<br>ITP: 6.2% |
| AIH type II | Thyroiditis | – | – |
| PBC | RA: 5.6%<br>SJS: 20.8%<br>Thyroiditis: 4.6%<br>UC: 1.3%<br>Raynaud's: 5.4% | Thyroiditis: 17%<br>SJS: 2% | Sicca syndrome: 11%<br>Thyroiditis: 11%<br>RA: 11% |
| PSC | UC: 20%<br>Crohn's disease: 5%<br>Chronic pancreatitis: 15%<br>Gallstone: 12% | – | – |
| AIC | SJS: 20% | Thyroiditis: 7% | – |

AIH: autoimmune hepatitis, PBC: primary biliary cirrhosis, PSC: primary sclerosing cholangitis, AIC: autoimmune cholangitis, RA: rheumatoid arthritis, SJS: Sjögren's syndrome, UC: ulcerative colitis, ITP: idiopathic thrombocytopenic purpura.

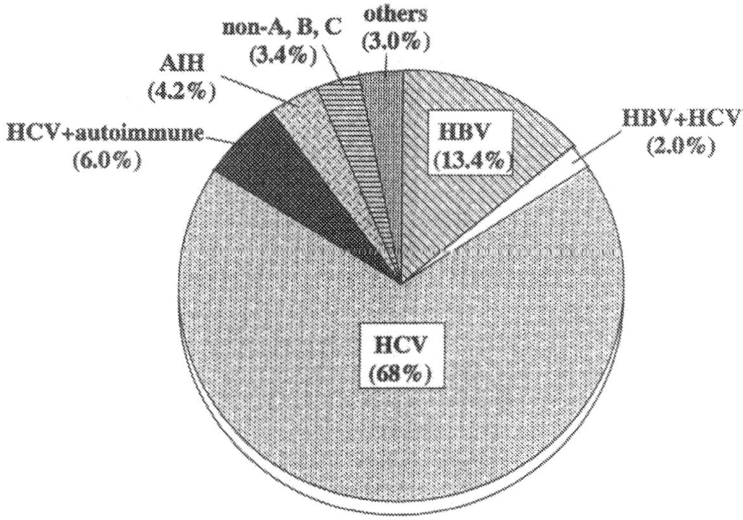


**Fig. 1** Aetiology of chronic hepatitis in Kagawa (1995–98)

questionnaires to more than 100 hospitals throughout Japan since 1978 to study the prevalence of AIH, its characteristics and its prognosis[5–7].

AIH in Japan seems infrequent. The estimated incidence of AIH in England, France, Austria and Japan is 0.1–0.2, 0.12, 1.2 and 0.08–0.015 cases per 100 000 persons per year, respectively[3]. In North America the incidence is uncertain, but it is likely to be similar to that in Western Europe, as reported by Czaja[8]. The low incidence of AIH in Japan may correspond to the characteristics in that country where HCV and HBV are common and there is a low prevalence of HLA-B8 and DR3 phenotypes. In Japan more than 90% of chronic hepatitis is caused by HCV and HBV infection[9]. The frequency of AIH is now estimated to be less than 5% of chronic hepatitis. Figure 1 shows the aetiology of chronic hepatitis in Kagawa Medical Hospital. AIH patients were found in 4.2% of those with chronic hepatitis.

## Deviation of age at onset in Japanese AIH patients

Since the initial report by Waldenström[10], it has been known that the majority of AIH patients are females between the ages of 10 and 30 years. However, the disease occurs in some postmenopausal women, and in men as well. In Japan the age at onset of AIH seems to be increasing. A retrospective analysis by Nishioka *et al.*[11] of 300 cases of AIH over 19 years (1966–85) demonstrated that the peak incidence in terms of age at onset was 50–59 years (108 cases among 300 cases), whereas in the period 1966–75 the peak was at 40–49 years. It is clear that in Japan the age at onset of AIH has shifted to 50–59 years from 40–49 years, particularly in postmenopausal females. This same age distribution was found in a national survey of AIH conducted in 1994[12].

The reason for the increase in the number of AIH patients among older people is unclear. The rare incidence of patients under 20 years of age in recent years may be a reflection of the rapidly increasing older population in Japan. We also noticed that the age at onset of AIH is shifting to 60–70 years.

## Types of autoimmune hepatitis

Autoantibodies specific for liver diseases such as antibody to liver/kidney microsome 1 antibody (anti-LKM-1) and antisoluble liver antigen antibody (anti-SLA) have been described[13]. Czaja[14] proposed a subclassification of AIH according to serological markers. AIH type I is a classical type of AIH positive for ANA. AIH type II is positive for anti-LKM-1, and is mainly found in children. AIH type III is positive for anti-SLA and is commonly seen in young women, but anti-SLA are also found in type I patients. There are no data on the frequency of AIH type II and III worldwide: thus, the validity of this classification has not yet been established, but there is merit in categorizing AIH patients for further epidemiological and clinical analysis.

In Japan AIH type II and III are very rare. Patients with anti-LKM-1 were found in Japan but they were usually associated with HCV infection. Miyakawa *et al.* confirmed that seven of eight AIH patients with anti-LKM-1 were positive for HCV-RNA[15]. We studied the frequency and significance of anti-P450IID6 in various diseases among adult patients. No AIH patient positive for anti-P450IID6 was identified[16].

Anti-P450IID6 was found in six of 235 patients (2.6%) with chronic hepatitis positive for HCV-RNA. They were younger and with lower gamma-globulin and IgG levels than patients without anti-P450IID6. Three of five patients with anti-P450IID6 responded well to interferon therapy, suggesting that HCV is associated with persistent hepatocyte destruction in these patients. One patient received prednisone, when interferon was ineffective[16]. Interestingly, only this patient was diagnosed as 'a definite' AIH according to the criteria proposed by the International Autoimmune Hepatitis Group (IAHG)[17]. A close association of HCV infection with anti-LKM-1 positivity is seen in high HCV endemic areas such as Japan[15,16] and Italy[18]. Recently we developed a sensitive ELISA for detecting anti-LKM1 using recombinant cytochrome P450IID6[19]. This sensitive test is now routinely used in Japan in place of immunofluorescence. This may help to study the epidemiology of patients with anti-LKM-1 in Japan.

It is uncertain if anti-SLA defines a valid subtype of AIH. We recently studied the significance of anti-SLA in patients with chronic liver disease using ELISA[20]. Anti-SLA was found in five of 78 patients (6.4%) with AIH (Table 4). There are no differences in clinical features, laboratory data or histological findings between these five AIH patients positive for anti-SLA and 26 AIH patients negative for anti-SLA (Table 5). Response to prednisone therapy in these patients was good, indicating that AIH type III is similar to AIH type I or a variant of AIH type I with different serological markers. Although the frequency of anti-SLA is very low in Japan, it seems specific for AIH, because of its infrequency in other liver diseases as well as collagen diseases.

**Table 4** Frequency of anti-SLA in various diseases

| | *No. of patients* | |
|---|---|---|
| *Diagnosis* | *Tested* | *Positive (%)* |
| Autoimmune hepatitis | 78 | 5 (6.4) |
| Chronic viral hepatitis | | |
| Hepatitis B virus | 73 | 1 (1.4) |
| Hepatitis C virus | 318 | 0 |
| Non-B, non-C hepatitis | 20 | 0 |
| PBC | 52 | 0 |
| Collagen diseases | 28 | 0 |
| Others | 31 | 0 |
| *Total* | 600 | 6 |

**Table 5** Characteristics of autoimmune hepatitis with anti-SLA

| | *Anti-SLA positive (n = 5)* | *Anti-SLA negative (n = 26)* | *P-value* |
|---|---|---|---|
| Clinical features | | | |
| Age (years) | 48.2 ± 3.2 | 55.4 ± 14.7 | <0.04 |
| Sex (male/female) | 0/6 | 2/24 | n.s. |
| Duration of illness (years) | 3.77 ± 3.9 | 4.19 ± 3.19 | n.s. |
| Laboratory data | | | |
| ALT (N <40 U/L) | 213.4 ± 183.0 | 301.2 ± 324.3 | n.s. |
| AST (N <33 U/L) | 263.4 ± 214.2 | 298.4 ± 338.2 | n.s. |
| $\gamma$-globulin (N < 1.5 mg/dl) | 3.26 ± 0.78 | 3.03 ± 0.84 | n.s. |
| IgG (N < 1.682 mg/dl) | 3.652 ± 951.5 | 3.342.8 ± 952.7 | n.s. |
| Histological findings | | | |
| CAH-2A (%) | 4 (80) | 8 (30.8) | n.s. |
| CAH-2B (%) | 0 | 14 (53.8) | |
| CPH (%) | 1 (20) | 0 | |
| LC (%) | 0 | 4 (15.4) | |

Data represent the mean ± SD.

## Clinical and histological features

AIH is typically of insidious onset in Japanese patients. An acute presentation such as acute or fulminant hepatitis is found in less than 10% of AIH patients. The typical symptoms at presentation in our patients were fatigue, malaise and abdominal discomfort[21]. These symptoms have been commonly seen in hospitals such as the Mayo Clinic[8] and King's College Hospital[22]. Easy fatiguability is the most common symptom, usually in combination with malaise, nausea and loss of appetite. However, almost 50% of our patients with AIH are asymptomatic[21]. They are introduced to a hospital because of abnormal liver function tests.

The discovery of HCV has enabled us to define the clinical entity of AIH more clearly. Therefore, clinical and histological analyses of current AIH patients should be performed, excluding patients with HCV infection. We conducted a nationwide survey of AIH in 1994 and collected data on 496 patients diagnosed as AIH on clinical and histological findings[12]. Most of the 496 fulfilled the criteria proposed in 1992 by the Japanese AIH Study Group[23] as shown in Table 6. These criteria make it possible to exclude many patients with HCV infection.

Symptoms at presentation in 472 AIH patients studied in this survey are shown in Table 7. It is important to note that more than 30% of the patients suffering from cirrhosis are asymptomatic, suggesting that AIH patients have chronic hepatitis or cirrhosis for a considerable period before they develop signs and symptoms. Relatively high frequencies of peripheral oedema, oesophageal varices and ascites could be found in patients with cirrhosis, compared with patients without cirrhosis. The age distribution of both sexes showed a single peak in the 50s. Concurrent immunological diseases were found in 132 (27%) of 417 patients with AIH, and chronic thyroiditis, rheumatoid arthritis and Sjögren's syndrome were seen frequently. These findings were similar to those of our previous survey[6].

In a histological analysis 92% of AIH patients had piecemeal necrosis. Bridging necrosis and plasma cell infiltration in the portal tract were observed in 60% and 50% of AIH patients, respectively.

**Table 6** Criteria for diagnosis of autoimmune hepatitis in Japan (Study Group of Japanese Ministry of Health and Welfare, 1992)

*General concept*
Increased prevalence in younger females, chronic active hepatitis with potential progression to cirrhosis, existence of autoimmune mechanisms in aetiology, exclusion of all other known specific causes of chronic hepatitis, such as viruses, alcohol, drugs, etc., good response to corticosteroid therapy (typical)

*I. Major findings*
1. Persistent elevation of serum aminotransferases
2. Hypergammaglobulinaemia of 2.5 g/dl or greater (or IgG concentration of 2.5 g/dl or greater)
3. Circulating autoantibody:(a) and/or (b)
   (a) LE test positive
   (b) ANA (antinuclear antibody) positive and/or LE test positive
4. IgM anti-HAV (hepatitis A virus) negative and absence of other evidence of HBV infection (HBs antigen negative, anti-HBs antibody negative or at low titres)
5. Absence of true-positive anti-HCV antibody or other evidence of HCV infection

*II. Minor findings*
1. Systemic manifestation such as fever, arthralgia and skin eruption
2. Complication of other autoimmune diseases including collagen disease
3. (a) and/or (b)
   (a) Accelerated ESR (erythrocyte sedimentation rate) at 30 mm/h or faster
   (b) C-reactive protein (CRP) positive

*III. Histology*
Chronic active hepatitis or cirrhosis with marked plasma cell infiltration and hepatocyte necrosis, absence of features of other specific diagnosis such as alpha-1-antitrypsin deficiency

*Diagnosis of autoimmune hepatitis*
1. Diagnostic: fulfil all criteria of I and III
2. Suggestive: fulfil all criteria of I and at least one of II
3. Possible: fulfil all criteria of I

**Table 7** Symptoms at presentation in 472 patients with autoimmune hepatitis in Japan

| | *No. of cases (%)* | | |
|---|---|---|---|
| *Symptoms* | *Total* | *Cirrhosis (–)* | *Cirrhosis (+)* |
| Asymptomatic | 180 (38.1) | 163 (38.4) | 17 (35.4) |
| Fatigue | 142 (30.1) | 134 (31.6) | 8 (16.7) |
| Jaundice | 86 (18.2) | 76 (17.9) | 10 (20.8) |
| Anorexia | 25 (5.3) | 21 (5.0) | 4 (8.3) |
| Pyrexia | 24 (5.1) | 23 (5.4) | 1 (2.1) |
| Common cold | 9 (1.9) | 7 (1.7) | 2 (4.2) |
| Peripheral oedema | 4 (0.8) | 1 (0.2) | 3 (6.3) |
| Abdominal fullness | 4 (0.8) | 4 (0.9) | – |
| Pyrexia | 2 (0.4) | – | 2 (4.2) |
| Malaise | 2 (0.4) | 1 (0.2) | 1 (2.1) |
| Ascites | 2 (0.4) | – | 2 (4.2) |
| Hepatic coma | 1 (0.2) | – | 1 (2.1) |
| *Total* | 472 | 424 | 48 |

## Virological markers

Anti-HCV and HCV-RNA are frequently positive in AIH patients, particularly in regions where there is a high prevalence of HCV infection. Sixty-two patients (12.5%) were positive for anti-HCV (C-100 or second-generation HCV antibody) in our nationwide survey in 1994[12]. Among these patients, all 50 patients examined were positive for serum HCV-RNA. Our national survey in 1998 interestingly revealed that 30 of 413 AIH patients (7.3%) were positive for anti-HCV and 16 patients (3.9%) were positive for HCV-RNA, indicating that approximately 7% of AIH patients are seropositive for the HCV marker in Japan.

Clinical findings in HCV-positive and -negative patients with AIH are shown in Table 8. Patients positive for HCV showed low serum levels of alanine aminotransferase (ALT), but were indistinguishable from patients without HCV-RNA in regard to age, sex, biochemical findings, ANA titres and HLA-DR4. In this context it is noted that frequencies of antibodies to recombinant nuclear antigens such as U1-RNP-A, U1-RNP-70, SSA-60 and SSA-50 are high in AIH

**Table 8** Clinical findings in HCV-positive patients and HCV-negative patients with autoimmune hepatitis

| | *Total* | *HCV-positive (%)* | *HCV-negative (%)* |
|---|---|---|---|
| No. of patients | 496 | 62 (13) | 434 (87) |
| Sex (male/female) | 61/435 | 6/56 (11) | 55/379 (15) |
| Age at onset | 50.8 ± 12.7 | 54.1 ± 8.3 | 50.4 ± 13.2 |
| ANA* (titre) | 320 | 320 | 320 |
| ALT (IU/L) | 301 ± 378 | 196 ± 167 | 314 ± 396 |
| IgG (mg/dl) | 3242 ± 1039 | 3362 ± 918 | 3143 ± 987 |
| HLA DR4 | 65/94 | 12/20 (60) | 53/74 (72) |
| AIH score (%)† | 48:46:6 | 3:66:31 | 54:43:3 |

* Median.
†Score by International AIH Study Group: definite: probable: others

**Table 9** Frequency of autoantibodies to recombinant nuclear antigens in autoimmune hepatitis

| | *No. of cases (%)* | |
|---|---|---|
| *Antibodies to* | *HCV-negative (n = 18)* | *HCV-positive (n = 17)* |
| U1-RNP-A | 4 (22) | 1 (6) |
| U1-RNP-70 | 5 (28) | 1 (6) |
| SS-A-60 | 4 (22) | 0 (0) |
| SS-A-52 | 7 (39) | 0 (0) |
| Cenp-B | 2 (11) | 3 (18) |

patients negative for HCV, as compared with the patients positive for HCV[24] (Table 9).

Recently, hepatitis G virus (HGV) has been identified. HGV is a RNA virus, transmissible through transfusion, and associated with acute and chronic infection. Since the virus may trigger the development of AIH, we studied the relationship of AIH with HGV. Serum HGV-RNA, measured by reverse transcription polymerase chain reaction (RT-PCR), was found in two out of 32 patients with AIH[25]. A similar frequency was seen in patients with chronic viral hepatitis, suggesting that HGV does not play a causal or ongoing role in the development of AIH.

AIH refers to chronic hepatitis not associated with active virus infection, drug or metabolic disorders. In our recent study on 68 patients diagnosed as AIH by criteria for Japanese AIH, 27 patients were positive for HCV, four for HBV, two for HGV, and two for TTV, as shown in Figure 2. Most patients positive for these hepatitis viruses could be considered as chronic viral hepatitis with AIH.

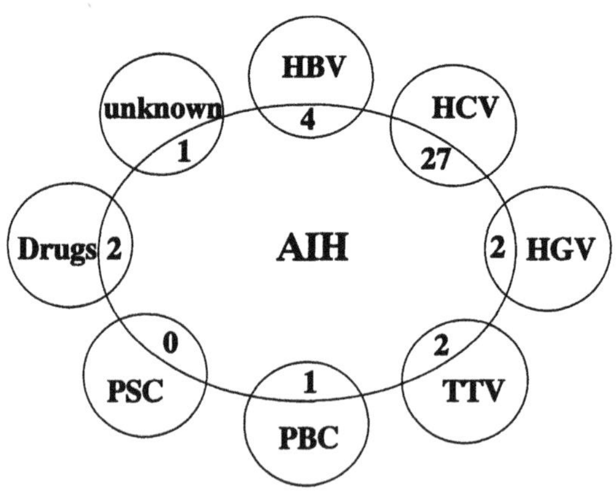


**Fig. 2** Overlap of viral hepatitis, drug-induced hepatitis, PBC and PSC in 68 patients with autoimmune hepatitis

Alternatively, it seems reasonable to include hepatitis virus as a possible aetiological factor in some patients with AIH.

## HLA phenotypes in Japan

It is well known that susceptibility of AIH is associated with the HLA DR3 and DR4. Differences in the prevalence of AIH in various regions may in part be explained by regional differences in the frequencies of HLA phenotypes[14]. In addition, these phenotypes may influence not only risk for AIH, but also the behaviour of the disease[14]. Patients with HLA DR4 seem to be older, and have higher levels of gamma-globulin than those with HLA DR3. Most AIH patients in Japan are associated with HLA DR4 and have characteristics of patients positive for HLA DR4. In our survey in 1994[12], HLA DR4 was found in 65 (69.1%) of 94 patients tested, as shown in Table 8. HLA DR2 seems to be an independent risk factor for AIH in Japan, but the significance of HLA DR2 is still unclear. Table 10 shows characteristics of AIH patients positive for DR2 or DR4 compared with American AIH patients.

## Validation of scoring systems in Japanese AIH patients

The scoring system proposed by the International AIH Study Group[17] was applied to all 496 patients surveyed in 1994[12]. Forty-eight per cent of patients originally diagnosed as having AIH by criteria proposed by the Japanese AIH Study Group (1992) had an aggregate score for definite AIH, as shown in Table 8. Forty six per cent of patients had a probable AIH and 6% were non-diagnostic, indicating that most of the AIH patients diagnosed as AIH by our Japanese criteria achieve a score for diagnosis of 'definite' or 'probable' AIH. Japanese criteria of AIH coincide with International criteria, as reported earlier[12]. When HCV-positive patients were excluded from the study group the percentages of definite and probable AIH were 54% and 43% respectively, as shown in Table 8. On the other hand, in patients positive for HCV, 3% of the patients were diagnosed as a definite AIH, 66% as probable AIH, and 31% as non-diagnostic, indicating that

**Table 10** Characteristics of AIH patients in relation to HLA phenotype

| | *Japan (Nishioka)* | | *USA (Czaja)* | |
|---|---|---|---|---|
| | *DR2 (n = 8)* | *DR4 (n = 16)* | *DR3 (n = 41)* | *DR4 (n = 44)* |
| Age (years), mean (range) | 52.8 (15–74) | 55.9 (28–78) | 38.2 | 51.0 |
| Sex (male/female) | 1/7 | 0/16 | 13/28 | * 5/39 |
| Immunological disorder | 25% | 56.3% | 26.8% | * 59% |
| AST (U/L) | 367 ± 486 | 220 ± 219 | 428 ± 52 | 536 ± 68 |
| IgG (g/dl) | 2.75 ± 0.25 | * 3.54 ± 1.14 | 2.73 ± 0.19 | * 3.30 ± 0.22 |
| ANA (≧ × 160) | 62.5% | 50% | 68.3% | 77.3% |

* $p < 0.05$.

this scoring system can exclude 30% of HCV-positive patients with autoimmune features. The scoring system was modified by the International AIH group in 1999[26]. The ability of the revised scoring system will be evaluated soon.

## Treatment and prognosis

AIH is generally responsive to immunosuppresive therapy in Japan. Corticosteroids can improve biochemical and histological abnormalities. In our survey in 1994 more than 80% of AIH patients were treated with corticosteroids and 89% of them responded well[12]. Only five patients were treated with azathioprine alone, resulting in normalization of serum transaminase. Interestingly, ursodeoxycholic acid (UDCA) was used in 8% of AIH patients; 51% of them showed improvement in biochemical data. UDCA seems to be an effective drug in some AIH patients.

In 62 patients with HCV infection in the survey, 37 were treated with corticosteroids. More than 80% of the patients showed a good response, indicating that there is no difference between HCV-positive and -negative patients in response to treatments with corticosteroids.

Interferon (IFN) treatment was carried out in 20 patients with HCV-RNA; 10 of them were responders. There was no difference in clinical data including age, gender, ALT levels, IgG levels and ANA titres between the patients who responded to IFN treatment and those who did not[12]. It seems impossible to predict the efficacy of IFN in those patients. Several new drugs such as cyclosporin and FK-506 are used in management of AIH, but those drugs are rarely tried in Japan.

Remission occurs in 80% of AIH patients after treatment. Prognosis of patients with cirrhosis is poor. In a previous study[6], 20 selected potential prognostic variables regarding clinical, biochemical and serological findings were subjected to univariate analysis[6]. Indocyanine green clearance and platelet count were found to be significantly related to prognosis. Regression equations were used to develop a prognostic index (PI) defined by the following equation: $PI = +0.0256 \log ICG + 0.0236 \log \text{platelet count} + 0.00055 \log ALT$. A higher prognostic index value was found to correlate with a higher risk of death and a worse prognosis.

## Acknowledgements

This study was carried out in collaboration with Professor Y. F. Liaw, Chang Gung Memorial Hospital, Taiwan; Professor C. Anuchit, Department of Medicine, Pramongkutklao Hospital, Bangkok, Thailand; and Dr K. Kurokohchi and Ms S Yoshino, Department of Internal Medicine, Kagawa Medical University, Kagawa, Japan. The research was supported in part by a grant from the Intractable Hepatitis Research Committee of the Health and Welfare Ministry of Japan.

## References

1. Krawitt EL. Medical progress: autoimmune hepatitis. N Engl J Med. 1996;334:897–903.
2. Mackay IR. Autoimmune diseases of the liver: chronic active hepatitis and primary biliary cirrhosis. In: Rose NR, Mackay IR, editors. The Autoimmune Diseases. Orlando, FL: Academic Press; 1985:291–337.

3. Nishioka M, Morshed SA, McFarlane IG *et al.* Geographical variation in the frequency and characteristics of autoimmune liver diseases. In: Krawitt EL, Wiesner RH, Nishioka M, editors. Autoimmune Liver Diseases, 2nd edn. Amsterdam: Elsevier; 1998;413–24.
4. Liaw YF. Viral hepatitis in Taiwan: status in the 1990s. In: Nishioka K, Suzuki H, Mishiro S, Oda T, editors. Viral Hepatitis and Liver Disease. Berlin: Springer-Verlag; 1994:419–21.
5. Monna T, Kuroki T, Yamamoto S. Autoimmune hepatitis: the present status in Japan. Gastroenterol Jpn. 1985;20:260–72.
6. Onji M, Nonaka T, Horiike N, Moriwaki H, Muto Y, Ohta Y. Present status of autoimmune hepatitis in Japan. Gastroenterol Jpn. 1993;28(Suppl. 4):134–8.
7. Ohta Y, Onji M. Clinical characteristics of autoimmune hepatitis in Japan. In: Nishioka M, Toda G, Zeniya M, editors. Autoimmune Hepatitis. Amsterdam: Elsevier; 1994:45–53.
8. Czaja AJ. Clinical aspects of autoimmune hepatitis in North America. In: Nishioka M, Toda G, Zeniya M, editors. Autoimmune Hepatitis. Amsterdam: Elsevier, 1994:27–43.
9. Nishioka M, Morshed SA. Viral hepatitis in Japan: update. J Gastroenterol Hepatol. 1997;12(Suppl.):S36-44.
10. Waldenström J. Leber, Blutprotein and Nahrungeiweiss. Dtsch Z Verdan Stoffwechselkz. 1950; 2:113–19.
11. Nishioka M, Morshed SA. Recent aspects of autoimmune hepatitis. In: Nishioka M, Toda G, Zeniya M, editors. Autoimmune Hepatitis. Amsterdam: Elsevier; 1994: 319–36.
12. Toda G, Zeniya M, Watanabe F *et al.* and the Japanese National Study Group of Autoimmune Hepatitis. Present status of autoimmune hepatitis in Japan – correlating the characteristics with international criteria in an area with a high rate of HCV infection. J Hepatol. 1997; 26: 1207–12.
13. Manns M, Gerken G, Kyriatsoulis A *et al.* Characterisation of a new subgroup of autoimmune chronic active hepatitis by autoantibodies against a soluble liver antigen. Lancet. 1987;1:292–4.
14. Czaja AJ. Autoimmune hepatitis: evolving concepts and treatment strategies. Dig Dis Sci. 1995; 40: 435–56.
15. Miyakawa H, Kako M, Nagai K *et al.* HCV-RNA in type 2 autoimmune hepatitis. Am J Gastroenterol. 1991;86:1688–9.
16. Nishioka M, Morshed SA, Kono K *et al.* Frequency and significance of antibodies to P450IID6 protein in Japanese patients with chronic hepatitis C. J Hepatol. 1997;26:992–1000.
17. Johnson PJ, McFarlane IG. Meeting Report: International Autoimmune Hepatitis Group. Hepatology. 1993;18:998–1005.
18. Lenzi M, Ballardini G, Fusconi M *et al.* Type 2 autoimmune hepatitis C virus infection. Lancet. 1990; 335: 258–9.
19. Hosomi N, Arima K, Kono K, Kurokohchi K, Watanabe S, Nishioka M. Establishment of a novel ELISA system to detect the anti-LKM1 antibody utilizing the recombinant cytochrome P450IID6 (CYP2D6) antigen. Acta Hepatol Jpn. 1998;39:366–73.
20. Matsuoka H, Ming C, Ando T *et al.* Frequency of antibody to soluble liver antigen in patients with chronic liver diseases and their characteristics. Acta Hepatol Jpn. 1997;38:152–8.
21. Nishioka M. Management of autoimmune hepatitis. Trop Gastroenterol. 1997;18:3–7.
22. McFarlane IG. Clinical spectrum and heterogeneity of autoimmune hepatitis: an overview. In: Meyer zum Büschenfelde KH, Hoofnagle JH and Manns M, editors. Immunology and Liver. Dordrecht: Kluwer; 1993:179–92.
23. Ohta Y. Report of the research subgroup of autoimmune hepatitis/primary biliary cirrhosis. Gastroenterol Jpn. 1993;28(Suppl.4):128–33.
24. Nishioka M. Nuclear antigens in autoimmune hepatitis. In: Meyer zum Büschenfelde KH, Hoofnagle JH, Manns M, editors. Immunology and Liver. Dordrecht: Kluwer; 1993:193–205.
25. Nishioka M, Morshed SA. Recent progress in autoimmune liver disease. In: Husband AJ, Beagly KW, Clancy RL, editors. Advances in Mucosal Immunology, vol. 1. Sydney: University of Sydney Press; 1997:425–37.
26. Alvarez F, Berg PA, Bianchi FB *et al.* International autoimmune hepatitis group report: review of criteria for diagnosis of autoimmune hepatitis. J Hepatol. 1999;31:929–38.

# 8
# Autoimmune hepatitis in South America

E. L. R. CANÇADO and G. PORTA

## INTRODUCTION

Autoimmune hepatitis (AIH) is a liver disease classically described in Caucasian patients from North America and Europe. There are very few publications regarding this disease in patients from South America. Doubts, however, arise as to whether there are the same similarities between the disease seen in patients from the former geographical areas and the disease seen in patients from the latter, especially regarding the following: clinical picture, onset of the disease, AIH serological markers, HLA association, and extrahepatic manifestations (mainly those related to other autoimmune diseases).

In Brazil, AIH is still considered an unusual disease, corresponding to 5–10% of liver diseases in the main medical centres of that country. In the Hospital das Clínicas of São Paulo Medical School, AIH corresponds to less than 5% of patients on the waiting list of liver transplantation. Of 247 cases transplanted only 6% had AIH.

One hundred and seventy-seven patients were followed by the authors, and 50 patients by other doctors from the staff of the hospital complex. The autoantibody and HLA determination were performed at the same laboratories.

## GENDER

The predominance of females is also evident among our patients, but the difference is less important for AIH than for primary biliary cirrhosis. If we take into account the total numbers of child and adult patients the female/male ratio is 4.7:1. In the group of patients with the serological marker anti-liver kidney microsome antibody type 1 (anti-LKM1), the ratio was greater than those observed in the group with anti-smooth muscle antibody (SMA) and antinuclear antibody (ANA), 9.6 : 1 and 4.2 : 1, respectively.

## AGE AT ONSET

Around 64% of patients experienced the onset of their diseases in childhood (≤ 15 years old). The majority of patients were ≤ 25 years old (76.5%), and we saw no evidence of a second peak of incidence after the menopause, as reported elsewhere.

Concerning patients with AIH and SMA with specificity to F-actin (SMA/AAA), although the majority were ≤ 15 years old, patients with this feature were found at all ages (3–69 years old). Patients with isolated antinuclear antibodies were more frequent in the adult range.

The youngest patients were those within the anti-LKM1 group (1–33 years old). Seventeen patients (53.1%) with type 2 AIH were ≤ 5 years old, as against 4.0% (7 in 177) in AIH type 1 AIH.

## SKIN COLOUR

The Brazilian population is very mixed in its composition. It is composed primarily of natives, Caucasian Europeans (from the Iberian Peninsula) and black Africans. Further there is an influence of French, Dutch, German, Italian and Japanese migration. It is really very difficult to define a Caucasian population in Brazil. Although the disease was more prevalent in the white population (53.7%), it was present in 33.5% of mulattos, in 11.4% of Afro-Brazilians and in 1.3% of Japanese descendants.

## CLINICAL PRESENTATION

The clinical manifestations at onset, in 70% of patients, resembled an acute viral hepatitis, with non-specific symptoms such as malaise, nausea/vomiting and anorexia, followed by choluria, faecal acholia and jaundice. However, other clinical evidence (splenomegaly, oedema, vascular spiders and palmar erythema); abnormal biochemical tests (hypergammaglobulinaemia, hypoprothrombinaemia, hypoalbuminaemia); abdominal ultrasonography; upper digestive endoscopy and liver histology pointed to a diagnosis of chronic liver disease. Some patients (4.8%) developed liver failure with a clinical feature of fulminant hepatitis. This form of presentation occurred in 18.8% of patients with serological markers of AIH-2, and less frequently with SMA/AAA (1.1%). Patients with similar forms of fulminant hepatitis, without any of the autoantibodies previously mentioned, account for 16.7% of the patients with AIH without serological markers. The summarized data of patients are displayed in Table 1.

Symptoms and signs of chronic hepatopathy comprised the second form of clinical presentation in around 15% of patients, constituting a large spectrum of clinical features such as upper digestive haemorrhage, ascites, epistaxis and splenomegaly.

Among the extrahepatic manifestations, arthralgia, usually without arthritis, and hormonal alterations in young women were the most common, and represented the initial symptoms in 8% of patients.

**Table 1** Clinical, biochemical, histological features, diagnostic criteria and therapeutic response of 277 patients with AIH

| *Features* | *Type 1* | *Type 2* | *Without markers* |
|---|---|---|---|
| Gender (F/M) | 143/34 | 29/3 | 15/3 |
| Skin colour | | | |
| White | 92 | 20 | 10 |
| Mulatto | 60 | 11 | 5 |
| Afro-Brazilian | 23 | 1 | 2 |
| Japanese descendant | 2 | 0 | 1 |
| Age of onset, median (range) | 12 (3–69) | 4 (1–33)* | 32 (6–52) |
| Clinical presentation | | | |
| Hepatitis | 125 | 22 | 12 |
| Chronic hepatopathy | 28 | 3 | 2 |
| Extrahepatic manifestations | 17 | 0 | 1 |
| Acute hepatitis | 5 | 0 | 0 |
| Fulminant hepatitis | 2 | 6 | 3 |
| Abnormal transaminases | 0 | 1 | 0 |
| ALT (×NV); mean (range)† | 18.3 (1.1–78) | 17.2 (1–58.4) | 19.4 (1.5–53.3) |
| AST (×NV); mean (range) | 22.5 (2–137) | 21.0 (1–70.2) | 23.5 (1.9–88.3) |
| ALP (×NV); mean (range) | 1.7 (1.0–8.0) | 1.4 (1.0–4.0) | 1.8 (1.0–4.6) |
| Albumin (g%); mean (range) | 3.3 (1.5–5.0) | 3.4 (1.6–5.0) | 3.4 (2.6–4.2) |
| Gammaglobulins (×NV); mean (range) | 2.9 (1–4.5) | 1.6 (1–3.0)* | 1.7 (1–3.6) |
| Total bilirubins (mg%) | 6.81 (0.6–36.8) | 10.9 (0.7–36.9) | 11.4 (0.5–37.5) |
| Histological findings | | | |
| Hepatic cirrhosis | 55 | 16 | 4 |
| Chronic hepatitis (stage 3) | 40 | 3 | 7 |
| Chronic hepatitis (stage 2) | 37 | 7 | 3 |
| Acute hepatitis | 10 | 2 | 3 |
| Chronic hepatitis (stage 1) | 1 | 0 | 0 |
| Not performed | 34 | 4 | 1 |

**Table 1** *(continued)*

| *Features* | *Type 1* | *Type 2* | *Without markers* |
|---|---|---|---|
| Chronic hepatitis (stage 1) | 1 | 0 | 0 |
| Hepatocarcinoma | 2 | 0 | 0 |

| *International score systems before and after treatment* | *1992* | *1998* | *1992* | *1998* | *1992* | *1998* |
|---|---|---|---|---|---|---|
| Definite → definite | 134 | 143 | 21 | 24 | 7 | 9 |
| Definite → probable | 29 | 24 | 7 | 5 | 1 | 1 |
| Probable → definite | 6 | 1 | 2 | 2 | 5 | 4 |
| Probable → probable | 8 | 9 | 2 | 1 | 5 | 4 |
| *Total* | 177 | 177 | 32 | 32 | 18 | 18 |

*$p < 0.001$ (comparison between AIH-1 and AIH-2).
†×NV – times upper the normal value.

**Table 2** Autoimmune manifestations in 227 patients with autoimmune hepatitis

| *Autoimmune manifestations* | *Total* |
|---|---|
| Thyroiditis | 6 |
| Vitiligo, coeliac disease | 4 |
| Mixed connective tissue disease, diabetes mellitus type 1 | 3 |
| Rheumatoid arthritis, polyserositis; autoimmune haemolytic anaemia, Raynaud, antiendomysium positive + intestinal biopsy without coeliac disease | 2 |
| Ulcerative colitis, arthritis, Weber Christian's paniculitis, asthma, focal glomerulosclerosis, interstitial pneumonitis; localized scleroderma | 1 |
| Total of autoimmune manifestations | 36 |
| Total of patients with autoimmune manifestations | 27 (11.9%) |
| Patients without autoimmune manifestations | 200 (88.1%) |

## AUTOIMMUNE MANIFESTATIONS

A broad spectrum of autoimmune diseases is present in patients with AIH and in their first-degree relatives; these diseases are listed in Table 2. Among the autoimmune manifestations the most common are thyroiditis, vitiligo and coeliac disease. Although the presence of a genetic marker represents a definite association between HLA of class II and the predisposition to several autoimmune diseases, it is highly significant that we did not document another case of AIH within the same family. On the other hand, we identified three cases of AIH, one as a daughter, one as a sister, and another as a niece of patients with primary biliary cirrhosis. Because of the rarity of autoimmune liver diseases in first-degree relatives of AIH patients, we do not routinely perform laboratory investigations in them.

## LABORATORY TESTS

The most important biochemical tests of patients with AIH are shown in Table 2. Usually the levels of transaminases are more than 10 times the normal value. Increases more than 50 times the normal value could be identified in both subtypes of AIH. Alkaline phosphatase was rarely more than 5 times the upper normal range.

The gammaglobulin levels were increased, especially in AIH with SMA/AAA and/or ANA more than in cases with anti-LKM1. Only 25% of patients with the latter autoantibody had gammaglobulins increased more than twice the normal range, contrasting with 67.2% of type 1 patients. IgA deficiency occurred more frequently in type 2 AIH, than in type 1.

The SMA is the most frequent autoantibody in our patients, usually in high titres, independent of whether or not the patient is an adult or a child. We always look for the specificity to antigens located on the microfilaments. The target of SMA is believed to be F-actin, and we consider that this specificity is important in order to homogenize the diagnostic criteria. A SMA with reactivity restricted to the vessels and/or to the gastric muscular layers in rodent tissue sections, and with lower titres (< 1/80) is not a marker for the great majority of patients with AIH. The pattern of a broad-spectrum SMA, with the reactivity in the stomach muscular layers, and in vessels, glomeruli and fibrils of the tubular cells of kidney sections, with higher titres (> 1/40) should be required in order to relate SMA with F-Actin[1]. This is the pattern frequently found in the majority of patients with AIH, before commencement their treatment, and with the correspondence of fluorescent microfilaments seen in human fibroblasts[2]. Around 10% of patients with isolated SMA did not exhibit reactivity to anti-microfilaments by way of indirect immunofluorescence in human fibroblasts. Unfortunately, there is no reliable technique to define F-actin specificity using a specific antigen by way of ELISA or blotting techniques.

The antinuclear antibody is the second most frequent antibody, present in approximately 50% of cases with SMA/AAA, and much less commonly in those with anti-LKM1. As an isolated serological marker it was found in 12% of AIH patients. This is a heterogeneous group of patients, usually with clinical manifestations starting as a rheumatological disease. Furthermore the ANA pattern is variable, suggesting different target antigens for this autoantibody. ANA was detected as homogeneous, speckled, nucleolar, centromeric, and with different associations among these patterns, especially the one between homogeneous and speckled.

All 32 patients with type 2 AIH (29 with anti-LKM1, and three with isolated anti-LC1) had negativity for anti-HCV. Using Western blotting 27 exhibited the 50 kDa band, three the 56 kDa, and four the 66 kDa. Two patients exhibited the latter band alone. Anti-LC1 was found also in five patients (17.2%) in association with anti-LKM1, and in one with SMA/AAA. As opposed to anti-LKM1, we have never seen anti-LC1 in patients with chronic hepatitis C. Although it can be identified by indirect immunofluorescence, when not associated with anti-LKM1, in all patients the specificity for 62 kDa human liver antigen, using Western blotting, was defined.

Although an autoantibody reactivity is an important parameter for the diagnosis of AIH, 14 out of 18 patients (77.8%) had a definite diagnosis of this disease in the absence of all the aforementioned antibodies. As we did not have the anti-soluble liver antigen tested, we cannot exclude the presence of this antibody in Brazilian patients.

Antimitochondria antibody is the hallmark of primary biliary cirrhosis. However, in our AIH patients it was detected in seven, including two young patients (6- and 16-year-old girls, at onset). All positive sera positive by immunofluorescence showed a reactivity to M2 antigens, confirmed using commercial pyruvate dehydrogenase and bovine heart antigen by way of Western blotting[3]. Usually the antimitochondria antibody was associated with antimicrofilament (in two cases), and with ANA (in six cases). However, one patient (a girl of 16 years of age) showed only the reactivity for anti-mitochondria antibody, and for statistical analysis she was considered as an AIH patient without any marker. In these patients there was no evidence of cholestasis, either biochemically or histologically, and six patients achieved complete therapeutic response under immunosuppression, with relapse after its suspension.

In two patients in the AIH group without autoantibody markers, antireticulin antibody was identified during the routine of antibody determination, and IgA antiendomysium antibody was further confirmed using human umbilical cord sections. Coeliac disease was then diagnosed by way of intestinal biopsies in these two adult patients without previous diagnosis, and with mild symptoms of flatulence and chronic iron-deficient anaemia. Although antiendomysium antibody was positive in four other patients with type 1 AIH, intestinal biopsy confirmed the diagnosis of gluten-induced enteropathy in half of them. According to these data and a recent publication regarding that association, coeliac disease should be borne in mind as an autoimmune disease associated with AIH, more frequently than we have diagnosed up to the present time[4].

## LIVER BIOPSY

Although liver biopsy should be performed before starting treatment in all patients, it is especially recommended in those patients without the classical forms of AIH (in men, in cases with elevated alkaline phosphatase, with gammaglobulin levels less than twice the upper normal levels, in the presence of antimitochondria antibody, and in the absence of any serological marker). The procedure was performed on 188 patients (82.8%). Structural alterations of lobular liver architecture were present in 55.1% (125 patients), in the first liver biopsy stages 3 and 4[5]. Definite cirrhosis was present in 60% of these patients (75 patients). Certainly these results would be more impressive if the liver biopsy could be performed in the remaining 39 patients, since in 27 patients there were clinical, laboratory, endoscopic or ultrasonographic data suggesting liver cirrhosis.

Even with acute presentation the histological findings are often of chronic liver diseases. Only 15 patients (6.6%) presented a liver biopsy of acute hepatitis, always with bridging or submassive necrosis. In these cases the periportal component was frequently present. At the time of the second liver biopsy, performed for therapeutic control, histological evidence of chronic hepatitis or cirrhosis was always present.

In this study we did not include patients with definite biliary duct damage, and we considered these cases as hybrid forms of AIH, either with primary sclerosing cholangitis or with autoimmune cholangitis, even if they obtained a score on the International Autoimmune Hepatitis Group scale showing of a definite diagnosis.

## HLA ASSOCIATION

Perhaps one of the most interesting findings concerning AIH in South America concerns those related to the disease association with HLA molecules. Susceptibility to AIH has been classically linked to HLA-DRB1*0301 and different DRB1*04 alleles in Europe, North America and Japan. Different HLA antigens were observed, however, in two distinct populations from South America[6,7]. In Brazil and Argentina, predisposition to AIH was primarily associated with HLA-DRB1*1301 and with DRB1*03 alleles in DRB1*1301-negative subjects. Age at onset was different between patients with either DRB1*13 or DRB1*03 antigens, and subjects with DRB1*03 from both countries were significantly older than their DRB1*13-positive counterparts. Interestingly, an association with HLA-DRB1*0405 was also shown in adult patients from Argentina. On the other hand, no increase in the frequency of DRB1*04 alleles was noted in Brazil, where the disease affects mainly children.

The majority of those studies were, however, performed in patients with type 1 AIH. In regard to type 2 AIH in Brazil, no increase in the frequencies of HLA-DR13 or DR4 was observed in 28 patients, and the haplotype DRB1*07/DRB4/DQB1*02 was present in the majority of patients. Furthermore, a secondary association with HLA-DRB1*03, found in most of the patients with AIH-2 from Europe, was also disclosed in DRB1*07-negative subjects. Analysis of relative risks conferred by these antigens suggested that the presence of either DRB1*07 or DRB1*03 was primarily associated with predisposition to this subtype of AIH.

## HYBRID FORMS OF AIH WITH CHOLESTASIS

Besides AIH with antimitochondria antibody, AIH patients can exhibit other features of cholestasis such as those of primary sclerosing cholangitis or autoimmune cholangitis. The clinical, biochemical, histological and radiological features, along with the treatment response in seven patients, are displayed in Table 3. AIH in adult men, in patients with ulcerative colitis, and in patients with high levels of alkaline phosphatase should raise suspicions of the presence of these hybrid forms. In these diagnoses we considered only patients with autoantibody markers of AIH (all had SMA/AAA, with or without ANA), with endoscopic retrograde cholangiography with features of primary sclerosing cholangitis or histological findings of a definite biliary duct injury.

## TREATMENT

The schedules of the treatment used in this study are summarized in Figure 1. Only patients followed up by the authors were included in these statistical analyses. In 177 patients the normalization of biochemical tests was achieved in 108 (61.0%), and in 26 (14.7%) it was associated with histological remission. Only in these 26 cases was drug therapy stopped, and relapse occurred in 20 (76.9%).

## INTERNATIONAL SCORE SYSTEMS

In order to follow the recommendations of the International AIH Group, the score system was always applied in patients with liver diseases which were considered for the diagnosis of AIH (Table 2). Regarding the Brighton consensus[8], 199 patients (87.7%) and 175 (77.1%) had definite AIH before and after the treatment, respectively. If we take into account the new proposition of the

**Table 3** Clinical, biochemical, histological features, diagnostic criteria and therapeutic response of seven adult patients with cholestatic hybrid forms with AIH

| *Features* | *Results* | |
|---|---|---|
| Gender (female/male) | 2/5 | |
| Skin colour | | |
| White/mulatto | 6/1 | |
| Age of onset, median (range) | 29 (16–61) | |
| Clinical Presentation | | |
| Abnormal transaminases | 2 | |
| Chronic hepatopathy | 2 | |
| Cholestasis | 1 | |
| Hepatitis | 1 | |
| Arthritis | 1 | |
| ALT (×NV); mean (range)* | 10.4 (1.5–18.2) | |
| AST (×NV); mean (range) | 10.4 (1.7–17.2) | |
| ALP (×NV); mean (range) | 3.2 (1.3–5.9) | |
| Gammaglobulins (×NV); mean (range) | 2.4 (1.4–4.1) | |
| Total bilirubins (mg%) | 3.6 (0.6–10.8) | |
| Autoantibodies | | |
| SMA–AAA/ANA | 7/6 | |
| Autoimmune diseases | | |
| Vitiligo | 2 | |
| Thyroid disease; ulcerative colitis; rheumatoid arthritis | 1 | |
| Histological findings | | |
| Interface hepatitis | 7 | |
| Bridging necrosis/Lobular component | 1/7 | |
| Lymphoplasmocytic infiltrate/rosettes | 4/2 | |
| Biliary duct injury | 5 | |
| ERCP† | | |
| Abnormal/normal | 4/2 | |
| Not performed | 1 | |
| HLA DRB1*13/DRB1*03/not performed | 6/0/1 | |
| Treatment | | |
| Complete response/partial | 3/4 | |
| Hepatocarcinoma | 1 | |
| *International score systems before and after treatment* | *1992* | *1998* |
| Definite → definite | 4 | 2 |
| Definite → probable | 0 | 0 |
| Probable → definite | 2 | 1 |
| Probable → probable | 1 | 4 |

×NV = Times upper normal value.
ERCP = Endoscopic retrograde cholangiopancreatography.

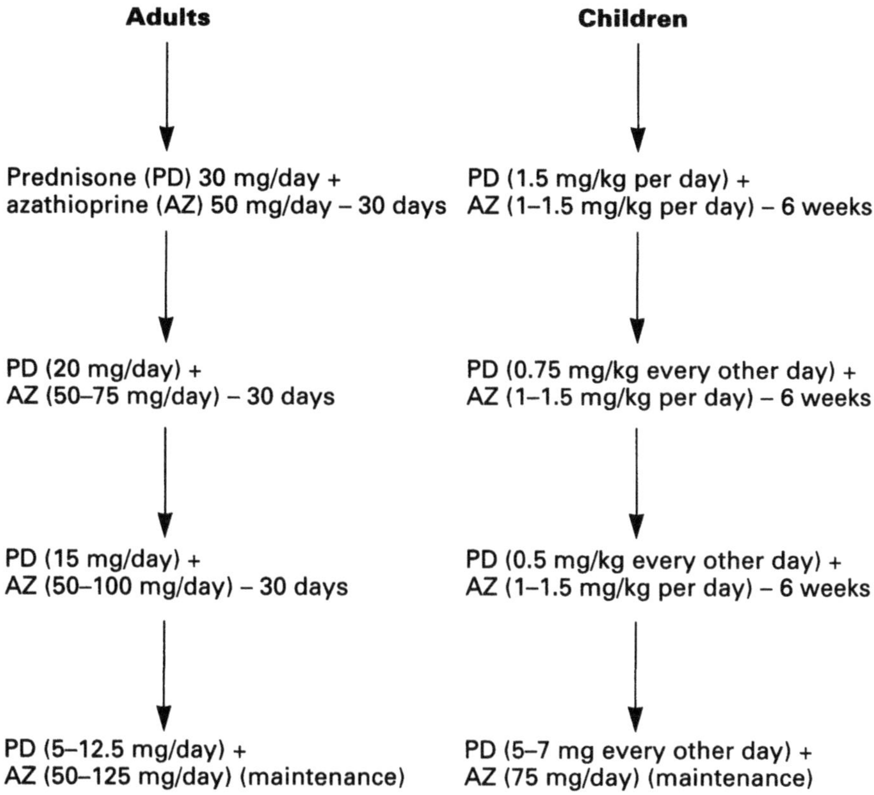


**Fig. 1** Schedules to treat autoimmune hepatitis in adults and children

Chicago Meeting[9], the respective figures would be 203 patients (89.4%) and 183 (80.6%).

We did not consider HLA for the diagnosis of AIH when we used the Brighton score system, because we had not performed class I HLA tests. When we classified our patients according to the Chicago consensus we had to make adjustments for our population. We considered a positive association for AIH-1, the presence of HLA-DR13 or -DR3, and for AIH-2, HLA-DR7 or DR3. Because of the low prevalence of DR4 in our patients its presence was not considered a positive association.

## Acknowledgment

We thank Luiz Caetano da Silva MD, Flair José Carrilho MD, Sérgio Mies MD, Paulo Lisboa Bittencourt MD, Alberto Queiroz Farias MD, Márcio Dias de Almeida MD, Bianca Della Guardia MD, Maíra Solange Câmara dos Santos MD, Marta Deguti MD, Márcia Kallas MD, Eloiza Helena Dias Quintela MD, Jorge Elias Kalil MD, Ana Carla Goldberg PhD, Clarice Pires Abrantes-Lemos BSc, Selma A Palacios BSc and Teresita Montersino, for their contributions to this chapter.

## References


1. Bottazzo GF, Florin-Christensen A, Fairfax A, Swana G, Doniach D, Groeschel-Stewart U. Classification of smooth muscle autoantibodies detected by immunofluorescence. J Clin Pathol. 1976;29:403–10.
2. Cançado ELR, Vilas-Boas LS, Abrantes-Lemos CP *et al.* Heat serum inactivation as a mandatory procedure for antiactin antibody detection in cell culture. Hepatology. 1996;16:1098–104.
3. Farias AQ. Estudo comparativo entre a reação de imunofluorescência indireta, immunoblotting, imunodifusão dupla e Elisa para detecção do anticorpo antimitocôndria. Dissertação de Mestrado, Faculdade de Medicina da Universidade de São Paulo, São Paulo, 1997.
4. Volta U, De Franceschi L, Molinaro N *et al.* Frequency and significance of anti-gliadin and anti-endomysial antibodies in autoimmune hepatitis. Dig Dis Sci. 1998;10:2190–5.
5. Desmet VJ, Gerber N, Hoofnagle JH, Manns M, Scheuer PJ. Classification of chronic hepatitis: diagnosis, grading and staging. Hepatology. 1994;19:1513–20.
6. Faiboim L, Marcos Y, Pando M *et al.* Chronic active autoimmune hepatitis in children. Strong association with a particular HLA-DR6 (DRB1*1301) haplotype. Hum Immunol. 1994;41:146–50.
7. Bittencourt PL, Goldberg AC, Cançado ELR *et al.* HLA-DR genetic susceptibility to autoimmune hepatitis type 2. Am J Gastroenterol. 1999;94:1906–13.
8. Johnson PJ, McFarlane IG. Meeting report: International Autoimmune Hepatitis Group. Hepatology. 1993;18:998–1005.
9. International autoimmune hepatitis group report: review of criteria for diagnosis of autoimmune hepatitis. J Hepatol. 1999;31:929–38.

# 9
# Autoimmune hepatitis in children

F. ALVAREZ

## INTRODUCTION

Autoimmune hepatitis (AIH) is a disease of unknown aetiology, in which a progressive destruction of the hepatic parenchyma occurs. This disease follows a chronic, but fluctuating course. AIH spontaneously progresses towards cirrhosis and liver failure, but often shows a relatively good response to immunosuppressive treatment[1]. It is characterized by a female preponderance, marked hypergammaglobulinaemia, circulating autoantibodies, low levels of complement factor 4 and a high prevalence of HLA B8 and DR3 and DR4 haplotypes[1]. Other autoimmune disorders are frequently found in patients with AIH as well as in first-degree relatives[1–3]. These clinical and laboratory observations led to the hypothesis that AIH is a multifactorial disease. Autoimmune associated disorders are of B and T lymphocyte origin, and other anomalies of the immune system, such as low levels of circulating IgA, are not uncommon. Two types of AIH are currently recognized according to the nature of the autoantibody detected in children at the time of diagnosis. Patients with AIH type 1 display anti-smooth muscle antibodies (SMA) and/or anti-nuclear antibodies (ANA) in their sera. AIH type 2 is characterized by anti-liver kidney microsome (LKM1) and/or anti-liver cytosol type 1 antibodies (LC1)[2,3].

## CLINICAL FEATURES

AIH is primarily a paediatric disease. Although the peak of incidence is in prepubertal females, autoimmune hepatitis has been diagnosed as early as 6 months of age[2–4]. In 40% of patients with AIH type 1 the disease was diagnosed in the paediatric age group; this percentage increases to 80% in the case of AIH type 2. Mean age at onset is around 10 and 6.5 years for AIH types 1 and 2, respectively. In both types the frequency of females being affected is between 70% and 90%, according to published series[2–5].

The most frequent modes of presentation are as an acute hepatitis, or with non-specific symptoms such as fatigue, anorexia and weight loss[2–5]. Rarely, AIH may present as a fulminant or subfulminant hepatitis[3,6–8]. In 10–15% of cases the finding of a hepatomegaly or an unexplained increase of transaminase levels leads to the diagnosis of AIH[2–5]. Less frequently, extrahepatic symptoms or the presence of other autoimmune disease leads to the discovery of an autoimmune process in the liver[2–5]. In a considerable number of patients a long delay exists between the onset of symptoms of the disease and the time of diagnosis. This unfortunately retards the institution of appropriate treatment. In AIH type 2 the presentation of acute liver failure occurs in very young patients, between 13 months and 4 years in those reported[6,7]. In contrast, in AIH type 1 patients, acute liver failure occurs mainly in the post-pubertal age group[8].

Most patients have firm hepatomegaly at diagnosis, and splenomegaly due to portal hypertension is seen in 50%[2,3]. Gastrointestinal bleeding secondary to portal hypertension is a rare event at the onset of the disease, as well as after initiating treatment[2,3]. Jaundice is present at the onset, or an episode of jaundice is recorded in more than 50% of the children[2,3]. Interestingly, only one-third of children have some sign orienting the clinician to the presence of a chronic liver disorder, such as spider naevi, palmar erythema, clubbing or ascites[2–5].

Extrahepatic autoimmune diseases are observed in 20–40% of children with AIH (Table 1)[2–3]. These are sometimes characteristic of a particular type of AIH, as in ulcerative colitis with or without sclerosing cholangitis, arthritis and vasculitis for AIH type 1 patients, and polyendocrinopathy, vitiligo and alopecia in AIH type 2 patients[2–3]. Rarely, AIH type 1 has been associated with an autoimmune enteropathy[9] or fibrosing alveolitis[10], and AIH type 2 to an autoimmune lymphoproliferative syndrome[11]. A history of autoimmune diseases in 20–40% of first-degree relatives might also lead one to a diagnosis of AIH in a child with suspected liver disease[2,3]. The kinds of autoimmune processes observed in the first-degree relatives do not differ from those observed in patients with AIH types 1 and 2. Rarely, AIH has already been diagnosed in another member of the family.

## LABORATORY DATA

The fluctuating course of AIH explains why plasma transaminase levels (ALT and AST) vary between 1.5 and 50 times normal values at the time of diagno-

**Table 1** Extrahepatic autoimmune diseases in children with AIH

| | *Common* | *Rare* |
|---|---|---|
| AIH type 1 (SMA and/or ANA) | Ulcerative colitis, sclerosing cholangitis, vasculitis, arthritis, autoimmune thrombocytopenia | Autoimmune enteropathy, fibrosing alveolitis |
| AIH type 1 and type 2 | Autoimmune haemolytic anaemia, glomerulonephritis, thyroiditis, diabetes | |
| AIH type 2 (LKM1 and/or LC1) | Polyendocrinopathy, vitiligo, alopecia | Autoimmune lymphoproliterative syndrome |

sis[2–5]. Gammaglutamyl transferase (GGT) and alkaline phosphatase (AP) are in general slightly increased. When plasma levels of GGT or AP are over 7–8 or 2–3 times the normal values, respectively, bile duct injury should be suspected and a cholangiography considered.

Assessment of plasma protein level is useful in the diagnosis of AIH and in evaluating liver function. Most patients are hypergammaglobulinaemic, due almost exclusively to markedly increased IgG, ranging between 13 and 73 g/L. The highest levels are observed in patients with AIH type 1[2–5]. Half of the patients display low levels of serum albumin and coagulation factors[2–5].

Determination of serum autoantibodies is of diagnostic value, as well as for follow-up (Table 2). SMA at titres of 1 : 100 to 1 : 500 000 are associated with ANA positivity at titres between 1 : 10 and 1 : 100 000 in 40–60% of patients with AIH type 1[2,3]. SMA are characteristically directed against actin filaments; ANA recognize a diversity of nuclear antigens. Currently, the more frequently used technique for the detection of these autoantibodies is indirect immunofluorescence on cryostat sections and cultured cells. LKM1 is detected in sera from patients with an AIH type 2 at dilutions between 1:10 and 1:100 000[2,3]. This autoantibody is directed against the cytochrome P450 2D6, an endoplasmic reticulum protein expressed mainly in liver and kidney. LC1 is also found in 50% of LKM1-positive sera, and is the only autoantibody present in the sera of 30% of patients with AIH type 2[12]. LC1 autoantibodies recognize a liver-specific enzyme called formiminotransferase cyclodeaminase[13]. In the near future, ELISA techniques for the detection of LKM1 or LC1 using recombinant proteins or synthetic peptides representing linear epitopes will become available. Anti-asialoglycoprotein receptor (ASGP-R) antibodies are thought to play a role in the pathogenesis of AIH. They are directed against a protein exposed to circulating antibodies on the hepatocyte sinusoidal membrane. In children with AIH the titres of anti-ASGP-R correlate with the level of hypergammaglobulinaemia, suggesting that these autoantibodies may be good markers of inflammatory activity. Interestingly, anti-ASGP-R antibodies have been found more frequently in sera from children with AIH type 1 (75% of cases) than in children with AIH type 2 (40% of cases) when tested by an ELISA using purified human liver ASGP-R as the antigen.

## HISTOPATHOLOGICAL FINDINGS

A key factor in the prognosis of AIH is the presence of cirrhosis at the time of diagnosis. The incidence of this complication varies widely from 38% to 89% of reported cases[2,3,14]. An explanation for this discrepancy is the methodology used in the diagnosis of cirrhosis. When only needle liver biopsies are analysed, cir-

**Table 2** Autoantibodies in children with AIH (percentage)

| *AIH type* | *SMA* | *ANA* | *SMA/ANA* | *LKM1* | *LC1* | *LKM1/LC1* |
|---|---|---|---|---|---|---|
| 1 | 90–100 | 0–10 | 40–60 | – | – | – |
| 2 | – | – | – | 40–45 | 20–25 | 35–40 |

rhosis has been observed in 50% of children with AIH. Adding laparoscopic examination to the initial evaluation demonstrates the presence of nodules on the liver surface in 90% of similar patients[14]. The subclinical and fluctuating course of AIH is probably responsible for the development of cirrhosis before symptoms or signs of inflammatory liver disease lead to the diagnosis. The presence of fibrosis at the liver biopsy is reversible in patients with AIH who have a satisfactory response to immunosuppressive treatment[15].

The fluctuating course of the disease is also reflected in the histological analysis of the portal, periportal and lobular inflammatory activity and aggressivity, described as mild or even absent in 10–40% of the patients in various reported series[2,3,5]. In patients with AIH type 2 a decrease of histological aggressiveness is generally observed in older patients[16].

About 10–20% of the liver biopsies obtained prior to initiating treatment reveal the presence of multinucleated giant hepatocytes[3]. In some cases electron microscopy has been carried out to look for viral particles. However, the results have been uniformly negative.

Recently a new type of histological picture has been associated with AIH, characterized by centrilobular necrosis and inflammation that almost completely spare the portal tracts[17,18]. This type of lesion is also compatible with toxic or hypoxaemic liver disease, such that these disorders should be eliminated before starting immunosuppressive treatment. These patients have been successfully treated with corticosteroids and azathioprine.

## TREATMENT

Treatment of AIH relies on immunosuppressive therapy, the favourable effects of which have been well established in large series of treated children. From the onset of the disease the combination of prednisone and azathioprine is the treatment of choice. Prednisone is given orally at a dose of 2 mg/kg per day (not exceeding 60 mg), and azathioprine at a dose of 1.5 to 2 mg/kg per day. Azathioprine as part of the initial treatment allows for a faster decrease of the prednisone dose. A satisfactory initial response seen in more than 80% of cases is evaluated by normalization of transaminase levels within 8–12 weeks from the beginning of the treatment[2,3,16]. Improvement of albumin and coagulation factor levels is also noted within a few weeks[2,3,16]. Nevertheless, in some patients persistence of abnormal transaminase activity despite normalization of plasma protein levels is observed, leading one to suppose that the inflammatory activity is only partially controlled. Most patients who present with fulminant liver failure show a poor response or no response to immunosuppressive treatment[6–8]. In addition, some children in liver failure at the onset of treatment do not recover a normal liver function. One can predict at the onset that between 10% and 20% of children will require a liver transplantation.

Prednisone therapy is usually necessary at high doses for prolonged periods of time. This is often responsible for many potentially serious complications, namely: (a) reduced growth velocity; (b) glucose intolerance; (c) Cushingoid facies and weight gain; (d) generalized osteoporosis; (e) striae; (f) psychiatric problems; (g) hypertension; (h) opportunistic infections; (i) cataracts. These side-effects are associated with elevated morbidity. Recently a pilot study has been conducted to try to avoid these problems. This trial has shown that cyclosporin can induce a biochemical remission of AIH in children with relatively few and well-tolerated side-effects[5]. These results have been obtained administering cyclosporin (Neoral[R]) orally at an initial dose of 4 mg/kg per day, divided into three daily doses. The dose is modified if necessary to maintain a whole blood concentration of the drug around 250 ng/ml for first 3 months, and around 200 ng/ml for the following 3 months. After 6 months of treatment cyclosporin is first overlapped and secondarily replaced by relatively low doses of prednisone and azathioprine. Thirty out of 31 treated children were noted to have normal transaminase levels at the end of the first year of treatment[5]. This protocol, using cyclosporin for a relatively short period of time, aims to avoid the long-term side-effects produced by the administration of this drug, such as renal failure or the development of cancer[5]. The use of cyclosporin should, however, be restricted to those centres with experience in the use of this drug.

Long-term follow-up of AIH shows that few children (10–15%) can completely stop all treatment[2,3]. Most of them relapse when the treatment is discontinued or if the doses of immunosuppressive drugs are diminished. Therefore, 70% of children with AIH receive long-term treatment until reaching adulthood[2,3]. About 15% of cases develop chronic liver failure and are transplanted before the age of 18 years.

In conclusion, the delay in the diagnosis of AIH and the lack of any specific immunosuppressive treatment compromise the outcome. Most patients already have cirrhosis at the time of diagnosis. Almost a third of children with AIH, in addition to those with acute and chronic liver failure, require a liver transplantation in the paediatric age group. Efforts leading to an early diagnosis, the understanding of the mechanisms responsible for the destruction of the liver, as well as the development of new therapies, will improve the quality of life and the survival of patients with immune-mediated disorders of the liver.

## References

1. Johnson PJ, McFarlane IG. Meeting report: International Autoimmune Hepatitis Group. Hepatology. 1993;18:998–1005.
2. Maggiore G, Verber F, Bernard O *et al.* Autoimmune hepatitis associated with anti-actin antibodies in children and adolescents. J Pediatr Gastroenterol Nutr. 1993;17:376–81.
3. Gregorio GV, Portmann B, Reid F *et al.* Autoimmune hepatitis in childhood: a 20-year experience. Hepatology. 1997;25:541–7.
4. Homberg JC, Abuaf N, Bernard O *et al.* Chronic active hepatitis associated with antiliver/kidney microsome antibody type 1: a second type of 'autoimmune' hepatitis. Hepatology. 1987;7:1333–9.
5. Alvarez F, Ciocca M, Cañero-Velasco C *et al.* Short-term cyclosporine induces a remission of autoimmune hepatitis in children. J Hepatol. 1999;30:222–7.
6. Maggiore G, Porta G, Bernard O *et al.* Autoimmune hepatitis with initial presentation as acute hepatic failure in young children. J Pediatr. 1990;116:280–2.
7. Porta G, Gayotto LC, Alvarez F. Anti-liver kidney microsome antibody-positive autoimmune hepatitis presenting as fulminant liver failure. J Pediatr Gastroenterol Nutr. 1990;11:138–40.
8. Herzog D, Rasquin-Weber AM, Debray D, Alvarez F. Subfulminant hepatic failure in autoimmune hepatitis type 1: an unusual form of presentation. Hepatol. 1997;27:578–82.
9. Lachaux A, Bouvier R, Cozzani E *et al.* Familial autoimmune enteropathy with circulating antibullous pemphigoid antibodies and chronic autoimmune hepatitis. J Pediatr. 1994;125:858–62.

10. Paul K, Wille L, Feist D, Kayser K. Fibrosing alveolitis in a 7-year-old girl with autoimmune hemolytic anemia and autoimmune hepatitis. Pneumologie. 1991;45:928–31.
11. Pesenti L, Costanzo A, Ianni A *et al.* Fas/AP01 mutations and autoimmune lymphoproliferative syndrome in a patient with type 2 autoimmune hepatitis. Gastroenterology. 1997;113:1384–9.
12. Martini E, Abuaf N, Cavalli F, Durand V, Johanet C, Homberg JC. Antibody to liver cytosol (anti-LC1) in patients with autoimmune chronic active hepatitis type 2. Hepatology. 1988;8:1662–6.
13. Lapierre P, Hajoui 0, Homberg JC, Alvarez F. Forminotransferase cyclodeaminase is an organ-specific autoantigen recognized by sera of patients with autoimmune hepatitis. Gastroenterology. 1999;116:1–6.
14. Vajro P, Hadchouel P, Hadchouel M, Bernard O, Alagille D. Incidence of cirrhosis in children with chronic hepatitis. J Pediatr. 1990;117:392–6.
15. Dufour JF, DeLellis R, Kaplan MM. Reversibility of hepatic fibrosis in autoimmune hepatitis. Ann Intern Med. 1997;127:981–5.
16. Maggiore G, Porta G, Bernard O *et al.* Autoimmune hepatitis with initial presentation as acute hepatic failure in young children. J Pediatr. 1990;116:280–2.
17. Pratt DS, Fawaz KA, Rabson A, Dellelis R, Kaplan MM. A novel histological lesion in glucocorticoid-responsive chronic hepatitis. Gastroenterology. 1997;113:664–8.
18. Te HS, Koukoulis G, Ganger DR. Autoimmune hepatitis: a histological variant associated with prominent centrilobular necrosis. Gut. 1997;41:269–71.

# 10
# Hepatitis in the polyendocrine syndrome type 1

P. OBERMAYER-STRAUB and M. P. MANNS

## INTRODUCTION

Autoimmune polyendocrine syndrome type 1 (APS1) is an autosomal recessive disorder, which is caused by mutations in a single gene, called autoimmune regulator (*AIRE*)[1,2]. The *AIRE* gene locus is located on the long arm of chromosome 21 and codes for a transcriptional regulator, which is expressed in thymus, lymph nodes, spleen and fetal liver[3]. The *AIRE* gene locus is believed to be involved in the establishment and maintenance of tolerance[3]. Absence of a functional AIRE protein results in a complex syndrome with mucocutaneous candidiasis and autoimmune diseases in a single patient[1,2]. Most patients with APS1 are affected by two to six different autoimmune diseases, most of which affect endocrine glands such as parathyroids, adrenals or ovaries[4]. Ectodermal disease components are found with a high prevalence such as hypoplasia of the dental enamel, nail dystrophy, keratopathy, alopecia and vitiligo[4]. Less frequent, but severe disease components are disease manifestations which affect the gastrointestinal tract, e.g. malabsorption and hepatitis. Malabsorption may interfere with the treatment of other autoimmune diseases and cause malnutrition in severe cases[5]. Hepatitis may be mild. However, repeatedly patients were reported who developed lethal fulminant hepatitis without signs of prewarning[4,6]. Many of the disease manifestations present in APS1 are also known as idiopathic autoimmune diseases. Since autoantibody patterns connected with autoimmune manifestations in APS1 and autoantibodies in idiopathic autoimmune diseases show significant overlap, APS1 may serve as a model to discover the genetic defects and mechanisms involved in the pathogenesis of idiopathic autoimmune diseases[7].

## GENETICS

The *AIRE* gene locus is located on the long arm of chromosome 21[8]. AIRE codes for a protein of 545 amino acids with a calculated isoelectric point of

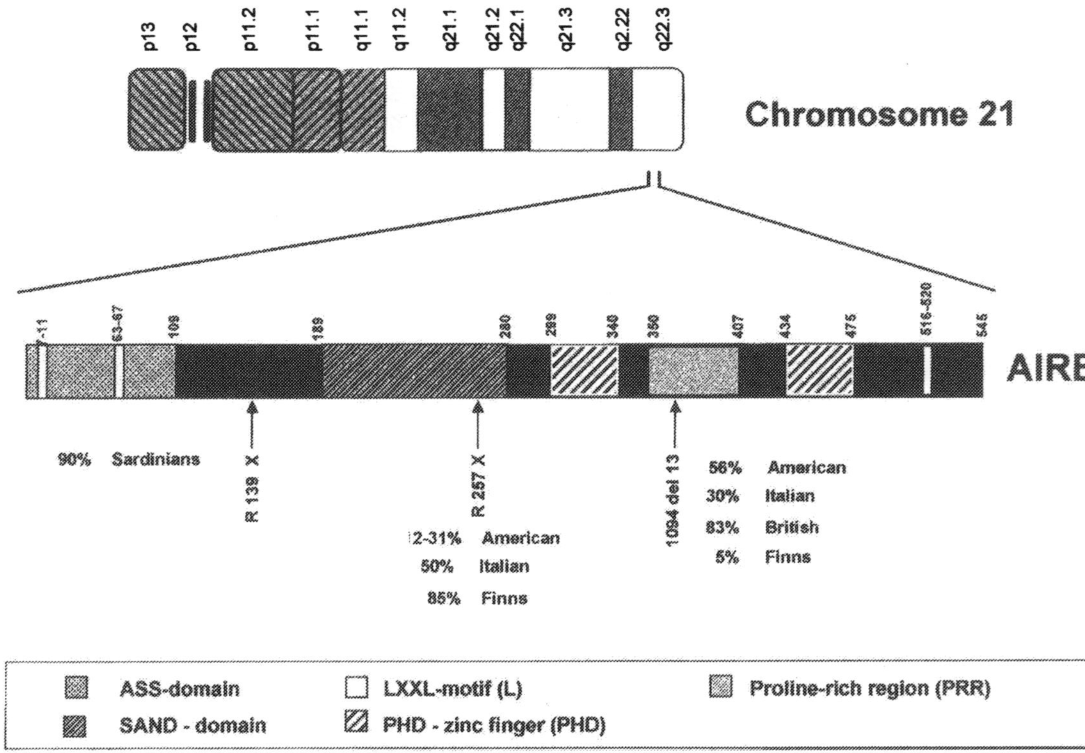


**Fig. 1** Location of *AIRE* gene locus on chromosome 21 and modular composition of the AIRE protein. Position of mutations detected with the highest prevalence in APS1

pH 7[2,8]. The AIRE protein is expressed in dotlike domains of the nucleus, called promyelocytic leukaemia protein nuclear bodies (PML). Several regions of the AIRE protein are homologous with domains typical for transcription factors such as two PHD zinc fingers, a LXXL nuclear binding domain, a nuclear translocalization signal (NLS), a DNA binding domain (SAND) and a proline-rich region (PRR) (Figure 1). The PHD fingers on the AIRE protein are cystein-rich domains, which share strong homology with the PHD finger motifs in nuclear proteins such as Mi-2[9,10] TIF1[11,12] and hKRIP-1[13].

The *AIRE* gene is approximately 12 kb in length and the coding sequence is split into 14 exons [14–16]. It contains several known transcription factor binding sites: binding sites for components essential for the basal transcriptional complex such as AP-4, an inverted CCAAT box and a typical TATA box; 2 binding sites for thymus-specific transcription factors ETS1 and GFI1; and 3 binding sites for transcription factors important in haematopoiesis[15]. In accordance with binding of thymus-specific transcription factors, AIRE expression is observed in rare cells of the thymus medulla, but also in thymic dentritic cells[3]. All AIRE-positive cells express high levels of class II HLA antigens and 20% of them furthermore express co-stimulatory molecules, indicating that they may be actively involved in antigen presentation[3]. As thymic medullary epithelial cells are believed to be involved in clonal deletion of a subset of high-affinity T cells and in induction of anergy in low-affinity subsets, AIRE may play an important role in these processes. Furthermore AIRE expression is detected in cells of the lymph node medulla and in paracortical regions. In lymph nodes 10–20% of AIRE positive cells were also characterized by the CD83 marker, indicating that they belong to the dendritic cell lineage. Similarly AIRE expression was detected in spleen and in fetal liver[2,3].

Multiple mutations in the *AIRE* gene have been described, which cause APS1, if both *AIRE* alleles code for mutated proteins. More than 20 different mutations, which are scattered along the entire coding sequence, are known to date. Populations with predominant single mutations are Finnish people, where a R257X mutation is found in 85% of APS1 patients[17], Sardinian people with a R139X mutation in 90% of APS1 patients[18], and British people with a 13 base-pair deletion at position 1094 present in approximately 80% of APS1 patients (Figure 1)[19]. Most of these mutations were generated by single mutational events. In contrast a broader spectrum of mutations are detected in other European countries and among Americans, and identical mutations were often generated by several mutational events. The 13 base-pair deletion at position 1094 was frequently found in both American and Italian APS1 patients with a prevalence of 56% and 30%, respectively[3,20,21]. Furthermore the major Finnish mutation was also detected with a high prevalence, namely 12–31% of American and 50% of Italian APS1 patients[3,20,21].

Recently the mouse homologue of the human *AIRE* gene was cloned. In the mouse the *AIRE* gene locus is located on a region of chromosome 10, which is homologue to the *AIRE* gene-containing region of the human chromosome 21. The *AIRE* gene is 13 kb in size and the coding sequence is split into 14 exons. The predicted protein has 552 amino acids and shares 71% sequence identity with the human AIRE protein. Structural motifs are similar in both human and murine AIRE proteins. Furthermore the promoters of both genes have conserved sites for several thymus-specific transcription factors and factors important for haematopoiesis [14–16].

## AUTOIMMUNE DISEASE COMPONENTS

### Hypoparathyroidism

Hypoparathyroidism is characterized by deficient parathyroid hormone secretion without an identified cause. Hypoparathyroidism is the most frequent endocrine disease component in APS1 and affects about 80–90% of all APS1 patients (Table 1)[4,22,23]. The incidence of hypoparathyroidism in very young children with APS1 is low; the rate of incidence rises sharply between 3 and 5 years of age[4]. Autoantibodies directed against a protein doublet of 120–140 kDa in parathyroid tissue are detected by Western blots and were identified as a calcium-sensing receptor[24]. The calcium-sensing receptor is involved in the response of parathyroid cells to changes in the concentration of calcium ions[25]. Using immunoprecipitation of *in-vitro* transcribed and translated protein (ITT assay), it could be shown that autoantibodies recognize the extracellular domain of the calcium-sensing receptor and that glycosylation is not necessary for binding[24]. Hypoparathyroidism is also found as idiopathic disease, where autoantibodies directed against the calcium-sensing protein are also detected[24].

### Adrenocortical insufficiency, gonadal failure and infertility

Another frequent endocrine disease component is adrenal failure, which affects more than 70% of APS1 patients[4,22,23]. Adrenal failure in APS1 is diagnosed from 4 to 41 years of age.[4,26]. Three autoantigens were identified in adrenal

**Table 1** Disease components in APS1

| *Disease components* | *Prevalence (%)* | | |
|---|---|---|---|
| | *Neufeld et al.*[23] | *Ahonen et al.*[4] | *Betterle et al.*[22] |
| *Endocrine components* | | | |
| Hypoparathyroidism | 76 | 79 | 93 |
| Adrenal failure | 100 | 72 | 73 |
| Insulin-dependent diabetes mellitus | 47 | 12 | 2 |
| Parietal cell atrophy | 13 | 13 | 15 |
| Autoimmune thyroid disease | 11 | 2 | 10 |
| Gonadal failure | 17 | 50 | 43 |
| *Non-endocrine components* | | | |
| Mucocutaneous candidiasis | 73 | 100 | 83 |
| Alopecia | 32 | 29 | 37 |
| Vitiligo | 8 | 13 | 15 |
| Keratoconjunctivitis | | 35 | 12 |
| Chronic hepatitis | 13 | 12 | 20 |
| Intestinal malabsorption | 22 | 18 | 15 |
| Enamel hypoplasia | | 77 | |
| Nail dystrophy | | 52 | |

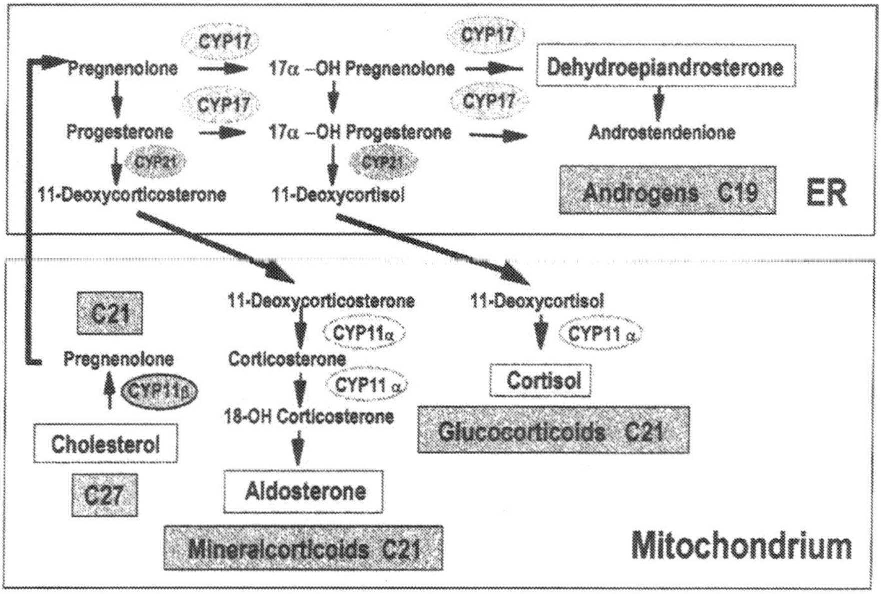


**Fig. 2** Adrenal and gonadal autoantigens in APS1 are involved in steroid biosynthesis. This figure was modified from Nebert and Gonzalez[61]

failure: CYP17, CYP11A1 and CYP21[27–29]. All three autoantigens are enzymes involved in steroid biosynthesis (Figure 2). In idiopathic Addison disease the major autoantigen associated with adrenal failure is CYP21, which is expressed only in adrenals[28]. In APS1, however, anti-CYP17 and/or anti-CYP11A1 autoantibodies are frequently associated[29,30]. Neither CYP17 or CYP11$\beta$ is restricted to adrenal expression; they are also expressed in gonads. Associated with adrenal and gonadal expression of autoantigens in APS1 is a high frequency (60%) of ovarian failure in females, which is not detected in idiopathic Addison disease[31]. It is interesting to note that testicular failure in men is found with a much lower prevalence (14%) than is ovarian failure in females[4]. This difference may indicate that the blood–testis barrier may provide an immunologically privileged zone. To date it is not clear whether these autoantibodies are of pathogenetic relevance; however, they are diagnostic markers and present risk factors for the development of adrenal and/or gonadal failures, when detected in the absence of disease in APS1 patients[26].

Male infertility in APS1 may not only be related to gonadal failure. A case of male infertility in APS1 was reported to be a result of antisperm antibodies. Immunosuppressive therapy was applied, resulting in a quantitative and qualitative improvement in semen parameters and fertility[32].

## Diabetes

Insulin-dependent diabetes mellitus (IDDM) is a chronic autoimmune disease, caused by a gradual destruction of pancreatic $\beta$ cells. A preclinical period characterized by various autoantibodies is followed by tissue infiltration with lymphocytes (insulitis) and destruction of insulin-containing $\beta$ cells by autoreactive T cells[33,34]. Typical autoantibodies associated with idiopathic IDDM are islet cell autoantibodies (ICA), insulin autoantibodies (IAA) and autoantibodies to glutamic acid decarboxylase (GAD65)[35,36]. High levels of GAD65 autoantibodies, especially when associated with ICA, are indicators for an increased risk of developing diabetes both in first-degree relatives of patients with idiopathic IDDM and in the general population[37,38]. In APS1 about 11% of patients develop diabetes[4]. In APS1 patients high levels of GAD65 autoantibodies are often present. Tuomi *et al.*[39] investigated 47 patients from Finland for GAD65 autoantibodies, eight of whom developed diabetes. Interestingly, in 51% of APS1 patients without diabetes, autoantibodies directed against GAD65, GAD67 or islet cells are detected. Of eight diabetic patients six were positive for anti-GAD65, four for ICA and one for anti-GAD67[39]. It is intriguing that in APS1, despite high titres of GAD65, only a few patients progress to diabetes.

Next to GAD65 a second islet cell autoantibody was identified with aromatic L-amino-acid decarboxylase (AADC)[40]. This enzyme catalyses the decarboxylation of aromatic L-amino acids, notably L-3,4-dihydroxyphenylalanine (dopa) and 5-hydroxytryptophane (5-HT)[41]. Both products are intermediates in the synthesis of catecholamine and indolamine neurotransmitters. It is interesting to note that in islet cells two enzymes, AADC and GAD65, are autoantigens, which are both involved in the synthesis of neurotransmitters, namely dopa, serotonin and GABA (Figure 3). This finding clearly underlines the neuron-like function of $\beta$ cells. Besides the products being neurotransmitters derived from amino acids, both enzymes catalyse a decarboxylation reaction and use pyridoxalphosphate as a cofactor. When patients with and without IDDM were analysed for AADC autoantibodies, however, the association of AADC with diabetes was not statistically significant[42]. AADC autoantibodies were detected in 78% of diabetic patients and in 47% of non-diabetic patients[42]. Furthermore AADC was also not found to be an autoantigen in patients with idiopathic diabetes[42]. However, in spite of this lack of correlation with IDDM an important autoantigen with high specificity for APS1 and expression in several organs, e.g. placenta, liver and kidney, was detected[40,42].

## Fat malabsorption

Intestinal dysfunction affects 25–30% of APS1 patients and is characterized by steatorrhoea, watery diarrhoea or constipation. Patients with malabsorption were reported, whose intestinal biopsies showed a seemingly normal architecture of the villi[43]. The pathogenetic mechanisms involved in this disease component remained unclear, until tryptophan hydroxylase was determined as a major autoantigen related to malabsorption[5]. Tryptophan hydroxylase is a tetrameric enzyme, composed of four monomers of 58 kDa, which catalyses the rate-limiting step in serotonin biosynthesis (Figure 3). Tryptophan hydroxylase is expressed in serotonin-producing cells in the central nervous system. However, most importantly this enzyme is also detected in the enterochromaffin cells of the intestinal mucosa and in neuronal cells in the submucosal myenteric plexus. Antibodies directed against tryptophan hydroxylase are detected in 90% of patients with fat malabsorption. Furthermore specific staining of enterochro-

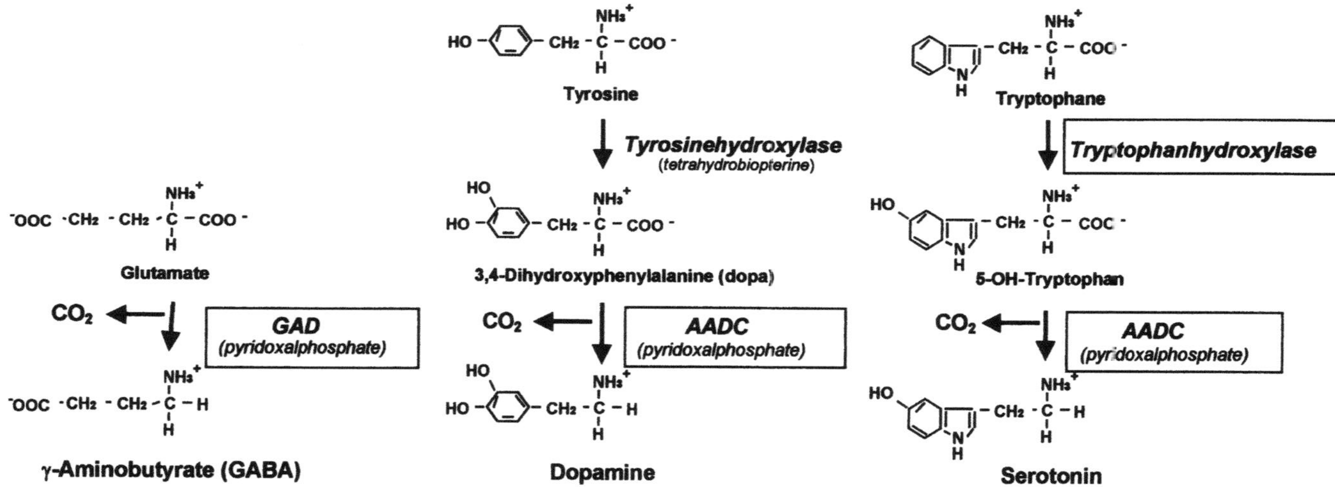


**Fig. 3** Glutamic acid dehydrogenase (GAD65), tryptophan hydroxylase and aromatic L-amino acid decarboxylase are active in the biosynthesis of neurotransmitters

maffin cells in the mucosa from APS1 patients revealed complete absence of enterochromaffin cells from duodenal biopsies[5,44]. In favour of the autoimmune nature of this disease component is a case report in which immunosuppressive therapy using cyclosporin was able to markedly improve fat malabsorption and diarrhoea [44].

## Vitiligo

Vitiligo is a dermal disorder characterized by destruction of melanocytes and loss of pigmentation in several areas of the skin. Vitiligo is frequently associated with endocrine disorders, APS1 and APS2[4,23,45,46]. Vitiligo therefore was early recognized as an autoimmune disease[46]. In accordance with an autoimmune nature of vitiligo, complement-fixing antimelanocyte autoantibodies were demonstrated in sera from vitiligo patients with APS1 or endocrine diseases[47–49]. A patient with APS1 was reported by Betterle *et al.*, who was positive for complement-fixing autoantibodies directed against melanocytes for a period of 6 years before onset of vitiligo[48]. This finding indicates that antimelanocyte antibodies may precede vitiligo and present a risk factor for the progression to vitiligo. In a patient treated with a combination therapy of prednisolone and azathioprine regression of vitiligo was noted after the onset of immunosuppressive treatment[50].

## Hepatitis

Chronic hepatitis is a serious disease component present in 10–18% of patients with APS1[4,51–53], and occasional deaths related to hepatitis are reported to occur in APS1 without prewarning[4,6]. Recently the first hepatic autoantigen in autoimmune hepatitis related to APS1 was identified as CYP 1A2[54]. Anti-CYP 1A2 autoantibodies may be detected by a predominant staining of the perivenous rat hepatocytes and a lack of staining of kidney tissue (Figure 4A). In Western blots with human liver microsomes anti-CYP 1A2 autoantibodies are characterized by a signal at 54 kDa; with human hepatic microsomes a band of 54 kDa is detected[55,56] (Figure 4B). A third characteristic of these autoantibodies is inhibition of CYP 1A2 enzymatic activity (Figure 4C)[56]. Anti-CYP 1A2 autoantibodies are specific for hepatitis in APS1, since none of a total of 60 sera from APS1 patients without hepatitis and none of 300 sera from patients with different liver diseases (AIH types 1–3, primary sclerosing cholangitis, primary biliary cirrhosis or viral hepatitis B, C or D), graft-versus-host disease, autoimmune rheumatic diseases or from healthy controls showed anti-CYP 1A2 autoantibodies. The only disease in which anti-CYP 1A2 autoantibodies were described in addition to APS1 is hepatitis induced by dihydralazine[57]. As only 55% of APS1 patients from Finland were CYP 1A2-positive, despite an excellent specificity of anti-CYP 1A2 autoantibodies for hepatitis in APS1, sensitivity of this autoantibody for the detection of APS1 patients with hepatitis is low.

A second hepatic autoantigen was identified by Rorsman *et al.* with AADC (Figure 3)[40]. AADC is expressed in the cytosol and was originally described as a $\beta$-cell autoantigen[40]. When 68 APS1 patients from Finland were screened for ADC autoantibodies, about 50% expressed anti-AADC autoantibodies. The prevalence of AADC autoantibodies was significantly increased in APS1

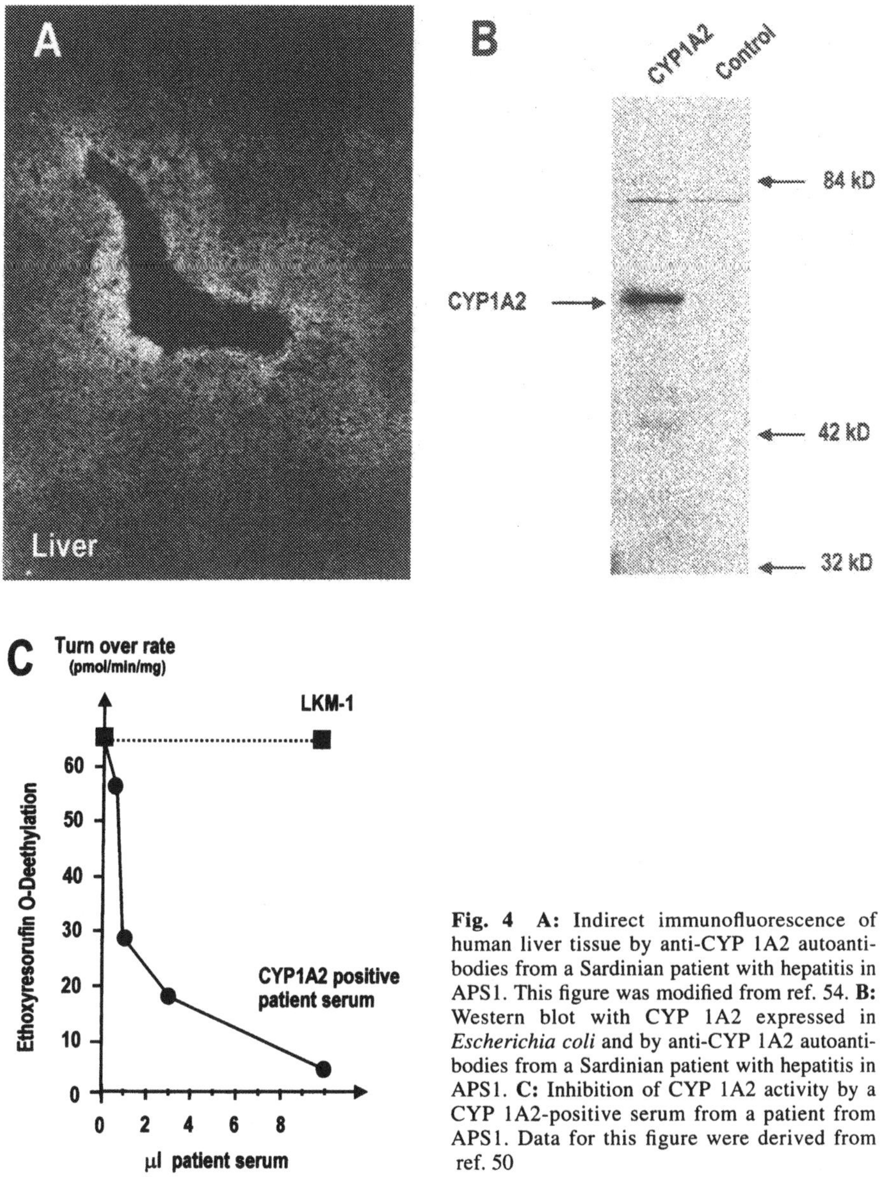


**Fig. 4** **A:** Indirect immunofluorescence of human liver tissue by anti-CYP 1A2 autoantibodies from a Sardinian patient with hepatitis in APS1. This figure was modified from ref. 54. **B:** Western blot with CYP 1A2 expressed in *Escherichia coli* and by anti-CYP 1A2 autoantibodies from a Sardinian patient with hepatitis in APS1. **C:** Inhibition of CYP 1A2 activity by a CYP 1A2-positive serum from a patient from APS1. Data for this figure were derived from ref. 50

patients with vitiligo and autoimmune hepatitis, 88% and 92% of patients were found to express AADC autoantibodies. So far AADC antibodies were reported only in APS1, and further work is needed to establish the role of IDDM in idiopathic autoimmune hepatitis type 2 and in vitiligo[42].

In several patients with APS1 autoantibodies directed against a second hepatic CYP were detected; however, the prevalence of hepatitis was not significantly

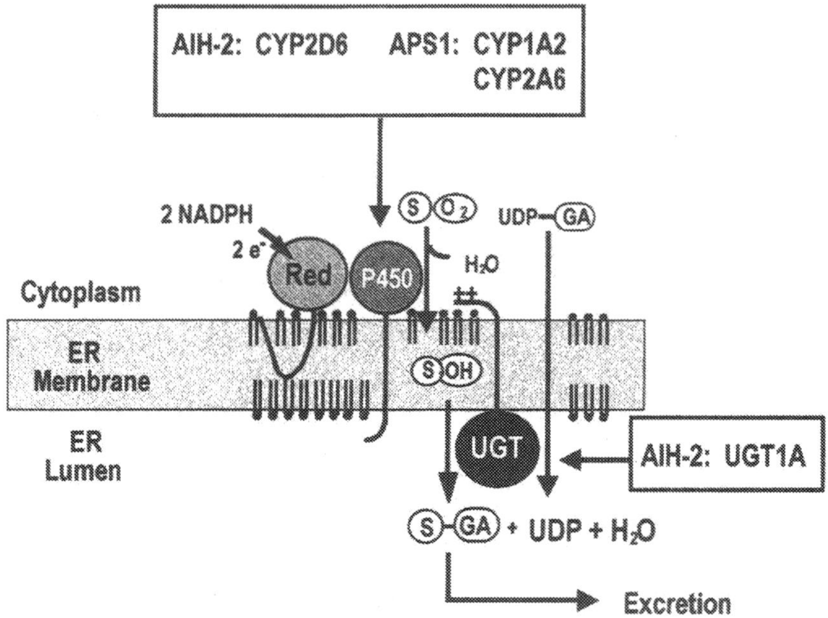


**Fig. 5** Drug-metabolizing enzymes are targets of hepatic autoimmunity in APS1 and in AIH type 2

increased in anti-CYP 2A6-positive patients. This result indicates that anti-CYP 2A6 may be indicators for a yet-unknown disease component in APS1.

Autoimmune hepatitis is also well known as an idiopathic disease. Autoimmune hepatitis type 2 (AIH type 2) shows some similarities to hepatitis in APS1. As seen in APS1 and in AIH type 2, patients are often affected in the paediatric age group. While patients from Finland, Sweden and Sardinia with hepatitis in APS1 produce autoantibodies directed against CYP 1A2, patients affected by AIH-2 are characterized by CYP 2D6 autoantibodies. CYP 2D6 is expressed both in liver and kidney, resulting in a liver–kidney microsomal staining pattern (LKM)[58]. Interestingly, regional differences were noted in the distribution of AIH type 2. While this disease accounts for approximately 10% of AIH patients in Germany and France, LKM-positive patients were not detected at all in Sweden, and were infrequent in the United States[59,60]. Regional differences in factors favouring LKM autoantibody induction, e.g. differences in viral infections and nutrition, may be responsible for different prevalences of AIH type 2. These regional differences may also explain our latest finding, which is anti-CYP 2D6 antibodies in a German patient with APS1 and hepatitis. This patient was characterized by mild hypoparathyroidism, adrenal insufficiency, chronic atopic gastritis (parietal cell antibodies positive), vitiligo, recurring idiopathic pancreatitis and 'autoimmune hepatitis type 2'. Another interesting finding was LKM1-positive hepatitis in the brother of an APS1 patient. Whether mild defects in the *AIRE* gene may also play a role in the pathogenesis of idiopathic autoimmune hepatitis type 2 remains to be established.

## References


1. The Finnish–German APECED Consortium. An autoimmune disease, APECED, caused by mutations in a novel gene featuring two PHD-type zinc finger domains. Nat Genet. 1970;17:399–403.
2. Nagamine K, Peterson P, Scott HS *et al.* Positional cloning of the APECED gene. Nature Genet. 1997;17:393–8.
3. Heino M, Peterson P, Kudoh J *et al.* Autoimmune regulator is expressed in the cells regulating immune tolerance in thymus medulla. Biochem Biophys Res Commun. 1999;257:821–5.
4. Ahonen P, Myllärniemi S, Sipilä I, Perheentupa J. Clinical variation of autoimmune polyendocrinopathy–candidiasis–ectodermal dystrophy (APECED) in a series of 68 patients. N Engl J Med. 1990;322:1829–36.
5. Ekwall O, Hedstrand H, Grimelius L *et al.* Identification of tryptophan hydroxylase as an intestinal autoantigen. Lancet. 1998;352:255–6.
6. Michele TM, Fleckenstein J, Sgrignoli AR, Tuluvath PJ. Chronic active hepatitis in the type I polyglandular autoimmune syndrome. J Postgrad Med. 1994;70:128–31.
7. Obermayer-Straub P, Manns MP. The autoimmune polyglandular syndromes. Baillières Clin Gastroenterol. 1999;12:293–315.
8. Aaltonen J, Börses P, Sandkuijl L, Perheentupa J, and Peltonen L. An autosomal locus causing autoimmune disease: autoimmune polyglandular disease type I assigned to chromosome 21. Nature Genet. 1994;8:83–7.
9. Seelig HP, Moosbrugger I, Fink T, Renz M, Genth E. The major dermatomyositis-specific Mi-2 autoantigen is a presumed helicase involved in transcriptional activation. Arthritis Rheum. 1995;38:1389–99.
10. Ge Q, Nilasena DS, O'Brien CA, Frank MB, Targoff I. Molecular analysis of a major antigenic region of the 240-kD protein of Mi-2 autoantigen. J Clin Invest. 1995;96:1730–7.
11. Le Douarin B, Nielsen AL, Garnier JM *et al.* The N-terminal part of TIF1, a putative mediator of ligand-dependent activation function (AF-2) of nuclear receptors is fused to B-raf in the oncogenic protein T18. EMBO J. 1995;14:2020–33.
12. Thenot S, Henriquet C, Rochefort H, Cavailles V. Differential interaction of nuclear receptors with the putative human transcriptional coactivator hTIF1. J Biol Chem. 1997;272:12062–8.
13. Kim SS, Chen YM, O'Leary E, Witzgall R, Vidal M, Bonventre JV. A novel member of the RING finger family, KRIP-q, associates with the KRAB-A transcriptional repressor domain of zinc finger proteins. Proc Natl Acad Sci USA. 1996;19:15299–304.
14. Blechschmidt K, Schweiger M, Wertz K *et al.* The mouse Aire gene: comparative genomic sequencing, gene organization, and expression. Genome Res. 1999;9:158–66.
15. Mittaz L, Rossier C, Heino M *et al.* Isolation and characterization of the mouse Aire gene. Biochem Biophys Res Commun. 1999;255:483–90.
16. Wang CY, Shi JD, Davoodi-Semiromi A, She X. Cloning of Aire, the mouse homologue of the autoimmune regulator (AIRE) gene responsible for autoimmune polyglandular syndrome type 1 (APS1). Genomics. 1999;55:322–6.
17. Björses P, Aaltonen J, Vikman A *et al.* Genetic homogeneity of autoimmune polyglandular disease type I. Am J Hum Genet. 1996; 59:879–86.
18. Rosatelli MC, Meloni A, Meloni A *et al.* A common mutation in Sardinian autoimmune polyendocrinopathy–candidiasis–ectodermal dystrophy patients. Hum Genet. 1998;103:428–34.
19. Pearce SHS, Cheetman T, Imrie H *et al.* A common and recurrent 13-bp deletion in the autoimmune regulator gene in British kindreds with autoimmune polyendocrinopathy type 1. Am J Hum Genet. 1998;63:1675–84.
20. Wang C-Y, Davoodi-Semiromi A, Connor E, Shi J-D, She J-X. Characterization of mutations in patients with autoimmune polyglandular syndrome type 1 (APS1). Hum Genet. 1998;103:681–5.
21. Scott HS, Heino M, Peterson P *et al.* Common mutations in autoimmune polyendocrinopathy–candidiasis–ectodermal dystrophy patients of different origins. Mol Endocrinol. 1998;12:1112–19.
22. Betterle C, Greggio NA, Volpato M. Autoimmune polyglandular syndrome type 1. J Clin Endocrinol Metab. 1998;83:1049–55.
23. Neufeld, M, Maclaren NK, Blizzard RM. Two types of autoimmune Addison's disease associated with different polyglandular autoimmune (PGA) syndromes. Medicine. 1980;60:355–62.
24. Li Y, Song YH, Rais N *et al.* Autoantibodies to the extracellular domain of the calcium sensing receptor in patients with acquired hypoparathyroidism. J Clin Invest. 1996;97:910–14.

25. Brown EM, Gamba G, Riccardi D *et al.* Cloning and characterization of an extracellular Ca2+-sensing receptor from bovine parathyroid. Nature. 1993; 366:575–80.
26. Ahonen P, Miettinen A, Perheentupa J. Adrenal and steroidal cell antibodies in patients with autoimmune polyglandular disease type I and risk of adrenocortical and ovarian failure. J Clin Endocrinol Metab. 1987;64:494–500.
27. Krohn K, Uibo R, Aavik E, Peterson P, Savilahti K. Identification by molecular cloning of an autoantigen associated with Addison's disease as steroid 17alpha-hydroxylase. Lancet. 1992;339:770–3.
28. Winqvist O, Karlsson FA, Kämpe O. 21-Hydroxylase, a major autoantigen in idiopathic Addison's disease. Lancet. 1992;339:1559–62.
29. Winqvist O, Gustafsson J, Rorsman F, Karlsson F, Kämpe O. Two different cytochrome P450 enzymes are the adrenal antigens in autoimmune polyendocrine syndrome Type 1 and Addison's disease. J Clin Invest. 1994;92:2377–85.
30. Uibo R, Aavik E, Peterson P, Perheentupa J, Aranko S, Pelkonen R, Krohn KJ. Autoantibodies to cytochrome P450 enzymes P450scc, P450c17, and P450c21 in autoimmune polyglandular disease types I and II and in isolated Addison's disease. J Clin Endocrinol Metab. 1994;78:323–8.
31. Winqvist O, Gebre-Mehedin G, Gustafsson J *et al.* Identification of the main gonadal autoantigens in patients with adrenal insufficiency and associated ovarian failure. J Clin Endocrinol Metab. 1995;80:1717–23.
32. Tsatsoulis A, Shalet SM. Antisperm antibodies in the polyglandular autoimmune (PGA) syndrome type I: response to cyclical steroid therapy. Clin Endocrinol Oxf. 1991;35:299–303.
33. Gorsuch AN, Spencer KM, Lister J *et al.* Evidence for a long prediabetic period in type I (insulin-dependent) diabetes mellitus. *Lancet.* 1981;2:1363–5.
34. Rossini AA, Greiner DL, Friedman HP, Mordes JP. Immunopathogenesis of diabetes mellitus. Diabetes Rev. 1993;1:43–75.
35. Baekkeskov S, Aanstoot HJ, Christgau S *et al.* Identification of the 64K autoantigen in insulin-dependent diabetes mellitus as the GABA-synthesizing enzyme glutamic acid decarboxylase. Nature. 1990;347:151–6.
36. Palmer JP. Insulin autoantibodies: their role in the pathogenesis of IDDM. Diabetes Metab. Rev. 1987;3:1005–15.
37. Bruining GJ, Molenaar JL, Grobbee DE *et al.* Ten-year follow-up study of islet-cell antibodies and childhood diabetes mellitus. Lancet. 1989;1:1100–3.
38. Greenbaum CJ, Brooks-Worrell BM, Palmer JP, Lermark A. Autoimmunity and prediction of insulin-dependent diabetes mellitus. In: Marshall H, Home PD, editors. The Diabetes Annual, vol. 8. Amsterdam: Elsevier; 1994: 21–52.
39. Tuomi T, Bjorses P, Falorni A *et al.* Antibodies to glutamic acid decarboxylase and insulin-dependent diabetes in patients with autoimmune polyendocrine syndrome type I. J Clin Endocrinol Metab. 1996;81:1488–94.
40. Rorsman F, Husebye ES, Winquist O, Björk E, Karlsson FA, Kämpe O. Aromatic L-aminoacid decarboxylase, a pyridoxal phosphate-dependent enzyme, is a beta-cell autoantigen. Proc Natl Acad Sci USA. 1995;92:8626–9.
41. Christenson JG, Dairman W, Udenfried S. On the identity of DOPA decarboxylase and 5-hydroxytryptophan decarboxylase (immunological titration-aromatic l-aminoacid decarboxylase–serotonin–dopamine–norepinephrine). Proc Natl Acad Sci USA. 1972;69:343–7.
42. Husebye ES, Gebre-Mehedin G, Tuomi T *et al.* Autoantibodies against aromatic-L-amino acid decarboxylase in autoimmune polyendocrine syndrome type 1. J Clin Endocrinol Metab. 1997;82:147–50.
43. Bereket A, Lowenheim M, Blethen SL, Kane P, Wilson TA. Intestinal lymphangiectasia in a patient with autoimmune polyglandular disease type I and steatorrhea. J Clin Endocrinol Metab. 1994;80:933–5.
44. Ward L, Paquette J, Seidman E *et al.* Severe autoimmune polyendocrinopathy–candidiasis ectodermal dystrophy in an adolescent girl with a novel AIRE mutation: response to immunosuppressive therapy. J Clin Endocrinol Metab. 1999;84:844–51.
45. McGregor BC, Katz HI, Doe RP. Vitiligo and multiple glandular insufficiencies. J Am Med Assos. 1972;219:724–5.
46. Bronstoff J. Autoantibodies in patients with vitiligo. Lancet. 1969;2:177–8.
47. Betterle CA, Pesserico A, Bersani G. Vitiligo and autoimmune polyendocrine deficiencies with autoantibodies to melanin-producing cells. Arch. Dermatol. 1979;115:364.

48. Betterle C, Caretto A, Pedini B, Rigon F, Bertoli P, Peserico A. Complement-fixing activity to melanin-producing cells preceding the onset of vitiligo in a patient with type 1 polyglandular failure [letter]. Arch Dermatol. 1992;128:123–4.
49. Hertz KL, Gazze C, Kirkpattrick C, Katz S. Autoimmune vitiligo. N Engl J Med. 1977;297:634–7.
50. Sacher M, Blümel P, Thaler H, Manns M. Chronic active hepatitis associated with vitiligo, nail dystrophy, alopecia and a new variant of LKM antibodies. J Hepatol. 1990;10:364–9.
51. Neufeld M, Maclaren N, Blizzard R. Autoimmune polyglandular syndromes. Pediatr Ann. 1980;9:154–62.
52. Perheentupa J. Autoimmune polyendocrinopathy–candidiasis–ectodermal dystrophy (APECED). Hormone Metab Res. 1996;28:353–6.
53. Riley WJ. Autoimmune polyglandular syndromes. Hormone Res. 1992;38(Suppl. 2):9–15.
54. Clemente MG, Obermayer-Straub P, Meloni A *et al.* Cytochrome P450 1A2 is a hepatic autoantigen in autoimmune polyglandular syndrome type 1. J Clin Endocrinol Metab. 1997;82:1353–61.
55. Clemente MG, Obermayer-Straub P, Meloni A *et al.* Cytochrome P450 1A2 as the hepatocellular autoantigen in autoimmune polyendocrine syndrome type 1. J Hepatol. 1995;23(Suppl.1):126.
56. Manns MP, Griffin KJ, Quattrochi L *et al.* Identification of cytochrome P450 IA2 as a human autoantigen. Arch Biochem Biophys. 1990;280:229–32.
57. Bourdi M, Larrey D, Nataf J, Bernuau J *et al.* Anti-liver endoplasmic reticulum antibodies are directed against human cytochrome P-450IA2. A specific marker of dihydralazine hepatitis. .J Clin Invest. 1990;85:1967–73.
58. Homberg JC, Abuaf N, Bernard O *et al.* Chronic active hepatitis associated with antiliver/kidney microsome type 1: a second type of 'autoimmune' hepatitis. Hepatology. 1987;7:1333–9.
59. Lindgren S, Braun HB, Michel G *et al.* Absence of LKM-1 antibody reactivity in autoimmune and hepatitis-C-related chronic liver disease in Sweden. Swedish Internal Medicine Liver Club. Scand J Gastroenterol. 1997;32:175–8.
60. Czaja AJ, Manns MP, Homburger HA. Frequency and significance of antibodies to liver/kidney microsome type 1 in adults with chronic active hepatitis. Gastroenterology. 1992;103:1290–5.
61. Nebert DW, Gonzalez FJ. Cytochrome P450 genes, structure, evolution and regulation. Annu Rev Biochem. 1987;56:945–93.

# Section III
# Pathogenesis of autoimmune liver diseases

# 11
# Genetics of autoimmune liver disease

P. T. DONALDSON

## INTRODUCTION

The dramatic variability in disease expression within populations is a clear indication of genes at work. Whilst our knowledge of single gene disorders is almost complete we are only just beginning to understand the genetics of complex diseases. Both autoimmune and viral diseases are subject to genetic influences. It has been suggested that up to half of the risk of autoimmunity may be genetically determined. These genetic associations reflect a staggering degree of genetic polymorphism within the human population and may be viewed in simple Darwinian terms. Genetic variability which increases resistance to viral disease has implications for survival of the species and increased susceptibility to autoimmune disease may be the price which we pay for this advantage.[1]

The genes which are associated with viral and autoimmune liver disease do not themselves cause these diseases, they are simply part of a multifactorial jigsaw and should be considered as risk factors with a potential to increase (i.e. susceptibility genes) or lower (i.e. resistance genes) the risk of disease. Genes may also determine disease expression through accelerated progression or severity of symptoms. It must be remembered that these genes are often present in a large number of non-affected individuals and that most are not defective under normal circumstances.

The greatest progress in understanding the genetics of complex disease has come from the field of immunogenetics, especially from studies of the HLA genes. The HLA system, encoded on chromosome 6p21.3, may be the most polymorphic genetic system in the human genome and is certainly the most studied. In this chapter I shall concentrate mostly on the relationship between HLA and the three autoimmune liver diseases, type 1 autoimmune hepatitis (AIH), primary sclerosing cholangitis (PSC) and primary biliary cirrhosis (PBC). However, as this subject has been reviewed elsewhere I shall restrict the discourse to the necessary background only, and limit the discussion to recent developments. Finally, in keeping with the new millennium, I shall briefly outline some exciting new areas for research, most of which lie outside the HLA region.

## GENETIC ORGANIZATION OF THE HLA REGION

The genetic structure and organization of the HLA region is reviewed extensively in the general literature, therefore I will endeavour to be brief and describe only those genes which are relevant to this chapter. The human MHC spans approximately 4 million base-pairs of DNA of chromosome 6p21.3.[2] By convention the region is divided into three subregions, reflecting a degree of functional and structural similarity of their gene products: HLA class I and class II at the opposite ends of the region and class III in the middle. An abridged gene map is given in Figure 1. The WHO nomenclature for HLA alleles is constantly reviewed and updated, and appears in a number of different journals including *Tissue Antigens, European Journal of Immunogenetics and Human Immunology* and also on the worldwide web. Currently there are over 456 class I (A, B and Cw) alleles and more than 400 (DRB, DQA DQB and DPB) alleles. Since this list would fill several pages I have chosen to list only the nomenclature of those HLA determinants referred to in the text of this chapter herein (Table 1) and advise the reader to seek the full and current nomenclature elsewhere.

## HLA class I genetics, structure and function

There are presently more than 100 genes or gene sequences mapped to the HLA class I region. We are concerned with only three: the classical HLA antigens, A, B and Cw. The HLA A, B and C genes are highly polymorphic with 124 recognized alleles of HLA-A, 258 of HLA-B and 74 of HLA-C.[3] Each gene encodes a single polypeptide $\alpha$-chain of 45 kDa which forms a non-covalent bond with a 12 kDa $\beta$2-microglobulin molecule (the $\beta$-chain, encoded on chromosome 15) and is expressed on all nucleated cells. The expressed HLA class I molecules form an $\alpha/\beta$ heterodimer spanning the plasma membrane with four extracellular domains, three from the $\alpha$-chain ($\alpha$1, $\alpha$2, and $\alpha$3) with $\beta$2-microglobulin providing the fourth ($\beta$1). The two domains closest to the cell membrane, namely $\alpha$3 and $\beta$1, form a supporting platform on top of which the remaining two domains ($\alpha$1 and $\alpha$2) are folded into a complex structure composed of criss-crossed $\beta$-pleated sheets surmounted by opposing $\alpha$-helices resulting in an enclosed groove 25 Å long, 10 Å wide and 11 Å deep.[4,5] This groove or cleft is the site at which antigenic peptides are bound for presentation to the T cell antigen receptor (TCR). Class I molecules present antigenic peptides derived from within the cell cytoplasm (endogenous antigens) to CD8-positive T cells. This interaction is favoured by the presence of a CD8 binding site on the $\alpha$3 domain of the class I molecule.

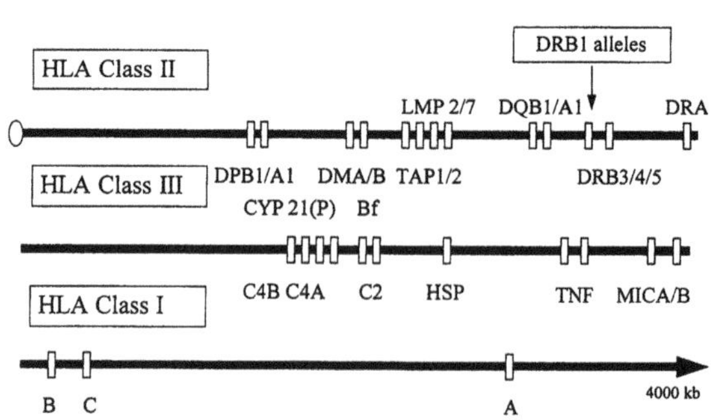


**Fig. 1** Human MHC (HLA region) chromosome 6p21.3

**Table 1** The past and present nomenclature for HLA antigens and genotypes used in this chapter

| | Serological Determinant | |
|---|---|---|
| *Old name* | *Current name* | *Allele* |
| HL-A1 | A1 | *A*0101, A*0104* |
| HL-A8 | B8 | *B*0801, B*0806* |
| | Cw7 | *C*0701* to *C*0712* |
| Dw2/Dw12[a] | DR2 | *DRB1*15011* to *DRB1*1508* |
| Dw3[a] | DR3[b] | *DRB1*03011* to *DRB1*0313* |
| Dw4,10,13,14,15 | DR4 | *DRB1*04011* to *DRB1*04012* |
| DRw6 | DR13 | *DRB1*1301* to *DRB1*1334* |
| DRw8 | DR8 | *DRB1*0801* to *DRB1*0821* |
| DRw52a/Dw24 | DR52 | *DRB3*0101* to *DRB3*0105* |
| Dw3/Dw7 | DQ2 | *DQB1*0201* to *DQB1*0203* |
| DQ3/Dw4,5,8,13 | DQ7 | *DQB1*03011, DQB1*03012, DQB1*0304* |
| DQ3/Dw4,10,13,14 | DQ8 | *DQB1*0302, DQB1*0305* |
| DQ4/Dw8,15 | DQ4 | *DQB1*0401 and DQB1*0402* |

[a]Specificities determined by mixed lymphocyte reaction (MLR).
[b]The common split of DR3 was called DRw17 later DR17 this term was not widely used before it was replaced by *DRB1*0301*. Current nomenclature is based on DNA sequencing data and is reviewed in ref. 3. In the current WHO nomenclature the first four letters represent the HLA locus, i.e. *DRB1*, *DQA1*, etc., and the first two numbers following the asterisk give the broad allelic group and are equivalent to the serologically defined antigen, thus *DRB1*03* = DR3. The last two numbers represent the specific allele and are based on DNA sequencing data. An additional number may be given to represent allelic variants which are usually silent changes or intron polymorphisms.

## HLA class II genetics, structure and function

The HLA class II region encodes more than 30 genes of which we are concerned with four: HLA *DRB*, *DQA*, *DQB* and *DPB*. However, several of the other genes encoded in this region are worthy of note, especially the genes encoding the intracellular proteins TAP (*TAP1* and *TAP2*), LMP (*LMP2* and *LMP*), and DM (*DMA* and *DMB*). The TAP and LMP proteins are required for antigen presentation by class I molecules and are important both in the production of antigenic peptide fragments and peptide transport within the cell, whereas DM is required for the transport of peptides associated with class II molecules.

The genetic arrangement of the HLA class II genes is more complex than that of HLA the class I region. In contrast to HLA class I, both the $\alpha$ and $\beta$ polypeptides of the HLA class II molecules are encoded on chromosome 6. The DR subregion has a single non-polymorphic *DRA* gene which encodes a 32 kDa $\alpha$-chain and nine *DRB* genes, five of which (*DRB2, DRB6, DRB7, DRB8, DRB9*) are not expressed (i.e. pseudogenes). The remaining four (*DRB1, DRB3, DRB4, DRB5*), each of which encodes a different 28 kDa $\beta$-chain, are all expressed. The number of *DRB* genes that an individual may possess depends on the parental haplotypes. In contrast to HLA DR each of the DQ and DP subregions encodes a single pair of functional A genes and B genes, both of which have extensive polymorphism. Presently there are more than 263 *DRB* alleles, 19 alleles of *DQA*, 39 alleles of *DQB*, 15 alleles of *DPA* and 84 alleles of *DPB*.[3]

HLA DR, DQ and DP molecules are expressed on specialized antigen-presenting cells, B cells, monocytes, tissue macrophages, dendritic cells and also to some extent on endothelial and bile-duct epithelial cells, but rarely if at all on hepatocytes. HLA class II molecules are expressed as $\alpha/\beta$ heterodimers with four extracellular domains ($\alpha$1, $\alpha$2, $\beta$1, and $\beta$2). X-ray crystallography reveals a similar antigen-binding groove to that of the class I molecules,[6]; however, whilst the HLA class I peptide-binding groove has closed ends favouring the binding of peptides of eight or nine amino acid residues, the class II groove is an open-ended structure allowing the linear binding peptides of up to 24 amino acid residues. Peptide binding to both class I and class II HLA molecules is further enhanced by specialized binding pockets at particular positions.[7,8]

Class II molecules present antigenic peptides which enter the cell through endocytosis and undergo proteolytic cleavage in acidic endosomes before binding newly synthesized class II antigens. Presentation of class II–peptide complexes to the TCR is enhanced by the presence of a CD4 binding site on the $\alpha$2 domain of the HLA class II molecule.

### HLA class III genetic structure and function

The HLA class III region encodes more than 70 genes amongst which there are a diverse array of genes encoding immunologically active proteins including: the complement proteins C2, C4 (A and B), factor B, tumour necrosis factor-$\alpha$ (TNF-$\alpha$) and lymphotoxin-$\alpha$ and $\beta$ (LT-$\alpha$ and LT-$\beta$), heat shock proteins (HSP-70, HSP-71, HSP-72) as well as a number of enzymes and pseudogenes. Of particular interest at present are two additional 'class I like' genes, *MIC A* and *B*, which map to between *HLA B* and *TNF*. There is strong evidence to suggest close associations between particular *MICA* alleles and both Behçet's disease and PSC. These genes are expressed on gut epithelium and control K (killer) and NK (natural killer) cell activity. In this chapter we are concerned with the class III complement genes, *TNF* and also *MICA*.

The complement proteins C2 and C4 are classical complement pathway polypeptides required for the conversion of C3 to C3d (C3 convertase) and C5 to C5d (C5 convertase). Factor B (Bf) has a similar catalytic function combining with C3b to form a C3 convertase in the alternative complement pathway (Figure 2). There are two isotypes of C4, C4A and C4B, which may have differing affinities for amino and carboxyl groups. The genes for *C2*, *C4A*, *C4B* and *Bf* are all polymorphic. Abnormal complement function has been demonstrated in chronic liver disease, though whether this is secondary to liver damage is uncertain. Individuals with null or non-expressed complement genes (either deleted or otherwise) are more likely to develop lupus-like illness and homozygous *C2* and *C4* nulls can lead to complement deficiencies and may be lethal.

## APPROACHES TO IDENTIFYING DISEASE GENES

Though most of this chapter is dedicated to describing the results of HLA–disease association studies, these studies are only part of a much larger

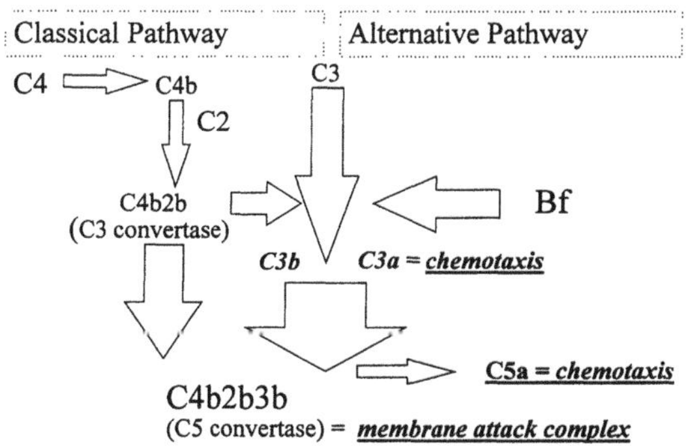


**Fig. 2** Functional relationships of the HLA class III region encoded complement proteins

undertaking to identify the genetic contribution to complex disease. Two different approaches may be used: (1) whole genome scanning, (2) candidate gene searches.

Whole genome scanning is useful in identifying large areas of the genome which may be involved in disease genesis, but does not focus on specific genes; nor does it allow insight into the relationship between the gene and the disease. Whole genome scanning studies with microsatellites have been used to determine which chromosomal locations are linked with diabetes and inflammatory bowel disease, but have not been applied in liver disease. Candidate gene searches are more focused, hypothesis-driven studies and may be based on families, limited sibships or populations. Two different types of studies are possible: linkage analysis which requires families or limited sibships, and association studies (case–control) which are based on groups of unrelated patients.

The major problem for investigators working on autoimmune liver disease is the relative rarity of families. Even transmission disequilibrium testing (TDT), which is a method enabling investigators to perform linkage studies on simplex (single cases), is difficult because of the requirement for DNA from parents. Since most of our subjects develop disease later in life it is often difficult or impossible to recruit parents to these studies, so the case–control (association) study has been the preferred method for most investigators of autoimmune liver disease. Candidate genes are shortlisted based on our knowledge of the disease, genetic polymorphisms are analysed and then the distribution/frequency of the different alleles compared with those of an appropriate, racially matched, control group. The quality of the results obtained is heavily dependent on absolute numbers. The greater the number tested the more powerful the statistical analysis and the greater the chance that any genetic association(s) described are true.

## INTERPRETATION OF HLA–DISEASE ASSOCIATION STUDIES

Early investigators of HLA and disease sought ever stronger genetic associations, but it was clear from the beginning that most of the diseases under investigation were not HLA-linked single gene disorders. Notable exceptions were hereditary haemochromatosis[9,10] and congenital adrenal hyperplasia due to 21-hydroxylase deficiency[11]. Few authors today would expect to find genes on the short arm of chromosome 6 whose inheritance leads directly to a disease state. Considering the number and variety of diseases with documented HLA associations it would be extraordinary if they all mapped to 621.3. These genetic associations are in most instances only part of a more complex multifactorial/ polygenic jigsaw[12].

As a result of the X-ray crystallography data (referred to above) and subsequent developments in immunological theory there has been a radical change in our perspective on HLA–disease associations. The key to understanding the significance of HLA polymorphism in terms of disease susceptibility and resistance lies in the observation that the majority of genetic variation between alleles is concentrated within three so-called hypervariable regions (HVR) within the second exon of the *DRB* gene. This part of the gene encodes amino acids at positions 9–14 (HVR1), 26–33 (HVR2) and 67–74 (HVR3) of the DR$\beta$-polypeptide which are located in the floor (HVR1 and HVR2) and on the $\alpha$-helix (HVR3) of the antigen-binding groove. Consequently most of the allelic variability results in amino acid substitutions in and around the antigen-binding groove. Substitution of one amino acid for another within this region may result in conformational changes which alter the antigen-binding characteristics of the molecule and also modify the interaction with the TCR resulting in HLA molecules with different peptide presenting characteristics.

Before we progress there are three other aspects of immunogenetics that require some explanation; these are the racial variation in gene distribution which is central to understanding the differences between studies, the statistical analysis which is applied to HLA studies and the phenomenon of linkage disequilibrium.

## Racial variation

In practice immunogenetic studies involve the comparison of gene frequencies between populations, i.e. population genetics. By comparing the frequencies of various polymorphic genes, either between one group of patients and another, or more commonly between patients and healthy controls, it is possible to identify alleles which may determine susceptibility or resistance to that disease. Alleles which are more common in the disease group are considered to be disease-susceptibility alleles, whilst those which are less common in the disease are considered to confer resistance to disease. The data derived from these studies may also be used to give information about disease severity and prognosis. As these genes are highly polymorphic it is essential that we compare like with like; thus controls should be drawn from the same racial group as the patients. There are marked differences in the distribution of HLA alleles between populations. These differences can be quite severe, e.g. the most common HLA haplotype in Britain and northern Europe (*A1-B8-DR3*) is almost absent in Japan. This is not unexpected between two such diverse racial groups. However, even within the same racial group there are often significant variations in allele frequencies with geography, e.g. the DR4 antigen is found in 25% of the French population and 40% of Britons. As a result there may be variation in the strength of genetic associations between populations. In addition different genes may be associated with the same disease in different populations. Frequently associations described reflect the gene distribution in the founder population: 'founder effect'. Thus in type 1 AIH the different *DR4* alleles associated with the disease are simply the most common *DR4* alleles in those populations; for example, *DRB1*0401* in Britain and *DRB1*0405* in Japan.

## Statistical analysis

HLA data are non-parametric and the chi-squared test and Fisher's exact probability test are the most commonly applied tests. Studies usually involve multiple comparisons, therefore probability values (*p*) must be corrected by multiplying *p* by the total number of antigen/alleles tested (*pc*) (i.e. Bonferroni's correction). The only exception to this rule is when there is an *a-priori* hypothesis, however, even in these circumstances correction for the number of alleles identified in the *a priori* hypothesis should be applied. In practice correction is rarely performed when data are being confirmed. Comparison at 'the phenotype level' (i.e. antigen frequencies or equivalent) is preferable to comparison of gene frequencies. The latter practice will increase the statistical power of the analysis without an increase in the total numbers studied, and may lead to type II statistical errors.

HLA association studies often quote a value referred to as relative risk (RR), which gives a crude means of comparing data from different studies. The value quoted in most cases is calculated from the cross-products ratio of the two-by-two contingency table used in chi-squared and Fisher's exact test, and is not the true relative risk. It is a rather crude approximation of the relative risk and should be more correctly referred to as the odds ratio (OR).

It is now becoming common to see studies in which secondary associations have been sought. Secondary associations are identified by reanalysing the distribution of the HLA alleles after correcting the data for those with the first identified susceptibility/resistance allele (primary association). This practice allows the investigator to identify associations which may be hidden by a strong positive or negative primary association.

Recent editorials in *Nature Genetics*[13] and the *Lancet*[14] suggest that candidate associations should be reproduced in a second patient group before being published. Replicate studies are an excellent idea; however, one of the two editorials above also emphasized the importance of large odds ratios and small probability values, suggesting that studies with *p* values close to 5% will be less favourably received whilst the other suggested that odds ratios as low as 1.4 may be important in disease and that *p* values are not absolute indicators of a study's worth.[14]

## Linkage disequilibrium

Linkage disequilibrium describes the non-random association of two genes encoded at different loci, i.e. when two or more HLA antigens/alleles occur together more often than predicted from the individual antigen/allele frequencies. The best example of linkage disequilibrium is the HLA *A1-B8-DR3* haplotype, which is present in 12–16% of northern European populations but would occur in less than 1–2% of the population if these alleles were independently assorted. The physical basis of this phenomenon is that two or more genes pass from generation to generation *en bloc* (i.e. as a discrete unit or haplotype) preventing equilibrium, and may result from strong selection effects.

## TYPE 1 AUTOIMMUNE HEPATITIS

Though there are a number of well-characterized subtypes of autoimmune hepatitis based on autoantibody profiles there is insufficient immunogenetic data to review all but type 1 AIH herein. The precise aetiology of type 1 autoimmune hepatitis (AIH) is unknown. The high female to male ratio and the now well-described HLA associations are clear evidence of a strong genetic component to this disease. However, the HLA associations described differ according to the populations studied.

In *northern European Caucasoid* patients early studies suggested that there is a strong genetic association with the HLA A1, B8 and Dw3 antigens (later called DR3)[15,16]. Subsequent investigations suggested that these three genes may be inherited as a single unit or haplotype, and that there may be a second association with DR4.[17,18] These two different HLA associations (A1-B8-DR3 and DR4) appeared to mark independent risk factors for AIH since those with *DR4* were mostly the older-onset patients with less severe disease. The 'dual association', A1-B8-DR3 and DR4, accounted for only 90% of patients studied and, in keeping with the philosophy of the time, it was suggested that the 'true' susceptibility allele may be a gene which lies close to DR3 and DR4, but that susceptibility is unlikely to be encoded by these genes themselves. However, further studies using DNA-based genotyping in these patients have failed to identify stronger associations in close proximity to the *DRB1* locus. None of the HLA class II *DQA1, DQB1* and *DPB1* alleles are more strongly associated with type 1 AIH[19–21]; nor are the HLA class III deleted complement *C4* null alleles[22] *TNF*A* locus promoter polymorphisms *TNF*A-238* and *TNF*A-308*,[23] or the HLA class I Cw alleles.[24] Furthermore, molecular genotyping data have led to a revision of the classical interpretation of these associations. Thus instead of considering the individual antigens or alleles these associations may be viewed in terms of molecular structures. The two susceptibility alleles *DR3* (*DRB1*0301*) and *DR4* (or *DRB1*0401* to be more precise) both encode specific six amino acid motif Leu-Leu-Glu-Gln-Lys-Arg (single-letter code LLEQKR) at positions 67–72 of the DR$\beta$-polypeptide.[19] This motif was found in all but 13 out of 205 (94%) patients and 64% of controls in two separate studies based at King's College Hospital (one of which was in collaboration with the Mayo Clinic)[19,20]. These amino acids are located on the edge of the $\alpha$-helix and are at a critical site for both antigen binding and interaction with the TCR. Further characterization of this 'shared epitope' model of susceptibility suggested that the critical amino acid is lysine (K) at position 71. The *DRB1*1501* allele, which is infrequent in patients with AIH and may have a protective effect being associated with low risk of disease, differs from *DRB1*0301* and *DRB1*0401* at only two positions within this motif: position 67 where there is an isoleucine residue (I) in place of leucine (L) and position 71 where there is an alanine residue (A) in place of lysine (K). The leucine residue at position 67 is a consensus amino acid and is encoded by a number of different *DRB* alleles, whereas alanine 71 is only encoded by the

**Table 2** Shared epitopes in AIH: Japanese and King's and King's/Mayo Clinic data

| *Allele* | *DR antigen* | *Position of amino acid* | | |
|---|---|---|---|---|
| | | *HVR1* | *HVR2* | *HVR3* |
| *DRB1** | | 9 – 14 | 26 only | 67 – 74 |
| 0101 | DR1 | W Q L L K F E | L | L L E Q R R A A |
| 1501 | DR2 | W Q L P K R E | F | I L E Q A R A A |
| 1502 | | W Q L P K R E | F | I L E Q A R A A |
| 1601 | | W Q L P K R E | F | F L E D R R A A |
| 1602 | | W Q L P K R E | F | L L E D R R A A |
| 0301 | DR3 | L E Y S T S E | **Y** | L L E Q **K** R G **R** |
| 0401 | DR4 | W E L V K H E | F | L L E Q **K** R A A |
| 0402 | | W E L V K H E | F | I L E D E R A A |
| 0403 | | W E L V K H E | F | L L E Q R R A E |
| 0404 | | W E L V K H E | F | L L E Q R R A A |
| 0405 | | W E L V K H E | F | L L E Q R R A A |
| 0406 | | W E L V K H E | F | L L E Q R R A E |
| 0407 | | W E L V K H E | F | L L E Q R R A E |
| 0408 | | W E L V K H E | F | L L E Q R R A A |
| *DRB3** | | | | |
| 0101 | DR52 | L E L R K S E | **Y** | L L E Q **K** R G **R** |
| 0201 | | L E L L K S E | F | L L E Q **K** R G Q |
| 0202 | | L E L L K S E | F | L L E Q **K** R G Q |
| 0301 | | L E L L K S E | F | L L E Q **K** R G Q |

The standard WHO single-letter code for amino acids has been used. Amino acids in bold are those associated with AIH in northern European and North American white AIH patients.[17,18] *Amino acids underlined are associated with AIH in Japanese patients.*[22]

*DRB1*15* alleles (*DRB1*1501, 1502*, and *1503*) and the less common of the *DRB5* alleles *DRB5*0201–0203* (illustrated in Table 2). However, we should not over-interpret these data, as both positions may be important. Structural models based on crystallographic studies[6] and complex computer modelling place both leucine 67 and lysine 71 over the seventh antigen-binding pocket (P7) of the HLA DR$\beta$ molecule separated by a single rotation of the $\alpha$-helix (personal communication with Paul Travers, June 1998).

The great advantage of this analysis over traditional analysis is that it offers a functional explanation for these genetic associations. *In-vitro* experiments confirm position 71 as a critical site in determining the peptide–MHC complex interaction with the T-cell receptor, whilst position 67 may be important in peptide binding (Doherty *et al.*, personal communication, March 1998). HLA alleles associated with increased susceptibility to autoimmune disease will be those which have both high affinities for autoantigenic peptides and favourable MHC-peptide complex interactions with the TCR.

Data based on *South American and Japanese AIH patients* appear to define different HLA-susceptibility alleles to those identified above. Thus, whilst this model of susceptibility fits the type 1 AIH patients from northern Europe and their descendants, it may need to be modified to accommodate data from South America and Japan. This is not surprising in relation to the Japanese, where the difference may be simply due to different genetic backgrounds in the two populations. In Japan, A1-B8-DR3 is almost absent and DR4 is associated with AIH.[25] Furthermore, the patients tend to present at a similar age to the older-onset European subgroup; however, the similarity ends there, because the predominant *DR4* allele associated with AIH in Japan is *DRB1*0405*. This allele has an arginine residue (R) at $\beta$71. Initial reports from Japan also suggested that DR2 may be a second risk factor for type 1 AIH. Consequently a model of susceptibility based on this observation which suggests that basic amino acids at position 13 of the DR$\beta$-polypeptide (encoded by all of the *DR2* alleles and also by *DRB1*0405*) has been developed.[26] However, the DR2 association has not been confirmed in a national study, and recent reports from Japan (Gotaro Toda, personal communication, September 1999) suggest that the model should be discarded in favour of arginine at $\beta$71. Since both arginine and lysine are highly charged polar amino acids they may have a similar effect on antigen binding by the class II molecule.

Surprisingly the data from South America suggest different models of susceptibility in adults and children with type 1 AIH. In adult patients from Argentina there is an increased frequency of *DRB1*0405*[27] and in patients from Mexico[28] *DRB1*0404* is most prevalent. Since both of these alleles encode arginine 71 the data are in keeping with the model above. In children from Argentina[29,30] and Brazil[31] there is a strong association with *DRB1*1301* and a weaker secondary association with *DRB1*0301. DRB1*1301* does not encode either lysine or arginine at $\beta$71, and a model based on valine 86 has been proposed.[30] This work is based on large series of genotyped patients, but may be flawed. These patients are referred to as 'white' or 'European' but their racial/ethnic background is not well defined, especially in Brazil and Mexico. In addition the disease in children may well have a different aetiology to that seen in adults. However, other series of paediatric cases have identified a high proportion of patients with the initial diagnosis of type 1 AIH having pathology similar to primary sclerosing cholangitis. The *DRB1*1301* allele is very strongly associated with primary sclerosing cholangitis in adults (see below). In the absence of endoscopic proof there will always be doubt about the diagnosis in these children. However, whatever the diagnosis is, type 1 AIH or autoimmune sclerosing cholangitis (ASC), the data from these studies are very strong.[29–31]

Differences in these genetic backgrounds for type 1 AIH in different populations, may simply reflect the genetic background of the founder populations or may reflect different underlying aetiologies and different initiating events – for example interaction with different viral triggers, etc. It is interesting to note that hepatitis A virus is endemic in Argentina and has been suggested as a potential trigger for type 1 AIH in children there.[30]

The $\beta$71 hypothesis, which provides a very convincing unifying hypothesis for HLA-encoded genetic susceptibility to type 1 AIH in adults, if not children, is simply a model and may not be correct. An alternative view of the data above suggests that, whilst the association with *A1-B8-DR3* may be limited to northern Europeans and their descendants, the common link in all three series is with DR4, albeit with three different *DR4* alleles. The *A1-B8-DR3* haplotype is very much a northern European phenomenon and is usually more common in Celtic and Anglo-Saxon populations than other European groups. In contrast this haplotype is almost absent in Japan and is considerably less frequent in southern Europe. If we ignore A1-B8-DR3 the data may suggest that there is a DR4 specific link with type 1 AIH, which has not yet been identified.

These DR4 associations may arise because DR4 is a marker for another 'true susceptibility gene' in close proximity to *DRB1*. The most plausible candidate for this role is the *DRB4* allele, *DRB4*0103*, which is found on all *DR4* haplotypes in the Mayo Clinic study,[20] but was not determined in any of the other studies cited above. With the exception of *DRB4*0103* other candidate genes are unlikely to be close to *DRB* since different *DQA* and *DQB* genes are associated with *DRB1*0401* in Europeans (*DQB1*0301* and *DQB1*0302*) and *DRB1*0405* in Japanese (*DQB1*04*)[25], but the possibility of a common shared allele elsewhere on the different *DR4* haplotypes cannot be ruled out, perhaps within the class III region for example: *TNF* or *C4*. Preliminary studies suggest a very strong link with complement *C4A* null alleles (*C4AQ0*) in children[32] and with *C4* deletions in adult patients[22,33], but these are in linkage disequilibrium with the *A1-B8-DR3* haplotype and have not been evaluated in the context of the shared epitope hypothesis and have only been studied in northern European patients or those of northern European origin. Further investigations are under way at present to determine whether TNF has an important role in AIH, and collaborative studies and shared analysis may help illuminate the *DR4* conundrum.

## Clinical correlates and disease severity

In rheumatoid arthritis (RA) it has been suggested that HLA may have 'more to do with disease severity than disease susceptibility'.[34] The data reviewed above explain the observations of increased susceptibility to AIH but not the earlier observation that the patients with DR4 tend to have later-onset disease than those with DR3. Perhaps a second HLA-linked gene may influence disease severity. Correlation between the clinical features of a disease and HLA genotype may be of value in patient management, especially in determining prognosis.

In adult AIH patients from King's and the Mayo Clinic those with B8 or DR3 presented earlier and were more likely to relapse whilst on treatment.[17,35,36] In addition, in an analysis of 38 children with AIH, only two (5%) had DR4 compared with an expected frequency of 39% in the general population,[37] and adult AIH patients with DR4 are more likely to have concurrent extrahepatic disease.[38,39] It remains to be seen whether susceptibility and disease severity in AIH are determined by the same or different HLA genes. In the study by Doherty *et al.*[19], although there is a common susceptibility determinant (lysine $\beta$71), those with *DRB1*0301* had more severe disease than those with *DRB1*0401*. One explanation for this observation is that genes in linkage with *DRB1*0401* and *DRB1*0301* determine severity and age of onset. Candidates for this role might include: HLA *A1, Cw*0701, B8, C4* null alleles, the *TNF-308* allele *A2,* the HLA class II alleles – *DQA1*0501* and *DQB1*0201*, or other polymorphic genes encoded on the haplotype – *TAP, LMP, DM,* for example.

An alternative possibility is that disease severity is determined by the number of lysine-DR$\beta$71 encoding genes. An individual may have from zero to four lysine DR$\beta$71 alleles (i.e. a maximum of two per chromosome). When the number of lysine 71 copies was evaluated in the above King's/Mayo Clinic series,[20] those with one or fewer lysine DRβ71 alleles had a low risk of developing AIH (one lysine β71 RR = 0.8, zero lysine β71 RR = 0.2) whilst those with two copies had a relative risk of 4.7 and those with four copies had a relative risk greater than 14. Additional analysis also noted two other amino acid substitutions were significantly associated with susceptibility to AIH (Table 3). These were tyrosine (single-letter code Y) at DRβ26 and an arginine (R) at DRβ74, both of which are encoded by the *DRB1*0301* and *DRB3*0101* alleles but not *DRB1*0401*. Whether these substitutions enhance the susceptibility effect of lysine β71 or determine disease severity is not known.

## PRIMARY SCLEROSING CHOLANGITIS

Unlike type 1 AIH PSC is a disease with a male predominance and does not easily fit the classic picture of an autoimmune disease. There are, however well-established strong HLA associations in PSC.

Four particular HLA haplotypes are associated with PSC. The mostly strongly linked haplotype is the *A1-B8-Cw7-TNF*2-DRB3*0101-DRB1*0301-DQA1*0501-DQB1*0201* haplotype. This is the same haplotype which is associated with type 1 AIH, and all components are associated with PSC, with the exception of A1 which is not significantly increased in PSC patients.[40–48] The second haplotype, *DRB3*0101-DRB1*1301-DQA1*0102-DQB1*0603*, is most strongly associated with PSC in Sweden, where the link with the first haplotype is weaker.[46] Since both of these two haplotypes carry the *DRB3*0101* allele it has been suggested that *DRB3*0101* forms the basis of HLA-encoded susceptibility in PSC.[44] However, this interpretation is not universally accepted[46] and does not necessarily stand up to review. The third haplotype, *DRB1*1501-DQB1*0602*, is

**Table 3** Significant associations with amino acids of the second exon of the DRβ-polypeptide from the pooled King's/Mayo Clinic AIH data

| *Amino acid residue* | *Position* | *Encoding alleles* | *Patients (n = 205)* | *Controls (n = 279)* | *Probability corrected (pc)* | *Relative risk* |
|---|---|---|---|---|---|---|
| Tyrosine (Y) | β26 | *DRB1*0301*<br>*DRB1*0901*<br>*DRB3*0101* | 61.4% | 31.2% | <0.000000001 | 3.52 |
| Lysine (K) | β71 | *DRB1*0301*[a]<br>*DRB1*0401*<br>*DRB1*0409*<br>*DRB1*0413*<br>*DRB1*0416*<br>*DRB1*1303*<br>*DRB3**[b] | 93.6% | 62.7% | <0.000000001 | 8.46 |
| Arginine (R) | β74 | *DRB1*0301*[a]<br>*DRB3*0101* | 60.5% | 29% | <0.000000001 | 3.74 |

[a]Includes the *DRB1*0301*, *DRB1*0302* and *DRB1*0303* alleles, but *DRB1*0301* was detected in this series.
[b]This amino acid is encoded by all of the *DRB3** alleles.

weakly associated with PSC in British patients.[43–45,47] Structural similarities between HLA DQ$\beta$ molecules encoded by the *DQB1*0602* and *DQB1*0603* alleles have been put forward as a unifying explanation for these racial differences, but have not been confirmed.[49] The fourth and final haplotype associated with PSC, *DRB1*0401-DQA1*03-DQB1*0302*, is thought to exert a protective effect, since it is found at a lower frequency in patients compared to controls. As with the other associations this is also controversial; in Sweden[46] and Norway[47] this *DR4* haplotype does not encode resistance, whereas in Finland[48], Britain[44,45,47] and the USA (Al Czaja, personal communication, September 1999), it does.

Additional controversy surrounds these associations, especially regarding the primary association. There are two distinct camps: on the one hand some suggest that *DRB1*0301* and *DRB1*1301* are the primary susceptibility genes, whereas others have suggested that susceptibility maps closer to the HLA *B-TNF* region of 6p21.3 than to *DRB1*.[50] More recently attention has been focused on the *MICA* locus in PSC with promising results. Early analysis indicates a strong link with the *MICA 008* allele. This may strengthen the case for *B-TNF* as the primary site of HLA-encoded susceptibility in PSC (Norris, personal communication, September 1999).

A second area of interest is the overlap between PSC and inflammatory bowel disease (IBD), mostly ulcerative colitis, which may occur in anything from 66% to 100% of patients with PSC. In contrast only 4% of IBD patients may develop PSC. Overall IBD is more common and more likely to occur in families than PSC, and linkage studies based on whole genome scanning with micro satellites have identified at least four chromosomal sites associated with either ulcerative colitis or Crohn's disease. Interestingly there appears to be very little genetic overlap between genes which encode susceptibility to PSC and those encoding susceptibility to IBD. HLA is not strongly linked with IBD. The question remains, however, whether IBD+PSC and IBD–PSC have the same aetiopathogenesis and underlying genetic susceptibility.

## PRIMARY BILIARY CIRRHOSIS

Whilst PBC, like type 1 AIH, fits the picture of a classical autoimmune disease it does not respond to corticosteroid therapy and the only confirmed HLA association, with DR8, is weak and of marginal significance.[50–54] Other genetic associations which have been described between PBC and chromosome 6p21.3 are most likely due to linkage with DR8.[55–57] As with DR4 in type 1 AIH, the specific *DR8* allele associated with PBC depends on the population studied and reflects the 'founder population'. Thus in Japan *DRB1*0803* is the primary HLA susceptibility allele[58–61], and in northern Europeans and their descendants *DRB1*0801* is the primary susceptibility allele.[52–54]

One feature of the different studies of PBC and HLA is the wide variation in the reported frequency of DR8. Recent reanalysis of the series from Newcastle suggests that this may be due to bias in the case-mix in some of these studies. In a study of 182 patients, 93 had stage 3 or stage 4 disease and 79 had stage 1 or 2 disease. Of the 93 with stage 3 or 4, 22 (24%) had DR8 *(DRB1*0801)*, whereas only four of 79 (5%) with stage 1 or 2 had DR8 ($p = 0.0007$). This has also been noted in recent studies of *TNF* genes in PBC.[62] Indeed Jones *et al.*[62] suggested that these genetic associations are less to do with susceptibility and more likely to reflect more rapid progression in those with DR8 or *TNF1/1*. Thus, patients series collected at tertiary referral centres such as the Mayo Clinic or King's College Hospital may be subject to ascertainment bias, and as a consequence may have higher DR8 frequencies than those patients series collected on a community basis, and this may explain variation between studies. Identifying genes associated with accelerated disease progression may prove more useful in the clinic than identifying 'susceptibility' genes.

## NEW GENES FOR INVESTIGATION AND THE FUTURE OF IMMUNOGENETICS

The technology for performing HLA studies and our understanding of the mechanisms by which HLA may determine disease susceptibility/resistance are advancing at a rapid pace. Yet HLA alone does not explain disease susceptibility, nor does HLA alone explain the variation in the clinical expression of these well-defined diseases. Other host factors and genes may also be important. Polymorphic genes which are prime candidates for this role include some of those which I have already mentioned, i.e. complement and TNF-$\alpha$ encoded on 6p21.3, and others, not on chromosome 6p21.3, e.g. the cytokine genes interleukins 1, 2, 4, 6, 10 and 12, which are all polymorphic or have polymorphic promoter genes, the adhesion molecules ICAM1, E-selectin, P-selectin, accessory molecules such as CTLA-4, growth factors such as TGF$\beta$1 and many drug-detoxifying enzymes such as thiopurine methyltransferase (TPMT), which is important in azathioprine detoxification. Studies of these genes in liver and other diseases are only now being performed. To date a number of these genes have been investigated in autoimmune liver disease, with mixed findings. Thus, although the interleukin-1 gene family (chromosome 2q13) including *IL-1B* (the gene for IL-1$\beta$) and *IL-1RN* (the gene for the IL-1 receptor antagonist) have been investigated in AIH and also in primary sclerosing cholangitis (PSC), neither is associated with disease[23] (Donaldson *et al.*, May 1999, unpublished observations), whilst *IL-1B* polymorphism is associated with disease progression/severity though not disease susceptibility in PBC (Donaldson *et al.*, May 1999, unpublished observations). In contrast none of three interleukin-10 promoter polymorphisms is associated with either type 1 AIH,[23] PSC (Donaldson *et al.*, May 1999, unpublished observations) or PBC.[63] There is a weak link between TNF-$\alpha$ and type 1 AIH, though this appears to be secondary to linkage with the *A1-B8-DR3* haplotype in contrast to the situation in PSC where the link with *TNFA*2* is stronger than the link with *DRB1*0301*.[50] Recent studies also suggest that the *CTLA-4* base-exchange polymorphism (chromosome 2q33) is associated with all three autoimmune liver diseases, type 1 AIH (Agarwal *et al.*, May 1999, unpublished observations), PSC[64] and PBC.[65] It seems that this latter polymorphism is universally associated with autoimmune diseases. Indeed a recent study suggested that up to 65% of genetic associations may be common to most autoimmune diseases, and that these genes may determine an increased propensity for autoimmune reactions rather than susceptibility to specific diseases.[66]

Two other, though less novel, genetic systems which should not be overlooked are the (TCR) and immunoglobulin genes (Ig). These two genetic systems are complex and difficult to study because much of the TCR and Ig variability arises through somatic mutation and gene rearrangement. However, there are germline polymorphisms encoded within both the TCR and Ig genome. These include the TCR constant (C) region genes (chromosome 7p14, 7p35) that may contribute to susceptibility to insulin-dependent diabetes mellitus, multiple sclerosis, rheumatoid arthritis and AIH,[67] and the immunoglobulin heavy chain constant region genes (Gm or *IGHG1* to *IGHG4*, chromosome 14q32)[68], which have been associated with AIH in two separate studies.[69,70] Both TCR and Ig play a very important role in disease, and it is only their complexity which has prevented these systems from being more thoroughly investigated in relation to disease susceptibility.

Finally it is pertinent to ask the question, what is the relationship between each disease and sex? After all, each one of these three diseases has a marked preponderance of one sex over the other. In PBC and type 1 AIH the majority of patients are female, whilst in PSC male patients predominate. What is the reason for this? This imbalance may reflect a difference in exposure to environmental risk between the sexes, hormonal differences or it may be genetic. At this time we can only speculate.

In conclusion, the story of genetic susceptibility and autoimmune liver disease is at present only half-written; there are many other polymorphic immunoregulatory genes which are potential candidates: *IL-2* (4q26), *IL-4* (5q23–31), *IL-4R* (16p12), *IL-6* (7p21), *IL-6R* (1q21), *IL-12B* (5q31–33), *ICAM-1* (19p13.2), *TGF-*gb-1* (19q13.2), *VCAM-1* (1p32), *ECAM-1* (1q22–25), etc. In the new millennium, as our collective interest and knowledge of other areas of the human genome develops, no doubt other polymorphic genes will be added to this list. Eventually it may be possible to predict disease profiles from genotypes, though at present this remains a distant prospect. Whilst we await this eventuality there may be great value in the short term from genetic studies which help define the disease aetiology and pathogenesis, and also enable more accurate prognostic models to be constructed for use in clinical practice.

## References


1. de Vries RRP. HLA and disease: from epidemiology to immunotherapy. Eur J Clin Invest. 1992;22:1–8.
2. Campbell D, Trowsdale J. A map of the human major histocompatibility complex. Immunology Today. 1997;18:43.
3. Bodmer JG, Marsh SGE, Albert ED, *et al.* Nomenclature for factors of the HLA system, 1998. Eur J Immunogenet. 1999;26:81–116.
4. Bjorkman PJ, Saper MA, Samraoui B, Bennett WS, Strominger JL, Wiley DC. Structure of human class I histocompatibility antigen, HLA-A2. Nature. 1987;329:506–12.
5. Bjorkman PJ, Saper MA, Samraoui B, Bennett WS, Strominger JL, Wiley DC. The foreign antigen binding site and T cell recognition regions of class I histocompatibility antigens. Nature. 1987;329:512–18.
6. Brown JH, Jardetzky TS, Gorga JC *et al.* Three-dimensional structure of the human class II histocompatibility antigen HLA-DR1. Nature. 1993;364:33–9.

7. Rammensee H-G. Chemistry of peptides associated with MHC class I and class II molecules. Curr Opin Immunol. 1995;7:85–96.
8. Madden DR. The three-dimensional structure of peptide–MHC complexes. Annu Rev Immunol. 1995;13:587–622.
9. Simon M, Pawlotsky Y, Bourel M, Fauchet R, Genetet B. Hemochromatose idopathique: maladie associee a l'antigene tissulaire HL-A 3. Nouv Presse Med. 1975;4:1432.
10. Feder JN, Gnirke A, Thomas W *et al.* A novel MHC class I-like gene is mutated in patients with hereditary haemochromatosis. Nature Genet. 1996;13;399–408.
11. Dupont B, Obersfield SE, Smithwick EM, Lee TD, Levine LS. Close genetic linkage between HLA and congenital adrenal hyperplasia (21-hydroxylase deficiency). Lancet. 1977;2:1309–12.
12. Todd JA, Bain SC. A practical approach to identification of susceptibility genes for IDDM. Diabetes. 1992;41:1029–34.
13. Freely associating. Nature Genet. 1999;22:1–2.
14. Todd JA. Interpretation of results from genetic studies of multifactorial disease. Lancet. 1999;354(Suppl. 1):15–16.
15. Mackay IR, Morris PJ. Association of autoimmune active hepatitis with HL-A1, 8. Lancet. 1972;2:793–5.
16. Oplez G, Votgen AGM, Summerskill WHJ, Schalm SW, Terasaki PI. HLA determinant in chronic active liver disease: a possible relation of HLA-Dw3 to prognosis. Tissue Antigens. 1977:9:36–40.
17. Donaldson PT, Doherty DG, Hayllar KM, McFarlane I, Johnson PJ, Williams R. Susceptibility to autoimmune chronic active hepatitis: human leucocyte antigens DR4 and A1-B8-DR3 are independent risk factors. Hepatology. 1991;13:701–6.
18. Williams RM, Martin S, Falchuk KR *et al.* Increased frequency of HLA-DRW4 in chronic active hepatitis. Vox Sang. 1978;35:366–9.
19. Doherty DG, Donaldson PT, Underhill JA *et al.* Allelic sequence variation in the HLA class II genes and proteins in patients with autoimmune hepatitis. Hepatology. 1994:19:609–15.
20. Strettell MJD, Donaldson PT, Thompson LJ *et al.* Allelic basis for HLA-encoded susceptibility to type 1 autoimmune hepatitis. Gastroenterology. 1997;112:2028–36.
21. Manabe K, Donaldson PT, Underhill JA *et al.* HLA A1-B8-DR3-DQ2-DPB1*0401 extended haplotype in autoimmune hepatitis. Hepatology. 1993;18:1334–7.
22. Doherty DG, Underhill JA, Donaldson PT *et al.* Polymorphism in the human complement C4 genes and susceptibility to autoimmune hepatitis. Autoimmunity. 1994;18:243–9.
23. Cookson S, Constantini PK, Clare M *et al.* Frequency and nature of cytokine gene polymorphisms in type 1 autoimmune hepatitis. Hepatology. 1999;30:851–6.
24. Strettell MDJ, Thomson LJ, Donaldson PT, Bunce M, O'Niell CM, Williams R. HLA-C genes and susceptibility to type I autoimmune hepatitis. Hepatology. 1997;26:1203–6.
25. Seki T, Ota M, Faruta S *et al.* HLA class II molecules and autoimmune hepatitis susceptibility in Japanese patients. Gastroenterology. 1992;103:1041–7.
26. Ota M, Seki T, Kiyosawa K *et al.* A possible association between basic amino acids at position 13 of *DRB1* chains and autoimmune hepatitis. Immunogenetics. 1992;36:49–55.
27. Marcos Y, Fainboim HA, Capucchio M *et al.* Two-locus involvement in the association of human leukocyte antigen with the extrahepatic manifestations of autoimmune chronic active hepatitis. Hepatology. 1994;19:1371–4.
28. Vasquez-Garcia MN, Alaez C, Olivo A *et al.* MHC class II sequences of susceptibility and protection in Mexicans with autoimmune hepatitis. J Hepatol. 1998;28:985–90.
29. Fainboim L, Marcos Y, Pando M *et al.* Chronic active autoimmune hepatitis in children: strong association with a particular HLA-DR6 (DRB1*1301) haplotype. Human Immunol. 1994;41:146–50.
30. Pando M, Larriba J, Fernandez GC *et al.* Paediatric and adult forms of type 1 autoimmune hepatitis in Argentina: evidence for differential genetic predisposition. Hepatology. 1999 (In press).
31. Bittencourt PL, Goldberg AC, Cancado ELR *et al.* Genetic heterogeneity in susceptibility to autoimmune hepatitis types 1 and 2. Am J Gastroenterol. 1999;94:1906–13.
32. Vergani D, Wells L, Larcher VF *et al.* Genetically determined low C4: a predisposing factor to autoimmune chronic active hepatitis. Lancet. 1985;2:294–8.
33. Scully LJ, Toze C, Sengar DPS, Goldstein R. Early-onset autoimmune hepatitis is associated with a C4A gene deletion. Gastroenterology. 1993;104:1478–84.
34. Ollier B. Shock revelations about HLA-DR4 a short cut to rheumatoid arthritis. Nature. 1996;2:279–80.

35. Czaja AJ, Rakela J, Hay JE, Moore SB. Clinical and prognostic implications of HLA B8 in corticosteroid-treated severe autoimmune chronic active hepatitis. Gastroenterology. 1990; 98:1587–93.
36. Czaja AJ, Strettell MDJ, Thomson LJ *et al.* Associations between alleles of the major histocompatibility complex and type 1 autoimmune hepatitis. Hepatology. 1997;25:317–23.
37. Gregorio GV, Portmann B, Reid F *et al.* Autoimmune hepatitis in childhood: a 20 year experience. Hepatology. 1997;25:541–7.
38. Czaja AJ, Carpenter HA, Santrach PJ, Moore SB. Genetic predisposition for the immunological features of chronic active hepatitis. Hepatology. 1993;18:816–22.
39. Czaja AJ, Carpenter HA, Santrach PJ, Moore SB. Significance of HLA DR4 in type 1 autoimmune hepatitis. Gastroenterology. 1993;195:1502–7.
40. Schrumpf E, Fausa O, Forre O, Dobloug J, Ritland S, Thorsby E. HLA antigens and immunoregulatory T cells associated with hepatobiliary disease. Scandinavian Journal of Gastroenterol. 1982;17:187–91.
41. Chapman R, Varghese Z, Gaul R, Patel G, Kokinon N, Sherlock S. Association of primary sclerosing cholangitis with HLA-B8. Gut. 1983;24:38–41.
42. Shepherd H, Selby W, Chapman R *et al.* Ulcerative colitis and persistent liver dysfunction. Q J Med. 1983;52:503–13.
43. Donaldson PT, Farrant JM, Wilkinson ML, Hayllar K, Portmann BC, Williams R. Dual association of HLA DR2 and DR3 with primary sclerosing cholangitis. Hepatology. 1991;13:129–33.
44. Farrant JM, Doherty DG, Donaldson PT *et al.* Amino acid substitutions at position 38 of the DR beta polypeptide confer susceptibility to and protection from primary sclerosing cholangitis. Hepatology. 1992;16:390–5.
45. Mehal W, Lo Y, Wordsworth B *et al.* HLA DR4 is a marker for rapid disease progression in primary sclerosing cholangitis. Gastroenterology. 1994;106:160–7.
46. Olerup O, Olsson R, Hultcrantz R *et al.* HLA-DR and HLA-DQ are not markers for rapid disease progression in primary sclerosing cholangitis. Gastroenterology. 1995;108:870–8.
47. Spurkland A, Saarinen S, Boberg KM, *et al.* HLA class II haplotypes in primary sclerosing cholangitis patients from five European populations. Tissue Antigens. 1999;53:459–69.
48. Färkkila M, Koskimes S, Karvonen A-L, Pikkarainen P, Nurmi H, Nuutinen H. HLA associations in primary sclerosing cholangitis (PSC): HLA DR4 has protective role? Gastroenterology. 1999;116:A1209 (Abstract L 0127).
49. Donaldson PT, Constantini PK, Underhill J *et al.* Remodelling the HLA associations with primary sclerosing cholangitis: novel association with phenylalanine at position 87 on DQb-polypeptide. Hepatology. 1998;28:403A (abstract 964).
50. Bernal W, Moloney M, Underhill J, Donaldson PT. Association of tumour necrosis factor polymorphism with primary sclerosing cholangitis. J Hepatol. 1999;30:237–41.
51. Gores GJ, Moore SB, Fisher LD, Powell FC, Dickson ER. Primary biliary cirrhosis: association with class II major histocompatibility complex antigens. Hepatology. 1987;7:889–92.
52. Underhill JA, Donaldson PT, Bray G, Doherty DG, Portmann BC, Williams R. Susceptibility to primary biliary cirrhosis is associated with the HLADR8–DQB1*0402 haplotype. Hepatology. 1992;16:1404–8.
53. Gregory W, Mehal W, Dunn AN *et al.* Primary biliary cirrhosis: contribution of HLA class II allele DR8. Q J Med. 1993;86:393–9.
54. Begovich AB, Klitz W, Moonsamy PV, Van de Water J, Peltz G, Gershwin ME. Genes within the HLA class II region confer both predisposition and resistance to primary biliary cirrhosis. Tissue Antigens. 1994;43:71–7.
55. Briggs DC, Donaldson PT, Hayes P, Welsh KI, Williams R, Neuberger JM. A major histocompatibility complex class III allotype C4B2 associated with primary biliary cirrhosis. Tissue Antigens. 1987;29:141–5.
56. Manns MP, Bremm A, Schneider PM *et al.* HLA DRw8 and complement C4 deficiency as risk factors in primary biliary cirrhosis. Gastroenterology. 1991;101:1367–73.
57. Mella J, Roschmann E, Maier K, Volk B. Association of primary biliary cirrhosis with the allele HLA DPB1*0301 in a German population. Hepatology. 1995;21:398–402.
58. Maeda T, Onoshi S, Saibara T, Iwasaki S, Yamamoto J. HLA DR8 and primary biliary cirrhosis. Gastroenterology. 1992;103:1118–19.
59. Seki T, Kiyosawa K, Ota M *et al.* Association of primary biliary cirrhosis with human leukocyte antigen DPB1*0501 in Japanese patients. Hepatology. 1993;18:73–8.

60. Mukai T, Kimura A, Ishibashi H *et al.* Association of HLA DRB1*0803 and *1602 with susceptibility to primary biliary cirrhosis. Int Hepat Commun. 1995;3:207–12.
61. Oguri H, Oba S, Ogina H *et al.* Susceptibility to primary biliary cirrhosis is associated with human leukocyte antigen DRB1*0803 in Japanese patients. Int Hepat Commun. 1994;2:263–70.
62. Jones DEJ, Watt FE, Grove J *et al.* Tumour necrosis factor-a promoter polymorphisms in primary biliary cirrhosis. J Hepatol. 1999;30:232–6.
63. Zappala F, Grove J, Watt FE *et al.* No evidence for involvement of the interleukin-10-592 promoter polymorphism in genetic susceptibility to primary biliary cirrhosis. J Hepatol. 1998;28:820–3.
64. Saarinen S, Broome U, Ligers A, Olsson R, Hultcrantz R, Olerup O. Cytotoxic T-lymphocyte antigen-4 the second susceptibility gene in primary sclerosing cholangitis. Gut. 1999 (In press).
65. Agarwal K, Grove J, Pearce S, Daly A, Jones DEJ, Bassendine MF. CTLA-4 gene polymorphism associated with primary biliary cirrhosis (PBC). J Hepatol. 2000;32:538–541.
66. Becker KG, Simon RM, Bailey-Wilson JE *et al.* Clustering of non-major histocompatibility complex susceptibility candidate loci in human autoimmune diseases. Proc Natl Acad Sci. 1998;95:9979–84.
67. Manabe K, Hibberd ML, Donaldson PT *et al.* T-cell receptor constant germ-line gene polymorphisms and susceptibility to autoimmune hepatitis. Gastroenterology. 1994;106:1321–5.
68. Propert ND. Detection of immunoglobulin polymorphisms. In: Simons MJ, Tait BD editors. Detection of Immune Associated Genetic Markers of Human Disease. London Churchill-Livingstone; 1984:65–81.
69. Krawitt EL, Kilby AE, Albertini RJ, Schanfield MS. Immunogenetic studies of autoimmune chronic active hepatitis: HLA, immunoglobulin allotypes and antibodies. Hepatology. 1987;7:1305–10.
70. Whittingham S, Mathews JD, Schanfield MS, Tait BD, Mackay IR. Interaction of HLA and Gm in autoimmune chronic active hepatitis. Clin Exp Immunol. 1981;43:80–6.

# 12
# The role of T cells in autoimmune hepatitis

**D. VERGANI and G. MIELI-VERGANI**

---

The typical histological picture of autoimmune hepatitis (AIH), characterized by a dense mononuclear cell infiltrate eroding the limiting plate and invading the parenchyma (periportal hepatitis), first suggested that autoaggressive cellular immunity may be involved in its causation[1,2]. Immunocytochemical studies have identified the phenotype of the infiltrating cells. T lymphocytes mounting the $\alpha/\beta$ T cell receptor predominate. Among the T cells a majority are positive for the CD4 helper/inducer phenotype and a sizeable minority for the CD8 cytotoxic/suppressor phenotype. Lymphocytes of non-T cell lineage are fewer and include, in decreasing order of frequency, killer/natural killer (K/NK) cells (CD16/CD56-positive), macrophages and B lymphocytes[3].

A powerful stimulus must be promoting the formation of the massive inflammatory cell infiltrate present at diagnosis. Whatever the initial trigger, it is most probable that such a high number of activated inflammatory cells cause liver damage. There are different possible pathways that an immune attack can follow to inflict damage on the hepatocyte (Figure 1). Liver damage is believed to be orchestrated by CD4-positive T lymphocytes recognizing a self antigenic peptide. To trigger an autoimmune response the peptide must be embraced by an HLA class II molecule and presented to uncommitted T helper (Th0) cells by professional antigen-presenting cells (APC), with the costimulation of ligand–ligand (CD28 on Th0, CD80 on APC) interaction between the two cells. Th0 cells become activated, differentiate into functional phenotypes according to the cytokines prevailing in the microenvironment and the nature of the antigen, and initiate a cascade of immune reactions determined by the cytokines they produce. Th1 cells, arising in the presence of the macrophage-produced interleukin 12, secrete mainly interleukin 2 and interferon-$\gamma$, which activate macrophages, enhance expression of HLA class I (increasing liver cell vulnerability to a cytotoxic attack) and induce expression of HLA class II molecules on hepatocytes, which then become able to present the autoantigenic peptide to Th cells, thus perpetuating the immune recognition cycle. Th2 cells, which differentiate from Th0 if the microenvironment is rich in interleukin 4, produce mainly interleukin 4, 5 and 10, which induce autoantibody production by B lympho-

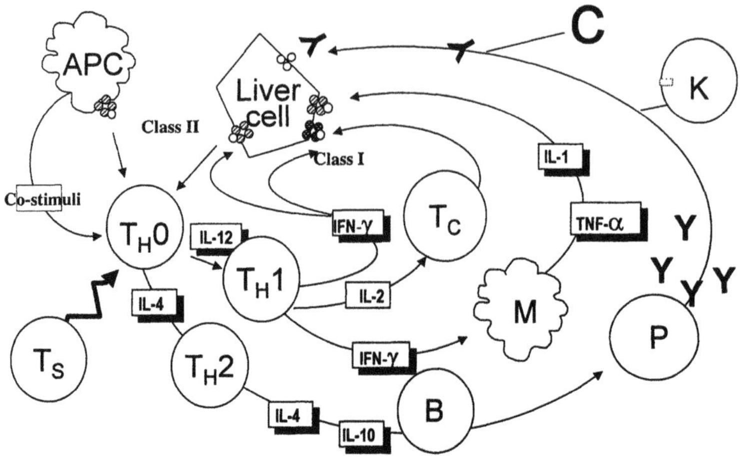


**Fig. 1** Autoimmune attack to the liver. A specific autoantigenic peptide is presented to an uncommitted T helper (Th0) lymphocyte within the HLA class II molecule of an antigen presenting cell (APC). Th0 cells become activated and, according to the presence in the microenvironment of interleukin (IL)-12 or IL-4 and nature of antigen, differentiate into Th1 or Th2 and initiate a series of immune reactions determined by the cytokines they produce: Th2 secrete mainly IL-4 and IL-10 and direct autoantibody production by B lymphocytes; Th1 secrete IL-2 and interferon-$\gamma$ (IFN-$\gamma$), which stimulate T cytotoxic (Tc) lymphocytes, enhance expression of class I and induce expression of class II HLA molecules on hepatocytes and activate macrophages; activated macrophages release IL-1 and tumour necrosis factor $\alpha$ (TNF-$\alpha$). If T 'suppressor' (Ts) lymphocytes do not oppose, a variety of effector mechanisms are triggered: liver cell destruction could derive from the action of Tc lymphocytes; cytokines released by Th1 and recruited macrophages; complement activation or engagement of killer (K) lymphocytes by the autoantibody bound to the hepatocyte surface

cytes. Physiologically Th1 and Th2 antagonize each other. The process of autoantigen recognition is strictly controlled by regulatory mechanisms. If these regulatory mechanisms fail, the autoimmune attack is perpetuated.

Over the past two decades different aspects of the above pathogenic scenario have been investigated.

An impairment of immunomodulatory mechanisms, which would enable the autoimmune response to develop, has been described in several reports. Children and young adults with AIH have low levels of T lymphocytes expressing the CD8 marker[4]. The notion of defective immunoregulation is supported by the finding that suppressor cell function is also impaired in AIH[5]. In addition it has been shown that patients with AIH have a specific defect in a subpopulation of T cells controlling the immune response to liver-specific membrane antigens[6].

Lobo-Yeo *et al.*[7] have shown that hepatocytes from patients with AIH, in contrast to normal hepatocytes, express HLA class II molecules. These hepatocytes, though lacking the antigen-processing machinery typical of APC, may present peptides through a bystander mechanism[8]. Whether presented by professional APC or by hepatocytes, the autoantigenic peptide is likely to be embraced by one of those HLA class II molecules conferring susceptibility to AIH and encoded by the genes DRB1*0301 and DRB3*0101.

Although there is no direct evidence as yet that an autoantigenic peptide is presented and recognized, activation of helper cells has been documented in

AIH[3,9]. These activated cells possess the CD4 phenotype and their numbers are highest when the disease is most active.

What triggers the immune system to react to an autoantigen is unknown. A lesson may be learned by the study of humoral autoimmune responses during viral infections. Recent studies aiming at determining the specificity of the LKM-1 antibody, present in both the juvenile form of AIH and in some patients with chronic hepatitis C virus (HCV) infection, have shown a high amino acid sequence homology between the HCV polyprotein and CYP 2D6, the molecular target of LKM 1, thus implicating a mechanism of molecular mimicry as a trigger for the production of LKM-1 in HCV infection[10,11]. It is therefore conceivable that an as-yet-unknown virus infection may be at the origin of the autoimmune attack in AIH.

Titres of antibodies to the liver-specific lipoprotein (LSP), a macromolecular complex present on the hepatocyte membrane, and to its well-characterized component asialoglycoprotein receptor (ASGPR) correlate with the biochemical and histological severity of AIH[12,13]. Recently antibodies to alcohol dehydrogenase (ADH), a second well-defined component of LSP, have been described in patients with AIH[14]. Immunofluorescence studies on monodispersed suspensions of liver cells obtained from patients with AIH showed that these cells are coated with antibodies *in vivo*[15]. A pathogenic role for these autoantibodies has been indicated by cytotoxicity assays showing that autoantibody-coated hepatocytes from patients with AIH are killed when incubated together with autologous[16] or allogeneic[15] lymphocytes. The effector cell was identified as a Fc receptor-positive mononuclear cell[16]. More recently, T cell clones obtained from the liver biopsy of children with AIH and expressing the $\gamma\delta$ T cell receptor have been shown to be cytotoxic to a variety of targets, but to exert preferential killing of liver-derived cells as opposed to cell lines derived from other organs[17].

A study in progress in our laboratory shows an elevation of the circulating levels of cytokines produced by both Th1 and Th2 cells at diagnosis of AIH, while Th1 cytokine levels significantly decrease and Th2 cytokines remain elevated during remission. This observation, implicating Th1 cytokines in the causation of liver damage, finds support in immunohistochemical studies showing a significantly higher number of interferon-$\gamma$ and interleukin 2-producing cells in the liver tissue of patients with active disease, while the number of interleukin 4- and interleukin 10-producing cells is similar in active and inactive biopsies (unpublished data).

The establishment of cell lines and clones has enabled Wen *et al.* [17,18] and Lohr *et al.* [19,20] to show that the majority of T cell clones obtained from the peripheral blood and a proportion of those from the liver of patients with AIH are CD4-positive and use the conventional $\alpha\beta$ T cell receptor. Some of these CD4-positive clones were further characterized and found to react with partially purified antigens, such as crude preparations of liver cell membrane or LSP[18], and with purified ASGPR [18,20] or recombinant CYP 2D6[19] and to be restricted by HLA class II molecules in their response. Since CD4 is the phenotype of helper T cells, both Wen *et al.* [18], and Lohr *et al.* [20] investigated whether these clones were able to help autologous B lymphocytes in the production of immunoglobulin in vitro, and found that their co-culture with B lymphocytes resulted in a dramatic increase in autoantibody production.

All the above experimental evidence suggests that cellular immune responses are involved in the liver damage of AIH, even though the evidence that the trigger is an autoantigen is still incomplete.

## References

1. De Groote J, Desmet VJ, Gedigk P *et al.* A classification of chronic hepatitis. Lancet. 1968;2:626.
2. Scheuer P. Chronic aggressive hepatitis. In: Liver Biopsy Interpretation, 2nd edn. London: Baillière Tindall; 1974:66–73.
3. Senaldi G, Portmann B, Mowat AP, Mieli-Vergani G, Vergani D. Immunohistochemical features of the portal tract mononuclear cell infiltrate in chronic aggressive hepatitis. Arch Dis Child. 1992;67:1447–53.
4. Nouri-Aria KT, Lobo-Yeo A, Vergani D, Mieli-Vergani G, Eddleston AL, Mowat AP. T suppressor cell function and number in children with liver disease. Clin Exp Immunol. 1985;61:283–9.
5. Nouri-Aria KT, Donaldson PT, Hegarty JE, Eddleston AL, Williams R. HLA A1-B8-DR3 and suppressor cell function in first-degree relatives of patients with autoimmune chronic active hepatitis. J Hepatol. 1985;1:235–41.
6. Vento S, Hegarty JE, Bottazzo G, Macchia E, Williams R, Eddleston AL. Antigen specific suppressor cell function in autoimmune chronic active hepatitis. Lancet. 1984;1:1200–4.
7. Lobo-Yeo A, Senaldi G, Portmann B, Mowat AP, Mieli-Vergani G, Vergani D. Class I and class II major histocompatibility complex antigen expression on hepatocytes: a study in children with liver disease. Hepatology. 1990;12:224–32.
8. Chen M, Shirai M, Liu Z, Arichi T, Takahashi H, Nishioka M. Efficient class II major histocompatibility complex presentation of endogenously synthesized hepatitis C virus core protein by Epstein–Barr virus-transformed B-lymphoblastoid cell lines to CD4(+) T cells. J Virol. 1998;72:8301–8.
9. Lobo-Yeo A, Alviggi L, Mieli-Vergani G, Portmann B, Mowat AP, Vergani D. Preferential activation of helper/inducer T lymphocytes in autoimmune chronic active hepatitis. Clin Exp Immunol. 1987;67:95–104.
10. Manns MP, Griffin KJ, Sullivan KF, Johnson EF. LKM-1 autoantibodies recognize a short linear sequence in P450IID6, a cytochrome P-450 monooxygenase. J Clin Invest. 1991;88:1370–8.
11. Vento S, Cainelli F, Renzini C, Concia E. Autoimmune hepatitis type 2 induced by HCV and persisting after viral clearance (letter). Lancet. 1997;350:1298–9.
12. Jensen D, McFarlane IG, Portmann B *et al.* Detection of antibodies directed against a liver-specific lipoprotein in patients with acute and chronic active hepatitis. N Engl J Med. 1978;299:1–7.
13. McFarlane BM, McSorley CG, Vergani D, McFarlane IG, Williams R. Serum autoantibodies reacting with the hepatic asialoglycoprotein receptor protein (hepatic lectin) in acute and chronic liver disorders. J Hepatol. 1986;3:196–205.
14. Ma Y, Gaken J, McFarlane BM *et al.* Alcohol dehydrogenase: a target of humoral autoimmune response in liver disease. Gastroenterology. 1997;112:483–92.
15. Vergani D, Mieli-Vergani G, Mondelli M, Portmann B, Eddleston AL. Immunoglobulin on the surface of isolated hepatocytes is associated with antibody-dependent cell-mediated cytotoxicity and liver damage. Liver. 1987;7:307–15.
16. Mieli-Vergani G, Vergani D, Jenkins PJ *et al.* Lymphocyte cytotoxicity to autologous hepatocytes in HBsAg-negative chronic active hepatitis. Clin Exp Immunol. 1979;38:16–21.
17. Wen L, Peakman M, Mowat AP *et al.* Gamma/delta+ T cell clones from liver biopsies of children with autoimmune chronic active hepatitis (aCAH) and primary sclerosing cholangitis (aPSC) are cytotoxic to human liver target cells. J Hepatol. 1991;13:S80.
18. Wen L, Peakman M, Lobo-Yeo A *et al.* T-cell-directed hepatocyte damage in autoimmune chronic active hepatitis. Lancet. 1990;336:1527–30.
19. Lohr H, Manns M, Kyriatsoulis A *et al.* Clonal analysis of liver-infiltrating T cells in patients with LKM-1 antibody-positive autoimmune chronic active hepatitis. Clin Exp Immunol. 1991;84:297–302.
20. Lohr H, Treichel U, Poralla T, Manns M, Meyer zum Buschenfelde KH. Liver-infiltrating T helper cells in autoimmune chronic active hepatitis stimulate the production of autoantibodies against the human asialoglycoprotein receptor *in vitro*. Clin Exp Immunol. 1992;88:45–9.

# 13
# 'ANCA' in liver diseases

B. TERJUNG and H. J. WORMAN

## INTRODUCTION

Antineutrophil cytoplasmic antibodies (ANCA) are heterogeneous autoantibodies directed against constituents of neutrophilic granulocytes. Since their first detection over 15 years ago, they have become valuable diagnostic tools for a variety of disorders. There is no doubt that ANCA play an important role in the diagnostic and therapeutic management of patients with systemic vasculitides such as Wegener's granulomatosis or microscopic polyangiitis. Recently, 'ANCA' have been described at particularly high frequencies in sera of patients with chronic inflammatory bowel diseases such as ulcerative colitis and Crohn's disease or autoimmune liver disorders such as primary sclerosing cholangitis and autoimmune hepatitis. However, the role of the so-called 'ANCA' in these disorders has still to gain consensus. With particular respect to this controversial discussion, this chapter aims to review the clinical and diagnostic relevance of such autoantibodies in autoimmune liver disorders.

## DEFINITION AND DETECTION METHODS FOR ANCA

ANCA are directed against constituents of neutrophils, or less frequently against proteins of monocytes. Indirect immunofluorescence microscopy has been established as the standard detection method for ANCA. With respect to the neutrophil-specific reactivity of these antibodies, slides with ethanol- or paraformaldehyde-fixed neutrophils are used as substrate and are incubated with the patient's serum. Bound ANCA are labelled with a fluorescein-conjugated secondary antibody and are then detected with a fluorescence microscope.

Two well-defined fluorescence patterns of ANCA can be distinguished on ethanol-fixed neutrophils: 'cANCA', which are characterized by a diffuse cytoplasmic staining of the neutrophils (Figure 1a) and 'pANCA', which show a fine rim-like staining of the perinuclear cytoplasm (Figure 1b). The pANCA fluorescence pattern represents an artifact due to the ethanol fixation. Strongly cationic proteins (e.g. myeloperoxidase), which have been released from azurophil or specific granules after neutrophil activation, migrate to the negatively charged

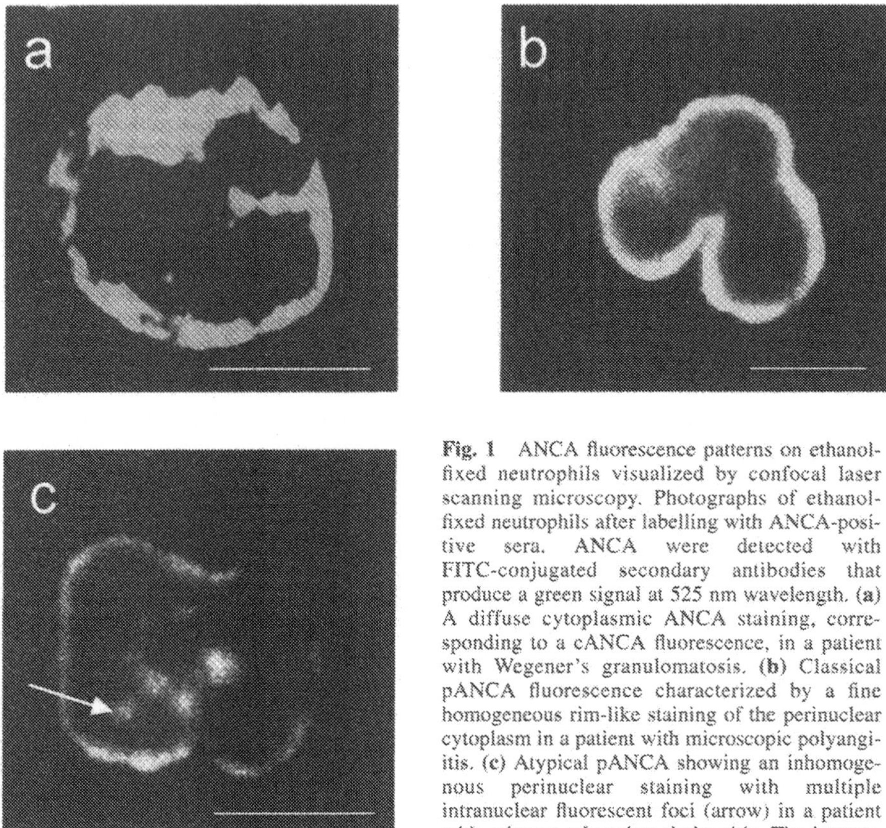


**Fig. 1** ANCA fluorescence patterns on ethanol-fixed neutrophils visualized by confocal laser scanning microscopy. Photographs of ethanol-fixed neutrophils after labelling with ANCA-positive sera. ANCA were detected with FITC-conjugated secondary antibodies that produce a green signal at 525 nm wavelength. (**a**) A diffuse cytoplasmic ANCA staining, corresponding to a cANCA fluorescence, in a patient with Wegener's granulomatosis. (**b**) Classical pANCA fluorescence characterized by a fine homogeneous rim-like staining of the perinuclear cytoplasm in a patient with microscopic polyangiitis. (**c**) Atypical pANCA showing an inhomogenous perinuclear staining with multiple intranuclear fluorescent foci (arrow) in a patient with primary sclerosing cholangitis. The intranuclear fluorescent spots correspond to infoldings of the nuclear envelope. Size bars indicate 10 $\mu$m

nuclear membrane and collapse in the perinuclear cytoplasm, giving the pANCA fluorescence. However, neutral or weakly cationic charged proteins (e.g. proteinase 3) are diffusely distributed in the neutrophils' cytoplasm after ethanol fixation yielding a cANCA staining pattern (Figure 2).

Recently a third subtype of ANCA, so called 'atypical pANCA', 'aANCA' or 'xANCA', has been classified. Contrary to the well-established staining patterns and antigen reactivities of cANCA and the classical pANCA, the significance of these atypical pANCA, their staining characteristics and association with a target antigen is rather controversial and has led to considerable confusion in the literature. Investigators still include heterogeneous staining patterns under the term atypical pANCA. Some describe a so-called 'snowdrift' fluorescence characterized by a combined cANCA and pANCA staining pattern[1]. Using high-resolution microscopy, recent reports have demonstrated that the perinuclear fluorescence of atypical pANCA in fact corresponds to a rim-like staining of the nuclear periphery (Figure 1c)[2,3]. In addition to the staining of the nuclear periphery, intranuclear fluorescent foci have been regularly found in atypical

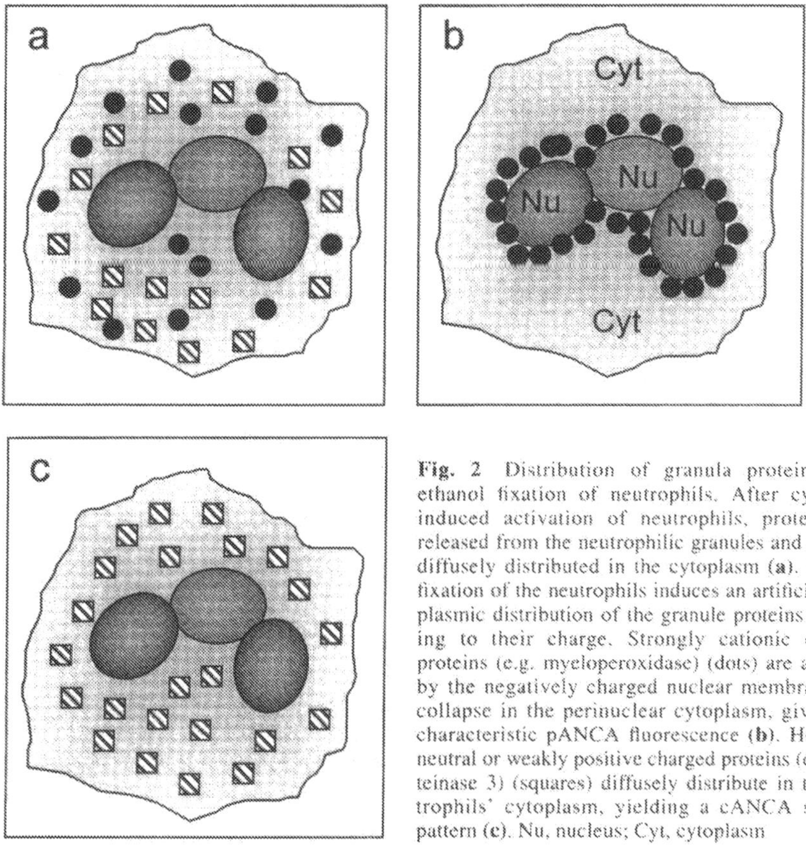


**Fig. 2** Distribution of granula proteins after ethanol fixation of neutrophils. After cytokine-induced activation of neutrophils, proteins are released from the neutrophilic granules and become diffusely distributed in the cytoplasm (**a**). Ethanol fixation of the neutrophils induces an artificial cytoplasmic distribution of the granule proteins according to their charge. Strongly cationic charged proteins (e.g. myeloperoxidase) (dots) are attracted by the negatively charged nuclear membrane and collapse in the perinuclear cytoplasm, giving the characteristic pANCA fluorescence (**b**). However, neutral or weakly positive charged proteins (e.g. proteinase 3) (squares) diffusely distribute in the neutrophils' cytoplasm, yielding a cANCA staining pattern (**c**). Nu, nucleus; Cyt, cytoplasm

pANCA. Studies using immunoelectron microscopy could attribute these intranuclear foci to infoldings of the nuclear envelope[4] (Terjung *et al.*, unpublished data). As high-resolution fluorescence microscopy cannot be used in the daily laboratory routine to distinguish between the staining of the perinuclear cytoplasm in classical pANCA and the labelling of the nuclear periphery in atypical pANCA, the characteristic focal intranuclear fluorescence of atypical pANCA might serve as a valuable tool.

## ANCA TARGET ANTIGENS AND ASSOCIATED DISORDERS

The three different ANCA subtypes – cANCA, classical pANCA and atypical pANCA – indicate a heterogeneity of the target antigens. In more than 90% of cANCA-positive sera, a reactivity to proteinase 3 (PR3), a major enzyme of the azurophil granules, can be detected (Table 1)[5,6]. This close association of ANCA staining pattern and target antigen is further enhanced as 80–95% of patients with Wegener's granulomatosis are positive for PR3-cANCA[7]. Therefore, some investigators suggested naming proteinase 3 the 'Wegener's

**Table 1** Contents of neutrophilic granules. Enzymes in italics are those which have been shown as putative target antigens of ANCA

| | *Azurophil granules* | *Specific granules* |
|---|---|---|
| Serine proteinases | *Azurocidin*<br>*Cathepsin G*<br>*Elastase*<br>*Proteinase 3* | |
| Acid hydrolases | *Beta-glucuronidase*<br>Beta-glycerophosphatase<br>N-acetyl-beta glucosaminidase<br>Cathepsin B<br>Cathepsin D | |
| Metalloproteinases | | Collagenase<br>Gelatinase |
| Other enzymes | *Bactericidal/permeability increasing protein (BPI)*<br>Defensins<br>*Lysozyme*<br>*Myeloperoxidase* | Histaminase<br><br>*Lactoferrin*<br>*Lysozyme*<br>Vitamin $B_{12}$-binding protein |

autoantigen'[8]. Recent studies showed that proteinase 3 antibodies only recognize a limited number of conformational epitopes of proteinase 3[9,10]. In only 5–20% of the patients with Wegener's granulomatosis was a pANCA fluorescence with reactivity to various other cytoplasmic proteins found.

A similar close association of an ANCA staining pattern observed by immunofluorescence microscopy and reactivity to a specific target protein was detected in sera positive for classical pANCA. The majority of those sera reacted to myeloperoxidase (MPO), a strongly cationic protein in the azurophil granules[11]. Similar to the PR3-cANCA and its close association with Wegener's granulomatosis, the MPO-pANCA was found in 60–80% of patients with pauci-immune necrotizing glomerulonephritis or microscopic polyangiitis. Various other putative target antigens of classical pANCA have also been identified, such as azurocidin[12], bactericidal/permeability increasing protein[13], beta-glucuronidase[14], cathepsin G, elastase, lactoferrin[15] or the lysosomal membrane protein h-lamp2[16]. However, reactivity to these proteins has been found in only a very small minority of sera from patients with microscopic polyangiitis and classical pANCA. Rarely, the aforementioned antigens also represented the target proteins of classical pANCA in patients with connective tissue disorders (20–35%) such as systemic lupus erythematosus, rheumatoid arthritis, Felty syndrome or in systemic vasculitides such as Churg–Strauss syndrome or polyarteritis nodosa[17].

Additional cytoplasmic constituents of the neutrophils, apart from the well-defined antigens of classical pANCA[18–22], have been proposed to be target proteins recognized by atypical pANCA. In this context, reactivity of atypical pANCA to actin[23], catalase and enolase[24, 25] or high-mobility group non-histone chromosomal protein (HMG 1/2)[26] has been reported. However, only 20–35% of the sera positive for atypical pANCA recognized one of these proteins as their target structure. Very few studies report higher percentages, but their value is limited due to small numbers of patients. The long list of putative target antigens of atypical pANCA reflects the heterogeneity of atypical pANCA as well as the fact that the predominant responsible antigen of atypical pANCA has not yet been identified.

Recent data discussed a nuclear localization of the target antigen recognized by atypical pANCA. A 50 kDa peripheral nuclear protein, epitopes of histone 1 anchoring the heterochromatin to the nuclear envelope as well as HMG 1/2, have been shown to be promising candidate proteins[2, 27–29]. We could demonstrate reactivity to a 50 kDa peripheral nuclear protein at particularly high percentages (92%) in patients with autoimmune liver disorders[27]. Antibodies to HMG 1/2 were found in 89% of patients with autoimmune hepatitis[26]. Studies on the frequencies of ANCA reacting with histone 1 are missing so far, but while interpreting these data, note that neither histones nor HMG 1/2 are neutrophil-specific proteins. Assuming a nuclear target antigen, the term ANCA, antineutrophil cytoplasmic antibodies, would be a misnomer and should be replaced by the more appropiate term ANNA, antineutrophil nuclear antibodies.

Atypical pANCA were exclusively detected in patients with chronic inflammatory bowel disorders such as ulcerative colitis (60–87%) or Crohn's disease (5–20%) as well as in autoimmune liver disorders such as primary sclerosing cholangitis (65–87%) or autoimmune hepatitis (50–96%)[2,30–38] (Table 2). Patients with other autoimmune hepatobiliary disorders such as primary biliary cirrhosis very rarely have atypical pANCA (5–29%)[35, 37–40].

## ANCA IN PRIMARY SCLEROSING CHOLANGITIS AND THEIR CLINICAL RELEVANCE

Atypical pANCA were first described in patients with chronic inflammatory bowel diseases (IBD). With respect to the fact that ulcerative colitis and Crohn's disease are associated with primary sclerosing cholangitis (PCS), and vice-versa, various studies were conducted to determine the presence of ANCA in patients with PSC. Prevalences from 33% up to 88% have been reported (Table 3), while the wide range of ANCA prevalences is most likely due to different detection techniques used. Besides the standard detection method, indirect immunofluorescence microscopy on ethanol-fixed neutrophils, some investigators either used a fixed neutrophil ELISA[19, 30, 41] or investigated their sera by immunohistochemistry using alkaline phosphatase- or immunoperoxidase-conjugated secondary antibodies[42, 43]. As to the association of PSC with either ulcerative colitis or Crohn's disease, the ANCA prevalence (65–80%) did not differ significantly between patients with PSC and associated IBD from those without associated IBD[30,32,35,44] (Table 3). Seibold and co-workers[45] were the only ones who reported a significantly higher presence of ANCA in patients with PSC without associated IBD compared to those with associated IBD. However, the value of this study is limited due to a relatively small study population. The overall results of these studies suggest that the presence of atypical pANCA in individuals with PSC is an independent phenomenon and is not merely due to

**Table 2** Association of the predominant ANCA fluorescence pattern and ANCA prevalence with the underlying disease

| *Disease* | *Predominant immunofluorescence pattern on ethanol-fixed neutrophils* | *Prevalence of ANCA(%)* | *Refs* |
|---|---|---|---|
| *Systemic vasculitides* | | | |
| Wegener's granulomatosis | cANCA | 80–90 | 5–7 |
| Microscopic polyangiitis | classical pANCA | 60–80 | 11, 15, 17 |
| Pauci-immune necrotizing glomerulonephritis | classical pANCA | 40–80 | 11, 15, 17 |
| Churg–Strauss syndrome | cANCA, classical pANCA | 10–20 | 17 |
| Polyarteritis nodosa | cANCA, classical pANCA | 10–20 | 17 |
| *Connective tissue disorders* | | | |
| Systemic lupus erythematosus | classical pANCA, rarely atypical pANCA | 15–30 | 17 |
| Rheumatoid arthritis | classical pANCA, rarely atypical pANCA | 20–40 | 17 |
| Felty syndrome | classical pANCA, rarely atypical pANCA | 40–50 | 17 |
| *Chronic inflammatory bowel diseases* | | | |
| Ulcerative colitis | atypical pANCA | 60–87 | 2, 30, 32, 33, 37, 43 |
| Crohn disease | atypical pANCA | 5–20 | 2, 30, 32, 33, 37 |
| *Autoimmune liver disorders* | | | |
| Primary sclerosing cholangitis | atypical pANCA | 65–87 | 2, 30, 32, 37, 38, 43, 44 |
| Autoimmune hepatitis | atypical pANCA | 50–96 | 2, 32, 34–38 |
| Primary biliary cirrhosis | classical pANCA, atypical pANCA | 5–29 | 35, 37–40 |

**Table 3** Overview of studies investigating the prevalence of ANCA in patients with primary sclerosing cholangitis

| *Study* | *Prevalence of ANCA (n)* | *ANCA detection technique*[a] |
|---|---|---|
| Snook *et al.*[42] | 84% (27/32) | Immunohistochemistry |
| Klein *et al.*[31] | 87% (26/30) | IIF |
| Duerr *et al.*[30] | 82%[b] (42/51)<br>79%[c] (11/14) | Fixed neutrophil ELISA, IIF |
| Lo *et al.*[43] | 77% (23/30) | Immunohistochemistry |
| Seibold *et al.*[45] | 88%[b] (15/17)<br>40%[c] (2/5) | IIF |
| Hardarson *et al.*[32] | 72%[b] (36/50)<br>76%[c] (22/29) | IIF |
| Peen *et al.*[19] | 33% (4/12) | Fixed neutrophil ELISA |
| Mulder *et al.*[33] | 79% (19/24) | IIF |
| Wilschanski *et al.*[60] | 38% (9/24) | IIF |
| Bansi *et al.*[35] | 65%[b] (41/61)<br>70%[c] (39/56) | IIF |
| Roozendaal *et al.*[44] | 67%[b] (46/69)<br>69%[c] (31/45) | IIF |

[a] ANCA detection techniques: IIF, indirect immunofluorescence microscopy using fluorescein-conjugated secondary antibodies. Immunohistochemistry, immunohistochemistry using alkaline phosphatase- or peroxidase-labelled secondary antibodies.
Fixed neutrophil ELISA, enzyme-linked immunosorbent assay using crude preparations of neutrophils which were coated onto microtitre plates and fixed with methanol.
[b] PSC without associated chronic inflammatory bowel disease (ulcerative colitis, Crohn's disease).
[c] PSC with associated chronic inflammatory bowel disease (ulcerative colitis or Crohn's disease).

individuals with PSC is an independent phenomenon and is not merely due to concomitant ulcerative colitis or Crohn's disease.

The responsible target antigen recognized by atypical pANCA in PSC remains elusive, as already discussed. Various neutrophil-specific cytoplasmic antigens with reactivity in about 20–30% of the PSC patients with atypical pANCA have been suggested. Table 4 gives an overview of the relevant studies focusing on this issue. Recently, our group demonstrated that 90% of sera from patients with PSC and atypical pANCA react with a neutrophil-specific 50 kDa protein of the nuclear periphery[27].

The clinical relevance of ANCA is well established in the diagnosis and management of patients with systemic vasculitides; however, the role of ANCA in autoimmune liver disorders is less well defined. Most investigators agree that titres of atypical pANCA in PSC do not correlate with clinical parameters such as disease activity, disease extent, disease duration and intake of medication such as ursodiol[30,38,44–46]. Very few studies observed a relationship between the presence of these autoantibodies and the disease severity. In this context, Pokorny *et al.*[47] detected biliary tract complications at higher percentages in ANCA-positive than in ANCA-negative PSC patients. Bansi and coworkers[35] reported that the presence of atypical pANCA in PSC correlated with the involvement of intra- as well as of extrahepatic biliary ducts, respectively. Mulder *et al.*[38] showed in a small collective of PSC patients that the presence of ANCA was correlated with liver cirrhosis due to PSC. Apart from these studies, which suggest a certain

**Table 4** Reactivity of ANCA to different target antigens in patients with primary sclerosing cholangitis

| *ANCA target antigen* | *Percentage reactivity to antigen (n)* | *Ref.* |
|---|---|---|
| BPI | 36% (13/36) | 20 |
| | 35% (13/37) | 22 |
| | 18% (5/28) | 13 |
| Cathepsin G | 23% (16/69) | 44 |
| | 50% (3/6) | 18 |
| | 16% (4/25) | 49 |
| Catalase | 60% (9/15) | 24 |
| Alpha-enolase | 27% (4/15) | 24 |
| Lactoferrin | 22% (15/69) | 44 |
| | 50% (6/12) | 19 |
| | 26% (5/19) | 38 |
| 50 kDa peripheral nuclear protein | 92% (21/22) | 27 |

clinical relevance of atypical pANCA in PSC, most investigators agree on the fact that atypical pANCA play a role as diagnostic parameter in PSC, but that atypical pANCA are not suitable parameters for the clinical management of patients with PSC.

Some controversy still exists whether atypical pANCA in PSC simply represent an epiphenomenon secondary to an inflammatory process of the bile ducts or whether atypical pANCA even play a role in the immunopathogenesis of PSC. The fact that atypical pANCA recur after removal of the inflamed organ by either liver transplantation for PSC or colectomy for associated ulcerative colitis convincingly defeats the theory of ANCA being simply an epiphenomenon. Unfortunately, only very few studies, mostly limited by a small number of study individuals and a relatively short follow-up period, have been conducted on this issue[48].

In conclusion, the high prevalence of atypical pANCA in PSC renders these autoantibodies a suitable seromarker for the diagnosis of PSC. The identification of the responsible antigen(s) will help to standardize the detection of atypical pANCA and to define a possible role of ANCA in the immunopathogenesis of PSC and associated disorders. As the titres of atypical pANCA in PSC do not correlate with any clinical parameters, they are not suited for the clinical management of those patients. The use of ANCA as a prognostic factor in PSC needs further investigation and long-term follow-up studies.

## ANCA IN AUTOIMMUNE HEPATITIS AND THEIR CLINICAL RELEVANCE

Since ANCA have been detected in PSC, patients with autoimmune hepatitis (AIH) were also tested for the presence of ANCA. Particularly high prevalences of ANCA have been reported for AIH ranging from 50% to 96%[32, 34, 35, 36, 40, 49] (Table 5). Based on the presence of serological immunomarkers, three different types of autoimmune hepatitis, although not accepted by all hepatologists, can be distinguished: AIH type 1 with high-titre antinuclear antibodies and/or anti-smooth muscle antibodies, AIH type 2 characterized by anti-liver/kidney microsomal type 1 antibodies and AIH type 3 defined by the presence of anti-liver cytosol type 1 antibodies. Most studies investigating the prevalence of ANCA in AIH focused on AIH type 1, comprising the vast majority of patients with AIH. Targan *et al* [34] reported the presence of high-titre atypical pANCA in 96% of the patients with AIH type 1, whereas other investigators detected atypical pANCA in only 50–75% of AIH type 1 patients[32, 33, 35]. Contrary to the high prevalence of atypical pANCA in AIH type 1, they are absent in AIH type 2 [36, 40]. Orth *et al.*[40] investigated a representative panel of patients with AIH type 3 for the presence of ANCA and were able to report atypical pANCA in 36% of the patients.

Similar to atypical pANCA in PSC, the identification of the target antigen in AIH remains elusive. Various proteins such as actin[23], bactericidal/permeability increasing protein[22], catalase[24, 25], cathepsin G[49], enolase[24, 25] and lactoferrin[38] have been described as putative target antigens of atypical pANCA in a minority of AIH patients (Table 6). In a very recent study, Sobajima *et al.*[26] reported a high prevalence (89%) of pANCA reacting with HMG 1/2 in AIH patients. However, it has to be considered that HMG 1/2 are not neutrophil-specific proteins.

The clinical significance of atypical pANCA in AIH has not been systematically studied. Orth *et al.*[23] reported a strong correlation between ANCA positivity and disease activity in AIH type 1, whereas this correlation could not be confirmed by others[34, 35, 38]. Reports on the recurrence of atypical pANCA after liver transplantation have only been reported as personal communications.

With respect to their high prevalence, atypical pANCA represent an important additional seromarker in the diagnosis of AIH. Some investigators even suggest officially including ANCA in the diagnostic criteria for AIH in addition to the

**Table 5** Overview of studies on the prevalence of ANCA in patients with autoimmune hepatitis

| *Study* | *Prevalence of ANCA (n)* | *Detection technique* |
|---|---|---|
| Hardarson *et al.*[32] | 50% (10/20) | IIF |
| Mulder *et al.*[38] | 88% (21/24) | IIF |
| Bansi *et al.*[35] | 50% (14/28) | IIF |
| Targan *et al.*[34] | 96% (100/104) | Fixed neutrophil ELISA |
| Orth *et al.*[23] | 75% (24/32)[a] | IIF |
| | 0% (0/15)[b] | |
| | 36% (10/28)[c] | |
| Zauli *et al.*[36] | 65% (30/46)[a] | IIF |
| | 0% (0/19)[b] | |
| Sobajima *et al.*[26] | 89% (25/28) | IIF |

For explanations and abbreviations of ANCA detection techniques see Table 3.
[a] Autoimmune hepatitis type 1.
[b] Autoimmune hepatitis type 2.
[c] Autoimmune hepatitis type 3.

**Table 6** Reactivity of ANCA to different target antigens in patients with autoimmune hepatitis

| *ANCA target antigen* | *Percentage reactivity to antigen (n)* | *Ref.* |
|---|---|---|
| Actin | 63% (20/32) | 23 |
| BPI | 29% (4/14) | 22 |
| Cathepsin G | 29% (5/17) | 38 |
| HMG 1/2 | 89% (25/28) | 26 |
| Lactoferrin | 8% (2/24) | 38 |
| 50 kDa peripheral nuclear protein | 92% (23/25) | 27 |

well-defined histopathological and serological characteristics[50]. At this point it should be emphasized that each patient's sera should be carefully investigated for the simultaneous presence of antinuclear antibodies (ANA) and ANCA. To reliably distinguish between both antibody types, sera should always be tested on Hep G2 cells for the presence of ANA as well as on ethanol-fixed neutrophils for the presence of ANCA. However, as ANA frequently also stain neutrophils, it has been decided that in case of simultaneous staining of ethanol-fixed neutrophils by ANA and ANCA, respectively, the titre of ANCA should be at least two-fold higher than the ANA titre.

## ANCA IN PRIMARY BILIARY CIRRHOSIS AND THEIR CLINICAL RELEVANCE

In contrast to PSC and AIH, only a minority of sera from patients with primary biliary cirrhosis (PBC) yields ANCA (5–29%)[35, 37–40]. A responsible target antigen of ANCA in PBC has not been identified. As to the low prevalence, studies concerning a putative correlation of ANCA with clinical parameters have not been undertaken. Compared to the high frequency of antimitochondrial antibodies in PBC, ANCA do not represent a suitable diagnostic seromarker.

## ANCA IN NON-AUTOIMMUNE LIVER DISORDERS AND THEIR CLINICAL RELEVANCE

Chronic hepatitis C virus infection (HCV) by itself as well as interferon-alpha therapy to treat the HCV infection are well known to induce various autoimmune reactions. Under these circumstances multiple low-titre autoantibodies (such as antinuclear antibodies, anti-smooth muscle antibodies, antibodies against thyreoglobulin) are frequently detected[51]. ANCA have also been found at low frequency (5–12%) in patients infected with HCV32[51]. The ANCA titers do not show any correlation with clinical parameters. Interestingly, we could demonstrate that the response rate to interferon therapy for patients with HCV infection was lower in ANCA-positive patients than in ANCA-negative patients[52]. However, interpretation of this observation was limited due to the small number of patients. To reliably decide whether ANCA represent a valuable prognostic marker for the response rate to interferon therapy in HCV patients, further studies are needed, also considering the combination therapy of interferon and ribavirin.

The prevalence of ANCA in chronic hepatitis B virus infection has not been systematically studied. However, preliminary data demonstrate the presence of ANCA in about 7–10% of patients with chronic hepatitis B[32]. The influence of ANCA on the response rate to interferon or lamivudine therapy has not been investigated.

Serum samples from patients with various non-autoimmune liver disorders such as alcoholic liver cirrhosis, cryptogenic liver cirrhosis or heamochromatosis served as disease controls in many studies. However, in none of these patients with non-autoimmune liver disorders have ANCA been found[32, 35, 38].

## ANCA AND THEIR ROLE IN IMMUNOPATHOGENESIS OF AUTOIMMUNE LIVER DISORDERS

The putative immunopathogenic role of ANCA has been extensively studied for patients with vasculitides such as Wegener's granulomatosis or microscopic polyangiitis. The so-called 'ANCA–cytokine-sequence-hypothesis' is accepted by many investigators and provides evidence for a role of ANCA in the immunoinflammatory processes of systemic vasculitides[53–56]. This hypothetical in-vitro model assumes an initial triggering infection, but the putative pathogens are not yet known. Neutrophils become activated after priming by proinflammatory cytokines such as interleukin 8 or tumour necrosis factor alpha. This activation of the neutrophils induces their granule proteins to be released from the azurophil and specific granules, and these proteolytic enzymes are then translocated and expressed on the neutrophils' surface. Circulating ANCA bind via neutrophil-specific FcγIII-receptors to their specific target antigen on the neutrophils' surface, which further enhances the oxidative burst and the degranulation of proteolytic proteins. However, these granule proteins are expressed not only on the neutrophils' surface, but also on the surface of endothelial cells, where they induce an enhanced expression of adhesion molecules (e.g. ICAM-1, intercellular adhesion molecule, ELAM-1, endothelial leukocyte adhesion molecule). Neutrophils are then attracted to the endothelial cells via the adhesion molecules, and this finally sets the stage for the disease-specific vascular injury.

Attempts to support a similar pathogenic role for atypical pANCA in autoimmune liver disorders have been fraught with problems such as the lack of convincing animal models. One exception may be an animal model suggested by Mizoguchi *et al.*[57] of T-cell receptor alpha negative mice which spontaneously developed an ulcerative colitis-like syndrome. ANCA were detectable in the serum of the T-cell receptor alpha negative, but not in T-cell receptor positive mice. Although these data do not provide evidence that atypical pANCA are pathogenic in these disorders, atypical pANCA may function as a marker antibody for a yet-unidentified dysregulation of the immune system[58].

This assumed alteration in the immune regulation inherent to autoimmune hepatobiliary disorders also represents one of the most likely explanations for the high prevalence of ANCA in so-called overlap syndromes (e.g. primary sclerosing cholangitis associated with autoimmune hepatitis, ulcerative colitis along with primary sclerosing cholangitis). In this context Boberg *et al.*[59] and we (unpublished data) could demonstrate atypical pANCA in patients with overlap syndromes at higher percentages (29/31; 97%) than they were found in patients with primary sclerosing cholangitis (77%), autoimmune hepatitis (81%) and ulcerative colitis (69%) without associated hepatobiliary disease. Although these high prevalences of ANCA in overlap syndromes do not provide any direct evidence for atypical pANCA being involved in the immunopathogenesis of these disorders, it seems unlikely that atypical pANCA merely represent an epiphenomenon secondary to inflammation in those disorders.

## RECOMMENDATIONS ON HOW TO USE ANCA IN THE DAILY CLINICAL ROUTINE

Contrary to the established role of cANCA and classical pANCA in the diagnosis and management of patients with systemic vasculitides, the role of atypical pANCA in autoimmune liver disorders has still to be defined. In this regard the identification of the target antigen(s) will be one of the most crucial steps. Currently, indirect immunofluorescence microscopy on ethanol- and/or paraformaldehyde-fixed neutrophils should be exclusively performed for the detection of atypical pANCA. Although various enzyme-linked immunosorbent assays for the detection of putative target antigens are commercially available, none of these test systems covers the entire panel of suggested target proteins. Furthermore, the test results are frequently characterized by a very high intra- and inter-test variability; therefore they should not be used in the daily laboratory routine. Contrary to ANCA in patients with systemic vasculitides, the titre of atypical pANCA in patients with autoimmune liver disorders does not correlate with the disease activity, the disease extent or duration. The ANCA titre is not altered by the intake of immunosuppressive drugs. Therefore, atypical pANCA in autoimmune liver disorders do not represent a suitable seromarker for the clinical and therapeutic management of these patients. However, atypical pANCA can be used as a valuable seromarker for the diagnosis of autoimmune liver disorders in addition to the disease-specific diagnostic criteria.

### References

1. Rump JA, Schölmerich J, Gross V *et al.* A new type of perinuclear anti-neutrophil cytoplasmic antibody (p-ANCA) in active ulcerative colitis but not in Crohn's disease. Immunobiology. 1990;181:406–13.
2. Terjung B, Herzog V, Worman HJ, *et al.* Atypical antineutrophil cytoplasmic antibodies with perinuclear fluorescence in chronic inflammatory bowel diseases and hepatobiliary disorders colocalize with nuclear lamina proteins. Hepatology. 1998;28:332–340.
3. Billing P, Tahir S, Calfin B, Gagne G, Cobb L, Targan S, Vidrich A. Nuclear localization of the antigen detected by ulcerative colitis-associated perinuclear antineutrophil cytoplasmic antibodies. Am J Pathol. 1995;147:979–87.

4. Fricker M, Hollinshead M, White N, Vaux D. Interphase nuclei of many mammalian cell types contain deep, dynamic, tubular membrane-bound invaginations of the nuclear envelope. J Cell Biol. 1997;136:531–44.
5. Goldschmeding R, van der Schoot CE, Ten Bokkel Huinink D *et al.* Wegener's granulomatosis autoantibodies identify a novel diisopropylfluorophosphate-binding protein in the lysosomes of normal human neutrophils. J Clin Invest. 1989;84:1577–87.
6. Lüdemann J, Utecht B, Gross WL. Anti-neutrophil cytoplasm antibodies in Wegener's granulomatosis recognize an elastinolytic enzyme. J Exp Med. 1990;171:357–62.
7. Woude van der FJ, Lobatto S, Permin H *et al.* Autoantibodies against neutrophils and monocytes: tools for diagnosis and marker of disease activity in Wegener's granulomatosis. Lancet. 1985;1:425–9.
8. Jenne DE, Tschopp J, Lüdemann J, Utecht B, Gross WL. Wegener's autoantigen decoded. Nature. 1990;346:520.
9. Sommarin Y, Rasmussen N, Wieslander J. Characterization of monoclonal antibodies to proteinase 3 and application in the study of epitopes for classical anti-neutrophil cytoplasm antibodies. Exp Nephrol. 1995;3:249–56.
10. Sun J, Fass DN, Viss MA, Hummel AM, Tang H, Homburger HA, Specks U. A proportion of proteinase 3 (PR3)-specific anti-neutrophil cytoplasmic antibodies (ANCA) only react with PR3 after cleavage of its N-terminal activation dipeptide. Clin Exp Immunol. 1998;114:320–6.
11. Falk RJ, Jennette JC. Anti-neutrophil cytoplasmic autoantibodies with specificity for myeloperoxidase in patients with systemic vasculitis and idiopathic necrotizing and crescentic glomerulonephritis. N Engl J Med. 1988;318:1651–7.
12. Zhao MH, Lockwood CM. Azurocidin is a novel antigen for anti-neutrophil cytoplasmic autoantibodies (ANCA) in systemic vasculitis. Clin Exp Immunol. 1996;103:397–402.
13. Zhao MH, Jones SJ, Lockwood CM. Bactericidal/permeability-increasing protein (BPI) is an important antigen for anti-neutrophil cytoplasmic autoantibodies (ANCA) in vasculitis. Clin Exp Immunol. 1995;99:49–56.
14. Martensson U, Nässberger L. Circulating autoantibodies directed against beta-glucuronidase (letter). Autoimmunity. 1992;11:213–14.
15. Lesavre P, Noel LH, Chauveau D, Geffriaud C, Grünfeld JP. Antigen specificities and clinical distribution of ANCA in kidney diseases. Klin Wochenschr. 1991;69:552–7.
16. Kain R, Matsui K, Exner M *et al.* A novel class of autoantigens of anti-neutrophil cytoplasmic antibodies in necrotizing and crescentic glomerulonephritis: the lysosomal membrane glycoprotein h-lamp-2 in neutrophil granulocytes and a related membrane protein in glomerular endothelial cells. J Exp Med. 1995;181:585–97.
17. Geffriaud-Ricouard C, Noel LH, Chauveau D, Houhou S, Grünfeld JP, Lesavre P. Clinical spectrum associated with ANCA of defined antigen specificities in 98 selected patients. Clin Nephrol. 1993;39:125–36.
18. Halbwachs-Mecarelli L, Nusbaum P, Noel LH *et al.* Antineutrophil cytoplasmic antibodies (ANCA) directed against cathepsin G in ulcerative colitis, Crohn's disease and primary sclerosing cholangitis. Clin Exp Immunol. 1992;90:79–84.
19. Peen E, Almer S, Bodemar G *et al.* Anti-lactoferrin antibodies and other types of ANCA in ulcerative colitis, primary sclerosing cholangitis, and Crohn's disease. Gut. 1993;34:56–62.
20. Stoffel MP, Csernok E, Herzberg C, Johnston T, Carrol SF, Gross WL. Anti-neutrophil cytoplasmic antibodies (ANCA) directed against bactericidal/permeability increasing protein (BPI): a new seromarker for inflammatory bowel disease and associated disorders. Clin Exp Immunol. 1996;104:54–9.
21. Walmsley RS, Zhao MH, Hamilton MI *et al.* Antineutrophil cytoplasm autoantibodies against bactericidal/permeability-increasing protein in inflammatory bowel disease. Gut. 1997;40:105–9.
22. Schnabel A, Csernok E, Schultz H *et al.* Bactericidal/permeability increasing protein (BPI)-ANCA markiert chronische entzündliche Darmerkrankungen und entzündliche hepatobiliäre Erkrankungen. Med Klin. 1997;92:389–93.
23. Orth T, Gerken G, Kellner R, Meyer zum Büschenfelde KH, Mayet WJ. Actin is a target antigen of anti-neutrophil cytoplasmic antibodies (ANCA) in autoimmune hepatitis type-1. J Hepatol. 1997;26:37–47.
24. Orth T, Kellner R, Diekmann O, Faust J, Meyer zum Büschenfelde KH, Mayet WJ. Identification and characterization of autoantibodies against catalase and $\alpha$-enolase in patients with primary sclerosing cholangitis. Clin Exp Immunol. 1998;112:507–15.

25. Roozendaal C, Zhao MH, Horst G *et al.* Catalase and $\alpha$-enolase: two novel granulocyte antigens in inflammatory bowel disease (IBD). Clin Exp Immunol. 1998;112:10–16.
26. Sobajima J, Ozaki S, Uesugi H *et al.* High mobility group (HMG) non-histone chromosomal proteins HMG1 and HMG2 are significant target antigens of perinuclear anti-neutrophil cytoplasmic antibodies in autoimmune hepatitis. Gut. 1999;44:867–73.
27. Terjung B, Spengler U, Sauerbruch T, Worman HJ. 'Atypical p-ANCA' in IBD and hepatobiliary disorders react with a 50 kD nuclear envelope protein of neutrophils and myeloid cell lines. Gastroeterology. (in press.)
28. Eggena M, Targan SR, Iwanczyk L, Vidrich A, Gordon LK, Braun J. Phage display cloning and characterization of an immunogenetic marker (perinuclear anti-neutrophil cytoplasmic antibody) in ulcerative colitis. J Immunol. 1996;156:4005–11.
29. Cohavy O, Eggena MP, Parseghian M *et al.* Histone H1, a candidate p-ANCA antigen in ulcerative colitis. Gastroenterology. 1997;112:A951.
30. Duerr RH, Targan SR, Landers CJ *et al.* Neutrophil cytoplasmic antibodies: a link between primary sclerosing cholangitis and ulcerative colitis. Gastroenterology. 1991;100:1385–91.
31. Klein R, Eisenburg J, Weber P, Seibold F, Berg PA. Significance and specificity of antibodies to neutrophils detected by Western blotting for the serological diagnosis of primary sclerosing cholangitis. Hepatology. 1991;14:1147–52.
32. Hardarson S, Labrecque DR, Mitros FA, Neil GA, Goeken JA. Antineutrophil cytoplasmic antibody in inflammatory bowel and hepatobiliary diseases. Am J Clin Pathol. 1993;99:277–81.
33. Mulder AHL, Broekroelofs J, Horst G, Limburg PC, Nelis GF. Anti-neutrophil cytoplasmic antibodies (ANCA) in inflammatory bowel disease: characterization and clinical correlates. Clin Exp Immunol. 1994;95:490–7.
34. Targan S, Landers C, Vidrich A, Czaja AJ. High-titer antineutrophil cytoplasmic antibodies in type-1 autoimmune hepatitis. Gastroenterology. 1995;108:1159–66.
35. Bansi D, Chapman R, Fleming K. Antineutrophil cytoplasmic antibodies in chronic liver diseases: prevalence, titre, specificity and Ig G subclass. J Hepatol. 1996;24:581–6.
36. Zauli D, Ghetti S, Grassi A *et al.* Anti-neutrophil cytoplasmic antibodies in type 1 and type 2 autoimmune hepatitis. Hepatology. 1997;25:1105–7.
37. Claise C, Johanet C, Bouhnik Y, Kapel N, Homberg JC, Poupon R. Antineutrophil cytoplasmic autoantibodies in autoimmune liver and inflammatory bowel diseases. Liver. 1996;16:28–34.
38. Mulder AHL, Horst G, Haagsma EB, Limburg PC, Kleibeuker JH, Kallenberg CGM. Prevalence and characterization of neutrophil cytoplasmic antibodies in autoimmune liver diseases. Hepatology. 1993;17:411–17.
39. Seibold F, Weber P, Schöning A, Mork H, Goppel S, Scheurlen M. Neutrophil antibodies (pANCA) in chronic liver disease and inflammatory bowel disease: do they react with different antigens? Eur J Gastroenterol Hepatol. 1996;8:1095–1100.
40. Orth T, Gerken G, Meyer zum Büschenfelde KH, Mayet WJ. Antineutrophil nuclear antibodies (ANNA) in primary biliary cirrhosis: their prevalence and antigen specificity. Z Gastroenterol. 1997;35:113–21.
41. Saxon A, Shanahan F, Landers C, Ganz T, Targan S. A distinct subset of antineutrophil cytoplasmic antibodies is associated with inflammatory bowel disease. J Allergy Clin Immunol. 1990;86:202–10.
42. Snook JA, Chapman RW, Fleming K, Jewell DP. Anti-neutrophil nuclear antibody in ulcerative colitis, Crohn's disease and primary sclerosing cholangitis. Clin Exp Immunol. 1989;76:30–3.
43. Lo SK, Fleming KA, Chapman RW. Prevalence of anti-neutrophil antibody in primary sclerosing cholangitis and ulcerative colitis using an alkaline phosphatase technique. Gut. 1992;33:1370–5.
44. Roozendaal C, van Milligen de Wit AWM, Haagsma EB *et al.* Antineutrophil cytoplasmic antibodies in primary sclerosing cholangitis: defined specificities may be associated with distinct clinical features. Am J Med. 1998;105:393–9.
45. Seibold F, Weber P, Klein R, Berg PA, Wiedmann KH. Clinical significance of antibodies against neutrophils in patients with inflammatory bowel disease and primary sclerosing cholangitis. Gut. 1992;33:657–62.
46. Lo SK, Fleming KA, Chapman RW. A 2-year follow-up study of anti-neutrophil antibody in primary sclerosing cholangitis: relationship to clinical activity, liver biochemistry and ursodeoxycholic acid treatment. J Hepatol. 1994;21:974–8.
47. Pokorny CS, Norton ID, McCaughan GW, Selby WS. Anti-neutrophil cytoplasmic antibody: a prognostic indicator in primary sclerosing cholangitis. J Gastroenterol Hepatol. 1994;9:40–4.

48. Haagsma EB, Mulder AHL, Gouw ASH, Meermann HG, Slooff MJH, Kallenberg CGM. Neutrophil cytoplasmic autoantibodies after liver transplantation in patients with primary sclerosing cholangitis. J Hepatol. 1993;19:8–14.
49. Lesavre P, Noel LH, Gayno S *et al.* Atypical autoantigen targets of perinuclear antineutrophil cytoplasm antibodies (p-ANCA): specificity and clinical associations. J Autoimmun. 1993;6:185–95.
50. Johnson PJ, McFarlane IG. Meeting report: International autoimmune hepatitis group. Hepatology. 1993;18:998–1005.
51. Heller J, Musiolik I, Homrighausen A, Sauerbruch T, Spengler U. Vorkommen und Bedeutung von Autoantikörpern im Rahmen der Interferontherapie der chronischen Hepatitis C. Deut Med Wochenschr. 1996;121:1179–83.
52. Terjung B, Musiolik I, Spengler U, Sauerbruch T. Antineutrophil cytoplasmic antibodies in hepatitis C indicate a poor response to interferon therapy. Gut. 1995;37:A114.
53. Gross WL, Schmitt WH, Csernok E. ANCA and associated diseases: immunodiagnostic and pathogenetic aspects. Clin Exp Immunol. 1993;91:1–12.
54. Reumaux D, Vossebeld PJM, Roos D, Verhoeven AJ. Effect of tumor necrosis factor-induced integrin activation on Fc$\gamma$receptorII-mediated signal transduction: relevance for activation of neutrophils by anti-proteinase 3 or anti-myeloperoxidase antibodies. Blood 1995;86:3189–95.
55. Brouwer E, Huitema MG, Klok PA *et al.* Anti-myeloperoxidase-associated proliferative glomerulonephritis: an animal model. J Exp Med. 1993;177:905–14.
56. Heeringa P, Brouwer E, Cohen Tervaert JW, Weening JJ, Kallenberg CGM. Animal models of anti-neutrophil cytoplasmic antibody associated vasculitis. Kidney Int. 1998;53:253–63.
57. Mizoguchi E, Mizoguchi A, Chiba C, Niles JL, Bhan AK. Antineutrophil cytoplasmic antibodies in T cell receptor $\alpha$-deficient mice with chronic colitis. Gastroenterology. 1997;113:1828–35.
58. Targan S. The search for pathogenic antigens in ulcerative colitis. Gastroenterology. 1998;114:1099–1100.
59. Boberg KM, Fausa O, Haaland G *et al.* Features of autoimmune hepatitis in primary sclerosing cholangitis: an evaluation of 114 primary sclerosing cholangitis patients according to a scoring system for the diagnosis of autoimmune hepatitis. Hepatology. 1996;23:1369–76.
60. Wilschanski M, Chait P, Wade JA *et al.* Primary sclerosing cholangitis in 32 children: clinical, laboratory, and radiographic features, with survival analysis. Hepatology. 1995;22:1415–22.

# 14
# Reactivity of autoimmune hepatitis sera with glutathione S-transferase

J. WĘSIERSKA-GĄDEK and E. PENNER

## INTRODUCTION

Autoimmune hepatitis (AIH)[1–4], an inflammatory liver disease, represents histologically and serologically a broad spectrum of characteristic features. The classification of AIH is primarily based on serological criteria. Type I AIH is defined by antibodies to nuclei (ANA) and eventually actin, while type II AIH is characterized by antimicrosomal antibodies recognizing cytochrome P450IID6[2–6]. Moreover, a substantial number of AIH patients[7–11] produce antibodies to a cytosolic soluble antigen[7–10], either alone or in combination with antinuclear and/or smooth muscle antibodies (SMA). One may assume that these patients represent a distinct AIH subgroup. However, two different cytosolic antigens have been described: liver–pancreas-specific antigen (LP)[12] and soluble liver antigen (SLA)[7]. From originally described characteristics and a careful comparison of the isolation procedure it can be deduced that the antigens are identical. Both antigens were defined as non-species-, non-organ-specific, despite their highest concentration being in the liver. According to the published protocols they were obtained as a supernatant after extensive ultracentrifugation of the tissue[9] homogenates, indicating their extremely high solubility. Moreover, both antigens represent a very heterogeneous fraction, consisting of at least 100 different proteins. Therefore, one might expect that human autoantibodies would exhibit specificity against more than a single antigen target.

In the present study we describe identification of three members of the glutathione *S*-transferase (GST) gene family as a major antigen for anti-SLA-seropositive AIH patients. GST, being highly expressed in liver, are primarily localized in the cytoplasm and represent key proteins mediating hepatic detoxification and acting as carrier proteins in biliary secretion.

## MATERIAL AND METHODS

### Patients

Sera were obtained from 31 untreated AIH patients seropositive for anti-SLA antibodies. Testing for anti-SLA followed the method described by Manns *et al.*[7]. Twenty-five of the patients were women (81%) with a mean age of 40 years (range 7–63), and seven (23%) had associated cirrhosis at the initial evaluation. Of these 31 patients, 12 sera reacted solely with SLA. Of the remaining 19 sera, 10 were also positive for ANA, four sera reacted with SMA, while five patients had both ANA and SMA. Anti-SLA-negative sera were obtained from patients with AIH type I ($n$ = 10), AIH type II ($n$ = 10), and from patients with chronic hepatitis C ($n$ = 10). Ten healthy individuals served as normal controls.

All patients with AIH type I, type II and anti-SLA-positive AIH fulfilled the criteria for definite disease[2,3,4,9], with aggregate scores >15. The patients with chronic hepatitis C had elevated serum aminotransferase concentrations, anti-HCV and HCV-RNA in serum, as well as chronic hepatitis on liver biopsy.

### Indirect immunofluorescence

All sera were tested by immunofluorescence microscopy for the presence of ANA and SMA using Hep-2 cells and rodent tissue preparations (Kallestad, Houston, TX). Sera were considered positive for ANA and for SMA at a dilution of ≥ 1:40.

### Isolation of SLA from rat liver

SLA was isolated from perfused rat liver according to a previously described protocol[7,13], in the presence of protease inhibitors. Briefly, liver was homogenized in a saccharose solution (0.25 M saccharose, 50 mM Tris/HCl, pH 7.4; 1 mM DTT, 1 mM PMSF, 100 $\mu$M Pefabloc). The homogenate was filtered to exclude cellular debris and fractionated by the successive centrifugation steps[13,14], yielding four subcellular fractions: (a) crude nuclei pelleted after 800 *g* for 15 min, (b) mitochondria after 8500 *g* for 15 min; (c) microsomes after 110 000 *g* for 2 h and (d) cytosol corresponding to the supernatant from the last centrifugation.

### Isolation of SLA from human liver

Post-resection liver specimens (3–4 g from one patient) were used for the preparation of SLA according to the above-described protocol.

### Immunodiffusion

For immunodiffusion biotinylated rat liver cytosol proteins (Amersham biotinylation kit) were mixed with their unmodified counterparts (20 mg/ml) in a ratio of 1:1000. Precipitin lines were excised, and eluted immune complexes were analysed.

## Immunoprecipitation

Biotinylated rat liver cytosol proteins (5–10 $\mu$g) or 0.5–1 $\mu$g biotinylated GST in a final volume of 100 $\mu$l was incubated with 10 $\mu$l patients' serum for 2 h at room temperature and then with 40 $\mu$l of prewashed Protein-G-Sepharose (Pharmacia Fine Chemicals, Uppsala, Sweden). Afterwards beads were washed stringently. Immune complexes eluted with SDS-sample buffer were electrophoretically separated and electroblotted onto membrane. Total proteins were visualized by Ponceau-S staining and biotinylated antigens were detected autoradiographically after incubation with streptavidin–horseradish peroxidase (HRP).

## Electrophoretic separation of proteins

Proteins were separated by one-dimensional SDS-PAGE as described by Laemmli[15], or by two-dimensional PAGE according to O'Farrell[16], and detected by Coomassie-blue R-250 staining.

## Immunoblotting

Immunoblotting was performed as described previously[17]. Separated proteins were transferred onto membranes and stained by Ponceau-S. The blots were probed with diluted sera (1:500), extensively washed and incubated with anti-human Ig-HRP (Amersham International, Little Chalfont, UK). The reactive antigens were detected by chemiluminescence using ECL kit (Amersham) and X-Omat S film (Eastman Kodak Co., Rochester, NY). Biotinylated antigens precipitated during immunodiffusion or immunoprecipitation were visualized autoradiographically after incubation of the blots with streptavidin-HRP and ECL kit.

## Microsequencing

For microsequencing, electrophoretically separated proteins were transferred on a polypropylene membrane (Selex-20; Schleicher & Schuell GmbH, Dassel), Coomassie-blue R-250 stained. Protein spots were excised and their N-terminal amino acid sequences were analysed on a HP G1005 A gasphase-sequenator.

## Glutathione-affinity chromatography

GST was purified from isolated SLA by glutathione-affinity chromatography[18]. The enzyme was eluted from the affinity column by competitive action of 10 mM glutathione in a buffer containing 50 mM Tris/HCl, pH 7.4 and 1 mM PMSF.

# RESULTS

Soluble liver antigen was prepared according to the original protocol described by Manns *et al.*[7]. Its electrophoretic analysis (Figure 1) revealed that this preparation consists of many proteins, the most prominent lying within the molecular weight range 20–50 kDa. In the first step we tested whether cytokeratins 8 and 18, previously reported as targets for anti-SLA activity, are present in the prepa-

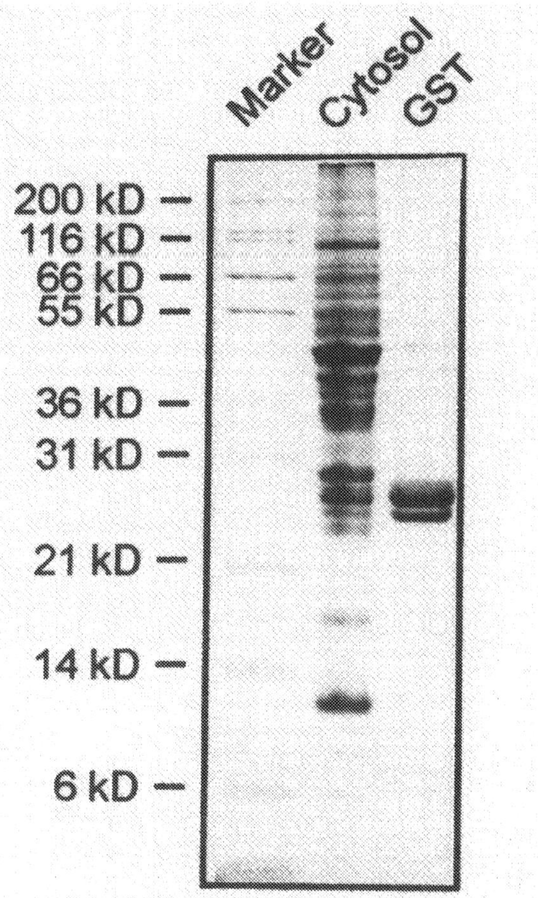


**Fig. 1** Analysis of soluble liver antigen (SLA) isolated from rat liver and purified glutathione *S*-transferase. Proteins separated on 15% SDS gel were stained with Coomassie-blue R-250. Molecular weight markers: myosin, 200 kDa; $\beta$-galactosidase, 116 kDa; phosphorylase b, 97 kDa; BSA, 66 kDa; glutamic dehydrogenase, 55 kDa; lactate dehydrogenase, 36 kDa; carbonic anhydrase, 31 kDa; trypsin inhibitor, 21 kDa; lysozyme, 14 kDa; aprotinin, 6 kDa

ration of liver cytosol. As shown in Figure 2, specific anticytokeratin monoclonals did not stain 48 kDa and 52 kDa protein bands in the sample of liver cytosol. However, corresponding recombinant antigens used as positive control were stained by the monoclonal antibodies, thereby proving the specificity of anticytokeratin antibodies and showing the absence of cytokeratins in the preparation of liver cytosol.

In the next step we characterized the serological profile of our AIH patient group. The presence of ANA, SMA and LKM was determined by immunofluorescence, whereas for evaluation of anti-SLA seropositivity immunodiffusion tests were performed. Thirty-one AIH sera were anti-SLA-positive and were used for further experiments. Screening of anti-SLA-positive sera by

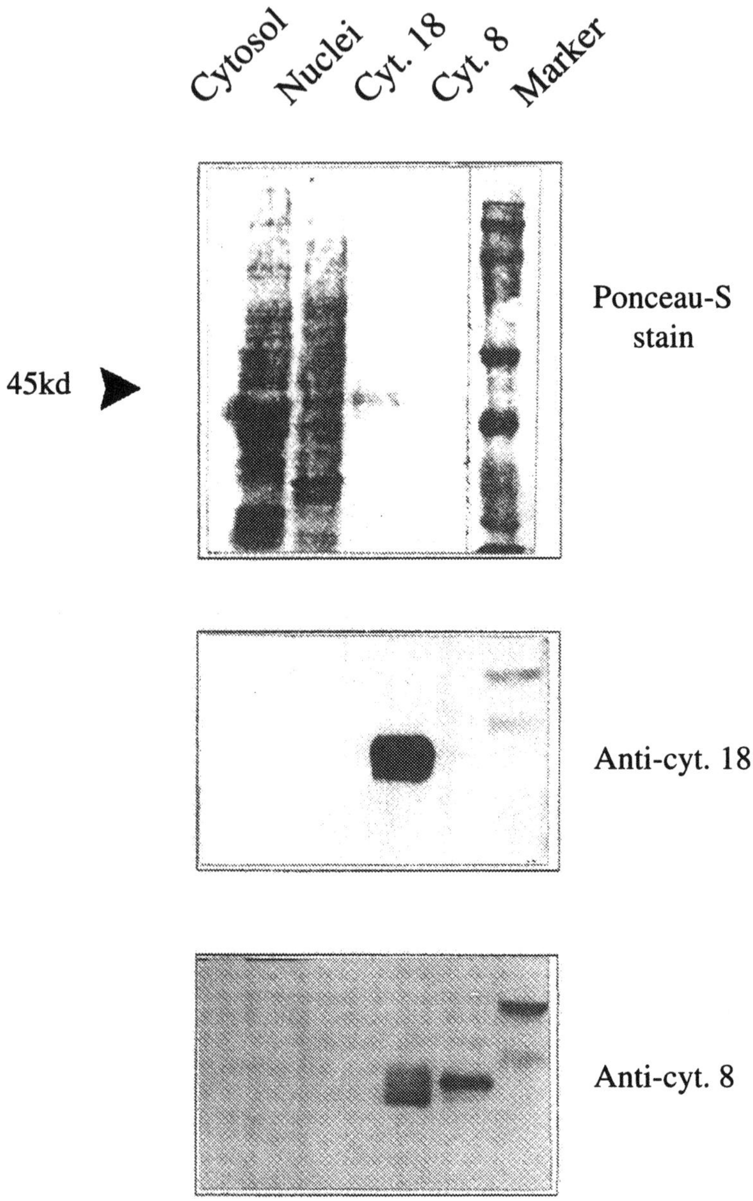


**Fig. 2** Testing of liver cytosol for the presence of cytokeratin 8 and 18. Proteins of soluble liver cytosol and nuclei (20 μg/lane) isolated from rat liver and recombinant cytokeratin 8 and 18 proteins were loaded on 10% SDS slab gel. Separated proteins were blotted onto a membrane, Ponceau-S stained and probed with anticytokeratin antibodies (Roche, 1:2000). Immune complexes were visualized by chemiluminescence using ECL + detection reagent from Amersham. Marker-Rainbow marker (Amersham)

immunoblotting on rat liver cytosol revealed positivity for several cytosol proteins. To characterize the target antigen(s) we used three different approaches. We first allowed immune complexes to form by immunodiffusion using rat liver cytosol as antigen source. To facilitate the discrimination between human serum proteins and immunoprecipitated antigens we biotinylated proteins of liver cytosol. After electrophoretic separation and transfer of immune complexes, total proteins encompassing a bulk of human serum proteins and liver antigens were stained by Ponceau-S. A sequential incubation of blots with streptavidin-HRP in the presence of an appropriate substrate visualized solely precipitated antigens. Of 31 anti-SLA-positive sera, 17 (55%) precipitated proteins in the molecular weight range 25–27 kDa. Depending on the human serum two or three precipitated peptides were detected (not shown).

In a second approach we performed immunoprecipitation using biotinylated proteins of rat liver cytosol. Immune complexes purified by affinity chromatography on Protein-G-Plus-Sepharose were electrophoretically separated and blotted onto membrane. By Ponceau-S total precipitated proteins, including a bulk of isolated immunoglobulins, were stained, whereas by autoradiography solely biotinylated antigens could be detected (Figure 3). Analysis of immune complexes revealed that the majority of anti-SLA-positive sera (25 of 31) precipitated one to three biotinylated proteins ranging between 25 and 27 kDa. If serum was omitted, or normal serum was applied, no biotinylated proteins could be detected, indicating that the reactivity was specific (Figure 3). Interestingly, by immunoprecipitation eight additional sera reactive with the low molecular antigens were detected, presumably due to the higher sensitivity of the assay.

Finally, we tested anti-SLA-positive sera by immunoblotting after separation of rat liver cytosol proteins by one-dimensional (Figure 4) and two-dimensional PAGE. Twenty-five anti-SLA-positive sera that immunoprecipitated proteins in the range 25–27 kDa stained on immunoblots at least one corresponding protein band.

An analysis of the results obtained by all methods revealed that the majority of the anti-SLA-positive AIH sera (81%) but none of normal controls (Figure 4) preferentially react with one to three proteins in the molecular weight range 25–27 kDa. To identify the autoantigens, reactive protein spots were excised from the membrane and submitted for protein sequencing. Microsequencing combined with mass spectrometry revealed that at least three subunits of glutathione *S*-transferase (GST): Ya (subunit 1), $Yb_1$ (subunit 3) and Yc (subunit 2), are the targets for autoantibodies to SLA. To unequivocally prove the identity of the autoantigens we next isolated GST from rat liver cytosol by affinity chromatography. As judged by Coomassie-blue (Figure 1) we purified to homogeneity a set of at least three related proteins that were not satisfactorily resolved by one-dimensional SDS-PAGE due to overlapping protein bands. Their separation by two-dimensional PAGE (IEF/SDS) revealed four spots differing slightly in their charges and molecular weights. They represented subunits Ya, $Yb_1$, $Yb_2$ and Yc. Immunoblotting using polyclonal antibodies specific for distinct GST subtypes confirmed their identity ascertained on the basis of $NH_2$-terminal sequence and characteristic charges.

Most of the anti-SLA-positive sera (25 of 31) immunoprecipitated purified enzyme (not shown) and reacted with it in immunoblotting tests (Figure 5).

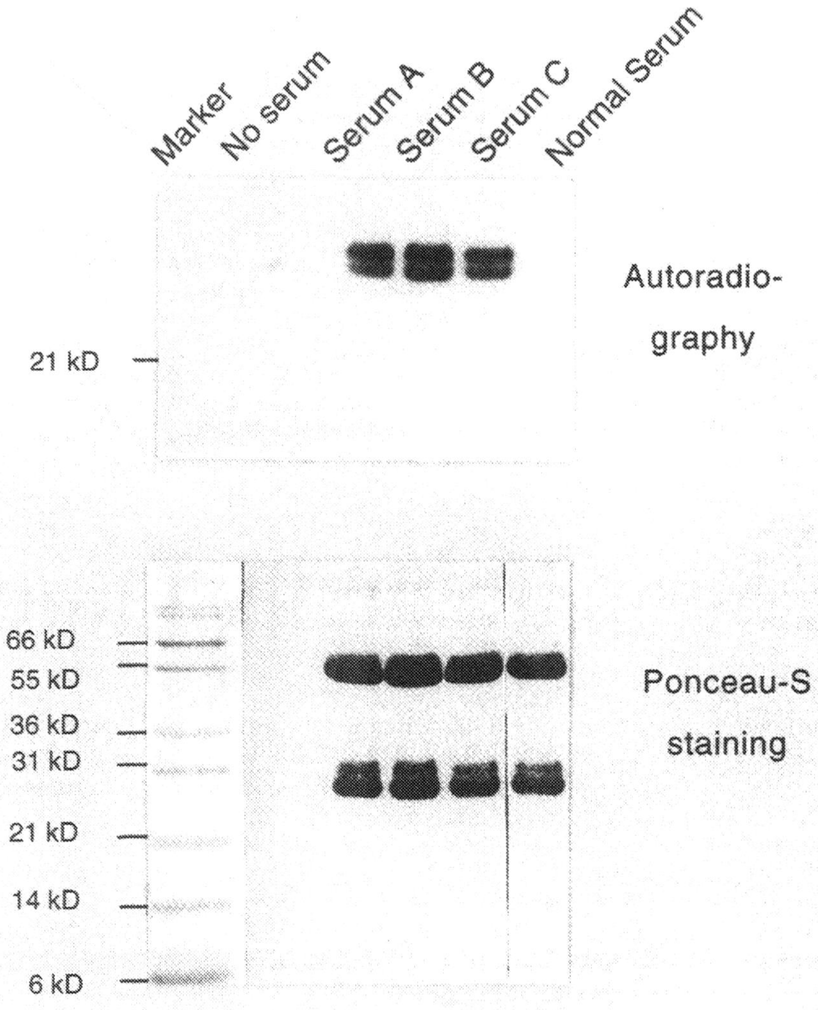


**Fig. 3** Immunoprecipitation of rat liver cytosol proteins by anti-SLA-positive sera. Immune complexes purified on Protein-G-Plus-Sepharose and separated on 15% SDS-gel were transferred onto nitrocellulose. Proteins were stained by Ponceau-S (lower panel) and biotinylated antigens were detected autoradiographically after overlay with streptavidin-HRP by chemiluminescence (upper panel). Molecular weight markers, see Figure 1. For control, human serum was omitted during incubation, or normal serum was used

Moreover, varying titres of antibodies and differing reactivity of individual sera towards several variants became apparent. Two-dimensional immunoblots allowing exact determination of the reactivity of the sera with individual subunits confirmed that three GST variants, Ya, $Yb_1$ and Yc, are targets for anti-SLA antibodies (not shown). Interestingly, one of 10 AIH type II sera has also recog-

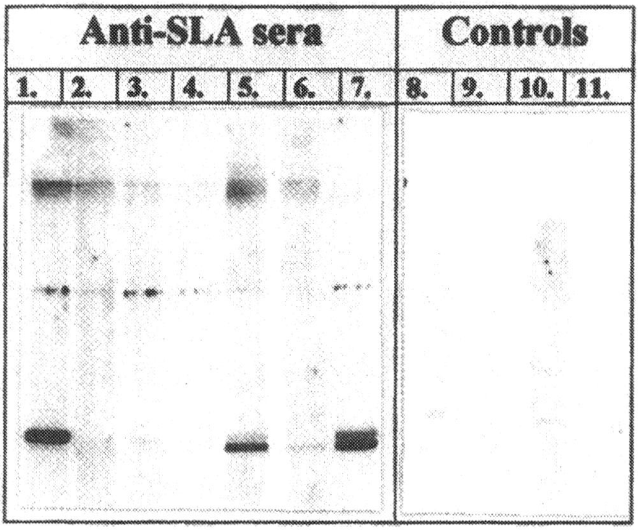


**Fig. 4** Testing of anti-SLA-positive sera for reactivity with antigens of rat liver cytosol. Normal sera were obtained from healthy individuals (lanes 8–11). Blot strips were incubated with patients' sera (1:500) and anti-human Ig-HRP (1:2000)[16]

nized GST (Table 1). We additionally proved whether the anti-GST-positive AIH sera exhibit the same reactivity with human GST. We isolated cytosol from human liver and additionally purified GST from human placenta by affinity chromatography. Interestingly, eight of 10 tested anti-SLA-positive sera reacted with 25–27 kDa proteins in the human SLA preparation but three out of 13 tested sera reacted weakly with human placental GST.

In summary, three approaches performed in our study with proteins of rat liver cytosol revealed that the majority of SLA-seropositive AIH patients recognize GST. Interestingly, about 20% of tested sera were GST-negative and reacted in immunoblots with other cytosolic antigens. Moreover, according to expectations, a few anti-GST-positive sera showed additional reactivity with another protein of SLA. Unfortunately, in our hands no prevalence of one distinct antigen could be observed.

## DISCUSSION

In the past at least two different groups described a subset of AIH patients characterized by the presence of circulating antibodies reactive with soluble antigens of liver cytosol. The preparations were originally defined as soluble liver antigen (SLA) and liver/pancreas antigen (LP). A comparison of the isolation protocol and definition of these antigens shows striking similarity. Both antigens were originally defined as a non-species-, non-organ-specific antigen despite its highest concentration in liver and kidney[7,12]. According to the published protocols both preparations were obtained as 100 000 *g* supernatant[7], indicating its

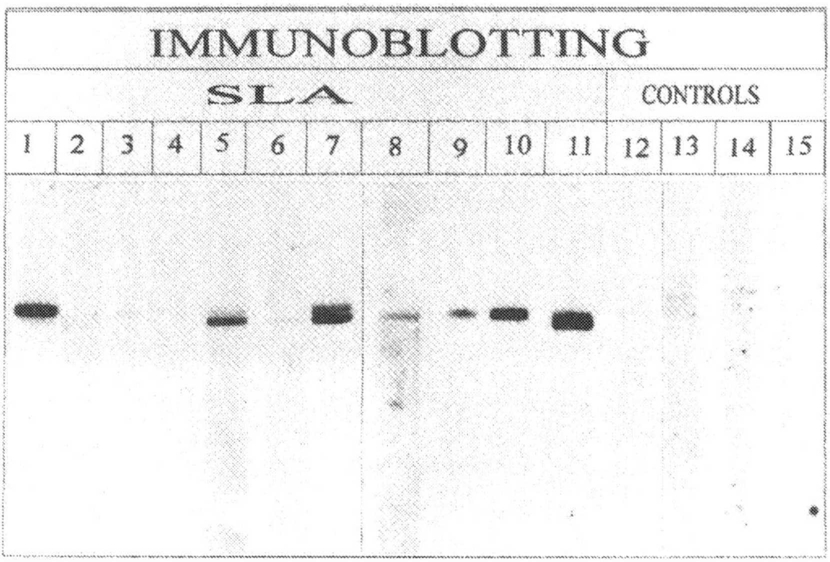


**Fig. 5** Immunoblotting using affinity-purified GST as antigen. Isolated GST were resolved on 15% SDS gel

**Table 1** Frequency of autoantibodies against GST, in SLA-seropositive AIH

| *Patients* | *n* | *SLA* | *GST* |
|---|---|---|---|
| Controls | 15 | 0 | 0 |
| AIH type I | 10 | 0 | 0 |
| AIH type II | 10 | 0 | 1 |
| SLA (+) AIH | 31 | 31 | 25 |
| Hepatitis C | 10 | 0 | 0 |

extremely high solubility. We have isolated both antigens according to the original protocols, and analysed them. Coomassie-blue staining of proteins separated on 10% and 15% SDS-slab gels revealed high similarity of the resolved proteins. Not only the number of separated proteins, but also the position and the intensity of distinct bands, was almost identical. We have excised a few prominent protein bands within the molecular weight range 25–27 kDa and at about 65 kDa from both samples, and submitted it for sequencing. The analysis of amino-terminal sequences revealed the identity of sequenced proteins in both antigen preparations. Four subtypes of GST were identified as low molecular weight proteins and the sequence EAHKSEIA was recognized as characteristic for rat albumin. Therefore, it seems obvious that the two antigen preparations are identical.

A few years ago Wächter *et al.*[19] identified that cytokeratins 8 and 18 are major targets of anti-SLA antibodies. Cytokeratins are components of cytoskeleton and, being intermediary filaments, are poorly soluble. This property is utilized for isolation of cytokeratins, which are readily pelleted after centrifugation for 20 min at 3500 *g*, even in the presence of non-ionic detergents and high salt[20,21]. Moreover, cytokeratins are known to be expressed in a cell- and tissue-specific manner[20,21]. Since the protocol used in our experiments for isolation of SLA is based on extensive ultracentrifugation steps that allow the separation of organelles and cytoskeleton from soluble cytosol proteins, it seems unlikely that cytokeratins represent the target antigen. Indeed, testing of the soluble cytosol preparations for the presence of cytokeratins revealed negative results, convincing us that cytoskeleton components were efficiently removed from the cytoplasm during the ultracentrifugation step. On the other hand our AIH sera tested consistently negative in immunoblots when probed with isolated cytoskeletal preparation as antigen target. On the other hand intermediate filaments undergo reorganization during mitosis and become soluble after hyperphosphorylation preceding the first events of cell division[22]. The disassembly of cytoskeleton in rat liver rarely occurs, since in adult rats the vast majority of hepatocytes are terminally differentiated and in a quiescent state. Thus, it became evident that cytokeratins are not the reactive antigens in SLA. Similar observations were recently reported by Stechenmesser *et al.*[23], who found no reactivity of liver–pancreas cytosol with monoclonal anticytokeratin antibodies.

Furthermore, careful examination of immunoblots shown by Wächter *et al.*[19] reveals the reactivity of all SLA-seropositive sera with a few antigens in the range 25–90 kDa. The molecular masses of three clearly discernible protein bands ranging between 25 and 27 kDa resemble those of GST subunits.

In the present study[30] we have characterized SLA and demonstrated that it belongs to the superfamily of GST, multifunctional enzymes with similar or overlapping specificities[24–29]. Mammalian GST are encoded by at least four gene families; cytosolic GST appear to be the product of three families, whereas microsomal GST is genetically distinct[26]. GST constitute more than 5% of the total rat liver proteins and provide several detoxification mechanisms against cytotoxic compounds and carcinogens[26,29]. Aside from the catalytic role, the enzymes may be considered as binding proteins that prevent genotoxic agents from interacting with DNA.

In the present study at least three distinct subunits were identified as antigen targets. The combination of electrophoretic separation, immunoblotting and microsequencing was crucial for the identification of the reactive antigen. Within the GST family the intra-class variations in primary structures are small and inter-class differences are extensive. Therefore, the determination of the amino-terminal sequences of GST was designed for its identification and classification. The differential reactivity of the sera with subunits suggests that autoantibodies are able to distinguish epitopes characteristic for distinct variants. On the other hand it is possible that patients' sera displaying the reactivity with three GST forms recognize an epitope exhibiting a high degree of sequence similarity between them. However, when tested against human placental GST, the majority of anti-GST-positive AIH sera were negative, thereby implicating narrow specificity of the autoimmune sera. Interestingly, the sequences encoding individual subunits are more distantly related to each other than are comparisons for the two interspecies subunits[26] (e.g. human and rat). Considering this aspect, it might well be that the reactivity of AIH type II serum with GST is due to cross-reaction with microsomal isoenzymes.

Since the GST are multifunctional proteins mediating hepatic detoxification of cytotoxic compounds, and acting as carrier proteins in biliary secretion, it seems important to test whether the patients' sera impair their enzymatic activity. Furthermore, it is necessary to determine the intra-individual differences in GST profiles and activity. There are reports of changes in the concentration of GST and their activity in liver disease[30].

Our data show that GST is the major but not exclusive autoantigen in SLA. The analysis of immunoblots performed with SLA shows occasional anti-SLA-positive sera reacting with proteins at about 50 and 100 kDa.

Recently Mackay[31] – considering the problems with definition of AIH and relation to stage of disease, overlaps and/or coexistence among autoimmune diseases and distinction of possible subtypes – suggested the necessity of further characterization of autoantibodies relevant for AIH. Our present study represents a further contribution for serological characterization of AIH.

## Acknowledgement

This work was supported in part by Jubileumsfond grant no. 6668 from the Oesterreichische Nationalbank.

## References

1. Mackay IR, Taft CO, Cowling DS. Lupoid hepatitis. Lancet. 1956;2:1323–6.
2. Czaja AJ. Autoimmune hepatitis. Evolving concepts and treatment strategies. Dig Dis Sci. 1995;40:435–56.
3. Czaja AJ. The variant forms of autoimmune hepatitis. Ann Intern Med. 1996;125:588–98.
4. Krawitt EL. Autoimmune hepatitis. N Engl J Med. 1996;334:897–903.
5. Smith MGM, Williams R, Walker R, Rizzetto M, Doniach D. Hepatic disorders associated with liver/kidney microsomal antibodies. Br Med J. 1974;2:80–4.
6. Homberg JC, Abuaf N, Bernard O *et al.* Chronic active hepatitis associated with anti-liver–kidney microsome antibody type 1: a second type of 'autoimmune' hepatitis. Hepatology. 1987;7:1333–9.
7. Manns M, Gerken G, Kyriatsoulis A, Staritz M, Meyer zum Büschenfelde KH. Characterization of a new subgroup of autoimmune chronic active hepatitis by autoantibodies against a soluble liver antigen. Lancet. 1987;1:292–4.
8. Johnson PI, McFarlane IG, McFarlane BM, Williams R. Autoimmune features in patients with idiopathic chronic active hepatitis who are seronegative for conventional autoantibodies. J Gastroenterol Hepatol. 1990;5:244–51.
9. Johnson PI, McFarlane IG. Meeting report: International Autoimmune Hepatitis Group. Hepatology. 1993;18:998–1005.
10. Czaja AJ, Carpenter HA, Manns MP. Antibodies to soluble liver antigen, P450IID6, and mitochondrial complexes in chronic hepatitis. Gastroenterology. 1993;105:1522–8.
11. McFarlane JG, Williams R. Historical overview. In: McFarlane JG, Williams R, editors. Molecular Basis of Autoimmune Hepatitis. Heidelberg: Springer-Verlag. 1996:1–21.
12. Stechenmesser E, Strienz J, Berg PA. Serological definition of a new subgroup of patients with autoimmune chronic active hepatitis. Lancet. 1987;1:683.
13. DeDuwe C, Pressman BC, Gianetto R, Wattiaux R, Appelmans F. Tissue fractionation studies. Intracellular distribution patterns of enzymes in rat liver tissues. Biochem J. 1955;60:604–10.
14. Tata JR. Isolation of nuclei from rat liver and other tissues. Methods Enzymol. 1974;31:253–62.
15. Laemmli UK. Cleavage of structural proteins during the assembly of the head of bacteriophage $T_4$. Nature. 1970;227:680–5.
16. O'Farrell PH. High resolution two-dimensional electrophoresis of proteins. J Biol Chem. 1975;250:4007–21.

17. Wesierska-Gadek J, Hohenauer H, Hitchman E, Penner E. Autoantibodies from patients with primary biliary cirrhosis preferentially react with the amino-terminal domain of nuclear pore complex glycoprotein gp210. J Exp Med. 1995;182:1159–62.
18. Simons PC, Vander Jagt DL. Purification of glutathione *S*-transferases from human liver by glutathione-affinity chromatography. Analyt Biochem. 1977;82:334–41.
19. Wächter B, Kyriatsoulis A, Lohse AW, Gerken G, Meyer zum Büschenfelde KH, Manns M. Characterization of liver cytokeratin as a major target antigen of anti-SLA antibodies. J Hepatol. 1990;11:232–9.
20. Franke WW, Schiller D, Moll R, Winter S, Schmid E, Engelbrecht I. Diversity of cytokeratins. Differentiation specific expression of cytokeratin polypeptides in epithelial cells and tissues. J Mol Biol. 1981;153:933–59.
21. Moll R, Franke WW, Schiller DL, Geiger B, Krepler R. The catalog of human cytokeratins: patterns of expression in normal epithelia, tumors and cultures cells. Cell. 1982;31:11–24.
22. Chou Y-H, Rosevear E, Goldman RD. Phosphorylation and disassembly of intermediate filaments in mitotic cells. Proc Natl Acad Sci USA. 1989;86:1885–9.
23. Stechenmesser E, Klein R, Berg PA. Characterization and clinical relevance of liver–pancreas antibodies in autoimmune hepatitis. Hepatology. 1993;18:1–9.
24. Bass NM, Kirsch RE, Tuff SA, Marks I, Saunders SJ. Ligand in heterogeneity: evidence that the two non-identical subunits are the monomers of the two distinct proteins. Biochim Biophys Acta. 1977;492:163–75.
25. Hayes JD. Purification and characterization of glutathione *S*-transferases P, S, and N. Isolation from rat liver of $Yb_1$ Yn protein, the existence of which was predicted by subunit hybridization *in vitro*. Biochem J. 1984;224:839–52.
26. Hayes JD, Pulford DJ. The glutathione *S*-transferase supergene family: regulation of GST* and the contribution of the isoenzymes to cancer chemoprotection and drug resistance. Crit Rev Biochem Mol Biol. 1995;30:445–600.
27. Pickett CB, Telakowski-Hopkins CA, Ding GJ-F, Argenbright L, Lu AYH. Rat liver glutathione *S*-transferases. Complete nucleotide sequence of a glutathione *S*-transferase mRNA and the regulation of the Ya, Yb, and Yc mRNA by 3-methylcholanthrene and phenobarbital. J Biol Chem. 1984;259:5182–8.
28. Telakowski-Hopkins CA, Rodkey JA, Bennett CD, Lu AYH, Pickett CB. Rat liver glutathione *S*-transferases. Construction of a cDNA clone complementary to a Yc mRNA and prediction of the complete amino acid sequence of a Yc subunit. J Biol Chem. 1985;260:5820–5.
29. Smith GJ, Ohl VS, Litwack G. Ligandin, the glutathione *S*-transferases, and chemically induced hepatocarcinogenesis: a review. Cancer Res. 1977;37:8–14.
30. Węsierska-Gądek J, Grimm R, Hitchman E, Penner E. Members of the glutathione S-transferase gene family are antigens in autoimmune hepatitis. Gastroenterology, 1996;114:329–35.
31. Hayes PC, Portmann B, Aldis PM, Williams R, Hayes JD. In: Mantle TJ, Pickett CB, Hayes JD, editors. Glutathione *S*-transferases and Carcinogenesis. London: Taylor & Francis; 1987;175–87.
32. Mackay IR. The grey edges of autoimmune hepatitis. Intern Hepatol Commun. 1996;5:191–200.

# Section IV
# Drug and hepatitis virus induced autoimmunity

# 15
# The cytochrome P450 supergene family: genetic organization and function

K.J. GRIFFIN and E.F. JOHNSON

## INTRODUCTION

At least eight human cytochrome P450s are recognized by autoantibodies associated with either alcoholic liver disease, autoimmune polyendocrinopathy, autoimmune hepatitis or drug-induced autoimmunity (Table 1). The polyspecific responses to both conformational and linear epitopes that have been characterized for autoantibodies to P450 2D6 in LKM-1-positive autoimmune hepatitis suggests that the autoimmune response is directed towards the P450[1–7]. Although the other P450 antigens listed in Table 1 have not yet received the same level of scrutiny, these enzymes nevertheless appear to be relatively specific targets for autoimmune responses.

**Table 1** Human P450s recognized by autoantibodies

| *P450* | *Condition* | *Ref.* |
|---|---|---|
| 1A2 | Idiopathic autoimmune hepatitis | 2, 80 |
| | Autoimmune polyglandular disease | 81 |
| | Drug-induced hypersensitivity (dihydralazine) | 82, 83 |
| | Drug-induced hypersensitivity (disulfiram) | 84 |
| 2A6 | Autoimmune polyglandular disease | 81 |
| 2C9 | Drug-induced hypersensitivity (tienilic acid) | 85–87 |
| 2D6 | Idiopathic autoimmune hepatitis | 36–38, 87–90 |
| 2E1 | Alchoholic liver disease | 41, 42 |
| 3A? | Drug-induced hypersensitivity (phenobarbital, phenytoin, carbamazepine) | 91, 92 |
| | Drug-induced hypersensitivity (disulfiram) | 84 |
| 11A1 | Addison's disease | 2, 93, 94 |
| | Autoimmune polyglandular disease | |
| 17 | Addison's disease | 2, 31, 93 |
| | Autoimmune polyglandular disease | |
| 21 | Addison's disease | 2, 30, 93 |
| | Autoimmune polyglandular disease | |

The focus of this brief review of the cytochrome P450 superfamily will be on general features and specific functional aspects of these membrane-bound, intracellular enzymes that may favour recruitment as autoantigens. In some cases, the capacity of P450s to activate substrates to highly reactive products that can bind covalently to cellular macromolecules, including the P450 catalysing the reaction, may be an initiating factor that fuels a misdirected immune response to the neoantigens created by adduct formation. In severe cases, the generation of reactive intermediates or exposure to toxic insult can lead to tissue damage or necrosis. This, in turn, can increase systemic exposure to these internal, cellular proteins which could potentially provoke elevated recognition by the immune system.

## P450 NOMENCLATURE

The cytochrome P450 enzymes constitute a diverse group of proteins that are thought to have evolved from a common ancestral gene. This lineage forms the basis for a widely used nomenclature based on sequence relatedness. Simple rules guide the naming of an individual P450 enzyme using a number–letter–number combination[8]. The first number designates a family of P450s that share 40% or greater amino acid sequence identity. There are currently 43, 46 and 25 recognized animal, plant and fungal P450 families, respectively[9]. A number–letter combination, e.g. P450 1B, denotes a particular subfamily within each family that contains P450s that are at least 55% identical; although subfamily members generally exhibit greater than 65–75% amino acid sequence identity within a species as well as between mammalian species. Not all P450 families exhibit subfamilies. However, others such as family 2 in mammals contain more than 10 subfamilies. The last number in the number–letter–number designation is used to identify specific P450 enzymes, e.g. P450 2C9. When a P450 gene is designated, the three-letter code, *CYP*, is used together with the number–letter–number name for the encoded protein, e.g. *CYP* 2C9.

Although the P450s that are associated with specific biological functions are more generally referred to by their enzymatic functions, e.g. the cholesterol side-chain cleavage enzyme, rather than P450 11B1, the uniform nomenclature provides a means of uniquely identifying enzymes that metabolize multiple, structurally distinct substrates such as the P450s that are involved in xenobiotic metabolism as well as orphan genes that encode P450s with as-yet-unidentified functions.

P450 subfamilies may be simple or complex. In subfamilies where there are multiple members for different species, the third number in the designation of the protein is generally unique for each enzyme in each species. As shown in Table 2, the number of members in each subfamily can vary between species.

**Table 2** P450 Families 1, 2, 3 and 4 are highly diverse

| | *1A* | *1B* | *2A* | *2B* | *2C* | *2D* | *2E* | *2F* | *2G* | *2J* | *2R* | *2S* | *3A* | *4A* | *4B* | *4F* | *4X* | *4Z* |
|---|---|---|---|---|---|---|---|---|---|---|---|---|---|---|---|---|---|---|
| Human | 2 | 1 | 3 | 1 | 4 | 1 | 1 | 1 | – | 1 | 1 | 1 | 3 | 1 | 1 | 5 | 1 | 1 |
| Mouse | 2 | 1 | 3 | 5 | 6 | 6 | 1 | 1 | 1 | 5 | – | 1 | 3 | 3 | 1 | 6 | – | – |
| Rat | 2 | 1 | 2 | 3 | 7 | 5 | 1 | 1 | 1 | 1 | – | – | 4 | 4 | 1 | 5 | – | – |

Subfamily designations are indicated across the top of the table. The number of known enzymes in each subfamily is given for the indicated species.

Many of these enzymes appear to reflect gene duplication and divergence that has occurred since the radiation of mammals. For example, the human P450 2C enzymes exhibit roughly 75% amino acid sequence identity with any rabbit P450 2C protein, whereas the sequence identity among rabbit 2C enzymes ranges from 68% to > 95%.

## GENETIC DIVERSITY OF HUMAN P450s

Based on current information combined from Genbank, the Human Genome Project and the Expressed Sequence Tag database, there are more than 50 human P450 genes encoding enzymes that can be grouped into 17 families. The general function of family members, as well as the number of subfamilies, is summarized in Table 3. Families 11, 24 and 27 encode mitochondrial P450s. The remaining gene families encode microsomal P450s. In addition, 14 pseudogenes have been identified, which do not encode functional proteins. Polymorphic forms of P450s in subfamilies 1A, 1B, 2A, 2C, 2D, 2E and 3A have also been identified[9]. Seemingly trivial amino acid substitutions can have a dramatic impact on enzyme function and thus on an individual's ability to metabolize specific drugs. Polymorphisms are defined as sequence differences that occur in at least 1% of a population. Rarer mutations are also evident.

## SHARED PROPERTIES OF P450 ENZYMES

The P450 monooxygenases utilize haem as a prosthetic group for the reduction of molecular oxygen. The P450 proteins exhibit a distinctive chromophore when the ferrous (reduced) enzyme binds carbon monoxide to the iron of the haem cofactor. The Soret band in the visible absorption spectrum of this enzyme–CO

**Table 3** Human P450 gene families

| *CYP* | *Functions* | *Subfamilies* | *Members* |
|---|---|---|---|
| 1 | Xenobiotic metabolism | 2 | 3 |
| 2 | Xenobiotic metabolism | 9 | 14 |
| 3 | Xenobiotic and steroid metabolism | 1 | 4 |
| 4 | Fatty acid and leukotriene $\omega$-hydroxylation | 5 | 9 |
| 5 | Thromboxane synthase | 1 | 1 |
| 7 | Cholesterol and steroid 7$\alpha$-hydroxylation | 2 | 2 |
| 8 | Bile acid (12$\alpha$-OH) and prostacyclin synthase | 2 | 2 |
| 11 | Steroid hormone synthesis (mitochondrial) | 2 | 3 |
| 17 | Steroid hormone synthesis | 1 | 1 |
| 19 | Aromatase (estrogen synthesis) | 1 | 1 |
| 21 | Steroid hormone synthesis | 1 | 1 |
| 24 | 1$\alpha$,25-Dihydroxyvitamin D3 inactivation (mitochondrial) | 1 | 1 |
| 26 | Retinoic acid inactivation | 1 | 1 |
| 27 | Vitamin D3 activation and bile acid synthesis (mitochondrial) | 2 | 2 |
| 39 | Orphan – no known function | 1 | 1 |
| 46 | Orphan – no known function | 1 | 1 |
| 51 | Lanosterol 14$\alpha$-demethylase | 1 | 1 |

The P450 gene families listed have been identified in the human genome. Most encode microsomal P450s with the exception of families 11, 24 and 27 that encode mitochondrial P450s.

complex exhibits a characteristic maximal absorbance at wavelengths around 450 nm leading to the designation P450 (pigment 450 nm)[10]. This distinctive spectrum reflects the unique ligation of the haem iron to a cysteinyl residue at the axial ligation site opposite from where carbon monoxide binds. This cysteine and adjacent residues form an amino acid sequence motif that is highly characteristic of P450s[11]. The three-dimensional structural components of P450s that form the haem binding site are highly conserved among P450s[12]. During catalysis these enzymes reductively cleave dioxygen to form a molecule of water and an oxygen species that remains bound at the active site[13]. The different P450s have evolved to control the reactivity of this powerful oxidant with a wide range of chemical substances. For the mammalian, microsomal P450s, the sequential reductions of the enzyme and the enzyme substrate complex to permit oxygen binding and to complete the reductive cleavage of oxygen is performed by a microsomal flavoprotein reductase that is reduced, in turn, by NADPH[13]. Although the microsomal P450s use the cytochrome P450 reductase (CPR), the mitochondrial P450s in mammals utilize different protein partners, adrenodoxin and adrenodoxin reductase, as a source of electrons. With the exception of the mitochondrial P450 11A1, the P450s that are recognized by autoantibodies are all microsomal enzymes.

Although the relatedness of various P450 enzymes is apparent when their amino acid sequences are aligned, they can exhibit extremely low (< 20%) amino acid sequence identity. Comparison of known structures of soluble prokaryotic P450s with a structure that we recently obtained for a mammalian P450 indicates that such significant sequence divergence does not disrupt the basic framework of these enzymes[12].

The majority of the mammalian monooxygenases are microsomal proteins synthesized with a leader sequence that targets the protein for co-translational insertion into the endoplasmic reticulum by signal recognition particle[14]. A stop-transfer signal following an N-terminal transmembrane domain, that is predicted to be a single helix, halts the translocation of the protein across the membrane. As a result, the protein is sequestered on the surface of the endoplasmic reticulum with the catalytic domain exposed to the cytoplasm[15–17]. The microsomal P450s also appear to contain additional membrane interaction sites as they bind to membranes following the deletion of the N-terminal transmembrane helix[18]. In most cases detergents are required to dissociate the truncated proteins from membrane fractions. However, in the case of truncated P450s 2C3 and 2C5, the binding of the catalytic domain to membranes is salt-dependent, suggesting that the binding interactions are monofacial rather than transmembrane[19]. A suitably modified form of truncated P450 2C5 has been crystallized, and the structure reveals a likely interaction surface for monofacial binding of the enzyme to membranes[95]. A hydrophobic surface is located near the site of attachment of the N-terminal transmembrane, leader sequence. The hydrophobicity of this surface suggests that this portion of the protein may be buried in the membrane's hydrophobic core. As a result, the entrance of the substrate access channel is also directly accessible to the membrane, which could facilitate the entry of hydrophobic substrates. In addition, this orients the surface of the enzyme that is proximal to the haem perpendicular to the plane of the membrane. This is likely to facilitate electrostatic interactions that guide CPR to interact with the P450 during catalysis. These results also indicate that the adaptation for membrane binding has occurred by the accumulation of changes in several discontinuous segments of the protein that form the hydrophobic surface.

Mammalian mitochondrial P450s are also synthesized with leader sequences that target them to mitochondria. These leaders are cleaved upon translocation to the inner mitochondrial membrane where the P450s bind to the matrix side of the membrane without the use of a transmembrane helix[20,21]. The molecular interactions that sequester the mitochondrial P450s to the membrane are unclear and may be similar to the mechanism that leads to the association of the truncated microsomal P450s with membranes.

Although microsomal P450s are predominantly localized in the endoplasmic reticulum, they have also been detected on the outer surface of the plasma membrane, and this could contribute to their ability to elicit autoantibodies[22–25]. It is generally thought that proteins that are expressed in the endoplasmic reticulum enter the vesicular transport system by default. The vesicles that bud off from the endoplasmic reticulum move proteins through the Golgi apparatus, and the proteins are eventually sorted into vesicles that transport proteins to specific organelles, such as lysosomes and secretory particles as well as the plasma membrane[26]. Proteins that remain resident in the endoplasmic reticulum are thought to contain features that either prevent their inclusion in the transport vesicles or that actively promote recycling back to the endoplasmic reticulum. The observation that microsomal P450s are expressed on the plasma membrane suggests that some of these P450s escape from the recycling and retention system. The N-terminal leader sequence and the cytoplasmic, catalytic domain appear to contain retention signals. However, P450s do not generally exhibit any of the known recognition sequences for retention in the endoplasmic reticulum, and the underlying mechanism for retention remains unclear[27–29].

## CATALYTIC DIVERSITY

Based on function, the mammalian P450 enzymes can be divided into two groups, biosynthetic and catabolic. The biosynthetic P450s are involved in many reactions that include the synthesis of thromboxane, androgens, steroid hormones, bile acids and the hormonal forms of vitamin D3. These enzymes have evolved to fill specific niches and can be distinguished by their specific catalysis of a single reaction. Three biosynthetic P450s have been described as autoantigens in patients with Addison's disease[30], and Addison's patients with autoimmune polyglandular syndrome[31] (Table 1). The side-chain cleavage enzyme (P450 11A1, scc) is found in mitochondria and catalyses the first step in steroid biosynthesis by converting cholesterol to pregnenolone. The 17$\alpha$-hydroxylase (P450 17) is expressed in tissues such as testes and ovaries where it catalyses a specific step in the synthesis of androgens and oestrogens. P450 17 is also expressed in the adrenal along with the adrenal steroid 21-hydroxylase (P450 21), where they contribute to cortisol production.

In contrast to the P450s that play vital but rather specific biosynthetic roles, the P450 enzymes that evolved to function in the detoxication of foreign compounds and the catabolism of endogenous fatty acids and sterols are more numerous and readily metabolize a variety of structurally dissimilar substrates. Moreover, there is often an overlap among different catabolic P450s in the metabolism of a particular substrate. This catalytic redundancy no doubt provides an important protective function, but makes it difficult to identify particular P450 enzymes by the specific reactions that they catalyse. These P450s participate in a variety of catabolic pathways for steroids, fatty acids and a wide range of foreign compounds. In general these P450s convert hydrophobic substrates to more soluble polar compounds[32]. The introduction of hydroxyl groups into the substrate or the unmasking of other functional groups by oxidation often leads to further metabolism by enzymes that conjugate the P450 catalysed reaction product with glutathione, glucuronic acid, or other molecules, which render the product more water-soluble and promote excretion. The catabolic P450s are found at many sites where environmental chemicals might gain access to the body, and many are expressed at relatively high concentrations in the liver, which plays a central role in the detoxication of foreign compounds. The P450s that are recognized by autoantibodies associated with autoimmune hepatitis and drug-induced autoimmunity are catabolic P450s.

The diversity of P450-catalysed reactions arises from structural differences in these proteins that discriminate between organic compounds and that orient substrates for reaction with the activated oxygen species formed at the haem prosthetic group. The surface of the haem on the side that binds oxygen forms the base of the binding site for the organic substrate. Six topological elements of P450 structures generally form the binding site for the organic substrates. These have been termed substrate recognition sites (SRS) 1–6 by Gotoh[33], who predicted the corresponding regions of family 2 enzymes based on the structure of a microbial enzyme, P450cam, using sequence alignments. Segments of the sequences of the mammalian family 2 enzymes surrounding residues that aligned with substrate contact residues in P450cam were identified as potential SRSs. Mutagenesis studies in family 2 enzymes have identified key residues that confer the catalytic activities or regiospecificities of hydroxylation from one enzyme to another, and these residues generally fall within the SRSs defined by Gotoh[33,34]. The amino acid substitutions in the SRS regions of family 2 enzymes are likely to account for the pronounced differences in substrate specificity and catalytic properties that are often exhibited by closely related P450s. In more distantly related P450s the three-dimensional topology of the SRS regions varies, which creates more dramatic changes in the substrate-binding cavity of different P450s[12].

The multiplicity that is apparent for the P450 enzymes most likely reflects a process of gene duplication and divergence. This process greatly expanded the catalytic capacity of the P450 system to metabolize a broad range of structurally distinct substrates, including recently created man-made chemicals for industrial and therapeutic uses[35]. The divergence of duplicated genes has also resulted in non-productive pseudogenes that encode defective alleles and polymorphic alleles encoding enzymes with altered metabolic capability.

The functional consequences of defective alleles are quite apparent in the CYP2D locus in humans, which encodes one of the P450 enzymes that is recognized by autoantibodies associated with autoimmune chronic active hepatitis, P450 2D6[36–38]. Defective alleles of 2D6 occur with a high frequency, leading to roughly 10% of Caucasians being deficient in this enzymatic capacity, and this results in impaired clearance of a wide variety of drugs[39]. This impaired metabolism affects bioavailability and, in some cases, can lead to unexpected toxic side-effects. Polymorphisms resulting in poor metabolizer phenotypes have also been identified for human P450s 2C19, 2E1 and 3A. The reduced ability to clear drugs is especially critical when there is a narrow range between the effective therapeutic dose and toxicity.

## GENERATION OF REACTIVE PRODUCTS

Several of the P450s listed in Table 1 are recognized by autoantibodies associated with drug-induced autoimmune responses that result from exposure to specific drugs that are substrates for the enzymes recognized by the autoantibodies. These drugs include the antihypertensive dihydralazine, tienilic acid, the anticonvulsants phenytoin and carbamazepine, the barbiturate, phenobarbital, and disulfiram, which is used to discourage alcohol consumption. The close linkage of P450 antigen recognition with exposure to a substrate suggests that a mechanistic relationship might exist between the autoimmune response, the drug and its metabolism by the P450. The reactive metabolites generated by P450 catalysis can modify proteins and lead to cytotoxicity[40].

Prolonged chemical exposure can also provoke changes that foster autoimmune responses. For example, alcoholic liver disease (ALD) is a common manifestation of chronic alcohol abuse, and this progressive disease is characterized by steatosis (fatty liver), hepatitis and/or fibrosis, and ultimately cirrhosis. The development of ALD is also associated with autoimmune reactions. In contrast to the other hypersensitivity reactions noted above that are relatively rapid, the delayed appearance of these autoantibodies suggests a less direct causation that may be related to the tissue damage resulting from constant insult. Patients with ALD display circulating antibodies that react with acetaldehyde and hydroxyethyl protein adducts. These radicals are both derived from the oxidation of ethanol, and their covalent binding to protein apparently forms neoantigens that are capable of initiating an immune response. P450 2E1 mediated ethanol oxidation is an important source of these radicals, and P450 2E1 adducts represent the major antigen for autoantibodies found in alcoholics[41,42]. The availability of P450 2E1-deficient mice will help to clarify the role of this enzyme in radical adduct formation, and provides a suitable model to examine immune responses[43,44]. Hepatic P450 2E1 expression levels are induced by ethanol exposure, suggesting that elevated levels of this enzyme could contribute to this process. Higher concentrations of hepatic CYP 2E1 resulting from exposure to certain other chemicals bioactivated by this enzyme, including agents such as halogenated anaesthetics, can also substantially increase the risk of developing ALD.

P450-generated electrophilic products can covalently modify cellular macromolecules, and this process appears to underlie the carcinogenicity of many chemicals that are otherwise rather inert[45,46]. Cytochrome P450s can catalyse the initial steps in either carcinogen activation or detoxication[47–49]. For instance, 2-acetylaminofluorene is metabolized by a number of rabbit

P450s to ring-hydroxylated products[50]. These products are readily excreted and are not thought to be carcinogenic. On the other hand, P450 1A2 catalyses the N-hydroxylation of 2-acetylaminofluorene[50], which can be subsequently sulphated. Alternatively, the N-acetyl group may migrate to form the N-acetoxy compound. The hydroxyl, sulphate and acetoxy moieties provide good leaving groups that are subject to displacement by cellular nucleophiles including nucleic acids. The resulting modification of cellular DNA is thought to generate mutations that, in turn, lead to neoplastic growth.

The relative balance between the detoxication pathways catalysed by some P450s versus the activation pathways catalysed by other P450 enzymes is likely to contribute to the relative risk of carcinogenesis[51]. This balance often differs between cell types, tissues and with age and diet due to the highly differentiated expression of various members comprising the P450 system. Moreover, this balance can be altered through the induction of specific P450s as a result of exposure to drugs and environmental chemicals.

## INDUCTION OF P450s BY ENVIRONMENTAL CHEMICALS

A variety of foreign chemicals can selectively increase the abundance of specific P450s. As indicated in Table 4, the principal mechanism of induction appears to be increased gene transcription. This has been shown experimentally by nuclear run-on assays for the induction of P450 2B enzymes by phenobarbital[52,53], of P450 1A enzymes by 2,3,7,8-tetrachlorodibenzo-*p*-dioxin (TCDD or dioxin)[54,55], of P450 3A enzymes by dexamethasone[56,57] and rifampicin[57], as well as of P450 4A enzymes by clofibrate[58]. In contrast, the induction of P450 2E enzymes by ethanol or heterocyclic compounds such as pyrazole or imidazole appears to reflect a

**Table 4** Receptor-mediated, conditional regulation of P450 gene expression

| *P450 gene* | *Receptor* | *Action* | *Ligands* |
|---|---|---|---|
| CYP1A1 | Ah-receptor | Induction of polynuclear aromatic hydrocarbon metabolism | Polynuclear aromatic hydrocarbons |
| CYP4A# | Peroxisome proliferator activated receptor $\alpha$ | Induction of fatty acid $\omega$-hydroxylation | Fatty acids, DHEA, fibrates |
| CYP2B# | Constitutive activated receptor | Induction of drug metabolism | Phenobarbital |
| CYP3A# | Pregnane X receptor | Induction of drug and steroid metabolism | Rifampicin, steroids |
| CYP26 | Retinoic acid receptor | Induction of retinoic acid degradation | Retinoic acid |
| CYP27B | Vitamin D3 receptor | Repression of hormone production | $1\alpha$, 25-dihydroxy-vitamin D3 |
| CYP24 | Vitamin D3 receptor | Activation of hormone degradation | $1\alpha$, 25-dihydroxy-vitamin D3 |
| CYP7 | Liver X receptor | Activation of bile acid synthesis | Oxysterols |
| CYP7 | Farnesoid X receptor | Repression of bile acid synthesis | Bile acids |

stabilization of the enzyme to turnover because the accumulation of protein is not preceded by an elevation of mRNA concentration[59,60]. P450 2E is also elevated in diabetic states, and in this case the abundance of mRNA is increased, but there is no evidence for an increase in transcription[61]. The induction of P450 3A enzymes by the antibiotics erythromycin and troleandromycin also reflects a contribution from protein stabilization as the half-life of P450 3A is increased by these drugs[62]. It is important to note that the spectrum of inducing agents may differ between species. For instance, rifampicin is an antibiotic that induces P450 3A enzymes in humans[63,64] and in rabbits[65], but it does not induce P450 3A in rats[66].

A member of the nuclear hormone receptor superfamily, the pregnane X receptor[67], generally mediates the transcriptional activation of CYP 3A genes in response to xenobiotics. Interestingly, the human[68,69] and rabbit[70,71] pregnane X receptors are activated by rifampicin, whereas the rat receptor is not[71,72]. Another member of the steroid hormone receptor family, the peroxisome proliferator activated receptor (PPAR)[73] mediates the induction of the CYP 4A genes by peroxisome proliferators[74]. In general these nuclear receptors bind directly to response elements in the target gene as a heterodimer with the retinoid X receptor. Ligand agonists alter the conformation of the receptors leading to the recruitment of co-activator proteins, and this multiprotein complex stimulates transcription of the target gene. The induction of P450 2B enzymes by phenobarbital is also mediated by a nuclear hormone receptor, the constitutive activated receptor. However, phenobarbital may alter the ability of the receptor to activate target genes by modulating its phosphorylation status and subsequently affecting its translocation from the cytosol to the nucleus[75]. The transcriptional activation of CYP 1A enzymes by polycyclic aromatic hydrocarbons and TCDD also reflects the actions of a cytosolic receptor, the dioxin or aryl hydrocarbon (Ah) receptor that is a protein oligomer composed of two non-identical subunits that contain basic helix–loop–helix and PAS domains[76–79]. Chronic exposure to inducers can greatly increase the P450 content of the endoplasmic reticulum and lead to an expansion of the membrane. It is possible that these changes alter the normal proteolytic processing of P450s and potentially lead to the presentation of new peptide fragments to the immune system that could contribute to the initiation of autoimmune responses.

## Acknowledgements

The authors acknowledge the support of NIH grants GM31001 and HD04445.

## References

1. Durazzo M, Philipp T, Van Pelt FNAM *et al.* Heterogeneity of liver–kidney microsomal autoantibodies in chronic hepatitis C and D virus infection. Gastroenterology. 1995;108:455–62.
2. Manns MP, Obermayer-Straub P. Cytochromes P450 and uridine triphosphate- glucuronosyltransferases: model autoantigens to study drug-induced, virus-induced, and autoimmune liver disease. Hepatology. 1997;26:1054–66.
3. Miyakawa H, Matsushima H, Narita Y *et al.* Differences in antigenic sites, recognized by anti-liver-kidney microsome-1 (LKM-1) autoantibody, between HCV-positive and HCV-negative sera in Japanese patients. J Gastroenterol. 1998;33:529–35.

4. Parez N, Herzog D, Jacqz-Aigrain E, Homberg JC, Alvarez F. Study of the B cell response to cytochrome P450IID6 in sera from chronic hepatitis C patients. Clin Exp Immunol. 1996;106:336–43.
5. Duclos-Vallée J-C, Hajoui O, Yamamoto AM, Jacqz-Aigrain E, Alvarez F. Conformational epitopes on CYP2D6 are recognized by liver/kidney microsomal antibodies. Gastroenterology. 1995;108:470–6.
6. Yamamoto AM, Cresteil D, Homberg JC, Alvarez F. Characterization of anti-liver–kidney microsome antibody (anti-LKM1) from hepatitis C virus-positive and -negative sera. Gastroenterology. 1993;104:1762–7.
7. Yamamoto AM, Cresteil D, Boniface O, Clerc FF, Alvarez F. Identification and analysis of cytochrome P450IID6 antigenic sites recognized by anti-liver-kidney microsome type-1 antibodies (LKM1). Eur J Immunol. 1993;23:1105–11.
8. Nebert DW, Nelson DR, Coon MJ *et al.* The P450 superfamily: update on new sequences, gene mapping, and recommended nomenclature. DNA Cell Biol. 1991;10:1–14.
9. Nelson DR. Cytochrome P450 and the individuality of species. Arch Biochem Biophys. 1999;369:1–10.
10. Omura T, Sato R. The carbon monoxide-binding pigment of liver microsomes. I. Evidence for its hemoprotein nature. J Biol Chem. 1964;239:2370–8.
11. Kalb VF, Loper JC. Proteins from eight eukaryotic cytochrome P-450 families share a segmented region of sequence similarity. Proc Natl Acad Sci USA. 1988;85:7221–5.
12. Graham SE, Peterson JA. How similar are P450s and what can their differences teach us? Arch Biochem Biophys. 1999;369:24–9.
13. White RE, Coon MJ. Oxygen activation by cytochrome P-450. Annu Rev Biochem. 1980;49:315–56.
14. Sakaguchi M, Katsuyoshi M, Sato R. Signal recognition particle is required for co-translational insertion of cytochrome P-450 into microsomal membranes. Proc Natl Acad Sci USA. 1984;81:3361–4.
15. Sakaguchi M, Mihara K, Sato R. A short amino-terminal segment of microsomal cytochrome P-450 functions both as an insertion signal and as a stop-transfer sequence. EMBO J. 1987;6:2425–31.
16. Szczesna-Skorupa E, Browne N, Mead D, Kemper B. Positive charges at the $NH_2$ terminus convert the membrane-anchor signal peptide of cytochrome P-450 to a secretory signal peptide. Proc Natl Acad Sci USA. 1988;85:738–42.
17. Monier S, Van Luc P, Kreibich G, Sabatini DD, Adesnik M. Signals for the incorporation and orientation of cytochrome P450 in the endoplasmic reticulum membrane. J Cell Biol. 1988;107:457–70.
18. Pernecky SJ, Larson JR, Philpot RM, Coon MJ. Expression of truncated forms of liver microsomal P450 cytochromes 2B4 and 2E1 in *Escherichia coli*: influence of $NH_2$-terminal region on localization in cytosol and membranes. Proc Natl Acad Sci USA. 1993;90:2651–5.
19. Von Wachenfeldt C, Richardson TH, Cosme J, Johnson EF. Microsomal P450 2C3 is expressed as a soluble dimer in *Escherichia coli* following modifications of its N-terminus. Arch Biochem Biophys. 1997;339:107–14.
20. DuBois RN, Simpson ER, Tuckey J, Lambeth JD, Waterman MR. Evidence for a higher molecular weight precursor of cholesterol side-chain-cleavage cytochrome P-450 and induction of mitochondrial and cytosolic proteins by corticotropin in adult bovine adrenal cells. Proc Natl Acad Sci USA. 1981;78:1028–32.
21. Ogishima T, Okada Y, Omura T. Import and processing of the precursor of cytochrome P-450(SCC) by bovine adrenal cortex mitochondria. J Biochem. 1985;98:781–91.
22. Loeper J, Descatoire V, Maurice M *et al.* Cytochromes P-450 in human hepatocyte plasma membrane: recognition by several autoantibodies. Gastroenterology 1993;104:203–16.
23. Loeper J, Le Berre A, Pompon D. Topology inversion of CYP2D6 in the endoplasmic reticulum is not required for plasma membrane transport. Mol Pharmacol. 1998;53:408–14.
24. Yamamoto AM, Mura C, De Lemos-Chiarandini C, Krishnamoorthy R, Alvarez F. Cytochrome P450IID6 recognized by LKM1 antibody is not exposed on the surface of hepatocytes. Clin Exp Immunol. 1993;92:381–90.
25. Yamamoto AM, Mura C, Morales MG, Bernard O, Krishnamoorthy R, Alvarez F. Study of CYP2D6 gene in children with autoimmune hepatitis and P450 IID6 autoantibodies. Clin Exp Immunol. 1992;87:251–5.

26. Rothman JE, Wieland FT. Protein sorting by transport vesicles. Science. 1996; 272:227–34.
27. Szczesna-Skorupa E, Ahn KS, Chen CD, Doray B, Kemper B. The cytoplasmic and N-terminal transmembrane domains of cytochrome P450 contain independent signals for retention in the endoplasmic reticulum. J Biol Chem. 1995;270:24327–33.
28. Murakami K, Mihara K, Omura T. The transmembrane region of microsomal cytochrome P450 identified as the endoplasmic reticulum retention signal. J Biochem (Tokyo). 1994;116:164–75.
29. Szczesna-Skorupa E, Kemper B. An N-terminal glycosylation signal on cytochrome P450 is restricted to the endoplasmic reticulum in a luminal orientation. J Biol Chem. 1993;268:1757–62.
30. Winqvist O, Karlsson FA, Kämpe O. 21-Hydroxylase, a major autoantigen in idiopathic Addison's disease. Lancet. 1992;339:1559–62.
31. Krohn K, Uibo R, Aavik E, Peterson P, Savilahti K. Identification by molecular cloning of an autoantigen associated with Addison's disease as steroid 17$\alpha$-hydroxylase. Lancet. 1992;339:770–3.
32. Alvares AP, Pratt WB. Pathways of drug metabolism. In: Pratt WB, Taylor P, editors. Principles of Drug Action: The Basis of Pharmacology, 3rd edn. New York: Churchill Livingstone; 1990:365–422.
33. Gotoh O. Substrate recognition sites in cytochrome P450 family 2 (CYP2) proteins inferred from comparative analyses of amino acid and coding nucleotide sequences. J Biol Chem. 1992;267:83–90.
34. Von Wachenfeldt C, Johnson EF. Structures of eukaryotic cytochrome P450 enzymes. In: Ortiz de Montellano PR, editor. Cytochrome P450: Structure, Mechanism, and Biochemistry (2nd edn). New York: Plenum Press; 1995:183–244.
35. Nebert DW, Gonzalez FJ. P450 genes: structure, evolution, and regulation. Ann Rev Biochem. 1987;56:945–93.
36. Zanger UM, Hauri H-P, Loeper J, Homberg J-C, Meyer UA. Antibodies against human cytochrome P-450db1 in autoimmune hepatitis type II. Proc Natl Acad Sci USA. 1988;85:8256–60.
37. Manns MP, Johnson EF, Griffin KJ, Tan EM, Sullivan KF. Major antigen of liver kidney microsomal autoantibodies in idiopathic autoimmune hepatitis is cytochrome P450db1. J Clin Invest. 1989;83:1066–72.
38. Gueguen M, Yamamoto AM, Bernard O, Alvarez F. Anti-liver kidney microsome antibody type 1 recognizes human cytochrome P450 dbl. Biochem Biophys Res Commun. 1989;159:542–7.
39. Caporaso NE, Shaw GL. Clinical inplications of the competitive inhibition of the debrisoquin-metabolizing isozyme by quinidine. Arch Intern Med. 1991;151:1985–92.
40. Boobis AR, Fawthrop DJ, Davies DS. Mechanisms of cell death. TIPS. 1989;10:275–80.
41. Clot P, Albano E, Eliasson E *et al.* Cytochrome P450 2E1 hydroxyethyl radical adducts as the major antigen in autoantibody formation among alcoholics. Gastroenterology. 1996;111:206–16.
42. Clot P, Bellomo G, Tabone M, Arico S, Albano E. Detection of antibodies against proteins modified by hydroxyethyl free radicals in patients with alcoholic cirrhosis. Gastroenterology. 1995; 108:201–7.
43. Ghanayem BI, Sanders JM, Chanas B, Burka LT, Gonzalez FJ. Role of cytochrome P-450 2E1 in methacrylonitrile metabolism and disposition. J Pharmacol Exp Ther. 1999;289:1054–9.
44. Bondoc FY, Bao Z, Hu WY *et al.* Acetone catabolism by cytochrome P450 2E1: studies with CYP2E1-null mice. Biochem.Pharmacol. 1999;58:461–3.
45. Miller EC. Some current perspectives on chemical carcinogenesis in humans and experimental animals: presidential address. Cancer Res. 1978;38:1479–96.
46. Heidelberger C. Chemical carcinogenesis. Annu Rev Biochem. 1975;44:79–121.
47. Wattenberg LW. Inhibitors of chemical carcinogenesis. Adv Cancer Res. 1978;26:197–226.
48. Conney AH. Induction of microsomal enzymes by foreign chemicals and carcinogenesis by polycyclic aromatic hydrocarbons: G.H.A. Clowes Memorial Lecture. Cancer Res. 1982;42:4875–917.
49. Guengerich FP. Metabolic activation of carcinogens. Pharmacol Ther. 1992;54:17–61.
50. McManus ME, Minchin RF, Sanderson N, Schwartz D, Johnson EF, Thorgeirsson SS. Metabolic processing of 2-acetylaminofluorene by microsomes and six highly purified cytochrome P-450 forms from rabbit liver. Carcinogenesis. 1984;5:1717–23.

51. Gillette JR. Activation systems – characteristics and drawbacks – comparisons of different organs, tissues, problems with toxication–detoxication balance in various tissues, extrapolation from *in vitro* to *in vivo*. Pharmacokinetics, absorption, distribution, excretion, metabolism. In: deSerres FJ, Fouts JR, Bend JR, Philpot RM, editors. In Vitro Metabolic Activation in Mutagenesis Testing. Amsterdam: Elsevier/North Holland; 1976:13–54.
52. Hardwick JP, Gonzalez FJ, Kasper CB. Transcriptional regulation of rat liver epoxide hydratase, NADPH-cytochrome P-450 oxidoreductase, and cytochrome P-450b genes by phenobarbital. J Biol Chem. 1983;258:8081–5.
53. Pike SF, Shephard EA, Rabin BR, Phillips IR. Induction of cytochrome P-450 by phenobarbital is mediated at the level of transcription. Biochem Pharmacol. 1985;34:2489–94.
54. Israel DI, Whitlock Jr JP. Regulation cytochrome P1-450 gene transcription by 2,3,7,8-tetrachlorodibenzo-*p*-dioxin in wild type and variant mouse hepatoma cells. J Biol Chem. 1984;259:5400–2.
55. Gonzalez FJ, Tukey RH, Nebert DW. Structural gene products of the Ah locus. Transcriptional regulation of cytochrome P1-450 and P3-450 mRNA levels by 3-methylcholanthrene. Mol Pharmacol. 1984;26:117–21.
56. Simmons DL, McQuiddy P, Kasper CB. Induction of the hepatic mixed-function oxidase system by synthetic glucocorticoids. J Biol Chem. 1987;262:326–32.
57. Potenza CL, Pendurthi UR, Strom DK *et al.* Regulation of the rabbit cytochrome P-450 3c gene: age dependent expression and transcriptional activation by rifampicin. J Biol Chem. 1989;264:16222–8.
58. Hardwick JP, Song B-J, Huberman E, Gonzalez FJ. Isolation, complementary DNA sequence, and regulation of rat hepatic lauric acid omega-hydroxylase (cytochrome P-450LAomega). J Biol Chem. 1987;262:801–10.
59. Song B-J, Gelboin HV, Park S-S, Yang CS, Gonzalez FJ. Complementary DNA and protein sequences of ethanol-inducible rat and human cytochrome P-450s. J Biol Chem. 1986;261:16689–97.
60. Porter TD, Khani SC, Coon MJ. Induction and tissue-specific expression of rabbit cytochrome P450IIE1 and IIE2 genes. Mol Pharmacol. 1989;36:61–5.
61. Song BJ, Matsunaga T, Hardwick JP *et al.* Stabilization of cytochrome P450j messenger ribonucleic acid in the diabetic rat. Mol Endocrinol. 1987;1:542–7.
62. Watkins PB, Wrighton SA, Schuetz EG, Maurel P, Guzelian PS. Macrolide antibiotics inhibit the degradation of the glucocorticoid-responsive cytochrome P-450p in rat hepatocytes *in vivo* and in primary monolayer culture. J Biol Chem. 1986;261:6264–71.
63. Combalbert J, Fabre I, Fabre G *et al.* Metabolism of cyclosporin A. IV. Purification and identification of the rifampicin-inducible human liver cytochrome P-450 (cyclosporin A oxidase) as a product of P450IIIA gene subfamily. Drug Metab Dispos. 1989;17:197–207.
64. Ged C, Rouillon JM, Pichard L *et al.* The increase in urinary excretion of 6β-hydroxycortisol as a marker of human hepatic cytochrome P450IIIA induction. Br J Clin Pharmacol. 1989;28:373–87.
65. Lange R, Larroque C, Balny C, Maurel P. Isolation and partial characterization of a rifampicin induced rabbit liver microsomal cytochrome P-450. Biochem Biophys Res Commun. 1985;126:833–9.
66. Wrighton SA, Schuetz EG, Watkins PB *et al.* Demonstration in multiple species of inducible hepatic cytochromes P-450 and their mRNAs related to the glucocorticoid-inducible cytochrome P-450 of the rat. Mol Pharmacol. 1985;28:312–21.
67. Kliewer SA, Moore JT, Wade L *et al.* An orphan nuclear receptor activated by pregnanes defines a novel steroid signaling pathway. Cell. 1998;92:73–82.
68. Blumberg B, Sabbagh WJ, Juguilon H *et al.* SXR, a novel steroid and xenobiotic-sensing nuclear receptor. Genes Dev. 1998;12:3195–205.
69. Bertilsson G, Heidrich J, Svensson K *et al.* Identification of a human nuclear receptor defines a new signaling pathway for CYP3A induction. Proc Natl Acad Sci USA. 1998;95:12208–13.
70. Savas Ü, Griffin KJ, Johnson EF. Molecular mechanisms of cytochrome P-450 induction by xenobiotics: an expanded role for nuclear receptors. Mol Pharmacol. 1999;56:851–87.
71. Savas U, Wester MR, Griffin KJ, Johnson EF. The rabbit pregnane X receptor is activated by rifampicin. Drug Metab Dispos. 2000;28:529–37.
72. Zhang H, LeCulyse E, Liu L *et al.* Rat pregnane X receptor: molecular cloning, tissue distribution, and xenobiotic regulation. Arch Biochem Biophys. 1999;368:14–22.

73. Issemann I, Green S. Activation of a member of the steroid hormone receptor superfamily by peroxisome proliferators. Nature. 1990;347:645–50.
74. Muerhoff AS, Griffin KJ, Johnson EF. The peroxisome proliferator activated receptor mediates the induction of CYP4A6, a cytochrome P450 fatty acid omega-hydroxylase, by clofibric acid. J Biol Chem. 1992;267:19051–3.
75. Kawamoto T, Sueyoshi T, Zelko I, Moore R, Washburn K, Negishi M. Phenobarbital-responsive nuclear translocation of the receptor CAR in induction of the CYP2B gene. Mol Cell Biol. 1999;19:6318–22.
76. Hoffman EC, Reyes H, Chu F-F *et al.* Cloning of a factor required for activity of the Ah (dioxin) receptor. Science. 1991;252:954–8.
77. Reyes H, Reisz-Porszasz S, Hankinson O. Identification of the Ah receptor nuclear translocator protein (Arnt) as a component of the DNA binding form of the Ah receptor. Science. 1992;256:1193–5.
78. Ema M, Sogawa K, Watanabe N *et al.* cDNA cloning and structure of mouse putative Ah receptor. Biochem Biophys Res Commun. 1992;184:246–53.
79. Burbach KM, Poland A, Bradfield CA. Cloning of the Ah-receptor cDNA reveals a distinctive ligand-activated transcription factor. Proc Natl Acad Sci USA. 1992;89:8185–9.
80. Manns MP, Griffin KJ, Quattrochi LC *et al.* Identification of cytochrome P450IA2 as a human autoantigen. Arch Biochem Biophys. 1990;280:229–32.
81. Clemente MG, Meloni A, Obermayer-Straub P, Frau F, Manns MP, De Virgiliis S. Two cytochromes P450 are major hepatocellular autoantigens in autoimmune polyglandular syndrome type 1. Gastroenterology. 1998;114:324–8.
82. Bourdi M, Gautier J-C, Mircheva J *et al.* Anti-liver microsomes autoantibodies and dihydralazine-induced hepatitis: Specificity of autoantibodies and inductive capacity of the drug. Mol Pharmacol. 1992;42:280–5.
83. Bourdi M, Tinel M, Beaune PH, Pessayre D. Interactions of dihydralazine with cytochromes P4501A: a possible explanation for the appearance of anti-cytochrome P4501A2 autoantibodies. Mol Pharmacol. 1994;45:1287–95.
84. Eliasson E, Stal P, Oksanen A, Lytton S. Expression of autoantibodies to specific cytochromes P450 in a case of disulfiram hepatitis. J Hepatol. 1998;29:819–25.
85. Beaune P, Dansette PM, Mansuy D *et al.* Human anti-endoplasmic reticulum autoantibodies appearing in a drug-induced hepatitis are directed against a human liver cytochrome P-450 that hydroxylates the drug. Proc Natl Acad Sci USA 1987;84:551–5.
86. Lecoeur S, André C, Beaune PH. Tienilic acid-induced autoimmune hepatitis: anti-liver and -kidney microsomal type 2 autoantibodies recognize a three-site conformational epitope on cytochrome P4502C9. Mol Pharmacol. 1996;50:326–33.
87. Philipp T, Straub P, Durazzo M, Tukey RH, Manns MP. Molecular analysis of autoantigens in hepatitis D. J Hepatol. 1995;22 Suppl. 1:132–5.
88. Abuaf N, Johanet C, Chretien P *et al.* Characterization of the liver cytosol antigen type 1 reacting with autoantibodies in chronic active hepatitis. Hepatology. 1992;16:892–8.
89. Lunel F, Abuaf N, Frangeul L *et al.* Liver/kidney microsome antibody type 1 and hepatitis C virus infection. Hepatology. 1992;16:630–6.
90. Manns MP. Viruses and autoimmune liver disease. Intervirology. 1993;35:108–15.
91. Riley RJ, Smith G, Wolf CR, Cook VA, Leeder JS. Human anti-endoplasmic reticulum autoantibodies produced in aromatic anticonvulsant hypersensitivity reactions recognise rodent CYP3A proteins and a similarly regulated human P450 enzyme(s). Biochem Biophys Res Commun. 1993;191:32–40.
92. Leeder JS, Riley RJ, Cook VA, Spielberg SP. Human anti-cytochrome P450 antibodies in aromatic anticonvulsant-induced hypersensitivity reactions. J Pharmacol Exp Ther. 1992;263:360–7.
93. Uibo R, Aavik E, Peterson P *et al.* Autoantibodies to cytochrome P450 enzymes P450scc, P450c17, and P450c21 in autoimmune polyglandular disease types I and II and in isolated Addison's disease. J.Clin Endocrinol Metab. 1994;78:323–8.
94. Winqvist O, Gustafsson J, Rorsman F, Karlsson FA, Kämpe O. Two different cytochrome P450 enzymes are the adrenal antigens in autoimmune polyendocrine syndrome type I and Addison's disease. J Clin Invest. 1993;92:2377–85.
95. Williams PA, Cosme J, Sridher V, Johnson EF, Mc Ree DE. The crystallographic structure of a mammalian microsomal cytochrome P450 monooxygenase: Structural adaptations for membrane binding and functional diversity. Mol Cell. 2000;5:121–132.

# 16
# Uridine diphosphate 5′-glucuronosyltransferases (UGT): genetic organization and function

C.P. STRASSBURG, M.P. MANNS and R.H. TUKEY

## INTRODUCTION

UDP-glucuronosyltransferases (UGT) are a superfamily of drug-metabolizing enzymes located in the inner membrane of the endoplasmic reticulum[1]. They perform a simple biochemical reaction which transforms lipophilic compounds such as dietary constituents, environmental toxins, carcinogens, and therapeutic drugs into water-soluble glucuronides[2]. Conjugation with glucuronic acid therefore facilitates renal and biliary elimination and almost always leads to inactive metabolites. UGT have evolved in vertebrate species, and the number of identified isoforms exceeds 50. The formation of glucuronides can proceed utilizing –O.R, –SR, –N.R′R″ or C.R chemical groups. This promiscuous property results in a broad range of chemically divergent xenobiotic and endobiotic compounds which are targeted for glucuronidation. In their ability to metabolize oxidized compounds, UGT complement the metabolic function of phase I enzymes including the cytochromes P450 (CYP), which are also located in the endoplasmic reticulum (external membrane) (Figure 1A). The considerable number and functional redundancy of the UGT supergene family indicates the importance of glucuronidation for homeostasis.

To date, 16 human UGT have been identified and cloned. Based on sequence homology data, UGT are divided into two families: UGT1 containing eight members and UGT2 containing seven members. The human *UGT1A* locus spans more than 150 kb on chromosome 2q37 and encodes UGT1A1[3], UGT1A3[4], UGT1A4[3], UGT1A5 (no mRNA expression detected so far), UGT1A6[5], UGT1A7[6], UGT1A8[7, 8], UGT1A9[9] and UGT1A10[6, 10, 11]. It is characterized by a unique genetic organization combining individual first exon cassettes at the 5′ end and common exons 2–5 at the 3′ end of the locus[12]. Individual transferase isoforms are generated by a strategy of exon sharing resulting in UGT1A gene products which share an identical carboxyterminal domain and differ in the aminoterminal portion (Figure 1B). Despite the shared carboxyterminal portion

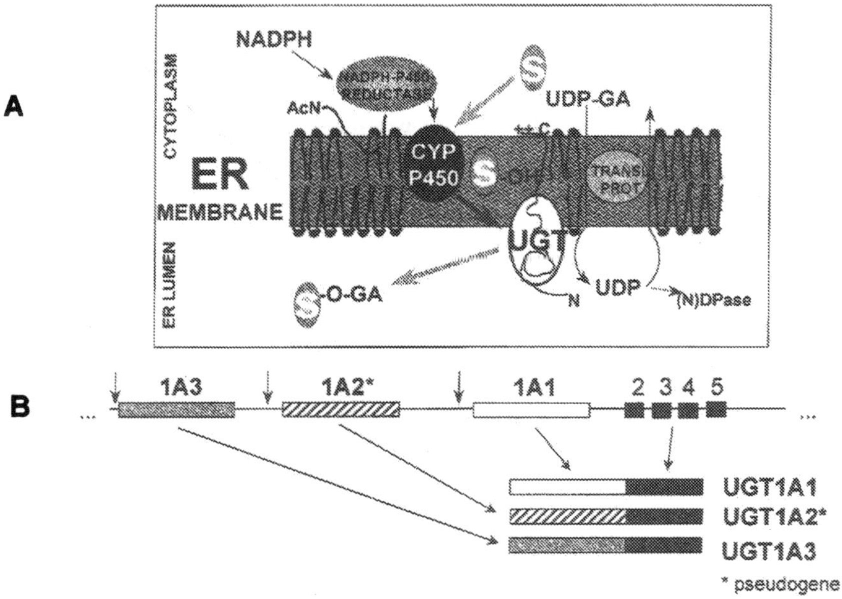


**Fig. 1** A: Schematic of the UGT membrane topology and function. The UDP-glucuronosyltransferases (UGT) are localized in the inner membrane of the endoplasmic reticulum (ER) and are anchored by a hydrophobic domain within the carboxyl terminus. Complementary metabolism of substrates (S) is performed with oxidative enzymes such as cytochromes (CYP). An unidentified, hypothetical transporter (Transl. Protein) shuttles UDP-glucuronic acid into the ER lumen. **B**: Schematic representation of the structure of the human *UGT1A* gene locus on chromosome 2. Individually variable exon 1 cassettes with appropriate promoter sequences (arrows) are numbered from the 3′ to the 5′ end of the locus. Common exons 2–5 are situated at the 3′ end of the gene locus which spans more than 150 000 bp. Individual UGT1A gene products are generated by exon sharing combining individual first exons with common exons 2–5. Transcription is initiated upstream of the exon 1 sequence and proceeds to the end of the locus. The sequence located between the donor splice site at the end of each exon 1 and the acceptor splice site at the beginning of exon 2 is then eliminated to form the individual UGT1A isoform mRNA. In this way up to nine functional UGT1A transcripts can be generated. UGT1A2 does not have an uninterrupted open reading frame and is therefore a pseudogene (*).

of 245 amino acids, UGT1A gene products are individually regulated and transcribed. In contrast to the *UGT1A* gene locus, *UGT2B* genes have been mapped to chromosome 4q13 and 4q28[13, 14]. *UGT2B* genes are encoded as individual genes and contain six exons. Transcripts of UGT2B4[15], UGT2B7[16], UGT2B10[17], UGT2B11[18], UGT2B15[14, 19], and UGT2B17[20] have been identified. In addition, UGT2A1[21], which is localized in olfactory tissue, has been cloned.

The human UGT span between 529 and 534 amino acids. Their sequences include conserved regions in the carboxyl terminus which anchors the protein into the endoplasmic reticulum membrane. The variable amino terminus is believed to define substrate specificity. In addition, all UGT apart from UGT1A10[6] have an N-terminal signal peptide domain which directs the protein to the endoplasmic reticulum.

While the initial studies of the physiological role of human glucuronidation relied on the isolation and purification of UGT proteins mainly from liver[22, 23], the introduction of molecular biological methods and tools has led to the identification of new isoforms, to the characterization of UGT catalytic function and to an elucidation of their role in different human diseases including unconjugated hyperbilirubinaemia, carcinogenesis and autoimmunity[3, 6, 7, 10, 24] (reviewed in ref. 1).

## BILIRUBIN METABOLISM AND UNCONJUGATED HYPERBILIRUBINAEMIA

The discovery of the human bilirubin UGT in 1991[3] has been the driving force of the discovery of the human *UGT1A* locus[9, 12]. Since 1991, 33 polymorphic alleles of the bilirubin transferase UGT1A1 have been identified and it has become evident that unconjugated hyperbilirubinaemia is the result of homozygous or compound heterozygous mutations of this isoform (reviewed in ref. 1). UGT1A1 is the only effective human bilirubin glucuronidating enzyme[25]. This is evident from the finding of mutations exclusively in the UGT1A1 exon 1 coding region which are capable of producing a complete absence of bilirubin glucuronides in the affected subjects. This event leaves all other UGT1A gene products intact. Clinically, the complete absence of UGT1A1 activity leads to fatal Crigler–Najjar type 1 disease, whereas a reduction of bilirubin activity to below 30% is compatible with Crigler–Najjar type 2 disease. In Gilbert's disease, mutations of the UGT1A1 promoter have been identified leading to a reduced expression of UGT1A1 gene products[26, 27]. From the analysis of the 32 known polymorphic UGT1A1 alleles it has been demonstrated that mutant alleles in both Crigler–Najjar type 1 and type 2 disease can affect all five exons. Different combinations of promoter mutations and homozygous or compound heterozygous combinations of coding region mutant alleles can lead to all three conditions (Figure 2). Based upon these findings, unconjugated hyperbilirubinaemia is not inherited in an autosomal dominant mode, but rather in an autosomal recessive mode.

## TISSUE-SPECIFIC REGULATION

Based on the discovery of the bilirubin UGT and the *UGT1A* locus glucuronidation was considered primarily to represent a metabolic pathway of the liver. This was substantiated by the cloning of UGT1A1, UGT1A3, UGT1A4, UGT1A6 and UGT1A9 from liver cDNA libraries. Additional UGT1A gene products were not detected. Based on the hypothesis, that UGT may function as a metabolic barrier, required to exist in tissues exposed to xenobiotic material such as the gastrointestinal tract, polymerase chain reaction (PCR)-based methodology was developed to identify individual UGT1A exons with high homology[6] (Figure 3). The main obstacle was the high homology of the UGT1A3-5 and UGT1A7-10 first exon cluster, which amounts to 94%. Specific discrimination of these gene products required the development of methods capable of detecting single base-pair differences. Previous studies had demonstrated that UGT

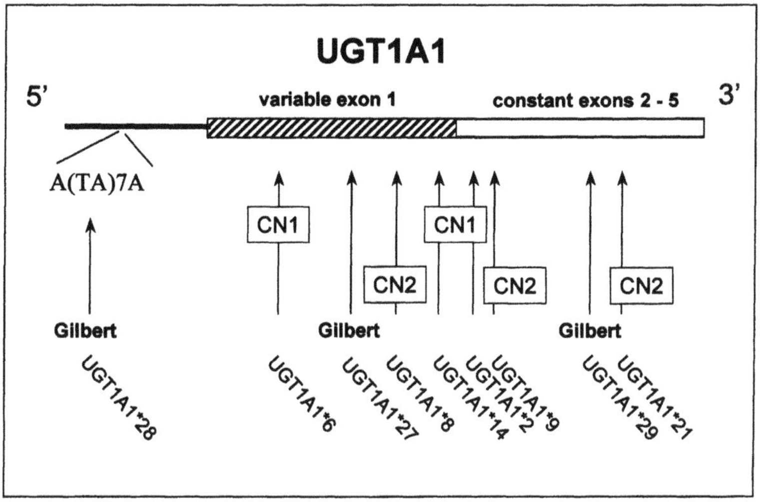


**Fig. 2** Human UGT1A1 is the only effective bilirubin-conjugating enzyme and variations of its function lead to unconjugated hyperbilirubinaemia. In Crigler–Najjar type 1 disease (CN1) UGT1A1 activity is absent, in Crigler–Najjar type 2 disease (CN2) UGT1A1 activity is reduced to under 30%, in Gilbert's disease hyperbilirubinaemia is the result of a less active UGT1A1 promoter variant and possibly additional mutant alleles. 32 mutant *UGT1A1* alleles have been identified. Contrary to early reports the mutant alleles can affect any of the five exons and lead to all three conditions. The presence of homozygous or compound heterozygous mutant alleles is required for a phenotype. Therefore, the mode of inheritance appears to be autosomal recessive. The schematic shows a selection of mutant alleles distributed throughout the *UGT1A1* gene and found in all three conditions

activity was present in kidney, intestine and colon but the precise repertoire of UGT1A transcripts had not been defined[28–30]. The analysis of oesophageal[31], gastric[32], biliary[6, 10] and colon tissue[6, 33] demonstrated the presence of UGT activity and of UGT1A mRNA expression in these organs with direct contact to ingested matter. A significantly lower level of overall UGT1A mRNA was detected in the extrahepatic tissues in comparison to liver epithelium[6]. Utilizing a detailed expression analysis by duplex reverse transcriptase PCR (DRT-PCR) we identified novel UGT1A mRNA not present in liver: UGT1A7 in oesophagus and stomach[6], UGT1A8 in oesophagus and colon[7, 31], and UGT1A10 (Figure 3) in all gastrointestinal tissues apart from liver[7]. These uniquely extrahepatic UGT1A gene products were cloned and expressed in heterologous expression systems for an analysis of their substrate specificities. The sequence analyses revealed typical UGT1A transcripts with divergent first exons and the consensus exons 2–5. Surprisingly, UGT1A10 lacked the N-terminal signal peptide domain present on all other UGT gene products, which is believed to target UGT proteins to the endoplasmic reticulum. Despite this abnormality, catalytic activity was demonstrated for recombinant UGT1A10 as well as for UGT1A7[7]. In comparison to the activity profile of other UGT isoforms both UGT1A10 and UGT1A7 were capable of glucuronidation of planar and complex phenolic substrates similar to the activities found with hepatic UGT1A6 and UGT1A9. However, UGT1A10 was identified to exhibit catalytic activity towards steroid hormones including $\beta$-oestradiol, oestrone and androsterone, all of which are

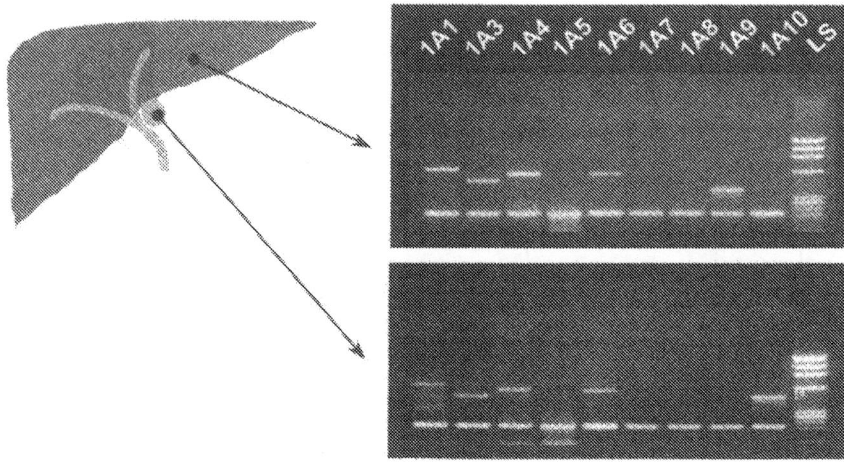


**Fig. 3** Example of the tissue-specific regulation of UGT1A transcripts. This experiment demonstrates the expression of UGT1A1, UGT1A3, UGT1A4, UGT1A6 and UGT1A9 in human liver and the absence of UGT1A5, UGT1A7, UGT1A8 and UGT1A10. In contrast, biliary epithelium does not express UGT1A9 and is characterized by UGT1A10 transcription. This experiment led to the identification and cloning of UGT1A10 which has now been found to be expressed in oesophagus, stomach, biliary epithelium and colon, but is absent from liver. The ethidium bromide-stained gels show duplex reverse transcriptase polymerase chain reaction products specifically amplified despite a high degree of sequence homology. Note that $\beta$-actin cDNA (lower band in each lane) was coamplified in every lane for quantification and quality purposes

not metabolized by UGT1A7. These data identify the novel extrahepatic UGT1A10 as only the second oestrone UGT and provide evidence for specific activity differences of UGT isoforms expressed in the liver and those present in extrahepatic tissues. In addition, both isoforms were capable of glucuronidating the tobacco carcinogen metabolites 7- and 8-hydroxy-benzo($\alpha$)pyrene. These findings conclusively demonstrate a quantitative and qualitative differential regulation of UGT in liver and the extrahepatic gastrointestinal tract. Differential regulation of UGT isoforms is therefore believed to represent the biochemical basis of tissue-specific glucuronidation activity in humans.

Studies of the catalytic activity in human liver and colon have demonstrated the individual catalytic profile of the two organs. While the overall hepatic activity rates of phenolic substrates were 96-fold higher for 4-nitrophenol and 64-fold higher for 4-isopropylphenol than those found in colon epithelium, a group of compounds including amitriptyline, desipramine, oestrone, imipramine and acetaminophen were conjugated with comparable rates in both tissues[33]. This catalytic behaviour clearly indicates a tissue-specific distribution of glucuronidation in human tissues and identifies the colon as a site of active metabolism likely to impact first-pass metabolism. Immunofluorescence analysis[33] has additionally localized UGT protein expression exclusively to the epithelial cell layer in colon tissue which is characterized by immediate contact to xenobiotic materials (Figure 4).

The expression pattern analysis of human gastric epithelium differed from the expression of UGT1A transcripts in liver and colon. Hepatic UGT1A expression

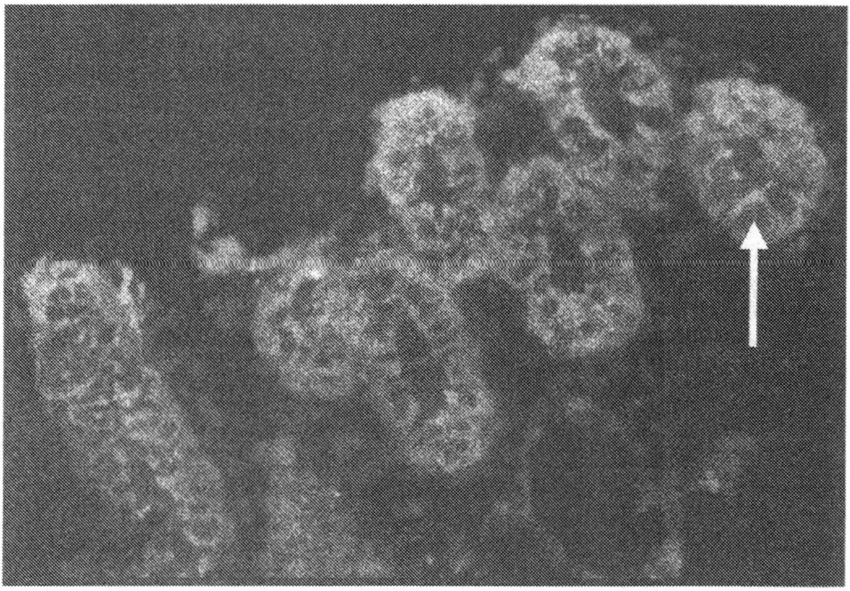

**Fig. 4** Immunofluorescence detection of UGT1A protein in the epithelial cell layer of sigmoid colon. Note the perinuclear pattern compatible with the localization of UGT in the endoplasmic reticulum. UGT1A protein was detected with a rabbit anti-human UGT exon 5 antibody diluted 1:160. This experiment documents that UGT1A proteins are located at the site of immediate xenobiotic contact of the digestive tract mucosa. Arrow – cell nucleus of a colon epithelial cell

is uniformly characterized by the presence of UGT1A1, UGT1A3, UGT1A4, UGT1A6 and UGT1A9[10] (Figure 3). In colon, UGT1A8 and UGT1A10 are expressed in addition to the hepatic isoforms[7]. When gastric epithelium was analysed a polymorphic mode of UGT1A gene product expression was detected. UGT1A7 and UGT1A10 transcripts were constitutively detected in all individuals but UGT1A1 (29%), UGT1A3 (21%), and UGT1A6 (36%) transcription was characterized by interindividual variation[32]. The functional impact of this finding was 2-4-fold interindividual variations of gastric microsomal UGT activity in addition to a qualitative variation of hyodeoxycholic acid glucuronidation between individuals. This regulatory polymorphism, which is different from the bimodally distributed genetic polymorphisms found in other drug-metabolizing enzymes, may represent the biochemical basis of interindividual differences in extrahepatic microsomal drug metabolism.

## UGT AND CARCINOGENESIS

The exposure to dietary and environmental carcinogens derived from combustion gases and tobacco smoke has been implicated in the aetiology of multiple human neoplasms. The human gastrointestinal tract is a common site of cancer development, and 9.7% of all newly diagnosed human cancers are found in the colon. A genoprotective and cytoprotective role for UGT has been proposed and their specific expression pattern in the human digestive system may link glucuronidation with neoplastic transformation[10, 34, 35]. In microsomal metabolism a tightly regulated balance of oxidative metabolism (i.e. by cytochrome P450 mono-oxygenases) and conjugation prevents the accumulation of reactive oxygen species which can result in DNA and protein adduct formation and may ultimately lead to carcinogenic initiation (Figure 5). Phenolic substrates can be oxidized to radicals such as epoxides, polyphenols, semiquinones and quinones; the latter can enter quinol/quinone redox cycling and result in the accumulation of radical oxygen species[34]. Phenols are targeted for glucuronidation by UGT1A gene products and glucuronidation may therefore prevent the generation of reactive nucleophiles and electrophiles. The presence of UGT1A proteins in the epithelial cell layers of organs with carcinogen exposure and gastrointestinal cancer development such as the oesophagus, the stomach, biliary tissue and the distal colon has been identified[6, 31, 33]. A significant observation is the considerable difference of UGT activity between human colon and liver tissue[28, 33]. In sigmoid colon the glucuronidation rate of 8-hydroxy-benzo($\alpha$)pyrene was 214-fold lower than in liver and the glucuronidation efficiency ($V_{max}/K_m$) was 70-fold lower[33]. Low glucuronidation rates for key metabolites coincide with the anatomical location of carcinogen-dependent neoplastic transformation in colon. The catalytic analysis of recombinant UGT proteins has shown that carcinogens such as primary amines, benzo($\alpha$)pyrene metabolites and the tobacco smoke carcinogen 2-hydroxyamino-1-methyl-6-phenylimidazo-(4, 5-$\beta$)pyridine (N-hydroxy PhIP) are substrates of a variety of human UGT including the newly identified extrahepatic human isoforms UGT1A7, UGT1A8 and UGT1A10[31].

The analysis of human hepatocellular carcinoma[10], cholangiocellular carcinoma[10], gastric carcinoma[32] and oesophageal carcinoma[31] has shown a pattern of differential down-regulation of UGT1A transcription in cancer tissue versus

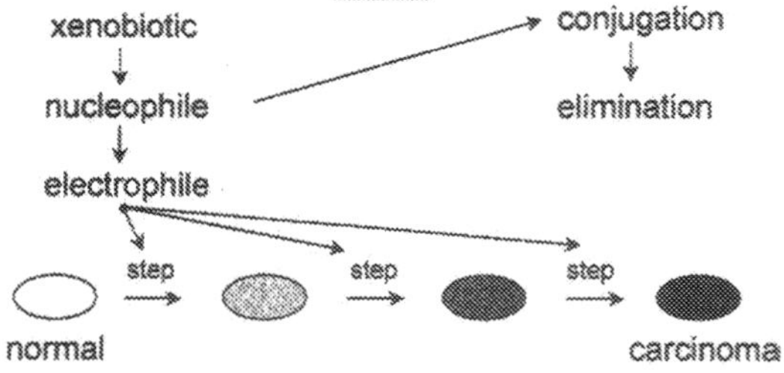


**Fig. 5** Hypothesis of chemically induced carcinogenesis. Oxidative metabolism leads to the generation of reactive metabolites such as epoxides, polyphenols, semiquinones and quinones. By conjugation of the original compound or the nucleophilic intermediate, subsequent cytotoxicity and genotoxicity can be prevented. In this respect UGT proteins may serve as a protective metabolic barrier in carcinogenesis

normal surrounding tissue. Although individual isoforms are selectively regulated in this process the general finding is that catalytic UGT activity towards carcinogens is significantly decreased in cancer tissue. In the example of hepaticellular carcinoma, differential down-regulation of the *UGT1A* locus was also detected at the early stage of adenomatous hyperplasia, indicating that UGT1A regulation may represent an early event of malignant tumorigenesis. Conversely, the analysis of benign focal nodular hyperplasia of the liver did not elicit regulation of UGT1A gene products.

In gastric tissue, in which a polymorphic regulation of UGT1A isoforms has been described, the interindividual variation of 7-hydroxy-benzo($\alpha$)pyrene glucuronidation was found to vary 4-fold between individuals[32]. In this respect polymorphic expression of UGT isoforms may not only represent the biochemical basis of individual drug metabolism but may also represent a carcinogenic risk factor.

In human oesophagus a very limited expression of four highly homologous UGT1A gene products was detected: UGT1A7, UGT1A8, UGT1A9 and UGT1A10. This tissue is therefore a model to study the catalytic effects of these mainly extrahepatic isoforms in the absence of the hepatic UGT1A1, UGT1A3, UGT1A4 and UGT1A6 gene products[31]. In squamous cell carcinoma of the oesophagus, down-regulation of UGT1A7 and UGT1A10 but not of UGT1A8 and UGT1A9 was detected. The resulting loss of 7-hydroxy-benzo($\alpha$)pyrene glucuronidation activity is therefore attributable to these isoforms and documents the role of extrahepatic UGT in carcinogen metabolism. This is particularly relevant in the oesophagus, which has been epidemiologically linked to tobacco smoke-derived carcinogen metabolites such as N-hydroxy PhIP and 7-hydroxy-benzo($\alpha$)pyrene, both of which are glucuronidated by recombinant UGT1A7 and UGT1A10[31].

The specific expression of unique UGT patterns in tissues with carcinogen-associated cancer, the localization of UGT specifically at the epithelial site of xenobiotic contact, the lower levels of UGT activity in the distal and proximal gastrointestinal tract in which cancer development is frequently detected, and the ability of UGT1A isoforms to conjugate and detoxify typical environmental carcinogens suggests a genoprotective role of UGT in human carcinogenesis.

## UGT AND AUTOIMMUNITY

In 1973 human autoantibodies directed against the endoplasmic reticulum in liver and the proximal renal tubules (liver-kidney microsomal autoantibodies, LKM) were detected[36], which have now been characterized to target microsomal drug-metabolizing enzymes. A clinically distinct second form of autoimmune hepatitis, termed autoimmune hepatitis type 2, was identified which exhibits anti-CYP2D6 autoantibodies (LKM-1 autoantibodies) as a serological marker[36–40]. A distinct type of LKM autoantibody was discovered in 1983 in patients with chronic hepatitis D[41]. These autoantibodies, designated LKM-3, were recently characterized to target family 1 UGT[42]. Beyond their occurrence as markers in about 10% of patients with hepatitis D infection, LKM-3 autoantibodies have been identified as serological markers in 10% of patients with

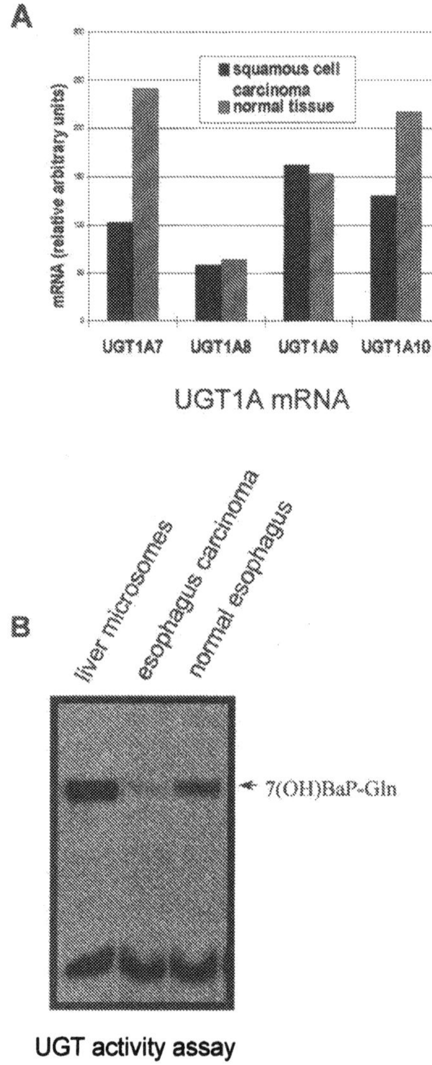


**Fig. 6** Example of differential down-regulation of UGT1A transcripts in human squamous cell carcinoma of the oesophagus in comparison to surrounding normal tissue from the same patient. A similar pattern of UGT1A down-regulation has been shown to exist in human hepatocellular carcinoma, gastric carcinoma and cholangiocellular carcinoma, but not in the benign tumour of focal nodular hyperplasia of the liver. **A**: In oesophagus only UGT1A7, UGT1A8, UGT1A9 and UGT1A10 are expressed, differential down-regulation is observed for UGT1A7 and UGT1A10. The expression of UGT2B isoforms in this tissue is negligible (not shown). The relative mRNA levels quantitated by duplex reverse transcription polymerase chain reaction are shown. **B**: In a catalytic activity assay, shown as the autoradiography of 14C-labelled glucuronides produced by tissue microsomal protein and separated by thin-layer liquid chromatography, down-regulation of 7-hydroxy-benzo($\alpha$)pyrene glucuronidation is demonstrated. This finding conclusively demonstrates that the activities of the human extrahepatic UGT1A7 and UGT1A10 isoforms play a role in carcinogen metabolism in tissues epidemiologically linked to carcinogen exposure. 7(OH)BaP-Gln, glucuronide of 7-hydroxy-benzo($\alpha$)pyrene

autoimmune hepatitis type 2[24]. In humans, LKM-3 autoantibodies have been identified to target UGT1A1, UGT1A6, UGT1A4 and rabbit UGT1A6, as well as a minor reactivity with UGT2B isoforms[24, 42]. The B-cell response in hepatitis C and hepatitis D virus infection is very specific and shows no overlap[24]. LKM-3/anti-UGT1A autoantibodies are not detected in autoimmune hepatitis type 1, or in hepatitis C virus infection. Conversely, LKM-1 anti-CYP2D6 autoantibodies are not detected in hepatitis D or autoimmune hepatitis type 2 but in hepatitis C virus infection. It is therefore an interesting speculation that CYP and UGT proteins may be at the interface of virus trigger and a specific endogenous immunological dysregulation, and these autoantigen targets may serve as models to study the mechanisms of the loss of self-tolerance underlying autoimmunity.

## SUMMARY

Recent molecular biological investigations have provided an important insight into the genetic organization and function of the human UGT supergene family. The multiplicity and functional redundancy of the 16 identified human UGT, as well as a highly tissue-specific differential regulation, indicates their intricate involvement in microsomal metabolism and their overall physiological significance for homeostasis. UGT are a key component of bilirubin metabolism, the absence of which is not compatible with life. UGT are implicated to contribute to individual drug metabolism, enterohepatic circulation, first-pass metabolism and the protection from genotoxic and cytotoxic metabolites. In their role as metabolic first line of defence in many tissues, UGT are likely to play a significant role in human gastrointestinal carcinogenesis. In addition, UGT proteins have been identified as autoantigen targets in liver disease. They serve as model autoantigens and are utilized for the serological detection of autoimmune hepatitis and hepatitis D-associated autoantibodies in clinical practice.

### Acknowledgements

This work was supported by Deutsche Forschungsgemeinschaft STR 493/3-1 (C.P.S.) and United States Public Health services Grant 49135 (R.H.T.)

### References

1. Tukey RH, Strassburg CP. Human UDP-glucuronosyltransferase: metabolism, expression and disease. Annu Rev Pharmacol Toxicol. 2000;40:3.
2. Dutton GJ. Glucuronidation of Drugs and other Compounds. Boca Raton, FL: CRC Press; 1980.
3. Ritter JK, Crawford JM, Owens IS. Cloning of two human liver bilirubin UDP-glucuronosyltransferase cDNAs with expression in COS-1 cells. J Biol Chem. 1991;266:1043–1047.
4. Mojarrabi B, Butler R, Mackenzie PI. cDNA cloning and characterization of the human UDP glucuronosyltransferase, UGT1A3. Biochem Biophys Res Commun. 1996;255:785–790.
5. Harding D, Fournel-Gigleux S, Jackson MR, Burchell B. Cloning and substrate specificity of a human phenol UDP-glucuronosyltransferase expressed in COS-7 cells. Proc Natl Acad Sci USA. 1988;85:8381–8385.
6. Strassburg CP, Oldhafter K, Manns MP, Tukey RH. Differential expression of the UGT1A locus in human liver, biliary, and gastric tissue: identification of UGT1A7 and UGT1A10 transcripts in extrahepatic tissue. Mol Pharmacol. 1997;52:212–220.

7. Strassburg CP, Manns MP, Tukey RH. Expression of the UDP-glucuronosyltransferase 1A locus in human colon. Identification and characterization of the novel extrahepatic UGT1A8. J Biol Chem. 1998;273:8719–8726.
8. Cheng Z, Radominska-Pandya A, Tephly TR. Cloning and expression of human UDP-glucuronosyltransferase (UGT) 1A8. Arch Biochem Biophys. 1998;356:301–305.
9. Wooster R, Sutherland L, Ebner T, Clarke D, Da Cruz e Silva O, Burchell B. Cloning and stable expression of a new member of the human liver phenol/bilirubin: UDP-glucuronosyltransferase cDNA family. Biochem J. 1991;278:465–469.
10. Strassburg CP, Manns MP, Tukey RH. Differential down-regulation of the UDP-glucuronosyltransferase 1A locus is an early event in human liver and biliary cancer. Cancer Res. 1997;57:2979–2985.
11. Mojarrabi B, Mackenzie PI. The human UDP glucuronosyltransferase, UGT1A10, glucuronidates mycophenolic acid. Biochem Biophys Res Commun. 1997;238:775–778.
12. Ritter JK, Chen F, Sheen YY *et al.* A novel complex locus UGT1 encodes human bilirubin, phenol, and other UDP-glucuronosyltransferase isozymes with identical carboxyl termini. J Biol Chem. 1992;267:32573–23579.
13. Mohaghan G, Clarke DJ, Povey S, See CG, Boxer M, Burchell B. Isolation of a human YAC contig encompassing a cluster of UGT2 genes and its regional localization to chromosome 4q13. Genomics. 1994;23:496–499.
14. Chen F, Ritter JK, Wang MG, McBride OW, Lubet RA, Owens IS. Characterization of a cloned human dihydrotestosterone/androstanediol UDP-glucuronosyltransferase and its comparison to other steroid isoforms. Biochemistry. 1993;32:10648–10657.
15. Jackson MR, McCarthy LR, Harding D, Wilson S, Coughtrie MW, Burchell B. Cloning of a human liver microsomal UDP glucuronosyltransferase cDNA. Biochem J. 1987;242:581–588.
16. Ritter JK, Sheen YY, Owens IS. Cloning and expression of human liver UDP-glucuronosyltransferase in COS-1 cells. 3,4-catechol estrogens and estriol as primary substrates. J Biol Chem. 1990;265:7900–7906.
17. Jin CJ, Miners JO, Lilywhite KJ, Mackenzie PI. cDNA cloning and expression of two new members of the human liver UDP-glucuronosyltransferase 2B subfamily. Biochem Biophys Res Commun. 1993;194:496–503.
18. Beaulieu M, Levesque E, Hum DW, Belanger A. Isolation and characterization of a human orphan UDP-glucuronosyltransferase, UGT2B11. Biochem Biophys Res Commun. 1998;248:44–50.
19. Green MD, Oturu EM, Tephly TR. Stable expression of a human liver UDP-glucuronosyltransferase (UGT2B15) with activity toward steroid and xenobiotic substrates. Drug Metab Dispos. 1994;22:799–805.
20. Beaulieu M, Levesque E, Hum DW, Belanger A. Isolation and characterization of a novel cDNA encoding a human UDP-glucuronosyltransferase active on C19 steroids. J Biol Chem. 1996;271:22855–22862.
21. Jedlitschky G, Cassidy AJ, Sales M, Pratt N, Burchell B. Cloning and characterization of a novel human olfactory UDP-glucuronosyltransferase. Biochem J. 1999;340:837–843.
22. Matern H, Lappas N, Matern S. Isolation and characterization of hyodeoxycholic-acid: UDP-glucuronosyltransferase from human liver. Eur J Biochem. 1991;200:393–399.
23. Peters WH, Jansen PL. Immunocharacterization of UDP-glucuronosyltransferase isoenzymes in human liver, intestine and kidney. Biochem Pharmacol. 1988;37:564–567.
24. Strassburg CP, Obermayer-Straub P, Alex B *et al.* Autoantibodies against glucuronosyltransferases differ between viral hepatitis and autoimmune hepatitis. Gastroenterology. 1996;111:1576–1586.
25. Bosma PJ, Seppen J, Goldhoorn B *et al.* Bilirubin UDP-glucuronosyltransferase 1 is the only relevant bilirubin glucuronidating isoform in main [published erratum appears in J Biol Chem. J Biol Chem. 1994;269:17960–17964.
26. Monaghan G, Ryan M, Seddon R, Hume R, Burchell B. Genetic variation in bilirubin UDP- glucuronosyltransferase gene promoter and Gilbert's syndrome. Lancet. 1996;347:578–581.
27. Bosma PJ, Chowdhury JR, Bakker C *et al.* The genetic basis of the reduced expression of bilirubin UDP-glucuronosyltransferase 1 in Gilbert's syndrome. N Engl J Med. 1995;333:1171–1175.
28. Peters WH, Kock L, Nagengast FM, Kremers PG. Biotransformation enzymes in human intestine: critical low levels in the colon? Gut. 1991;32:408–412.
29. McDonnell WM, Hitomi E, Askari FK. Identification of bilirubin UDP-GTs in the human alimentary tract in accordance with the gut as a putative metabolic organ. Biochem Pharmacol. 1996;51:483–488.

30. Matern S, Matern H, Farthmann EH, Gerok W. Hepatic and extrahepatic glucuronidation of bile acids in man. Characterization of bile acid uridine 5′-diphosphate-glucuronosyltransferase in hepatic, renal, and intestinal microsomes. J Clin Invest. 1984;74:402–410.
31. Strassburg CP, Strassburg A, Nguyen N, Li Q, Manns MP, Tukey RH. Regulation and function of family 1 and family 2 UDP-glucuronosyltransferase genes (UGT1A, UGT2B) in human oesophagus. Biochem J. 1999;338:489–498.
32. Strassburg CP, Nguyen N, Manns MP, Tukey RH. Polymorphic expression of the UDP-glucuronosyltransferase UGT1A gene locus in human gastric epithelium. Mol Pharmacol. 1998;54:647–654.
33. Strassburg CP, Nguyen N, Manns MP, Tukey RH. UDP-glucuronosyltransferase activity in human liver and colon. Gastroenterology. 1999;116:149–160.
34. Lilienblum W, Bock-Hennig BS, Bock KW. Protection against toxic redox cycles between benzo($\alpha$)pyrene-3,6-quinone and its quinol by 3-methylcholanthrene-inducible formation of the quinol mono- and diglucuronide. Mol Pharmacol. 1985;27:451–456.
35. Bock KW. UDP-glucuronosyltransferases and their role in metabolism and disposition of carcinogens. Adv Pharmacol. 1994;27:367–383.
36. Rizzetto M, Swana G, Doniach D. Microsomal antibodies in active chronic hepatitis and other disorders. Clin Exp Immunol. 1973;15:331–344.
37. Manns MP, Johnson EF, Griffin KJ, Tan EM, Sullivan KF. Major antigen of liver kidney microsomal antibodies in idiopathic autoimmune hepatitis is cytochrome P450db1. J Clin Invest. 1989;83:1066–1072.
38. Homberg JC, Abuaf N, Bernard O *et al.* Chronic active hepatitis associated with antiliver/kidney microsome type 1: a second type of ‘autoimmune’ hepatitis. Hepatology. 1987;7:1333–1339.
39. Guenguen M, Yamamotoh AM, Bernard O, Alvarez F. Anti-liver kidney microsome antibody type 1 recognizes human cytochrome P450 db1. Biochem Biophys Res Comm. 1989;159:542–549.
40. Zanger UM, Hauri HP, Loeper J, Homberg JC, Meyer UA. Antibodies against human cytochrome P-450db1 in autoimmune hepatitis type 2. Proc Natl Acad Sci USA. 1988;85:8256–8260.
41. Crivelli O, Lavarini C, Chiaberge E *et al.* Microsomal autoantibodies in chronic infection with HBsAg associated delta (delta) agent. Clin Exp Immunol. 1983;54:232–238.
42. Philipp T, Durazzo M, Trautwein C *et al.* Recognition of uridine diphosphate glucuronosyl transferases by LKM-3 antibodies in chronic hepatitis D. Lancet. 1994;344:578–581.

# 17
# Allergic and autoimmune reactions to xenobiotics: how do they evolve?

M. WULFERINK, P. GRIEM and E. GLEICHMANN

## INTRODUCTION

Immune reactions to xenobiotics (i.e. drugs, metals, industrial and naturally occurring chemicals) can give rise to allergy and autoimmunity. These reactions are frequent and encompass a broad spectrum of different diseases and organs. In order to decrease the health risks associated with exposure to xenobiotics, it is important to understand the pathogenic mechanisms involved and to identify human populations at risk. In view of the striking clinicopathological similarity between adverse immune reactions to xenobiotics and graft-versus-host reactions, there is little doubt that adverse reactions to xenobiotics are initiated and maintained by T cells[1]. For immunologists a major difficulty in trying to study T-cell reactions to sensitizing xenobiotics is the fact that the ultimate neoantigens formed by xenobiotics are not known, even though considerable progress has recently been made in this respect using the classical hapten trinitrophenyl (TNP)[2,3] and 3-pentadecyl-catechol, a representative catechol derivative in urushiol, the sensitizing component of poison ivy[4]. In extension of these findings it is assumed that adverse immune reactions to other xenobiotics also involve formation of protein adducts (in the toxicological terminology) or hapten–carrier conjugates (in the immunological terminology).

Reactive organic compounds most often bind covalently; that is, their electrophilic properties enable them to react with protein nucleophilic groups such as thiol, amino and hydroxyl groups (reviewed in ref. 5). Examples of such reactive, haptenic compounds that frequently lead to sensitization after dermal contact or inhalation are toluene diisocyanate, trimellitic anhydride, phthalic anhydride, benzoquinone, formaldehyde, hexyl cinnamic aldehyde, ethylene oxide, dinitrochlorobenzene, picryl chloride, penicillins, and *D*-penicillamine. Sensitizing metal ions react somewhat differently in that they oxidize proteins or form stable protein–metal chelate complexes by undergoing multipoint binding with several amino acid side-chains (Figure 1). Since all of these compounds have long been known as sensitizers, protection measures are being taken in order to decrease the risk of sensitization (e.g. at workplaces).

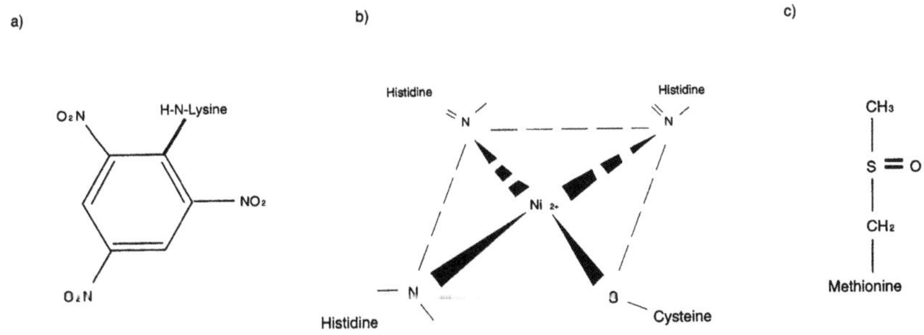


**Fig. 1** Haptens comprise organic compounds as well as metal ions and bind to proteins forming either covalent bonds (**a**) or coordination complexes (**b**). These two types of chemical bond differ in the amount of energy required to break the bond (bond strength). (**a**) Organic haptens forming covalent bonds bind to a single amino acid side-chain. Depicted is the covalent binding of trinitrophenyl (TNP) to lysine. (**b**) Metal complexes consist of a centre-placed metal ion and a set of atoms, ions or small molecules, regarded as ligands. These ligands are aligned in a characteristic geometric form, e.g. a plane square or an octagon. The interactions between a metal ion and ligands allow the electron-rich ligands to transfer part of their electron density to the positively charged metal ion (coordination bond) in order to increase complex stability. Depicted is a square planar complex of nickel with three histidines and one cysteine. (**c**) Alternatively, certain reactive chemicals can irreversibly oxidize protein side-chains, such as those of cysteine and methionine. Shown is a methionine sulphoxide

In contrast to haptenic compounds, most xenobiotics eliciting adverse immune reactions are unable to bind to proteins when entering the body; however, they can do so after conversion to reactive metabolites (Table 1). These xenobiotics can be considered as prohaptens. Hence, this chapter takes into account that neoantigen formation by prohaptens involves an initial pharmaco-toxicological phase that is determined by metabolic conversion of prohapten into hapten. This phase precedes the T-cell-sensitization phase, and this, in turn, is followed by an immune-effector phase that leads to the various clinicopathological manifestations of adverse immune reactions to xenobiotics. There are several model xenobiotics for each phase in this pathogenic cascade. The reader should be aware, however, that no single xenobiotic has yet been analysed so extensively that it could serve as a universal example for the entire cascade. Therefore, different xenobiotics will have to illustrate the individual phases described.

## PREIMMUNOLOGICAL PHASE

### Hepatic metabolism of xenobiotics

As the main organ for metabolism of xenobiotics the liver is well equipped with xenobiotic-metabolizing enzymes and is prepared for detoxifying reactive metabolites. This might be one of the reasons why, compared with its high metabolic activity, adverse immune reactions in the liver are relatively rare. Nevertheless, such reactions do occur; one example being the autoimmune hepatitis caused by long-term treatment with the diuretic drug tienilic acid (a prohapten). This side-effect is associated with the production of autoantibodies

**Table 1** Examples of adverse immune reactions to xenobiotics that involve reactive metabolites [a]

| *Parent compound* | *Adverse immune reaction* | *Candidate metabolite involved* | *Ref.* |
|---|---|---|---|
| Procainamide | Drug-induced lupus | *N*-Hydroxyprocainamide (M,H) | 15, 70 |
| Propylthiouracil | Vasculitis, drug-induced lupus | Propyluracilsulphonic acid (M,H) | 16, 71 |
| Halothane | Autoimmune hepatitis | Trifluoroacetylchloride (R,H) | 8, 72 |
| Tienilic acid | Autoimmune hepatitis | Thiophene sulphoxide (H) | 7 |
| Dihydralazine | Drug-induced lupus, autoimmune hepatitis | Hydralazine radical (R,H) | 9 |
| Gold(I) antirheumatics | Dermatitis, glomerulonephritis | Gold(III) (M,H) | 17, 73 |
| Practolol | Oculomucocutaneous syndrome | Practolol epoxide (H) | 74 |
| Urushiol | Contact dermatitis | 3-pentadecyl-*o*-quinone (M) | 4 |
| *p*-Phenylenediamine | Contact dermatitis | Bandrowski's base (H) | 14 |

[a] The adverse immune reactions listed in the table were observed in humans, while identification of candidate metabolites was achieved in: M, mice; R, rats; H, humans.

directed against the cytochrome P450 (CYP) isoenzyme 2C9 (CYP 2C9), and interestingly this is the very enzyme that catalyses hepatic metabolism of the prohapten to its reactive metabolite[6,7]. This short-lived, haptenic metabolite was found to bond covalently to CYP 2C9. A similar mechanism is assumed for other cases of drug-induced autoimmune hepatitis, such as those caused by halothane[8] or dihydralazine[9]; here, too, autoantibodies are directed against the enzymes converting these prohaptens to the respective haptens (CYP 2E1 and CYP 1A2, respectively). T-cell recognition of the haptenated enzymes in drug-induced hepatitis is likely, but has not been formally demonstrated.

## Extrahepatic metabolism of xenobiotics

In quantitative terms, extrahepatic metabolism of xenobiotics is less important than hepatic metabolism. However, as far as adverse immune reactions to prohaptens are concerned, extrahepatic metabolism appears to play a crucial role. Rather than being metabolized to reactive, haptenic metabolites in the liver, and subsequently travelling to distant extrahepatic sites such as the skin, lung, or bone marrow, it is likely that reactive metabolites are formed at the very sites where adverse immune reactions to xenobiotics manifest themselves. Hence, the xenobiotic-metabolizing capacity of extrahepatic tissues merits special attention in the present context. One example here is the skin, a barrier organ which has both a considerable metabolic capacity and immunological competence, and is often involved in adverse immune reactions to xenobiotics, be it after dermal or systemic application[10]. Interestingly, dermal Langerhans cells contain CYP 1A isoenzymes and are able to metabolize prohaptenic xenobiotics, such as the polyaromatic hydrocarbon dimethylbenz-[*a*]-anthracene, to haptens. They can activate specific T cells that mediate contact hypersensitivity, presumably by presentation of haptenated peptides[11]. Similarly, urushiol, a mixture of allergenic 3-alkyl and 3-alkenyl catechols from the plants poison ivy and poison oak, can be oxidized in the skin to reactive *o*-quinones that can elicit specific T-cell responses after adduct formation with protein[4,12,13]. Another chemical frequently involved in allergic contact dermatitis is *p*-phenylenediamine, which is oxidized to a reactive metabolite termed Bandrowski's base. Specific T-cell reactions to this hapten have been demonstrated *in vitro:* peripheral mononuclear cells of sensitized patients responded to Bandrowski's base, but not to the prohapten *p*-phenylenediamine[14].

## Xenobiotic metabolism in phagocytes

Phagocytes include polymorphonuclear leukocytes (PMN), monocytes, macrophages, and resident Langerhans cells. While the latter three can themselves act as antigen-presenting cells (APC), PMN die after they have been activated at inflammatory sites; the dead cells and debris are phagocytosed and processed by APC. Hence, the capacity of phagocytes to metabolize xenobiotics is particularly relevant in the present context. For instance, there is indirect evidence that metabolism in phagocytic cells may be involved in systemic adverse immune reactions caused by procainamide (PA)[15], propylthiouracil[16] and disodium gold(I) thiomalate[17]. Whereas the respective parent compounds, or prohaptens, themselves proved unable to elicit T-cell reactions in mice, their reactive metabolites generated in macrophages were able to do so.

Generation of reactive metabolites in neutrophils and monocytes has been attributed to metabolizing enzymes with a broad substrate specificity, such as myeloperoxidase (MPO), prostaglandin H synthase, and various CYP isoenzymes[10,18–20]. For PA it has been shown in mice that T cells sensitized to the reactive metabolite *N*-hydroxy-PA, which can easily be further oxidized to nitroso-PA (another reactive, unstable metabolite), recognized macrophages incubated with the non-reactive parent compound (i.e. the prohapten), indicating generation of the hapten and hapten–protein adducts in these cells[15]. Additionally, *in vivo* bioactivation of PA in macrophages to *N*-hydroxy-PA and nitroso-PA was indirectly demonstrated by successful restimulation of *N*-hydroxy-PA-primed T cells with peritoneal cells of long-term PA-treated mice[15] (Figure 2). Similar findings were obtained with a chemically different compound, the antirheumatic drug gold(I) thiomalate. Using gold(III)-specific T cells as detection probes in *in vivo* and *in vitro* assays, indirect evidence was provided for the generation of the short-lived, reactive metabolite gold(III) in macrophages[17,21]. Hence, in view of the multiple functions they can fulfil, macrophages, and presumably other types of APC, appear to serve as a connecting link between the preimmunological phase, which includes regional xenobiotic bioactivation and neoantigen formation, and the phase of T-cell sensitization to these neoantigens.

## Genetic polymorphisms of xenobiotic-metabolizing enzymes

Metabolism of xenobiotics can be divided into two phases. Phase I reactions, such as those carried out by CYP isoenzymes, usually lead to insertion of functional groups into xenobiotics, or lead to demasking of such groups, and thus can result in formation of reactive metabolites (some of which can act as haptens). In phase II reactions, metabolites are conjugated with small endogenous molecules, such as glucuronic acid, glutathione, acetate, or sulphate in order to increase water-solubility and facilitate elimination from the body. Unlike larger haptenated peptides, these conjugates are too small to make stable contact with the MHC binding groove and thus are unable to cause sensitization.

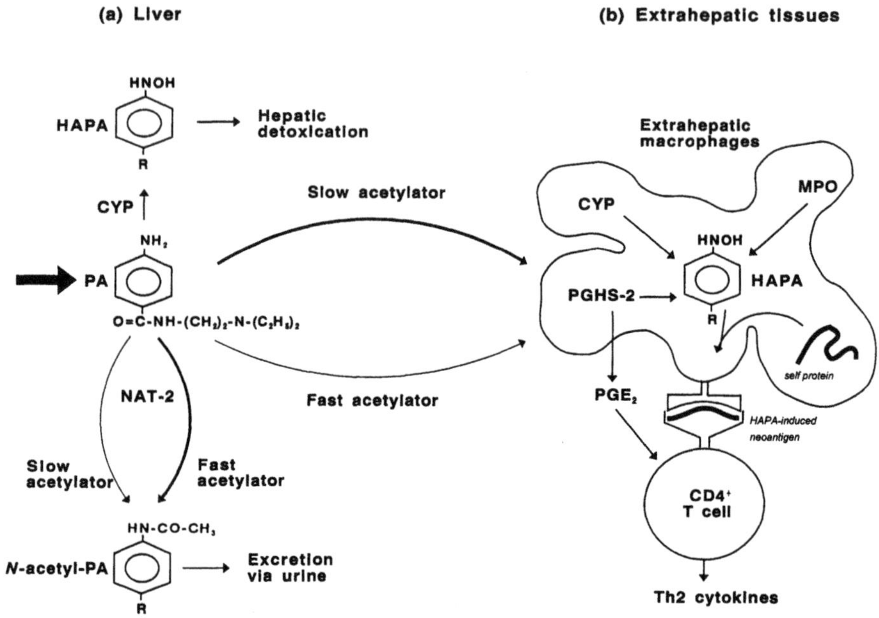


**Fig. 2** Hypothetical scheme of the initial immunotoxic steps underlying PA-induced SLE, based on experimental results[15,80]. (**a**) Hepatic metabolism of the arylamine PA consists of two competing pathways[26,27]. *N*-acetylation of the amino group, catalysed by NAT-2, leads to formation of *N*-acetyl PA, a stable metabolite that can be eliminated. By contrast, oxidation of the amino group by CYP isoenzymes yields HAPA and, through further oxidation, yields nitroso-PA (not shown); the latter can haptenate proteins and thus can induce the adverse immune reactions seen in PA-induced SLE. However, in the liver, probably due to its high detoxicating capacity, PA-induced adverse immune reactions fail to develop. Because of genetic polymorphism, individuals differ in their NAT-2 activity, resulting in the slow- and fast-acetylator phenotype. In slow-acetylator individuals, hepatic acetylation of PA is reduced, thereby increasing the amount of substrate available for extrahepatic PA metabolism. (**b**) Extrahepatic metabolism of PA can occur in phagocytic cells containing enzymes with a broad substrate specificity, such as PGHS-1, PGHS-2, MPO and CYP isoenzymes[10,18–20]. Importantly, phagocytic cells, like monocytes and macrophages, which are capable of oxidizing PA to HAPA and further to nitroso-PA, can process proteins and present hapten-conjugated peptides to T cells. Interestingly, PA was shown to induce expression of PGHS-2 in mouse macrophages, and thus can probably enhance its own oxidation to HAPA and nitroso-PA. Moreover, the PA-induced enhancement of the generation of $PGE_2$ by PGHS-2 might skew the immune reaction towards a Th2-type response[81], thereby favouring formation of (auto)antibodies.

Abbreviations: CYP, cytochrome P450 isoenzyme; HAPA, *N*-hydroxylamine PA; MPO, myeloperoxidase; NAT-2, *N*-acetyl transferase 2; PA, procainamide; $PGE_2$, prostaglandin $E_2$; PGHS, prostaglandin H synthase; SLE, systemic lupus erythematosus; Th2, T helper 2

Several genetic polymorphisms of xenobiotic-metabolizing enzymes have been identified, some of which cause expression of defective enzymes, or enzymes with a reduced (or increased) metabolic activity[22]. These inter-individual differences in the generation of reactive metabolites among humans may influence formation of protein adducts and, hence, may result in a different susceptibility to chemically induced allergy and autoimmunity.

Whether a genetic polymorphism of a xenobiotic-metabolizing enzyme has clinical relevance depends on its functional role in the metabolism of a given compound (i.e. its bioactivation or detoxication), and on whether other enzymes can compensate for the defect. Individuals carrying certain genetic polymorphisms, especially combined phase I and phase II defects, might be at higher risk for allergic and autoimmune disorders induced by xenobiotics[23–25]. However, it should be noted that, besides genetic determination, the individual activity of xenobiotic-metabolizing enzymes can also be influenced by non-genetic factors such as drugs, diet, alcohol, smoking and cytokines.

Table 2 presents selected examples of polymorphic enzymes that metabolize drugs associated with adverse immune reactions in humans. Thus far, the clearest association between a genetic polymorphism and adverse immune reactions to certain drugs has been found for *N*-acetyltransferase-2 (Figure 2). Approximately half of the Caucasian population is homozygous for the mutant alleles and thus exhibits the slow-acetylator phenotype. In individuals exhibiting the slow-acetylator phenotype, the incidence of dihydralazine- or PA-induced systemic lupus erythematosus (SLE) is higher or the disease starts earlier than in those exhibiting the fast-acetylator phenotype[26,27]. Furthermore, of patients developing severe erythema multiforme variants (Stevens–Johnson syndrome

**Table 2** Polymorphisms of xenobiotic-metabolizing enzymes[a]

| *Enzyme* | *Substrates associated with adverse (immune) reactions* |
|---|---|
| **Phase I enzymes** | |
| CYP1A2[h] | Aromatic amines[b,e] |
| CYP2A6[g] | Coumarin[b] |
| CYP2C9[g] | Non-steroidal anti-inflammatory drugs (diclofenac[b], tienilic acid[d,], piroxicam[b,c], tenoxicam[b,c], ibuprofen[b], naproxen[b]), phenytoin[b,b,e], tolbutamide[b,c] |
| CYP2C19[g] | Omeprazol[b], proguanil[b,c], propranolol[b,c], imipramine[b,c], citalopram[b], moclobemide[b], diazepam[b], hexobarbital[b] |
| CYP2D6[g] | Antiarrhythmics[f], beta-blockers[f], antihypertensives[f], neuroleptics[f], tricyclic antidepressants[f], MAO inhibitors[f], analgesics[f], miscellaneous agents[f] |
| CYP2E1[g] | Dapsone[b,c,e], carbamazepine[b,e], quinidine[e], acetaminophene[b], halothane[d] |
| **Phase II enzymes** | |
| *N*-Acetyltransferase-2[g] | Isoniazid[b,e], dihydralazine[e], procainamide[e], dapsone[b,c,e], sulphasalazine[c,e] |
| Glutathione-*S*-transferases M1 and T1[g] | Halothane[d] |
| NAD(P)H-quinone reductase[g] | Azo dyes[b], nitroaromates[b], quinones[b] |
| Phenolsulphotransferase (P-PST)[h] | Aromatic hydroxylamines[b] |

[a] Data are from refs 22, 75 and 76; selected adverse (immune) reactions to single drugs or certain, not necessarily all, members of classes of compounds are as follows: [b] skin reactions (e.g. exanthema, urticaria, dermatitis); [c] haematological adverse effects (aplastic anaemia, leukopenia, agranulocytosis); [d] autoimmune hepatitis; [e] drug-induced lupus; [f] chemically heterogeneous drugs with versatile adverse effects. Polymorphisms influencing enzyme activity as as follows: [g] characterized at molecular level; [h] mutation not discovered yet, described by distinct phenotypes.

Abbreviations: CYP, cytochrome P450 isoenzyme; MAO, monoamine oxidase; NAD(P)H, reduced form of nicotinamide adenine dinucleotide or nicotinamide adenine dinucleotide phosphate.

and toxic epidermal necrolysis) following sulphonamide treatment, 90% compared with 45% in controls exhibited the slow-acetylator phenotype[28]. It remains to be studied whether or not adverse immune effects caused by the other xenobiotics listed in Table 2 are also associated with certain polymorphisms of the metabolizing enzymes listed. As far as idiopathic autoimmune diseases are concerned, associations with genetic polymorphisms of xenobiotic-metabolizing enzymes would indirectly point to xenobiotics as aetiological agents of such diseases and provide information as to the type of chemical compound to be searched for.

## SENSITIZATION PHASE

Only few of the different hapten–protein conjugates formed in the body will induce clinically manifest allergy or autoimmunity. Whether an immune response is initiated depends on several factors such as dose, metabolism, protein binding, type and activation state of APC, antigen processing and peptide density on APC, some of which will be discussed in more detail.

T cells are activated when they receive both signal 1 and signal 2[29, 30]. Signal 1 is triggered by T-cell recognition of peptides embedded in major histocompatibility complex (MHC) molecules on the surface of APC and involves signal transduction via the T-cell receptor (TCR)-associated CD3 complex and coreceptors such as CD4. Signal 2 is an abstract, generic term for a variety of different costimulatory signals transmitted during T cell–APC interaction. During this crosstalk, exchange of signal 1 and signaling via the CD40–CD40L interaction, up-regulates membrane molecules on the APC, such as intercellular adhesion molecule 1 (ICAM-1), CD80 and CD86, that contribute to signal 2 for T-cell activation.

Dendritic cells residing in tissues must be activated in order to migrate to lymph nodes and prime T cells. While residing in non-lymphoid organs, dendritic cells, such as dermal Langerhans cells, efficiently take up and process material, including haptenated protein, from their vicinity, but their T-cell-stimulating capacity during this developmental stage is poor. Specific signals, such as tumour necrosis factor $\alpha$ (TNF-$\alpha$) and interleukin 1 (IL-1), which may originate, for example, from activated or damaged keratinocytes, can switch the functional state of dendritic cells. Dendritic cells then migrate to the draining lymph nodes, lose their capacity to take up and process antigen, up-regulate MHC class I and class II molecules as well as accessory molecules on the cell surface, and thereby differentiate into immunostimulatory dendritic cells that can efficiently trigger naive T cells[30,31]. The necessity of costimulation for T-cell priming might be another reason why there are, considering the drug metabolizing capacity of the liver, relatively more extrahepatic than hepatic adverse immune reactions to drugs. It is known that hepatic APC cannot effectively prime T cells, because of their poor capacity to provide signal 2.

### Activation of dendritic cells following exposure to xenobiotics

The two-signal requirement for T-cell activation poses the interesting question of how sensitizing xenobiotics can activate dendritic cells. Dendritic-cell maturation might be triggered by a casual infection at the site of exposure, implicating activation of APC by bacterial or viral toxicants, such as lipopolysaccharide, glycans, double-stranded RNA and *N*-formylmethionyl peptides[31]. In all likelihood, however, xenobiotics themselves can act in a similar way by inducing keratinocytes to produce TNF-$\alpha$, IL-1$\alpha$, IL-6 and other cytokines. Keratinocyte activation could be achieved by cytotoxicity of the sensitizing chemical itself or a locally generated reactive metabolite[19], or by concomitant exposure to chemical or physical noxae, such as sodium dodecyl sulphate, dimethylsulphoxide, phorbol myristate acetate, and ultraviolet light[31–33]. In addition to exerting unspecific toxic effects, sensitizing xenobiotics may lead to activation of dendritic cells and more efficient costimulation of T cells by more specific mechanisms (Table 3). Having outlined how xenobiotics can activate dendritic cells (i.e. elicit signal 2 for T-cell activation) this chapter will now discuss signal 1 – the manner in which T cells 'see' xenobiotics or, more exactly, their footprints on self-proteins.

## T-cell reactions to haptenated peptides

Activation of $\alpha\beta$ T cells that recognize peptides in the context of MHC class I or class II molecules involves signalling through the TCR. This requires the three-dimensional structure of its antigen-binding site to be complementary to that of the peptide–MHC complex, and thus allows ionic, dipole, aromatic and hydrophobic interactions. Bonding of a xenobiotic to a peptide–MHC complex alters its structure and the number, type and distribution of possible interactions with the TCR. A neoantigen is thus created and can be specifically recognized by T cells.

TNP derivatives were the first haptens for which T-cell reactions against haptenated peptides presented by MHC class I or class II molecules were demonstrated[2,3,34–36]. These studies clearly demonstrated that both MHC class I- and class II-restricted, hapten-specific T cells recognize TNP-conjugated peptides irrespective of the exact amino acid sequence of the peptides. The only requirements were: (1) that the haptenated peptides carried appropriate side-chains for anchoring in the MHC groove and (2) that the TNP-coupled lysine side-chain of the peptide was correctly positioned relative to these anchors so that TNP could make contact with the TCR. The first requirement by definition is fulfilled by all self-peptides presented and the second requirement is apparently met by a

**Table 3** Selected examples of how xenobiotics can contribute to costimulation of T cells

| *Chemical* | *Effects observed* | *Ref.* |
|---|---|---|
| TNCB, DNCB | Induction of IL-1$\beta$ mRNA in Langerhans cells, induction of IL-1$\alpha$ and TNF-$\alpha$ mRNA in keratinocytes | 32 |
| DNFB, nickel sulphate | Induction of IL-1$\beta$ in Langerhans cells | 77 |
| Nickel sulphate | Stabilizing TNF-$\alpha$ mRNA in keratinocytes | 33 |
| Nickel sulphate, Cobalt sulphate | Expression of adhesion molecules on endothelial cells | 78 |
| Mercuric chloride | Secretion of IL-1 from macrophages | 79 |

Abbreviations: DNCB, dinitrochlorobenzene; DNFB; dinitrofluorobenzene; IL-1, interleukin 1; mRNA, messenger ribonucleic acid; TNCB, trinitrochlorobenzene; TNF-$\alpha$, tumour necrosis factor $\alpha$.

variety of different self-peptides. Thus, after exposure to trinitrobenzene sulphonic acid (TNBS) or trinitrochlorobenzene (TNCB), both of which form TNP–protein conjugates, a large pool of MHC-bound, haptenated self-peptides becomes available for T-cell recognition[2,36]. A recent publication suggests that some TNP-specific human T cells can even recognize TNP in context of different MHC class II molecules[36]. Taken together, these findings may explain the extraordinary strength of immune reactions against TNP derivatives, which are comparable with those seen in alloreactions[2]. T-cell reactions to the 3-alkyl and 3-alkenyl catechols contained in urushiol follow the same rules laid down for TNP, namely recognition of the correctly positioned hapten irrespective of the amino acid sequence of the peptide[4].

Specific reactions of human T cells from patients with drug allergies have been shown for a large number of drugs, such as $\beta$-lactam antibiotics (penicillin)[37–40], sulphonamides, non-steroidal anti-inflammatory drugs, and aromatic anticonvulsants such as phenytoin and carbamazepine[41]. There is evidence that the TCR of penicillin-specific T cells can interact with both the thiazolidin ring, which is common to all $\beta$-lactam antibiotics, and the penicilloyl side-chain, which is specific for a particular antibiotic[38–40]. T-cell reactions to structurally defined haptenated peptides have also been shown for diazotized *p*-aminobenzene arsonic acid[42] and photoreactive azido compounds[43]. Interestingly, in some autoimmune disorders, T-cell responses against endogenously haptenated peptides, i.e. physiological protein modifications, were found[44,45]. MHC-restricted recognition of noncovalently bound organic xenobiotics is rare and has so far been proposed only for sulphamethoxazole[46].

Despite the fact that various metal salts can induce hypersensitivity and/or autoimmune reactions[47], knowledge of how metal ions elicit the specific T-cell reactions underlying these conditions is very limited. Although there is indirect experimental evidence that nickel(II)[48,49], beryllium(II)[50], gold(I)[51] and some other metals might act as haptens in that they are recognized as metal–peptide complexes, demonstration of T-cell recognition of a structurally defined metal-peptide–MHC complex is still lacking. Theoretically, reactive chemicals and metal ions could also elicit specific T-cell responses by binding to the MHC molecule itself rather than to an embedded peptide. Beryllium ions are good candidates for such alloreactive-like T-cell reactions: it has been proposed that beryllium ions might bind directly to the critical glutamate residue in position 69 of the HLA-DPB1*0201 molecule, which shows a strong positive correlation with berylliosis[50]; but again conclusive experimental proof is lacking.

## T-cell reactions to cryptic peptides uncovered by xenobiotics

Chemical modification of self-proteins can change their processing in APC and lead to presentation of cryptic peptides that may elicit autoimmune T-cell reactions. While T-cell reactions to cryptic peptides are known to occur in humans, the induction of T-cell responses to cryptic peptides by xenobiotics has so far been demonstrated only in mouse models. Analysis of T-cell hybridomas prepared after immunization of mice with phosphorylcholine-conjugated hen egg lysozyme revealed that some clones reacted against a cryptic lysozyme peptide such that modification of the protein led to presentation of a novel peptide which itself was not haptenated[52]. The same peptide was presented when lysozyme was pretreated with other diazotized aromatic amines, all of which bind to tyrosine side-chains, but not when lysine-reactive fluorescein isothiocyanate was used.

Similar results were obtained following investigation of the murine T-cell response to bovine ribonuclease A that had been pretreated with gold(III), this being the reactive metabolite of gold(I)-containing antirheumatic drugs[21]. T-cell hybridomas reacting specifically against gold(III)-pretreated ribonuclease recognized one of two cryptic peptides of this protein. When these clones were tested with ribonuclease pretreated with other metals, they only showed crossreactivity with palladium(II), palladium(IV), nickel(IV), and platinum(IV) salts, indicating these metals, but not others, induced presentation of the same cryptic peptides to T cells. The envisaged conformational change of ribonuclease A treated with the crossreacting metals was detectable, indeed, using circular dichroism spectroscopy, suggesting that these changes are the molecular basis for the observed alteration of antigen processing (P. Griem, K. Panthel, S.L. Best, P.J. Sadler, and C.F. Shaw III, unpublished).

Experimental evidence suggests that *in vivo* treatment with mercury(II) can lead to the presentation of cryptic peptides of fibrillarin[53], a nucleolar protein recognized by autoantibodies of mice treated with mercury(II), gold(I), or silver(I), and also by autoantibodies of scleroderma patients[47]. The observation that mercury(II) can alter the protein structure of fibrillarin[54], could explain the presentation of cryptic fibrillarin peptides.

By definition, T cells recognizing cryptic self-peptides are autoreactive and, moreover, some hapten-specific T cells also recognize the non-haptenated peptide after priming[35]. Hence, the possibility arises that an immune response may be extended and lead to overt autoimmunity, even if the offending xenobiotic has been cleared from the body. On the other hand some xenobiotics, especially metals, can persist for years in the body and might continuously activate T cells through specific alteration of self-protein.

## $CD4^+$ versus $CD8^+$ T-cell responses to xenobiotics

Defining rules as to whether a given xenobiotic will predominantly activate $CD4^+$ or $CD8^+$ T cells is a difficult task. From current knowledge concerning hapten recognition by T cells, we can conclude that reactivity and lipophilicity of xenobiotics will determine in which extra- or intracellular compartment haptenated proteins will be formed and which presentation pathway these will enter. Reactive xenobiotics that can directly bind to proteins and modify peptide–MHC complexes seem to induce both $CD4^+$ and $CD8^+$ T-cell responses, as has been observed for TNP derivatives[2,55], penicillins[37] and nickel[48,49]. Likewise, non-reactive xenobiotics, such as urushiol, that can be converted into reactive metabolites non-enzymatically or extracellularly, were found to activate both $CD4^+$ and $CD8^+$ T cells[4,13].

Xenobiotics such as PA and propylthiouracil, that can be metabolized inside APC by enzymes localized along the exogenous processing pathway, might be preferentially presented in the context of MHC class II molecules. The same is true for xenobiotics that can be metabolized extracellularly, such as during the oxidative burst of phagocytes[18], and then bind to extracellular proteins or membrane proteins. This explanation might account for $CD4^+$ T-cell help to B cells and thus for the production of autoantibodies. However, other drugs such as sulphonamides, carbamazepine and phenytoin, which can also be metabolized via myeloperoxidase-dependent oxidation in phagocytes, have been shown to induce specific activation of both $CD4^+$ and $CD8^+$ T cells[41].

Xenobiotics that are lipophilic enough to cross the cell membrane and are metabolized inside the cell (e.g. by CYP isoenzymes at the endoplasmic reticulum) tend to modify proteins inside the cytoplasm that preferentially enter the class I-processing pathway. Examples of this type of xenobiotic are polyaromatic hydrocarbons[11]. Similarly, tienilic acid is metabolized by CYP 2C9 into reactive metabolites that haptenate this CYP isoenzyme. Considering the intracellular localization of the CYP 2C9 isoenzyme at the endoplasmic reticulum, one would expect involvement of $CD8^+$ T cells in the immune reactions against tienilic acid. However, in tienilic acid-induced autoimmune hepatitis, anti-CYP 2C9 IgG autoantibodies were found, implying participation of $CD4^+$ T helper cells and the class II-processing pathway[6,7]. The proposed involvement of $CD4^+$ T cells in this situation could result from hepatocytes that were killed by highly reactive, toxic metabolites of tienilic acid or by hapten-specific $CD8^+$ cells, and that were subsequently taken up by APC, thus entering the class II pathway.

### Direct recognition of xenobiotics by $\gamma\delta$ and $\alpha\beta$ T cells?

Recent investigation of the antigen recognition of T cells expressing $\gamma\delta$ TCR revealed that these cells, unlike conventional $\alpha\beta$ T cells, recognize antigens in an immunoglobulin-like fashion. Interestingly, human $\gamma\delta$ T cells can react to non-proteinaceous microbial components, such as isopentenyl pyrophosphate and $\gamma$-substituted 5′-triphosphorylated thymidine[56]. Moreover, it has been established that human $CD4^-$ $CD8^-$ (double-negative) $\alpha\beta$ T cells can also react to hydrophobic non-peptide antigens, such as lipoarabinomannan and mycolic acids bound to MHC-related CD1 molecules on APC56. These findings open up the possibility that T cells might also recognize 'free' xenobiotics, which are not reactive enough to bind covalently to proteins. This hypothesis is supported by recent publications describing human $\gamma\delta$ T cells specific for lidocain[57] and human $CD8^+$ $\alpha\beta$ T cells recognizing a pollen antigen-derived carbohydrate[58].

## EFFECTOR PHASE IN ADVERSE IMMUNE REACTIONS TO XENOBIOTICS

Specific T-cell reactions to xenobiotic-induced neoantigens comprise both T helper 1 (Th1) and Th2 responses and can trigger an array of effector mechanisms that are not different from those of immune reactions to conventional protein antigens. As with protein antigens, factors such as the route of administration, dose and genetic background of individuals play a role in determining the type of effector mechanisms triggered by xenobiotics. Some examples underlining the importance of these factors will be mentioned below.

## Administration route

It has long been known that cutaneous sensitization of mice to the classical hapten dinitrofluorobenzene (DNFB) does not occur if the animals were orally pretreated with DNFB[59], and the same is true for Ni(II)[60]. In contrast to feeding DNFB to normal littermates, feeding of either MHC class II-deficient or CD4-depleted mice with DNFB did not tolerize but primed to the hapten[61]. This indicates that oral application of DNFB, and possibly of other haptens as well, generates both hapten-specific $CD8^+$ T cells, which act as effector cells in contact hypersensitivity, and hapten-specific $CD4^+$ T cells, which suppress activity of the $CD8^+$ T cells in normal mice so that tolerance results. This is in line with other studies on contact hypersensitivity to DNFB and oxazolone showing that cutaneous application of sensitizing doses of these haptens induces two opposing T-cell populations: interferon $\gamma$ (IFN-$\gamma$)-producing Th1-like $CD8^+$ T cells as effector cells; and IL-4- and IL-10-producing $CD4^+$ Th2 cells as down-regulatory cells[62].

## Dose

The type of effector mechanism induced by xenobiotics is also dose-dependent: while cutaneous application of sensitizing doses of oxazolone induces effector mechanisms leading to contact hypersensitivity in mice, cutaneous application of low, subsensitizing doses of oxazolone induces tolerance that is solely mediated by specific $CD8^+$ cells expressing a Th2-like cytokine pattern[63]. It has been proposed that this mechanism may also be valid for other xenobiotics, and that this might explain why most individuals fail to show signs of sensitization after continuous exposure to low concentrations of xenobiotics on the skin although an immune response is induced. By contrast, exposure to relatively high concentrations of xenobiotics would break tolerance and lead to sensitization.

## Genetic background

The genetic background also influences the risk of immune reactions and the kind of immunopathological lesions ensuing. The importance of polymorphisms of xenobiotic-metabolizing enzymes and the HLA association of the beryllium-induced lung[50] have already been mentioned. Another example is the striking MHC dependence of susceptibility to the systemic autoimmune syndrome that can be induced by mercury and gold salts in mice and rats[1,47,65]. Treatment with mercuric chloride or the antirheumatic drug gold(I) thiomalate induces a Th2-like effector response in susceptible $H\text{-}2^s$ mice and Brown Norway rats, causing production of autoantibodies and increased levels of serum IgG1, IgG2a and IgE. In contrast, resistant $H\text{-}2^d$ mice showed a Th1-like response[1,64]. Unlike Brown Norway rats, Lewis rats do not develop the Th2-dependent systemic autoimmune disease, presumably due to the fact that their activated T cells produce tumour necrosis factor $\beta$[66]. Furthermore, susceptibility of Brown Norway rats to gold-induced systemic autoimmunity correlates with a polymorphism in a putative enhancer element in the second intron of the IL-4 gene[67].

## OUTLOOK

In chemically induced carcinogenesis the role of reactive metabolites acting as ultimate carcinogens has been firmly established decades ago. Accordingly, metabolite-generating systems are used in mutagenicity screening tests. By analogy, reactive metabolite-generating systems that can render prohaptens into haptens should be used in tests designed to detect the sensitizing potential of xenobiotics. For instance, liver microsomes have been successfully used for bioactivation of some non-reactive xenobiotics to haptens in the lymphocyte transformation test in humans[10] and in the popliteal lymph node assay[68]. Conceivably, the blood monocytes present in the lymphocyte transformation test fulfil a similar function within the limits of their xenobiotic-metabolizing capacity. The development of prognostic tools, based on genetic polymorphisms of xenobiotic-metabolizing enzymes, could help protect people with an increased risk for adverse immune reactions to certain classes of xenobiotics that are substrates of those enzymes.

Interestingly, immune responses to xenobiotics, just like those to conventional antigens, can be subject to tolerance induction. In mouse models, tolerance was induced by oral administration of DNCB[59] and nickel[60], parenteral treatment with a peptide haptenated with 3-pentadecyl catechol from urushiol[4] and topical application of low doses of oxazolone[63]. Furthermore, TNP-specific T cells could be inhibited by altered peptide ligands carrying alterations either in the peptide sequence or the hapten[69]. In view of these findings, new therapeutic approaches such as tolerance induction and modulation of immune responses by altered peptide ligands might also be feasible with xenobiotics.

### Acknowledgements

This chapter is reprinted with alterations from P. Griem, M. Wulferink, B. Sachs, J. B. Gonzalez and E. Gleichmann, 'Allergic and autoimmune reactions to xenobiotics: how do they arise?', *Immunology Today*, **19**, 133–141, copyright 1998, with permission from Elsevier Science. The work of the authors is supported by project C1 (granted to E.G.) of SFB 503 'Molecular and cellular mediators of exogenous noxae'.

### References

1. Goldman M, Druet P, and Gleichmann E. (1991) Immunol. Today. 1991;12:223–7.
2. Kohler J, Martin S, Pflugfelder U, Ruh H, Vollmer J, Weltzien HU. Eur J Immunol. 1995;25:92–101.
3. Cavani A, Hackett CJ, Wilson KJ, Rothbard JB, and Katz, SI. J Immunol. 1995;154:1232–8.
4. Gelber C, Gemmell, L, McAteer D. *et al.* J Immunol. 1997;158:2425–34.
5. Roberts DW, Lepoittevin J-P. In: (Lepoittevin J-P, Basketter DA, Goosens A, Karlberg A-T, editors. Allergic Contact Dermatitis. Berlin: Springer Verlag;1998:81–116.
6. Lecoeur S, Bonierbale E, Challine D. *et al.* Chem Res Toxicol. 1994;7:434–42.
7. Lecoeur S, Andre C, Beaune PH. Mol Pharmacol. 1996;50:326–33.
8. Eliasson E, Kenna JG. Mol Pharmacol. 1996;50:573–82.
9. Bourdi M, Tinel M, Beaune PH, Pessayre D. Molec Pharmacol. 1994;45:1287–95.
10. Merk HF, Lepoittevin J-P, Basketter DA, Goosens A, Karlberg A-T, editors. Allergic Contact Dermatitis. Berlin: Springer Verlag; 1998:68–80.
11. Anderson C, Hehr A, Robbins R *et al.* J Immunol. 1995;155:3530–7.
12. Liberato DJ, Byers VS, Ennick RGD, Castagnoli N. J Med Chem. 1981;24:28–33.

13. Kalish RS, Wood JA, LaPorte A. J Clin Invest. 1994;93:2039–47.
14. Krasteva M, Nicolas JF, Chabeau G *et al.* Int Arch Allergy Immunol. 1993;102:200–4.
15. Kubicka-Muranyi M, Goebels R, Goebel C, Uetrecht JP, Gleichmann E. Toxicol Appl Pharmacol. 1993;122:88–94.
16. Von Schmiedeberg S, Hanten U, Goebel C, Schuppe HC, Uetrecht J, Gleichmann, E. Clin Immunol Immunopathol. 1996;80:162–70.
17. Goebel C, Kubicka-Muranyi M, Tonn T, Gonzalez J, Gleichmann E. Arch Toxicol. 1995;69:450–60.
18. Uetrecht JP. Drug Metab Rev. 1992;24:299–366.
19. Jiang X, Khursigara G, Rubin RL. Science. 1994;266:810–13.
20. Eling TE, Thompson DC, Foureman GL, Curtis JF, Hughes MF. Annu Rev Pharmacol Toxicol. 1990;30:1–45.
21. Griem P, Panthel K, Kalbacher H, Gleichmann E. Eur J Immunol. 1996;26:279–87.
22. Daly AK. J Mol Med. 1995;73:539–53.
23. Von Schmiedeberg S, Fritsche E, Rönnau AC *et al.* Exp Toxicol Pathol (Suppl.); 1996:349–53.
24. Flockhart DA, Clauw DJ, Buchert-Sale E, Hewett J, Woosley RL. Clin Pharmacol Ther. 1994;56:398–405.
25. Ollier W, Davies E, Alldersea J, Fryer A, Jones P, Strange R. Arthritis Rheum. 1996;39:1763–4.
26. Weber WW. The Acetylator Genes and Drug Response. Oxford: Oxford University Press; 1987.
27. Woosley RL, Drayer DE, Reidenberg MM, Nies AS, Carr K, Oates JA. New Engl J Med. 1978;298:1157–9.
28. Wolkenstein P, Carriere V, Charue D *et al.* Pharmacogenetics. 1995;5:255–8.
29. Matzinger P. Annu Rev Immunol. 1994;12:991–1045.
30. Cella M, Sallusto F, Lanzavecchia A. Curr Opin Immunol. 1997;9:10–16.
31. Ibrahim MAA, Chain BM, Katz DR. Immunol Today. 1995;16:181–6.
32. Enk AH, Katz SI. Proc Natl Acad Sci USA. 1992;89:1398–402.
33. Lisby S, Muller KM, Jongeneel CV, Saurat JH, Hauser C. Int Immunol. 1995;7:343–52.
34. Ortmann B, Martin S, von Bonin A, Schiltz E, Hoschutzky H, Weltzien HU. J Immunol. 1992;148:1445–50.
35. Martin S, von Bonin A, Fessler C, Pflugfelder U, Weltzien HU. J Immunol. 1993;151:678–87.
36. Kohler J, Hartmann U, Grimm R, Pflugfelder U, Weltzien HU. J Immunol. 1997;158:591–7.
37. Brander C, Mauri-Hellweg D, Bettens F, Rolli H, Goldman M, Pichler WJ. J Immunol. 1995;155:2670–8.
38. Mauri-Hellweg D, Zanni M, Frei E *et al.* J Immunol. 1996;157:1071–9.
39. Padovan E, Mauri-Hellweg D, Pichler WJ, Weltzien HU. Eur J Immunol. 1996;26:42–8.
40. Padovan E, Bauer T, Tongio MM, Kalbacher H, Weltzien HU. Eur J Immunol. 1997;27:1303–7.
41. Mauri-Hellweg D, Bettens F, Mauri D, Brander C, Hunziker T, Pichler WJ. J Immunol. 1995;155:462–72.
42. Nalefski EA, Rao A. J Immunol. 1993;150:3806–16.
43. Romero P, Casanova JL, Cerottini JC, Maryanski JL, Luescher IF. J Exp Med. 1993;177:1247–56.
44. Champion BR, Page KR, Parish N *et al.* J Exp Med. 1991;174:363–70.
45. Michaelsson E, Broddefalk J, Engstrom A, Kihlberg J, Holmdahl R. Eur J Immunol. 1996;26:1906–10.
46. Schnyder B, Mauri-Hellweg D, Zanni M, Bettens F, Pichler WJ. J Clin Invest. 1997;100:136–41.
47. Griem P, Gleichmann E. Curr Opin Immunol. 1995;7:831–8.
48. Sinigaglia F, Scheidegger D, Garotta G, Scheper R, Pletscher M, Lanzavecchia A. J Immunol. 1985;135:3929–32.
49. Moulon C, Vollmer J, Weltzien HU. Eur J Immunol. 1995;25:3308–15.
50. Richeldi L, Sorrentino R, Saltini C. Science. 1993;262:242–4.
51. Romagnoli P, Spinas GA, Sinigaglia F. J Clin Invest. 1992;89:254–8.
52. Jang YS, Lim KH, Kim BS. Eur J Immunol. 1991;21:1303–10.
53. Kubicka-Muranyi M, Griem P, Lübben B *et al.* Int Arch Allergy Immunol. 1995;108:1–10.
54. Pollard KM, Lee DK, Casiano CA, Bluthner M, Johnston MM, Tan EM. J Immunol. 1997;158:3521–8.
55. Kempkes B, Palmer E, Martin, S *et al.* J Immunol. 1991;147:2467–73.
56. Porcelli SA, Morita CT, Modlin RL. Curr Opin Immunol. 1996;8:510–16.
57. Zanni MP, Mauri-Hellweg D, Brander C *et al.* J Immunol. 1997;158:1139–48.

58. Corinti S, De Palma R, Fontana A, Gagliardi C, Pini C, Sallusto F. J Exp Med. 1997;186:899–908.
59. Bour H, Peyron E, Gaucherand M *et al.* Eur J Immunol. 1995;25:3006–10.
60. Van Hoogstraten IM, Boos C, Boden D, von Blomberg ME, Scheper RJ, Kraal G. J Invest Dermatol. 1993;101:26–31.
61. Desvignes C, Bour H, Nicolas JF, Kaiserlian D. Eur J Immunol. 1996;26:1756–61.
62. Xu H, Diiulio NA, Fairchild RL. J Exp Med. 1996;183:1001–12.
63. Steinbrink K, Sorg C, Macher E. J Exp Med. 1996;183:759–68.
64. Doth M, Fricke M, Nicoletti F *et al.* Clin Exp Immunol. 1997;109:149–56.
65. Hanley GA, Schieffenbauer J, Soebel E. Clin Immunol Immunopathol. 1997;84:328–37.
66. Bridoux F, Badou A, Saoudi A *et al.* J Exp Med. 1997;185:1769–75.
67. Kermarrec N, Dubay C, De Gouyon B *et al.* Genomics. 1996;31:111–14.
68. Katsutani N, Shionoya H. J Immunopharmacol. 1992;14:681–6.
69. Preckel T, Grimm R, Martin S, Weltzien HU. J Exp Med. 1997;185:1803–13.
70. Uetrecht JP, Sokoluk B. Drug Metab Dispos. 1992;20:120–3.
71. Waldhauser L, Uetrecht JP. Drug Metab Dispos. 1991;19:354–9.
72. Kharasch ED, Hankins D, Mautz D, Thummel K. Lancet. 1996;347:1367–71.
73. Verwilghen J, Kingsley GH, Gambling L, Panayi GS. Arthritis Rheum. 1992;35:1413–18.
74. Davies GE. In: Turk JL, Parker D, editors. Drugs and Immune Responsiveness. London: Macmillan; 1979:199–211.
75. Yung RL, Johnson KJ, Richardson BC. Lab Invest. 1995;73:746–59.
76. Gleichmann E, Kimber I, Purchase IFH. Arch Toxicol. 1989;63:257–73.
77. Rambukkana A, Pistoor FH, Bos JD, Kapsenberg ML, Das PK. Lab Invest. 1996;74:422–36.
78. Goebeler M, Meinardus-Hager G, Roth J, Goerdt S, Sorg C. J Invest Dermatol. 1993;100:759–65.
79. Zdolsek JM, Soder O, Hultman P. Immunopharmacology. 1994;28:201–8.
80. Goebel C, Vogel C, Wulferink M *et al.* Chem Res Toxicol. 1999;12:488–500.
81. Hilkens CMU, Snijders A, Vermeulen H, Vandermeide PH, Wierenga EA, Kapsenberg ML. J Immunol. 1996;156:1722–7.

# 18
# Immune (T cell) response in viral hepatitis

**J.T. GERLACH, N. GRUENER, H. DIEPOLDER, M.-C. JUNG and G.R. PAPE**

## INTRODUCTION

The immune system is of central importance in the course of viral diseases and increasing evidence suggests that this is also true for viral hepatitis B and C. On the one hand immune responses to viral antigens are believed to be responsible for viral clearance in acute hepatitis B and C, and on the other hand, if they fail to eliminate or control the virus, they most likely cause chronic inflammatory liver disease. The uncompromised human immune system is equipped with humoral and cellular components, that in most viral infections can eliminate the virus or at least achieve viral control. In the natural course of viral hepatitis, however, persistence of the infecting virus is common and numerous observations suggest that both viral and host factors may contribute to viral persistence. Since HBV and HCV are non-cytopathic viruses, liver tissue damage in chronic hepatitis is the result of a permanent inflammatory process within the liver mediated by effector cells of the immune system which obviously cannot eliminate the virus-infected hepatocytes and therefore cannot terminate infection. The decisive role of the immune system becomes evident in acute hepatitis B and C virus infection when the immune system of the infected host holds the key to decide whether there will be viral clearance or control and self-limited disease or viral persistence and chronic hepatitis. Although acute infection displays similar features in hepatitis B and C there are numerous and not only virologically important differences in the course of both viral infections. In acute hepatitis B infection, at least in healthy adults, only a minority (5–10%) of infected individuals will develop chronic disease. In acute hepatitis C infection the majority will run an asymptomatic course of disease that in about 85% will progress to chronic hepatitis. Only those patients who display symptomatic acute hepatitis C, however, clear the infection in about 50%, suggesting that a vigorous immune response contributes to viral clearance in these patients.

Medical strategies have focused on prevention, and sophisticated antiviral treatment has been developed for both virus infections. Potent prophylactic vaccines for hepatitis B are increasingly available all over the world and, as shown by results from research into antiviral immune responses, first trials with therapeutic T cell vaccines in patients with chronic HBV infection are being conducted.

A decade after the identification of hepatitis C virus as the causative agent of most cases of transfusion-associated and community-acquired non-A non-B hepatitis, research efforts in different fields from laboratories throughout the world have contributed towards a substantial improvement in our knowlege of HCV, and have helped to prevent new infections. However, a protective vaccine for HCV remains to be developed.

This chapter will introduce the participants of the immune response in viral hepatitis, but will focus on the key players in acute and chronic viral hepatitis, the virus-specific T lymphocytes.

## IMMUNOLOGICAL EFFECTOR MECHANISMS

### Antibodies

Virus-specific antibodies of different immunoglobulin subclasses to distinct viral proteins define the course of infection with hepatitis B virus and enable us to differentiate between acute, chronic and self-limited infection. In contrast antibodies against anti-HCV are detectable during the chronic course of HCV to each – structural and non-structural – protein. However, there is no pattern of anti-HCV antibodies known so far which indicate the stage of infection (acute vs chronic) or confer immunity. This is consistent with the observation of HCV reinfection in chimpanzees after viral challenge with the same strain (See ref. 23). The presence of antibodies directed against certain epitopes within the hypervariable region 1 (HVR1) of the E2 protein have been shown to principally display neutralizing activity in patients and chimpanzees, but their neutralizing capacity and their contribution to viral clearance or evolution of disease is still under debate[1–3]. Finally the decline of HCV core-specific IgM antibody titres during successful interferon-alpha-induced viral elimination argues against a decisive role of antibodies in viral elimination[4].

### Antigen presenting cell

The cellular components of the immune response (Figure 1) consist of specific antigen-presenting cells, B and T lymphocytes. In order to induce a strong immune response antigens have to be presented by antigen-presenting cells (APC). The most potent APC appear to be the highly specialized dendritic cells (DC) which present antigen as peptides to $CD4^+$ T helper cells via HLA class II molecules or to $CD8^+$ cytoxic T cells via HLA class I[5] in combination with co-signals. DC are classified according to their stage of development into immature and mature DC. Immature DC are present in most tissues and capture antigen in a very effective manner (e.g. by phagocytosis, endocytosis, and by viral infection). Antigen itself supports the maturation process of immature DC which then migrate into the T cell areas of lymphoid tissues (i.e. lymph nodes) and complete their maturation. Mature DC attract and prime T cells and may be of great importance for the maintenance of a long-lasting T cell response.

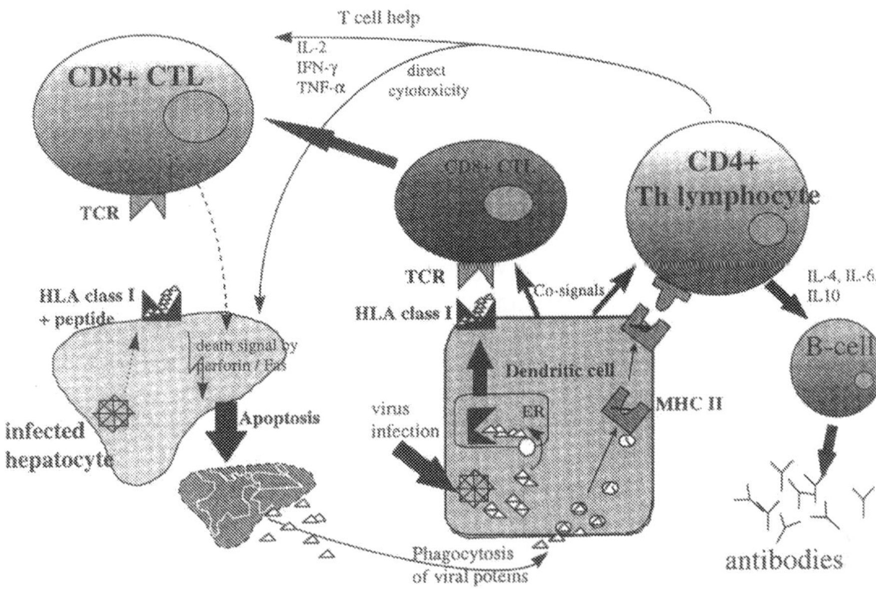


**Fig. 1** Cellular immune response in viral infection. APC (e.g. dendritic cells) present viral antigen on HLA class I or class II molecules to CD8+ or CD4+ T lymphocytes, respectively. After priming the antigen-specific CD8+ T lymphocytes recognize viral antigen presented on infected hepatocytes and deliver a death signal (e.g. perforin/Fas) to the infected cells. CD4+ T cells provide T cell help to CD8+ cytotoxic T cells via Th1 type cytokines (IL-2, IFN-δ and TNF-α, alpha) while CD4+ Th2 lymphocytes secrete IL-4, IL-5, IL-6 and IL-10 and support B cells

## CD4+ T cells

Extracellular antigens such as HBV or HCV proteins from destroyed hepatocytes are taken up by the DC and enter the endocytic pathway. After phagocytosis and proteolytic cleavage of proteins into peptides of about 12–25 amino acids' length, HLA class II molecules are loaded with the peptides and are presented as HLA–antigen complexes on the surface of the APC to virus-specfic CD4+ T helper lymphocytes. The T cell receptor of the specific CD4+ T cell recognizes viral peptide in the binding groove of the HLA class II molecule and differentiation, secretion of cytokines and clonal expansion of the T cell is initiated. Multiple cofactors influence the interaction of virus-specific T cells and APC; i.e. number of HLA molecules expressed on the APC, amount of antigen, affinity of antigen to the T cell receptor, co-signalling, etc. The secretion of distinct cytokine profiles characterizes the subgroups of T helper (Th) cells[6] and crucially influence the direction of the immune response: Th1 cells secrete interleukin 2 (IL-2), interferon (IFN)-γ and tumour necrosis factor (TNF)-α while Th2 lymphocytes secrete IL-4, IL-5, IL-6 and IL-10. While Th2 lymphokines support the humoral response, i.e. production of antibodies by B lymphocytes and thus support humoral immunity, Th1 lymphokines of virus-specific CD4+ T cells provide help to the cellular immune response, i.e. the virus-specific CD8+ cytotoxic T cells. Th1 cytokines exert antiviral effects on infected cells and may even induce viral elimination in several viral diseases. Although CD4+ T cells usually have regulatory functions and direct the immune response, activated CD4+ T cells may display cytotoxic properties and kill infected cells.

## CD8+ T cells

CD8+ cytotoxic T lymphocytes (CTL) are supposed to be a major force of the immune system in the fight against viral infection. CTL recognize short (eight to 12 amino acid residues) peptides bound to the binding groove of HLA class I molecules. In contrast to peptides presented on HLA class II molecules, antigen presented to CD8+ T cells is generated endogenously, most likely by infection of the APC. Cytosolic protein is cleaved proteolytically and is translocated into the endoplasmic reticulum via the TAP I and II transporters. Finally the HLA class I – antigen complex is newly assembled and transported to the surface of the APC. For activation of the virus-specific CTL the T cell receptor of the CD8+ T cell has to recognize a binding motif within the presented peptide[7,8]. These antigen-specific activated cytotoxic T cells can kill virus-infected cells very effectively by inducing cell death directly by cellular interaction, but are also capable of viral elimination by secretion of antiviral cytokines without killing the infected cell[9]. This capability enables even low numbers of virus-specific T cells to cure large numbers of infected hepatocytes. During acute and chronic hepatitis CTL have been shown to be involved directly or indirectly in the increase of transaminases and tissue damage.

## T cell response in HBV

Immune responses to HBV have been studied in peripheral blood mononuclear cells (PBMC) in acute and chronic hepatitis B. These studies revealed distinct patterns of the immune response in order to achieve viral clearance in contrast to evolution of chronic disease in animal models and in natural infection in humans. In acute HBV virus-specific CD4+ T cells are detected in peripheral blood and respond vigorously, mainly against HBV core antigen[10]. This Th cell response is broadly specific even if immunodominant epitopes are frequently recognized. CD4+ T cells are of Th1 type and support a readily detectable strong peripheral and intrahepatic CTL response, which is thought to be the mainstay of the antiviral immune response and ultimately clears the viral infection. Experimentally this was confirmed in transgenic mice that express HBV envelope on their hepatocytes; the transfer of HLA class I restricted HBV surface-specific CD8+ T cells initiated, in these mice, an acute hepatitis histologically characterized by Councilman bodies and bearing a striking resemblance to the picture in human hepatitis. In the course of the murine hepatitis hours after the adoptive transfer viral titres decreased and only few hepatocytes within the liver were killed (about 5%) favouring additional non-cytopathic mechanisms for viral elimination[9,11]. In a second phase of the immune response necroinflammation and jaundice occurs, about 12 hours after adoptive T cell transfer when host-derived inflammatory cells accumulate in the liver and destroy additional hepatocytes. HBV-specific CTL reduced viral expression significantly, which was mediated by cytokines since it could be inhibited by prior application of antibodies against IFN-$\gamma$ or TNF-$\alpha$ and was still detectable after application of perforin-deficient CTL[12].

The CD8+ cytotoxic T cell response in humans is polyclonal, multispecific for HBV envelope, capsid and polymerase antigens[13,14] and is maintained, probably indefinitely, after recovery. Interestingly, minute amounts of HBV DNA antigen persist even in the face of strong antiviral CTL responses over decades, probably replicating actively and generating viral antigen which maintains a continuous virus-specific CTL response[15,16]. In chronic HBV infection the CTL response is weak, narrowly focused insufficient to control the virus but sufficient to cause permanent liver disease. In those patients with chronic HBV infection who succeed in clearing the virus spontaneously, or following treatment with IFN-$\alpha$ the CTL[17] and Th cell response[18] increases during seroconversion, clinically manifested as so-called flare-up, and reaches levels comparable to those with self-limiting acute hepatitis. The cytokine profile of the liver-infiltrating CTL and Th cells in chronic HBV was mainly Th0[19], whereas the cytokine profile in acute HBV is only known in PBMC and displayed a Th1/Th0 type.

## HBV persistence

The detailed mechanisms leading to chronic HBV infection are still unknown. Numerous theories including viral and host factors exist as to how a virus evades the immune response or may become less visible for the immune system, i.e. hypoimmunogenic. The most common cause of chronic HBV worldwide, neonatal infection, leads to tolerance with a high risk for the development of hepatocellular carcinoma. A high viral load was suggested to overwhelm the immune response and exhaust the T cell response before a significant decrease of virus is achieved. Mechanisms of viral persistence comprise induction of tolerance or anergy[20]. Additionally, since hepatocytes are not professional APC, they do not deliver co-signals required for activation, thus antigen presentation by infected hepatocytes could induce anergy rather than activation of specific T cells. The striking influence of the immune system on the course of HBV is also outlined by the observation of an association of MHC class II molecules and the outcome of infection[21]. This suggests that innate conditions of our immune system favour subgroups of individuals in combating viral hepatitis. Since presentation of antigen could be disturbed not only by the innate MHC class I or II molecules and its interaction with the specific antigen, but also by mutations within the viral epitope or the T cell receptor, the complex process of antigen recognition could be an ideal target for viral escape strategies. Mutations within the viral epitope can alter functions of specific T cells in various ways; for example they could serve as T cell receptor antagonists for CTL specific for the mutated epitope, or as so-called altered peptide ligands they could differentially turn down or shut off proliferation or cytokine production of CD4+ T cells[22]. However, since the antiviral response is multispecific and polyclonal and redundant, the *in vivo* relevance of these escape mutations needs to be shown. Perhaps they are less important in reducing viral persistence, but more involved in the maintenance of viral persistence in the chronically infected individual.

## T cell response in HCV

The experience from immunological research in HBV could rapidly be transferred to HCV infection. In contrast to HBV only a minority of patients display clinically apparent acute hepatitis C and initial studies focused on chronic HCV infection and on patients during IFN-$\alpha$ induced viral clearance. The distinct clinical appearance of HCV showing a high percentage of chronic courses without spontaneous viral clearance resembles infection with HIV that is also characterized by only exceptional viral clearance. In the absence of an appropriate small animal model important information on the immune response was obtained in experimental HCV infections in chimpanzees. In these studies chimpanzees mounted no protective antiviral antibody response to HCV during or after viral clearance of acute HCV infection[23], but *in vitro* immunization of the HVR1 region of E2 prevented infection with the identical, but neutralized, viral inoculum[1]. In a similar study infected chimpanzees generated HCV-specific CTL responses that were associated with viral clearance rather than with specific antibody responses[24]. In chronic infection in humans, antibodies are found to any viral protein in high titres but decrease in titre during successful viral clearance[4].

Human studies have initially focused on virus-specific CTL and on the proliferative CD4+ T cell response in chronic HCV infection and in seropositive healthy subjects. While the impact of CTL responses in acute HCV infection in humans is just beginning to be explored, studies of cytotoxic T cell responses in chronically infected patients have detected CTL epitopes in all viral proteins[25–27]. The strength of the CTL response was in between cytotoxic responses in chronic HBV and acute HBV infection, probably due to a lower precursor frequency of HCV-specific CTL corresponding to a lower level of antigen in chronic HCV compared to HBV. Comparable to the compartmentalization of HCV-specific CD4+ T cells to the liver the number of intrahepatic virus-specific CD8+ cytotoxic T lymphocytes seems to be higher than in the peripheral blood, since PBMC, in contrast to intrahepatic T cells, have to be restimulated with specific antigen before cytotoxicity can be detected[25]. Definition of CTL epitopes mainly focused on the restriction element HLA A2, that is frequent in the Caucasian population (approximately 45%), but in addition principally revealed viral epitopes restricted to a vast spectrum of HLA class I molecules indicating a broad immune response. It is unknown, however, why HCV persists in the face of HCV-specific CTL responses. Such evasion from the immune response has been described for other viruses before and could include for example interference of HCV with antigen processing and antigen presentation or viral mutations leading to specific CTL antagonism[28] and altered peptide ligands which could impair the cellular immune response.

In patients with chronic HCV CD4+ T cells revealed a multispecific polyclonal immune response against all HCV proteins[29–32]. Although studies were conducted with various proteins the HCV core protein was more frequently recognized and a core-specific proliferative response was associated with a benign course of disease[33]. Proliferative responses to HCV proteins were also noted in patients being successfully treated with IFN-$\alpha$[34] and immunodominant epitopes in the core protein have been defined. A protective property of HCV-specific CD4+ T cells was also suggested by proliferative responses detected in healthy spouses of chronically infected patients[35]. However, the most vigorous and sustained

CD4+ T cell responses were observed in patients with self-limiting acute symptomatic HCV. The identification and detailed study of these patients showed the existence of a protective antiviral immune response in humans that occurred in the initial weeks after infection and determined the outcome of infection. This CD4+ T cell response was directed predominantly against non-structural proteins (NS) of the virus. Particularly NS3 and NS4 were targets of a strong virus-specific T cell response[36,37]. Within NS3 an immunodominant epitope could be defined that was recognized in association with five different HLA class II alleles and promiscuously binds 10 of the 13 most common HLA class II alleles worldwide[38]. The importance of NS4 had already been suggested by the observation that NS4-specific CD4+ T cells providing strong help to polyclonal immunoglobulin (Ig)A production by B cells predominantly compartmentalize to the liver in chronic HCV[39]. Patients with symptomatic acute HCV infection generally exhibited a more benign course of disease, with self-limitation in approximately half of the individuals, than patients with asymptomatic acute infection that leads to chronic disease in the vast majority of cases. During sustained viral absence a HCV-specific CD4+ T cell response was maintained for up to 20 years in patients who were acutely infected by a contaminated batch of anti-D immunoglobulins, whereas all patients who failed to mount a significant T cell response developed chronic disease. Moreover, loss of an initial CD4+ T cell response which 'eliminated' the virus in acute hepatitis was unequivocally followed by viral recurrence and led to chronic evolution of disease[40]. The cytokine profile of virus-specific CD4+ T helper lymphocytes was confined to a Th1 profile with specific secretion of IFN-$\gamma$. It has also been reported that the cytokine profile of PBMC from patients with acute hepatitis who failed to eliminate HCV and developed chronic disease was confined to a Th2 type[41]. The long persistence of antiviral T cell responses over a very long period suggests an immunological memory that, similar to HBV, could be perpetuated by persistent low-level viral replication[16] and could indicate viral control rather than viral elimination.

The causes for the high rate of chronicity of HCV infection are still not understood. However, all experimental data to date indicate that virus-specific T cells are involved in viral clearance and control. Important tools comprising animal models, *in vitro* models and infectious clones of the virus have recently been generated, and will open up new avenues to elucidate mechanisms of viral elimination and persistence.

## OUTLOOK

The clinical appearance of hepatitis B and C strongly suggests that the outcome of these infections is determined by the individual antiviral immune response. To achieve the ultimate goal of viral clearance and termination of infection all participants involved in the immune response have to cooperate. Protective antibodies have to be generated to neutralize the virus and to minimize the spread of viral load. CD8+ CTL responses would – in a cytopathic manner by killing infected hepatocytes and in a non-cytopathic manner by secreting antiviral cytokines ('kill and cure') – mediate antiviral defence. The CD4+ T cell response orchestrates and coordinates the humoral and cytotoxic immune response and is of critical importance to terminate HBV and HCV infection and convey permanent control. Assuming that the discussed immunological concept of hepatitis B and C, is correct, strategies designed to alter an inefficient antiviral T cell response should be able to terminate infection. Thus the development of a T cell vaccine can crucially influence future therapeutic strategies in chronic viral hepatitis.

## References


1. Farci P, Shimoda A, Wong D *et al.* Prevention of hepatitis C virus infection in chimpanzees by hyperimmune serum against the hypervariable region 1 of the envelope 2 protein. Proc Natl Acad Sci. 1996;93:15394–9.
2. Prince AM, Brotman B, Lee DH, Ren L, Moore BS, Scheffel JW. Significance of the anti-E2 response in self-limited and chronic hepatitis C virus infections in chimpanzees and in humans. J Infect Dis. 1999;180:987–91.
3. Zibert A, Kraas W, Ross RS *et al.* Immunodominant B-cell domains of hepatitis C virus envelope proteins E1 and E2 identified during early and late time points of infection. J Hepatol. 1999;30:177–84.
4. Nagayama R, Miyake K, Tsuda F, Okamoto H. IgM antibody to a hepatitis C virus core peptide (CP14) for monitoring activity of liver disease in patients with acute or chronic hepatitis C. J Med Virol. 1994;42:311–17.
5. Cella M, Sallusto F, Lanzavecchia A. Origin, maturation and antigen presenting function of dendritic cells. Curr Opin Immunol. 1997;9:10–16.
6. Mosmann TR, Cherwinski H, Bond MW, Giedlin MA, Coffman RL. Two types of murine helper T cell clone. I. Definition according to profiles of lymphokine activities and secreted proteins. J Immunol. 1986;136:2348–57.
7. Rammensee H-G, Falk K, Rötzschke O. Peptides naturally presented by MHC class I molecules. Annu Rev Immunol. 1993;11:213–44.
8. Bertoletti A, Ferrari C, Fiaccadori F *et al.* HLA class I-restricted human cytotoxic T cells recognize endogenously synthesized hepatitis B virus nucleocapsid antigen. Proc Natl Acad Sci USA. 1991;88:10445–9.
9. Guidotti LG, Rochford R, Chung J, Shapiro M, Purcell R, Chisari FV. Viral clearance without destruction of infected cells during acute HBV infection. Science. 1999;284:825–9.
10. Jung MC, Spengler U, Schraut W *et al.* Hepatitis B virus antigen-specific T-cell activation in patients with acute and chronic hepatitis B. J Hepatol. 1991;13:310–17.
11. Guidotti LG, Ando K, Hobbs MV *et al.* Cytotoxic T lymphocytes inhibit hepatitis B virus gene expression by a noncytolytic mechanism in transgenic mice. Proc Natl Acad Sci USA. 1994;91:3764–8.
12. Guidotti LG, Ishikawa T, Hobbs MV, Matzke B, Schreiber R, Chisari FV. Intracellular inactivation of the hepatitis B virus by cytotoxic T lymphocytes. Immunity. 1996;4:25–36.
13. Nayersina R, Fowler P, Guilhot S *et al.* HLA A2 restricted cytotoxic T lymphocyte responses to multiple hepatitis B surface antigen epitopes during hepatitis B virus infection. J Immunol. 1993;150:4659–71.
14. Rehermann B, Fowler P, Sidney J *et al.* The cytotoxic T lymphocyte response to multiple hepatitis B virus polymerase epitopes during and after acute viral hepatitis. J Exp Med. 1995;181:1047–58.
15. Michalak TI, Pasquinelli C, Guilhot S, Chisari FV. Hepatitis B virus persistence after recovery from acute viral hepatitis. J Clin Invest. 1994;93:230–9.
16. Rehermann B, Ferrari C, Pasquinelli C, Chisari FV. The hepatitis B virus persists for decades after patients' recovery from acute viral hepatitis despite active maintenance of a cytotoxic T-lymphocyte response. Nat Med. 1996;2:1104–8.
17. Rehermann B, Lau D, Hoofnagle JH, Chisari FV. Cytotoxic T lymphocyte responsiveness after resolution of chronic hepatitis B virus infection. J Clin Invest. 1996;97:1655–65.
18. Jung MC, Diepolder HM, Spengler U *et al.* Activation of a heterogeneous hepatitis B (HB) core and e antigen-specific CD4+ T-cell population during seroconversion to anti-HBe and anti-HBs in hepatitis B virus infection. J Virol. 1995;69:3358–68.

19. Bertoletti A, D'Elios MM, Boni C *et al.* Different cytokine profiles of intrahepatic T cells in chronic hepatitis B and hepatitis C virus infections. Gastroenterology. 1997;112:193–9.
20. Diepolder HM, Jung M-C, Wierenga EA *et al.* Anergic hepatitis B virus core-specific TH1 clones as immunoregulators during viral clearance. J Hepatol. 1995;23(Suppl.1):S24.
21. Thursz MR, Kwiatkowski D, Allsopp CEM, Greenwood BM, Thomas HC, Hill AVS. Association between an MHC class II allele and clearance of hepatitis B virus in the Gambia. N Engl J Med. 1995;332:1065–9.
22. Bertoletti A, Sette A, Chisari FV *et al.* Natural variants of cytotoxic epitopes are T-cell receptor antagonists for antiviral cytotoxic T cells. Nature. 1994;369:407–10.
23. Farci P, Alter HJ, Govindarajan S *et al.* Lack of protective immunity against reinfection with hepatitis C virus. Science. 1992;258:135–40.
24. Cooper S, Erickson AL, Adams EJ *et al.* Analysis of a successful immune response against hepatitis C virus. Immunity. 1999;10:439–49.
25. Koziel MJ, Dudley D, Wong JT *et al.* Intrahepatic cytotoxic T lymphocytes specific for hepatitis C virus in persons with chronic hepatitis. J Immunol. 1992;149:3339–44.
26. Battegay M, Fikes J, Di Bisceglie AM *et al.* Patients with chronic hepatitis C have circulating cytotoxic T cells which recognize hepatitis C virus-encoded peptides binding to HLA-A2.1 molecules. J Virol. 1995;69:2462–70.
27. Cerny A, McHutchison JG, Pasquinelli C *et al.* Cytotoxic T lymphocyte response to hepatitis C virus-derived peptides containing the HLA A2.1 binding motif. J Clin Invest. 1995;95:521–30.
28. Chang KM, Rehermann B, McHutchison JG *et al.* Immunological significance of cytotoxic T lymphocyte epitope variants in patients chronically infected by the hepatitis C virus. J Clin Invest. 1997;100:2376–85.
29. Botarelli P, Brunetto MR, Minutello MA *et al.* T-lymphocyte response to hepatitis C virus in different clinical courses of infection. Gastroenterology. 1993;104:580–7.
30. Leroux-Roels G, Esquivel CA, DeLeys R *et al.* Lymphoproliferative responses to hepatitis C virus core, E1, E2, and NS3 in patients with chronic hepatitis C infection treated with interferon alfa. Hepatology. 1996;23:8–16.
31. Ferrari C, Valli A, Galati L *et al.* T-cell response to structural and nonstructural hepatitis C virus antigens in persistent and self-limited hepatitis C virus infections. Hepatology. 1994;19:286–95.
32. Schupper H, Hayashi P, Scheffel J *et al.* Peripheral-blood mononuclear cell responses to recombinant hepatitis C virus antigens in patients with chronic hepatitis C. Hepatology. 1993;18:1055–60.
33. Lechmann M, Ihlenfeldt HG, Braunschweiger I *et al.* T- and B-cell responses to different hepatitis C virus antigens in patients with chronic hepatitis C infection and in healthy anti-hepatitis C virus-positive blood donors without viremia. Hepatology. 1996;24:790–5.
34. Hoffmann RM, Diepolder HM, Zachoval R *et al.* Mapping of immunodominant $CD4^+$ T lymphocyte epitopes of hepatitis C virus antigens and their relevance during the course of chronic infection. Hepatology. 1995;21:632–8.
35. Bronowicki JP, Vetter D, Uhl G *et al.* Lymphocyte reactivity to hepatitis C virus (HCV) antigens shows evidence for exposure to HCV in HCV-seronegative spouses of HCV-infected patients. J Infect Dis. 1997;176:518–22.
36. Diepolder HM, Zachoval R, Hoffmann RM *et al.* Possible mechanism involving T-lymphocyte response to non-structural protein 3 in viral clearance in acute hepatitis C virus infection. Lancet. 1995;346:1006–7.
37. Missale G, Bertoni R, Lamonaca V *et al.* Different clinical behaviors of acute hepatitis C virus infection are associated with different vigor of the anti-viral cell-mediated immune response. J Clin Invest. 1996;98:706–14.
38. Diepolder HM, Gerlach JT, Zachoval R *et al.* Immunodominant $CD4^+$ T-cell epitope within nonstructural protein 3 in acute hepatitis C virus infection. J Virol. 1997;71:6011–19.
39. Minutello MA, Pileri P, Unutmaz D *et al.* Compartmentalization of T lymphocytes to the site of disease: Intrahepatic $CD4^+$ T cells specific for the protein NS4 of hepatitis C virus in patients with chronic hepatitis C. J Exp Med. 1993;178:17–25.
40. Gerlach JT, Diepolder HM, Jung M-C *et al.* Recurrence of hepatitis C virus after loss of virus-specific $CD4^+$ T-cell response in acute hepatitis C. Gastroenterology. 1999;117:933–941.
41. Tsai SL, Liaw YF, Chen MH, Huang CY, Kuo GC. Detection of type 2-like T-helper cells in hepatitis C virus infection: implications for hepatitis C virus chronicity. Hepatology. 1997;25:449–58.

# 19 Autoimmune response in hepatitis C and D

F.B. BIANCHI, D. ZAULI, M. LENZI, F. CASSANI and L. MURATORI

Infection with hepatitic DNA viruses such as HBV is infrequently associated with the occurrence of autoantibodies which, if present, are detectable only at low titre. On the other hand, infection with RNA viruses such as HCV and HDV may lead to the emergence of a spectrum of autoantibodies which are in part similar to those detected in autoimmune hepatitis.

In the course of chronic HDV infection two major autoreactivities have been reported. The most frequent is that directed to an antigen present in epithelial cells such as the cells of the basal layer of rat forestomach (basal cell layer antibodies – BCLA) and the stellate epithelial cells of rat thymus (stellate epithelial cell antibodies – SECA). The reported prevalence of BCLA/SECA in HDV-positive patients was 50% in all the histological subgroups studied[1]. HDV-negative cases were consistently negative. Because of the similarity between the pattern of positivity of BCLA/SECA and that of monoclonal antibodies directed against acidic cytokeratins, the hypothesis was made that the autoantigen was indeed a cytokeratin[2]. A Spanish group from Barcelona confirmed our data and added the information that the target antigen is represented by a 46 kDa protein whose molecular identity is still unknown[3].

In 1983 Crivelli *et al.* from Turin described, in a small proportion of HDV-positive patients, an autoantibody giving an immunomorphological pattern similar to that of liver kidney microsomal antibody type 1 (LKM1), and called anti-LKM3 such a reactivity[4]. More than a decade later, the group of Michael Manns characterized the autoantibody and identified its target antigen as uridine diphosphate glucurosyl transferase 1. Occasional sera from patients with autoimmune hepatitis type 2 were also reported to be reactive with the same recombinant protein[5].

Far more relevant, both in quantitative and qualitative terms, is the autoreactivity detected in HCV-infected patients. The frequent emergence of B-cell autoreactivity in chronic HCV infection could be due to the binding of the E2 protein of HCV to the CD81 molecule expressed on B lymphocytes. This event might reduce B cells' activation threshold in genetically predisposed individuals and give rise to both polyclonal and monoclonal responses[6].

In our experience the prevalence of autoantibody positivity in chronic hepatitis C is 30%. By univariate analysis autoantibody-positive patients are more often females with higher values of AST, ALT and IgG and higher score of portal–periportal necroinflammation according to the Scheuer index; by stepwise logistic regression both female gender and ALT values maintain a statistical significance[7]. Thus, autoantibody positivity appears to be associated with a higher activity of liver disease. This is somehow confirmed by the observation that the prevalence of serum autoantibodies is significantly higher in a series of hospitalized HCV-positive patients (with abnormal ALT values in most cases) than in HCV-positive patients detected in a random sample of the general population of Sersale (a small town of southern Italy) most of whom showed normal ALT (unpublished observations).

HCV-related autoreactivity is largely confined to anti-nuclear (ANA), anti-smooth muscle (SMA) and LKM1 antibodies, which are also the accepted markers of autoimmune hepatitis type 1 and type 2. However, ANA with a 'homogeneous' pattern of positivity (ANA-H) and SMA reacting with a component of 'microfilaments' (SMA-MF), which are frequently detected in autoimmune hepatitis type 1, are rarely found in HCV-infected patients, where their titre is significantly lower. In particular, SMA-MF appears to be more sensitive and specific than ANA-H for the diagnosis of autoimmune hepatitis type 1. In our experience the association of ANA-H and SMA-MF rules out HCV infection[8].

In 1990 Lenzi *et al.* were the first to report a strikingly high prevalence of anti-HCV positivity in patients suffering from so-called type 2 autoimmune hepatitis[9], a rare subset of the disease diagnosed on the basis of cryptogenic aetiology and positivity for liver kidney microsomal antibody type 1 (LKM1)[10]. The demonstration of HCV RNA sequences in such patients corroborated further the genuine viral nature of the liver disease[11]. Michel *et al.*[12] and Lunel *et al.*[13] confirmed our previous findings, and introduced the important observation that LKM1 can be detected in two different clinical settings: on one hand, *true* type 2 autoimmune hepatitis, a cryptogenic, severe and progressive liver disease without markers of HCV infection, which mostly affects young girls and is responsive to immunosuppression, according to Homberg's original report[10]; on the other hand, anti-HCV positive/HCV RNA positive chronic hepatitis, a viral liver disease with features of autoreactivity.

In 1985 it was reported that, by immunoblotting, autoimmune LKM1 reacts with a 50 kDa microsomal protein extracted from rat liver[14], but in the late 1980s two groups independently identified the molecular target of the autoimmune LKM1 reactivity as CYP2D6, the isoform 2D6 of the cytochrome P450 family[15,16]. This notion became the starting point for subsequent studies which aimed at defining the immunological target of the HCV-related LKM1. Diego Vergani's group was the first to remark that autoimmune and HCV-related LKM1 react differently with recombinant CYP2D6 expressed in bacteria[17,18]. A systematic analysis and comparison of the LKM1 reactivity in autoimmune and HCV-related liver disease allowed us to appreciate that autoimmune sera react more frequently with the recombinant protein and particularly with its immunodominant epitope spanning amino acids 257–269 of CYP2D6, whereas the spectrum of reactivities against the native microsomal antigens extracted from rat and human liver microsomes was substantially the same[19]. The interpretation of these findings was that autoimmune sera react with linear epitopes more often than sera from patients with HCV infection. When eukaryotically expressed CYP2D6 was used as antigen in a radioligand assay, the reactivity of LKM1-positive sera with the CYP2D6 conformational epitopes was the same both for autoimmune and viral patients[20,21].

In our epidemiological context the prevalence of LKM1 in chronic hepatitis C is 6% in the adult population with chronic hepatitis C[7], but can be as high as 10% in children[22]. In other geographical areas such as the United States[23,24] or Sweden[25] the occurrence of LKM1 in association with HCV infection seems to be a much rarer event.

The reason for the occurrence of LKM1 in a proportion of patients with chronic hepatitis C is still a matter of opinion and speculation. The observation of the *de-novo* appearance of LKM1 in a patient with chronic hepatitis C after an ALT flare during interferon therapy[26] or after HCV infection acquired following a liver transplantation[27] or an accidental needle stick injury[28] suggests that the virus may play a critical role in the disruption of the immunological tolerance to CYP2D6, a self antigen. One of the most intriguing mechanisms which could explain LKM1 appearance in the course of HCV infection is the *molecular mimicry* hypothesis. Michael Manns reported a striking homology between E1 and NS5, two regions of the HCV polyprotein, and CYP2D6[29] which could account for the appearance of LKM1 in HCV-infected patients, but experimental evidence to support this hypothesis is still lacking.

As far as the virus is concerned, no association was observed between LKM1 occurrence and a particular HCV genotype[30,31]. However, it is worth noting that LKM1-positive patients have a significantly lower HCV viraemia despite liver disease severity similar to that of patients without such an autoreactivity. It is therefore likely that in LKM1-positive patients with chronic hepatitis C in addition to HCV-related mechanisms, an autoimmune process is also involved in the pathogenesis of the disease.

LKM1 is a partially liver-specific autoantibody, since its main target CYP2D6 is expressed both in the liver and in the kidney, although renal distribution is limited to the distal region of the proximal tubules. Most of CYP2D6 is indeed located within the endoplasmic reticulum of the hepatocyte, but some evidence indicates that CYP2D6 is also physiologically expressed on the outer surface of the hepatocyte plasma membrane. In 1984 we described a membrane-like positivity given by LKM1-positive sera incubated with viable rabbit hepatocytes, and immunoelectronmicroscopy with colloidal gold showed a discrete membranous positivity[32]. Recently, with laser confocal microscopy, we demonstrated that both autoimmune and HCV-related LKM1 sera recognize CYP2D6 molecules expressed on the surface of non-permeabilized rat hepatocytes as discrete clumps[33].This observation, which confirms our previous findings, proves that CYP2D6 is accessible to circulating LKM1, and supports the notion that anti-CYP2D6 humoral (and possibly cellular) autoreactivity might be operative in the progression and perpetuation of liver cell damage both in type 2 autoimmune hepatitis and in LKM1-positive chronic hepatitis C.

## References


1. Zauli D, Fusconi M, Crespi C *et al.* Close association between basal cell layer antibodies and hepatitis B virus-associated chronic delta infection. Hepatology. 1984;4:1103–6.
2. Zauli D, Crespi C, Bianchi F *et al.* Preliminary characterisation of autoantibodies associated with chronic hepatitis delta virus infection. In: Zuckerman AJ, editor. Viral Hepatitis and Liver Disease. New York: Alan R. Liss; 1988:412–14.
3. Amengual MJ, Catalfamo M, Pujol A *et al.* Autoantibodies in chronic delta virus infection recognize a common protein of 46 kD in rat forestomach basal cell layer and stellate thymic epithelial cells. Clin Exp Immunol. 1989;78:80–4.
4. Crivelli O, Lavarini C, Chiaberge E *et al.* Microsomal autoantibodies in chronic infection with the HBsAg associated delta (delta) agent. Clin Exp Immunol. 1983;54:232–8.
5. Philipp T, Durazzo M, Trautwein C *et al.* Recognition of uridine diphosphate glucuronosyl transferases by LKM-3 antibodies in chronic hepatitis D. Lancet. 1994;344:578–81.
6. Pileri P, Uematsu Y, Campagnoli S *et al.* Binding of hepatitis C virus to CD81. Science. 1998;282:938–41.
7. Cassani F, Cataleta M, Valentini P *et al.* Serum autoantibodies in chronic hepatitis C: comparison with autoimmune hepatitis and impact on the disease profile. Hepatology. 1997;26:561–6.
8. Cassani F, Muratori L, Manotti P *et al.* Serum autoantibodies and the diagnosis of type-1 autoimmune hepatitis in Italy: a reappraisal at the light of hepatitis C virus infection. Gut. 1992;33:1260–3.
9. Lenzi M, Ballardini G, Fusconi M *et al.* Type 2 autoimmune hepatitis and hepatitis C virus infection. Lancet. 1990;335:258–9.
10. Homberg JC, Abuaf N, Bernard O *et al.* Chronic active hepatitis associated with antiliver/kidney microsome antibody type 1: a second type of (autoimmune) hepatitis. Hepatology. 1987;7:1333–9.
11. Garson JA, Lenzi M, Ring C *et al.* Hepatitis C viraemia in adults with type 2 autoimmune hepatitis. J Med Virol. 1991;34:223–6.
12. Michel G, Ritter A, Gerken G *et al.* Anti-GOR and hepatitis C virus in autoimmune liver diseases. Lancet. 1992;339:267–9.
13. Lunel F, Abuaf N, Frangeul L *et al.* Liver/kidney microsome antibody type 1 and hepatitis C virus infection. Hepatology. 1992;16:630–6.
14. Alvarez F, Bernard O, Homberg JC *et al.* Anti-liver–kidney microsome antibody recognizes a 50,000 molecular weight protein of the endoplasmic reticulum. J Exp Med. 1985;161:1231–6.
15. Gueguen M, Yamamoto AM, Bernard O *et al.* Anti-liver–kidney microsome antibody type 1 recognizes human cytochrome P450 db1. Biochem Biophys Res Commun. 1989;159:542–7.
16. Manns MP, Johnson EF, Griffin KJ *et al.* Major antigen of liver kidney microsomal autoantibodies in idiopathic autoimmune hepatitis is cytochrome P450db1. J Clin Invest. 1989;83:1066–72.
17. Ma Y, Peakman M, Lenzi M *et al.* Case against subclassification of type II autoimmune chronic active hepatitis. Lancet. 1993;341:60.
18. Ma Y, Peakman M, Lobo-Yeo A *et al.* Differences in immune recognition of cytochrome P4502D6 by liver kidney microsomal (LKM) antibody in autoimmune hepatitis and chronic hepatitis C virus infection. Clin Exp Immunol. 1994;97:94–9.
19. Muratori L, Lenzi M, Ma Y *et al.* Heterogeneity of liver/kidney microsomal antibody type 1 in autoimmune hepatitis and hepatitis C virus related liver disease. Gut. 1995;37:406–12.
20. Ma Y, Gregorio G, Gaken J *et al.* Establishment of a novel radioligand assay using eukaryotically expressed cytochrome P4502D6 for the measurement of liver kidney microsomal type 1 antibody in patients with autoimmune hepatitis and hepatitis C virus infection. J Hepatol. 1997;26:1396–402.
21. Yamamoto AM, Johanet C, Duclos-Vallee JC *et al.* A new approach to cytochrome CYP2D6 antibody detection in autoimmune hepatitis type-2 (AIH-2) and chronic hepatitis C virus (HCV) infection: a sensitive and quantitative radioligand assay. Clin Exp Immunol. 1997;108:396–400.
22. Bortolotti F, Vajro P, Balli F *et al.* Non-organ specific autoantibodies in children with chronic hepatitis C. J Hepatol. 1996;25:614–20.
23. Reddy KR, Krawitt EL, Homberg JC *et al.* Absence of anti-LKM-1 antibody in hepatitis C viral infection in the United States of America. J Viral Hepatol. 1995;2:175–9.
24. Clifford BD, Donahue D, Smith L *et al.* High prevalence of serological markers of autoimmunity in patients with chronic hepatitis C. Hepatology. 1995;21:613–19.

25. Lindgren S, Braun HB, Michel G *et al.* Absence of LKM-1 antibody reactivity in autoimmune and hepatitis-C-related chronic liver disease in Sweden. Swedish Internal Medicine Liver Club. Scand J Gastroenterol. 1997;32:175–8.
26. Muratori L, Zauli D, Giostra F *et al.* LKM1 appearance in a HLA-DR3+ patient with chronic hepatitis C during interferon treatment. J Hepatol. 1993;18:259–60.
27. Mackie FD, Peakman M, Yun M *et al.* Primary and secondary liver/kidney microsomal autoantibody response following infection with hepatitis C virus. Gastroenterology. 1994;106:1672–5.
28. Vento S, Cainelli F, Renzini C *et al.* Autoimmune hepatitis type 2 induced by HCV and persisting after viral clearance. Lancet. 1997;350:1298–9.
29. Manns MP, Griffin KJ, Sullivan KF *et al.* LKM-1 autoantibodies recognize a short linear sequence in P450IID6, a cytochrome P-450 monooxygenase. J Clin Invest. 1991;88:1370–8.
30. Gerotto M, Pontisso P, Giostra F *et al.* Analysis of the hepatitis C virus genome in patients with anti-LKM-1 autoantibodies. J Hepatol. 1994;21:273–6.
31. Michitaka K, Durazzo M, Tillmann HL *et al.* Analysis of hepatitis C virus genome in patients with autoimmune hepatitis type 2. Gastroenterology. 1994;106:1603–10.
32. Lenzi M, Bianchi FB, Cassani F *et al.* Liver cell surface expression of the antigen reacting with liver–kidney microsomal antibody (LKM). Clin Exp Immunol. 1984;55:36–40.
33. Muratori L, Parola M, Ripalti A *et al.* Liver/kidney microsomal antibody type 1 targets CYP2D6 on hepatocyte plasma membrane. Gut. 2000;46:553–61.

# Section V
# Primary biliary cirrhosis, primary sclerosing cholangitis and overlap syndromes

# 20
# Histological classification of autoimmune cholestatic liver diseases

S.G. HÜBSCHER

## INTRODUCTION

A number of diseases may be associated with immune-mediated bile duct damage (Table 1). In practice the term *autoimmune* cholestatic liver disease can be applied to three main syndromes: primary biliary cirrhosis (PBC); primary sclerosing cholangitis (PSC); and overlap syndromes involving PBC, PSC and autoimmune hepatitis (AIH) in varying combinations. The use of the term *autoimmune* in this context is somewhat unsatisfactory, as there is no conclusive evidence to indicate that the autoantibodies which characterize these syndromes play a major pathogenetic role in mediating damage to biliary epithelial cells. Bile ducts are also targets for alloimmune damage in liver allograft rejection and graft versus host disease. Inflammatory bile duct lesions can also be seen in a number of other conditions such as sarcoidosis, hepatitis C infection and drug reactions, in which immune mechanisms may also be involved. It has also been suggested that some cases of so-called 'idiopathic' adult ductopenia may represent examples of small duct PSC or autoimmune cholangitis in which the usual diagnostic markers are no longer present[1].

**Table 1** Diseases associated with immune-mediated bile duct damage

| | |
|---|---|
| Autoimmune | Primary biliary cirrhosis<br>Primary sclerosing cholangitis<br>Overlap syndromes (PSC/PBC/AIH) |
| Alloimmune | Liver allograft rejection<br>Graft versus host disease |
| Other | Sarcoidosis<br>Hepatitis C<br>Drug reactions<br>Idiopathic adult ductopenia |

In this chapter the histological features of PBC and PBC will be described, concentrating initially on the bile duct lesions which enable a definitive histological diagnosis to be made[2]. Other histological changes which may be important in the diagnosis and classification of autoimmune cholestatic liver diseases will also be considered. These include: inflammatory lesions, principally involving portal/periportal regions, but also, to a lesser degree, the liver parenchyma; features relating to chronic cholestasis such as bile ductular proliferation and cholate stasis; and progressive liver fibrosis resulting eventually in cirrhosis[2].

Problems with the histological classification of autoimmune cholestatic liver disease fall into two main categories. First, there are problems with sampling variation in small needle biopsy specimens. Secondly, considerable confusion exists regarding the classification of autoimmune overlap syndromes. Changing concepts regarding the diagnosis of autoimmune overlap syndromes are discussed in another chapter. However, a brief consideration of this subject from a histological perspective will be given here.

## BILE DUCT LESIONS IN PBC AND PSC

PBC is characterized by inflammatory lesions, which mainly involve small (interlobular) bile ducts. Inflammatory lesions may be seen less frequently in larger bile ducts. By contrast, PSC is a disease which affects bile ducts of all sizes, both intra- and extrahepatic.

A number of effector cells have been implicated in mediating bile duct damage in PBC. These include lymphocytes (mainly CD8-positive T cells), plasma cells which may be involved in humoral-mediated damage, histiocytes which are involved in granuloma formation, eosinophils and neutrophils[3–7]. In practice two main patterns of damage are seen histologically. The first is lymphocytic infiltration of bile ducts, which is associated with degenerative changes in biliary epithelium including swelling, cytoplasmic vacuolation and fragmentation of the basement membrane (Figure 1). Secondly there is granulomatous bile duct destruction (Figure 2). This is generally regarded as the most characteristic bile duct lesion seen in PBC. However, granulomatous cholangitis has also been described in other conditions including sarcoidosis[8] and chronic hepatitis C infection[9]. Granulomatous cholangitis is also seen in so-called 'autoimmune cholangitis', although the relationship of this entity to PBC will be discussed later. Portal granulomas can also be seen in other diseases associated with bile duct damage. These include PSC, in which portal tract granulomas have been reported in up to 10% of cases[10,11], drug reactions[12], liver allograft rejection[13], Langerhans cell histiocytosis[14] and Hodgkin's lymphoma[15,16]. However, in contrast with PBC, portal granulomas in these other conditions are not usually directly associated with bile duct damage.

The characteristic bile duct lesion in PSC is a fibrous obliterative cholangitis. In the early stages this is characterized by oedema and loose concentric periductal fibrosis (Figure 3). As the disease progresses there is more dense periductal fibrosis associated with compression and atrophy of the biliary epithelium (Figure 4). Eventually the bile duct is completely replaced by a nodular scar

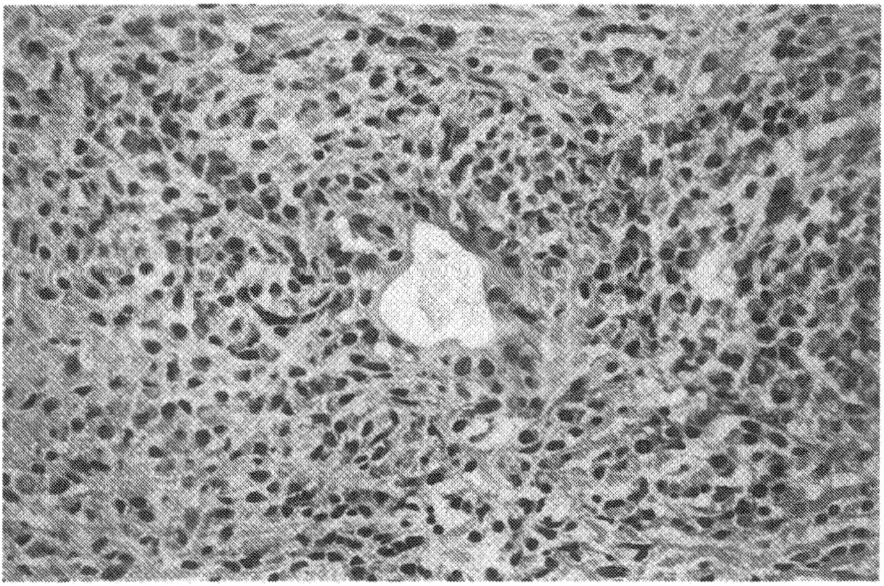

**Fig. 1** Lymphocytic bile duct lesion in PBC. A small (interlobular) bile duct shows infiltration and effacement by a dense lymphoid infiltrate. Haematoxylin and eosin

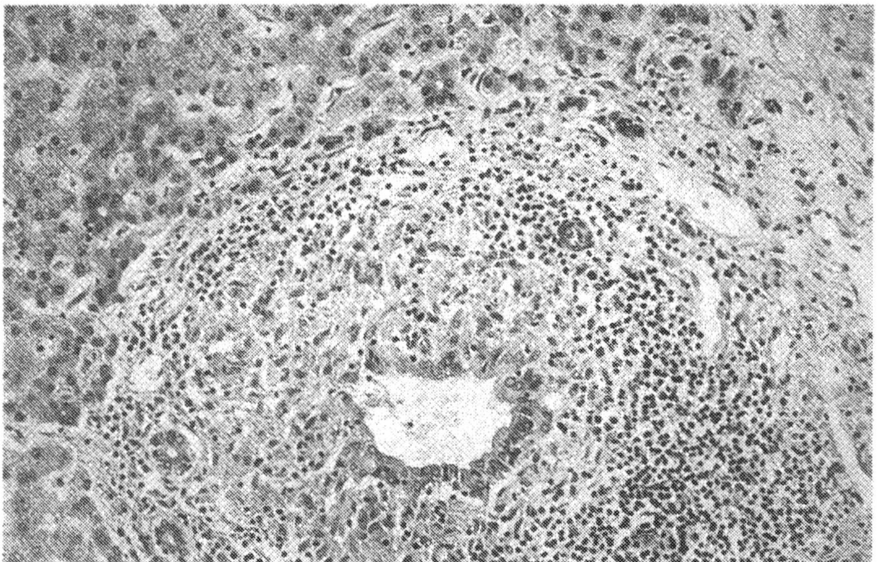

**Fig. 2** Granulomatous bile duct lesion in PBC. A medium-sized (septal) bile duct is surrounded by a granulomatous infiltrate, associated with disruption of the biliary epithelium. This 'florid duct lesion' is generally regarded as a characteristic feature of early (stage 1) disease. However, the bile duct shown in this illustration was present in a cirrhotic hepatectomy specimen obtained at liver transplantation, indicating that active bile duct damage can be seen at all stages of the disease. Haematoxylin and eosin

(Figure 5). Studies of hepatectomy specimens obtained at liver transplantation have shown that fibro-obliterative lesions mainly affect medium-sized (septal) ducts[17] and therefore they may not be seen in needle biopsy specimens which sample smaller bile duct branches. However, a small duct variant of PSC has been described, in which typical histological features of PSC are present in liver biopsy specimens in the absence of radiological abnormalities of large ducts on cholangiography[18,19]. The incidence of small duct PSC is difficult to determine, due to problems with different criteria which have been used to make the diagnosis, but it probably occurs in less than 5% of cases[20]. An association between small duct PSC and AIH was postulated in one study[21]. The large duct lesions which are detected by cholangiography are usually only seen pathologically when hepatectomy specimens become available for examination at liver transplantation (Figures 6 and 7)[17,22]. Bile ducts affected show dilatation with inflammation and fibrosis in the duct wall, extensive ulceration of the mucosa and inspissation of biliary sludge.

It is worth noting that histological features indistinguishable from PSC can be seen in a number of other conditions (Table 2). Bile ducts receive a single blood supply derived from branches of the hepatic arterial system, and are therefore susceptible to ischaemic damage caused by hepatic arterial inclusion. Arterial causes of bile duct injury include hepatic artery thrombosis, traumatic injury, intra-arterial infusions (e.g. chemotherapeutic agents or ethanol embolization for the treatment of hepatic neoplasms) and vasculitis (e.g. polyarteritis nodosa). It has also been postulated that the bile duct loss which

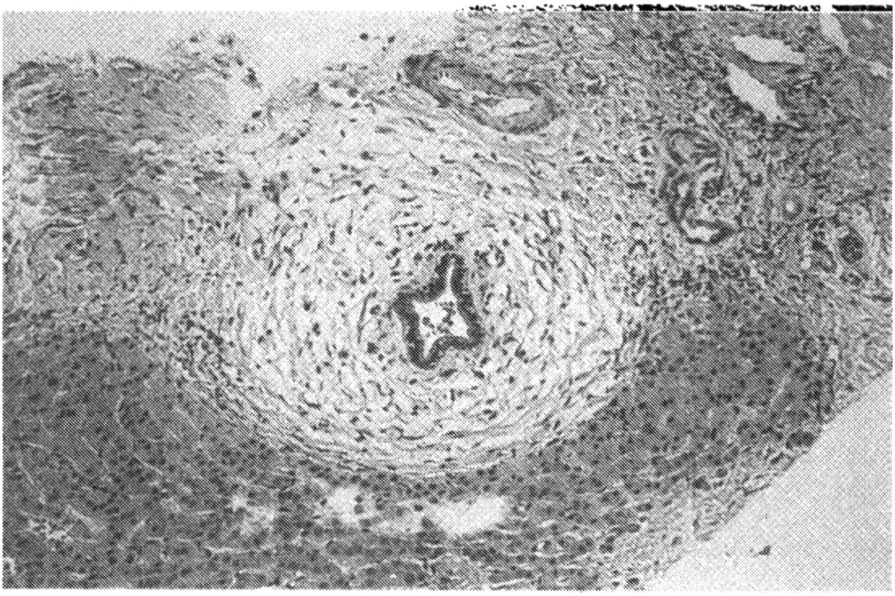

**Fig. 3** Early bile duct lesion in PSC. Bile duct is surrounded by a zone of oedema and loose concentric periductal fibrosis. A light infiltrate of inflammatory cells is also present in this area. Haematoxylin and eosin

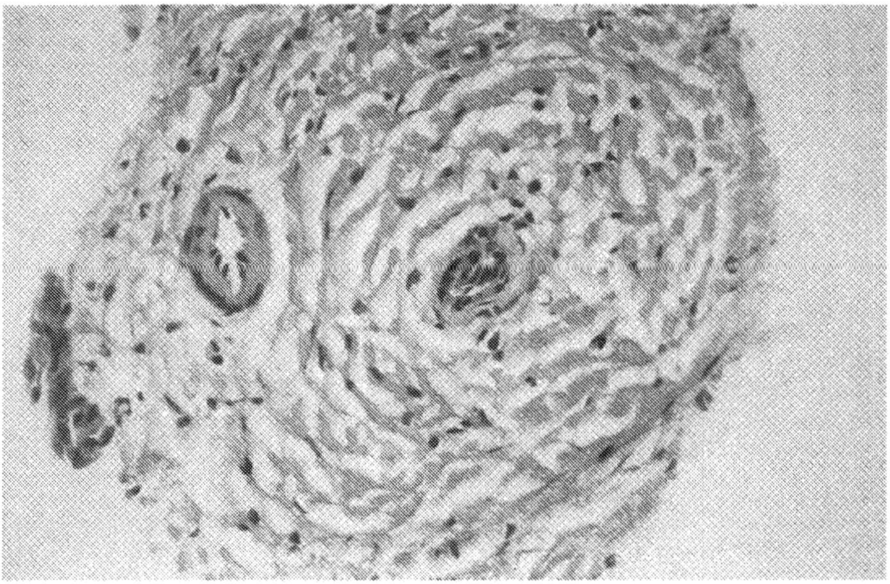

**Fig. 4** Sclerosing bile duct lesion in PSC. Bile duct is surrounded by a zone of dense concentric fibrosis. This is associated with compression and atrophy of biliary epithelium. Haematoxylin and eosin

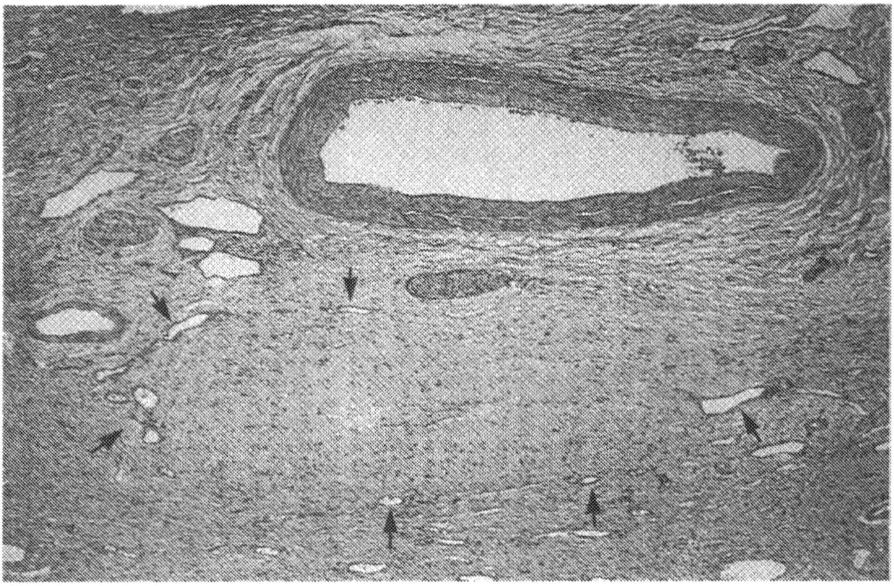

**Fig. 5** Fibro-obliterative scar in PSC. This slide shows the remnant of a medium-sized (septal) bile duct which has been replaced by a nodular fibrous scar. Remnants of the peribiliary vascular plexus can still be seen (arrows). Haematoxylin and eosin

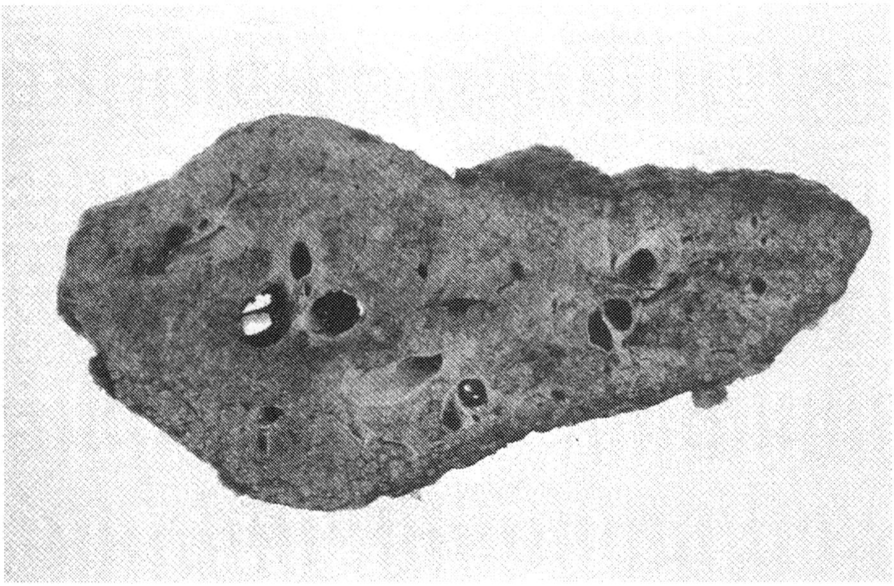

**Fig. 6** Large bile duct lesions in PSC. In this specimen, obtained at liver transplantation, there are several dilated ducts containing inspissated biliary sludge. These are responsible for producing the characteristic beading pattern seen at cholangiography

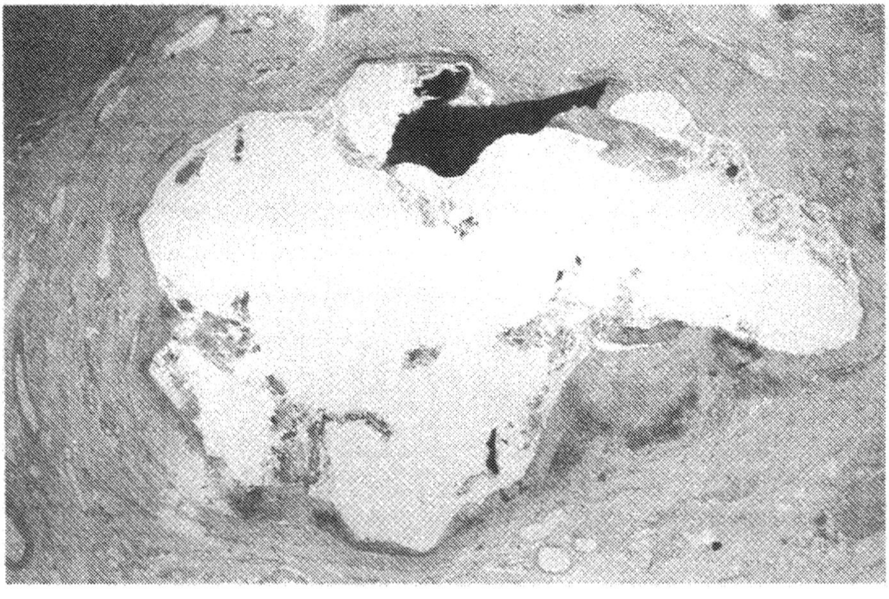

**Fig. 7** Large bile duct lesion in PSC. Same case as Figure 6. Dilated large (hilar) duct shows inflammation in the wall, extensive mucosal ulceration and fragments of biliary sludge in the lumen. Haematoxylin and eosin

**Table 2** Sclerosing cholangitis – other causes

| | |
|---|---|
| Vascular | Hepatic artery occlusion<br>Portal vein occlusion (rare) |
| Infective | Bacterial<br>Viral<br>Protozoal |
| Neoplastic | Langerhans cell histiocytosis<br>Systemic mastocytosis |
| Idiopathic | Idiopathic adult ductopenia |

The vascular, infective and neoplastic diseases listed here can produce histological and radiological changes indistinguishable from PSC. Some cases of so-called 'idiopathic adult ductopenia' may represent examples of burnt-out PSC.

occurs in chronic liver allograft rejection may partly have an ischaemic basis, secondary to the obliterative ateriopathy which occurs in this condition[23,24]. However, typical sclerosing bile duct lesions are rarely seen in chronic rejection. Portal venous obstruction more rarely gives rise to problems involving the biliary tree. However, a PSC-like syndrome ('pseudosclerosing cholangitis') has been reported in association with portal vein thrombosis, possibly reflecting compression of bile ducts due to choledochal varices[25]. Minor degrees of periductal fibrosis and bile duct loss have also been documented in association with the obliterative portal venopathy occurring in non-cirrhotic portal hypertension[26]. Bacterial infection of the biliary tree in ascending cholangitis may rarely be associated with inflammatory bile duct destruction[27]. Coloniation of the biliary tree by viral agents such as cytomegalovirus (CMV) or protozoa (e.g. cryptosporidia or microsporidia) has been implicated in the pathogenesis of AIDS-associated sclerosing cholangitis[28,29]. A sclerosing cholangitis-like picture has also been reported in association with neoplastic infiltration of portal tracts in Langerhans cell histiocytosis[14,30] and in systemic mastocytosis[31].

In a post-mortem study by Terada and Nakanuma, cholangiographic changes resembling PSC were seen in a number of other conditions including non-biliary cirrhosis, submassive hepatic necrosis, and primary and metastatic hepatic neoplasms[32]. Varying degrees of periductal fibrosis and inflammation were noted histologically in these cases. However, advanced fibro-obliterative lesions (nodular scars) were not described.

As a consequence of the bile duct lesions described above there is destruction of small, and in the case of PSC, sometimes larger, bile ducts ('vanishing bile duct syndrome') (Figure 8). At this stage the lesions that caused bile duct destruction may no longer be present, and it is then not possible to decide if the changes seen are due to PBC, PSC or other causes of intrahepatic bile duct loss. In a study carried out by Wiesner *et al.* only seven (12%) of 60 biopsies obtained from PSC patients had diagnostic features of fibrous cholangitis and only 85 (32%) of 258 biopsies from PBC patients had diagnostic lesions of granulomatous cholangitis[33].

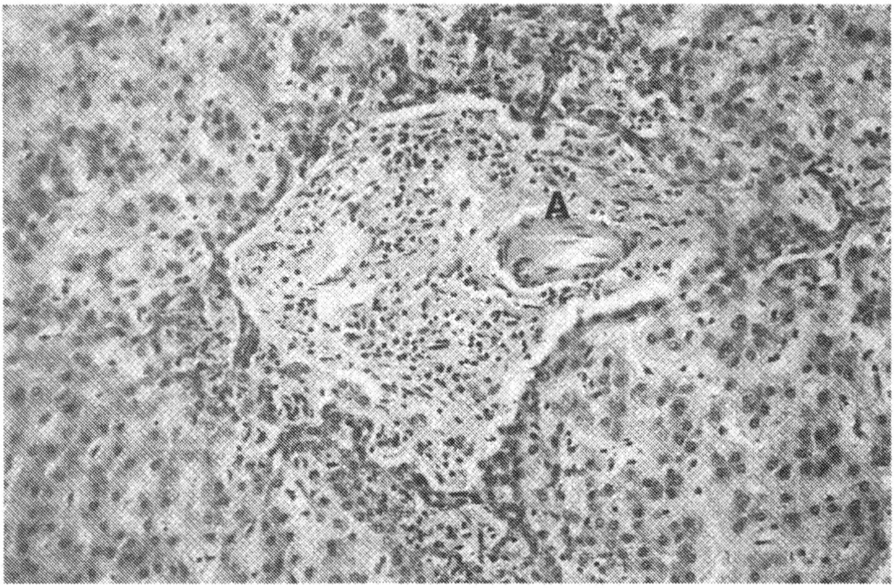


**Fig. 8** Bile duct loss in PBC. This portal tract contains a small arterial branch (**A**), without an accompanying bile duct. Ductular transformation is seen at the periphery of the portal area. In the absence of a diagnostic bile duct lesion, histological distinction from PSC or other causes of 'vanishing bile duct syndrome' is not possible. Haematoxylin and eosin

## OTHER HISTOLOGICAL FEATURES OF PBC AND PSC

### Portal and parenchymal inflammation

Portal inflammation is commonly seen in PBC and PSC and is frequently accompanied by varying degrees of interface hepatitis. In cases where interface hepatitis is marked and is associated with a prominent component of plasma cells, the possibility of an overlap syndrome with AIH should be considered (Figure 9) (see later). There is also increasing evidence to suggest that periportal inflammatory infiltration is an important mechanism in the pathogenesis of fibrosis in chronic cholestatic liver diseases. In a recent study of paired liver biopsies obtained at 4-year intervals from 54 PBC patients, the presence of lymphocytic piecemeal necrosis in the initial biopsies was strongly predictive for the development of progressive fibrosis in the follow-up biopsies[34]. In liver biopsy specimens interface hepatitis is frequently associated with a deposition of new collagen fibres (Figure 10).

Mild spotty parenchymal inflammation is commonly seen in PBC, and may include occasional epithelioid granulomas. In a small proportion of cases there may be more severe inflammation associated with confluent zone 3 necrosis and the development of zone 3 fibrosis[35]. In the study of paired liver biopsies from PBC patients by Degott *et al.*[34] the presence of lobular inflammation and necro-

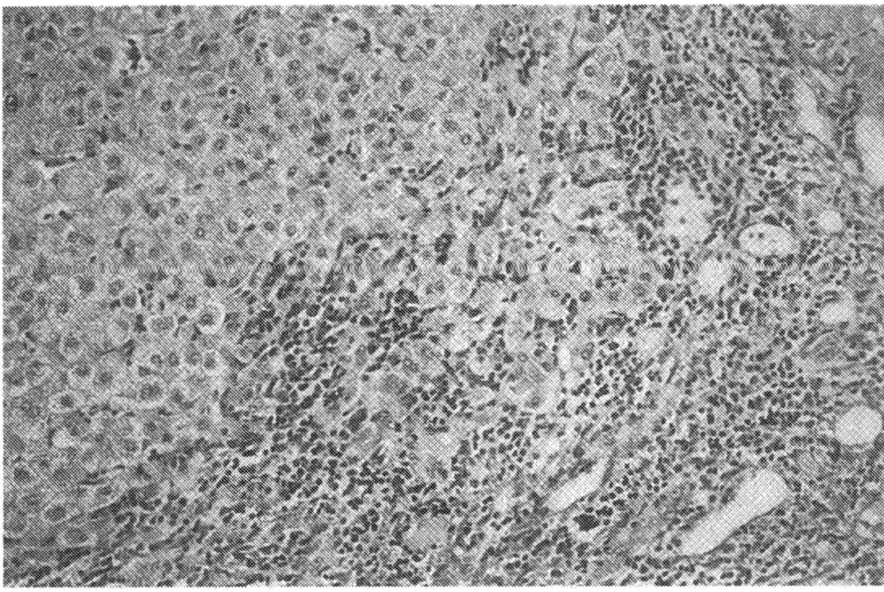

**Fig. 9** Severe interface hepatitis in PBC. Portal and periportal inflammation are commonly seen in PBC and PSC. However, in cases such as this where interface hepatitis is severe and includes a prominent component of plasma cells, the possibility of an overlap syndrome with autoimmune hepatitis should be considered. Haematoxylin and eosin

sis in initial biopsies was also strongly predictive for the development of progressive fibrosis in follow-up biopsies obtained 4 years later. Minor degrees of parenchymal inflammation can also be seen in cases of PSC.

## Bile ductular proliferation and cholate stasis

Bile ductular proliferation (also known as ductular reaction or ductular metaplasia)[36,37] and cholate stasis are two lesions which are frequently seen in combination in chronic cholestatic liver diseases associated with loss of intrahepatic bile ducts.

Bile ductular proliferation is typically seen at the periphery of portal tracts (Figure 11) and may have a protective role in ductopenic syndromes, enabling resorption of bile and recirculation within the liver (cholehepatic cycling) when the normal pathway of enterohepatic circulation is blocked due to bile duct loss. Three main sources of bile ductular proliferation have been postulated (see Table 3). Of these, ductular metaplasia of periportal hepatocytes is thought to be the most important mechanism in chronic cholestatic liver diseases such as PBC and PSC. Immunohistochemical studies have shown that periportal hepatocytes in these conditions express antigens that are confined to bile ducts in the normal liver. These include bile duct cytokeratins (cytokeratins 7 and 19), blood group antigens, tissue plasminogen activator (TPA), neuroendocrine markers (e.g. chromogranin), bile duct integrins (VLA 2, 3 and 6), and other bile duct-specific antibodies (e.g. human epithelial antigen 125) (Figure 12). Studies using three-

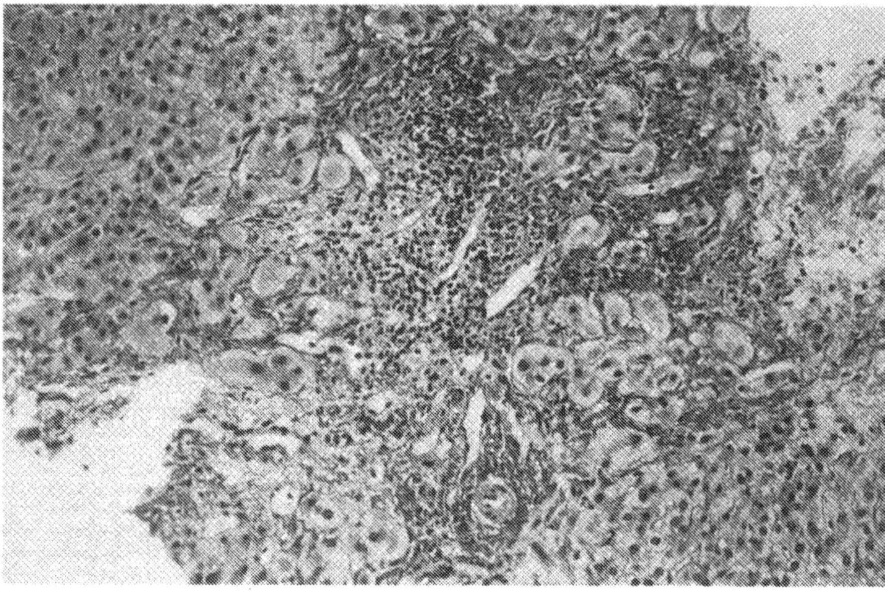

**Fig. 10** Periportal inflammation and fibrosis in PBC. This portal tract contains a moderately dense infiltrate of lymphoid cells. There is interface hepatitis associated with deposition of collagen fibres surrounding periportal hepatocytes. Haematoxylin van Gieson

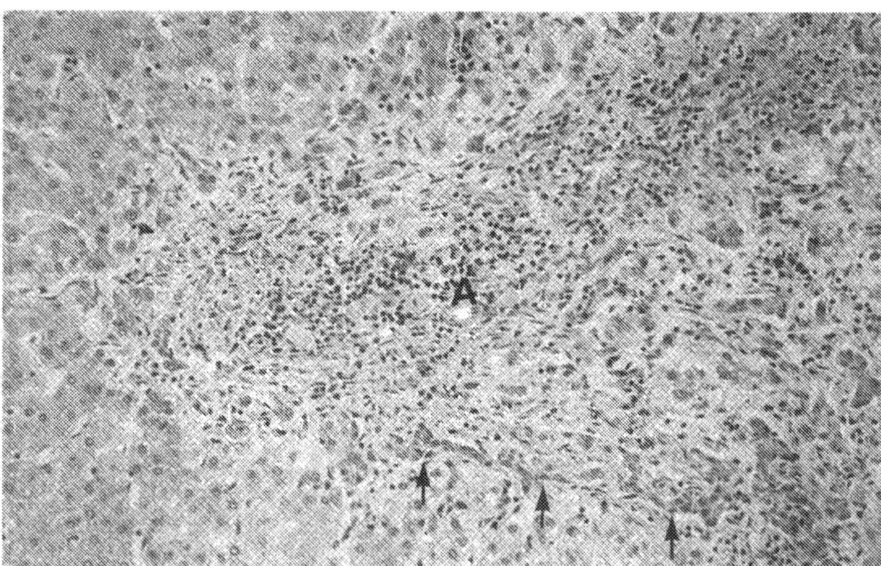


**Fig. 11** Bile ductular proliferation in PBC. This portal tract contains an artery (A) without an accompanying bile duct. At the periphery of the portal area there is an area of bile ductular proliferation (arrows). Haematoxylin and eosin

**Table 3** Sources of proliferating bile ductules in different types of liver disease

| *Histological type* | *Source of ductules* | *Associated diseases* |
|---|---|---|
| 1. Typical ductular proliferation | Pre-existing bile ductules | Extrahepatic biliary obstruction |
| 2. Atypical ductular proliferation | Periportal hepatocytes (ductular metaplasia) | Chronic cholestatic diseases |
| 3. Oval cell proliferation | Oval cells | Experimental hepatocarcinogesis |

dimensional reconstruction have demonstrated that periportal hepatocytes showing features of biliary metaplasia are in continuity with ductular structures at the periphery of portal areas[38]. Recent immunohistochemical studies using antibodies to the rat oval cell marker OV6 have suggested that oval cells may also be involved in the ductular reaction which occurs in cholestatic liver diseases including PBC and PSC[39–41].

The term cholate stasis is used to describe a range of degenerative changes in periportal (zone 1) hepatocytes probably related to toxic effects of retained bile acids. Changes seen include hepatocyte ballooning and feathery degeneration,

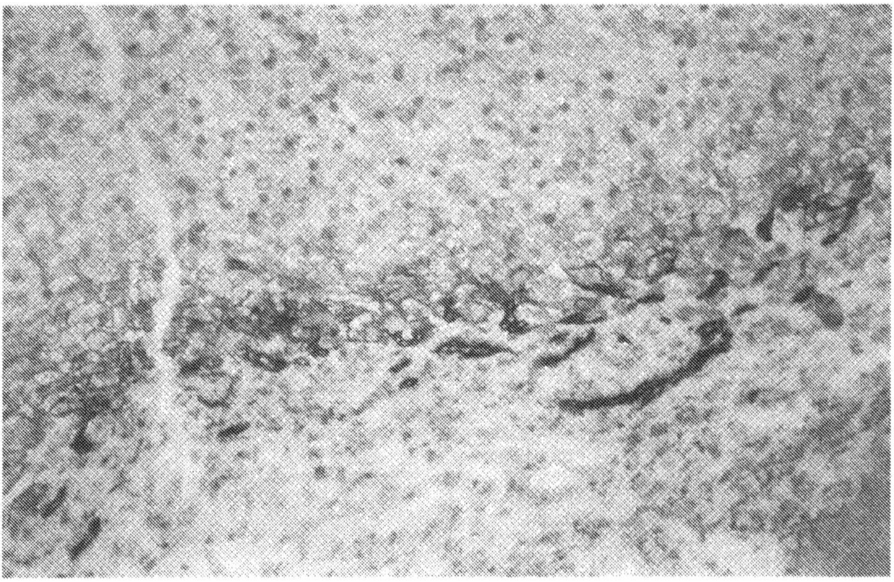

**Fig. 12** Ductular metaplasia of periportal hepatocytes in PBC. This slide has been stained with an antibody to HEA-125, which recognizes a biliary-specific glycoprotein in the normal liver. HEA immunoreactivity is present both in bile ductules at the periphery of an expanded portal area and, with a membranous pattern, in adjacent periportal hepatocytes. Immunoalkaline phosphatase

disruption of the cytoskeleton resulting in formation of Mallory's hyaline, and deposition of copper-associated protein. Bilirubinostasis may also be seen in periportal hepatocytes, although this usually occurs as a late event. Lipid-laden macrophages (xanthoma cells) and hepatocytes (psuedoxanthoma cells) are also commonly seen in periportal regions.

Bile ductular proliferation and cholate stasis are important lesions to recognize histologically, because they enable a diagnosis of chronic cholestatic liver disease to be made, even if diagnostic bile duct lesions are not present. In addition, there is increasing evidence to suggest that ductular proliferation is another important factor driving the development of periportal fibrosis in chronic biliary disease. Factors involved in this process include the recruitment of an inflammatory infiltrate rich in neutrophils (cholangiolitis) (Figure 13), direct production of basement membrane-related proteins (e.g. collagen type 4 or laminin) by bile ductules themselves (ductular fibrosis) and the release of cytokines (e.g. transforming growth factor beta, TGF-$\beta$) which can stimulate portal/periportal fibroblasts or myofibroblasts to produce fibrous tissue. In liver biopsy specimens a delicate framework of new collagen fibres can frequently be seen around neocholangioles in diseases where marginal ductular reaction occurs (Figure 13). Further evidence for the role of bile ductular proliferation as an important mechanism for the development of periportal fibrosis comes from observations made in bile duct losing diseases in which ductular proliferation is not seen. Two good examples of this phenomenon are chronic liver allo-

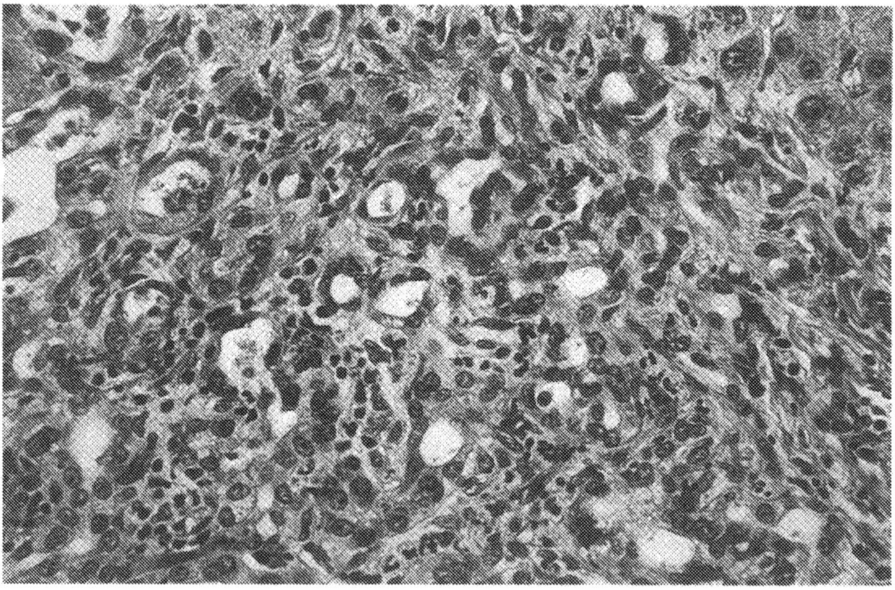

**Fig. 13** Cholangiolitis and ductular fibrosis in PBC. Section taken from the edge of a portal tract shows numerous irregular bile ductules associated with a dense infiltrate of neutrophils (cholangiolitis) and deposition of collagen fibres. Haematoxylin van Gieson

graft rejection and Alagille's syndrome, in which advanced bile duct loss is seen in normally sized portal tracts with no accompanying ductular reaction or periportal fibrosis.

## Fibrosis and staging in PBC and PSC

As a consequence of the necroinflammatory lesions and bile ductular proliferation described above there is progressive fibrosis, leading in some cases to the development of a true cirrhosis. Fibrosis can be divided into three main phases. First, there is fibrous portal expansion (periportal fibrosis). This is followed by the formation of linkages between vascular structures (mainly portal–portal, some portal–central). Normal vascular relationships are still retained at this stage. Finally, there is the development of a true cirrhosis with nodular regeneration and loss of the normal liver architecture.

Another important aspect of histological classification in chronic cholestatic liver disease is the staging of progressive liver injury. A number of staging systems have been described in PBC. Four of the more commonly used ones are summarized in Table 4[42–45]. A similar approach has been advocated for staging liver disease in PSC[46]. All four systems shown in Table 4 agree that early (stage 1) disease is characterized by bile duct damage and/or portal inflammation and that late (stage 4) disease is defined by the presence of an established cirrhosis. However, varying criteria are used to define the intermediate stages (stages 2 and 3). Bile ductular proliferation, interface hepatitis (periportal hepatitis) and fibrosis are all used to varying degrees. In line with the concepts which have been developed for the histological classification of chronic hepatitis, in which a distinction is made between necroinflammatory activity as a histological *grade* and fibrosis as a histological *stage*, it might be more appropriate to adopt a simplified staging system, which is based purely on the degree of fibrosis present[47,48]. An example of such a system is also included in Table 4.

**Table 4** Summary of four staging systems which have been used in the histological assessment of PBC. A simplified system, based purely on the extent of fibrosis, is also included for comparison

| | *Rubin et al. (1965)*[42] | *Scheuer (1967)*[43] | *Popper and Schaffner (1970)*[44] | *Ludwig et al. (1978)*[45] | *Simplified system* |
|---|---|---|---|---|---|
| **Stage 1** | Bile duct damage | Florid duct lesion | Cholangitis | Portal hepatitis | No fibrosis |
| **Stage 2** | Ductular proliferation | Ductular proliferation | Ductular proliferation and destruction | Periportal hepatitis | Periportal fibrosis |
| **Stage 3** | Ductular proliferation | Scarring | Precirrhotic stage | Bridging necrosis and/ or fibrosis | Bridging fibrosis |
| **Stage 4** | Cirrhosis | Cirrhosis | Cirrhosis | Cirrhosis | Cirrhosis |

## SAMPLING VARIATION IN NEEDLE BIOPSIES

As discussed earlier, the characteristic bile duct lesions of PBC and PSC are patchy in distribution and may not be sampled in small needle biopsy specimens. However, the presence of bile duct loss associated with bile ductular proliferation, degenerative changes in periportal hepatocytes (cholate stasis) and deposits of copper-associated protein in periportal hepatocytes enable a diagnosis of chronic cholestatic liver disease to be made even if diagnostic bile duct lesions are not seen. In practice, most patients having these histological features will eventually turn out to have PBC or PSC. In the absence of diagnostic bile duct lesions, two features which favour a diagnosis of PBC rather than PSC are the presence of portal lymphoid aggregates, which may mark the site of former bile ducts ('tombstone aggregates') (Figure 14) or the presence of portal granulomas. However, the results of other investigations, in particular antimitochondrial antibodies and endoscopic retrograde cholangiopancreatography (ERCP), are required before a definite diagnosis can be made.

There is also considerable variation in the severity of fibrosis in the livers of patients with chronic biliary diseases. This problem has been highlighted by the examination of hepatectomy specimens obtained at liver transplantation, in which areas of established cirrhosis may be seen in close proximity to areas in which there is a normal architecture with little or no periportal fibrosis (Figure 15). In a study by Garrido and Hübscher only 10 (20%) of 50 hepatectomy spec-

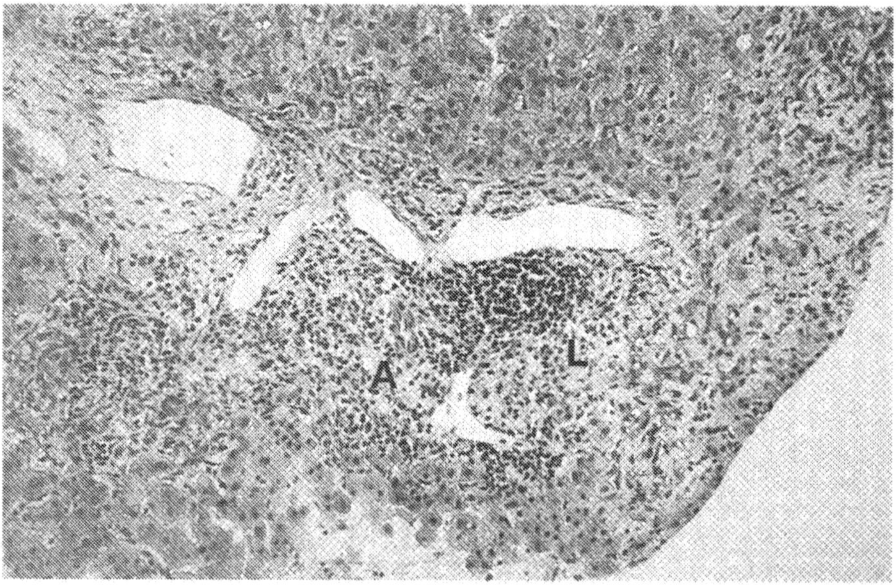


**Fig. 14** Bile duct loss and portal lymphoid aggregate in PBC. Portal tract contains an arterial branch (A) without an accompanying bile duct. A lymphoid aggregate (L) marks the site where the bile duct possibly once was. Lymphoid aggregates seen in this situation are sometimes referred to as 'tombstone aggregates'. Haematoxylin and eosin

imens obtained at liver transplantation had the same stage throughout the liver[48]. Of the remaining 40 cases 23 (46%) varied by one stage, 14 (28%) by two stages and three (6%) by three stages. A similar, though less marked, variation in histological stage was observed in a study of paired needle biopsies from patients with PSC[49]. On the basis of these observations it would seem reasonable to suggest that histological staging is not appropriate for the assessment of disease progression in individual patients. However, staging may still be relevant in the context of clinical trials in which the presence of large numbers of specimens may overcome some of the problems associated with sampling variation.

## OVERLAP SYNDROMES IN AUTOIMMUNE LIVER DISEASE

The concept of overlap syndromes in autoimmune liver disease has been recognized fairly recently. These syndromes may involve PBC, PSC and AIH in any combination. The diagnosis of an overlap syndrome can be based on any of the main diagnostic criteria which are used to diagnose the individual disease entities (biochemistry, immunology, radiology or histology). In most cases overlapping features present simultaneously. However, there are also cases in which patients present initially with features of one disease (e.g. AIH) and then present after an interval of several months or years with typical features of another syndrome (e.g. PBC or PSC)[50–54]. Temporal dissociation appears to be more common with overlap syndromes involving AIH and PSC than with syndromes involving AIH and PBC.

Two main forms of autoimmune overlap syndromes can be recognized, as illustrated by the two examples presented in Table 5. Patient 1 has serological, biochemical and histological features which would be compatible both with a diagnosis of AIH and with a diagnosis of PBC. This could be regarded as an example of a true overlap syndrome. Patient 2 has a 'crossover' syndrome in which the serological profile is typical of AIH (with negative antimitochondrial antibodies), but the biochemical and histological features suggest PBC as the most likely diagnosis. The term autoimmune cholangitis has been used to describe this combination of findings[55,56].

One of the main problems relating to the classification of overlap syndromes concerns the criteria which are used to make the diagnosis. For example, in a hypothetical patient who is antimitochondrial antibody (AMA) positive, with a raised serum alkaline phosphatase and histological findings compatible with PBC, what additional features are required to make a diagnosis of overlap syndrome? Should it be based on the presence of hepatitic biochemistry (if so, what level of transaminitis is required?), positive autoantibodies (if so, which antibodies and at what titre?), or on the presence of necroinflammatory changes in the liver biopsy? As far as the latter are concerned, portal and periportal inflammation are commonly seen in PBC and to a lesser extent in PSC, and it is not clear what degree of interface hepatitis or lobular necroinflammatory activity is required in order for a diagnosis of overlap syndrome to be made. In two recent studies 9% and 19% of patients with an initial diagnosis of PBC were considered to have overlap features of AIH, based on a combination of biochemical, serological and histological findings[57,58]. A higher proportion of patients with PSC

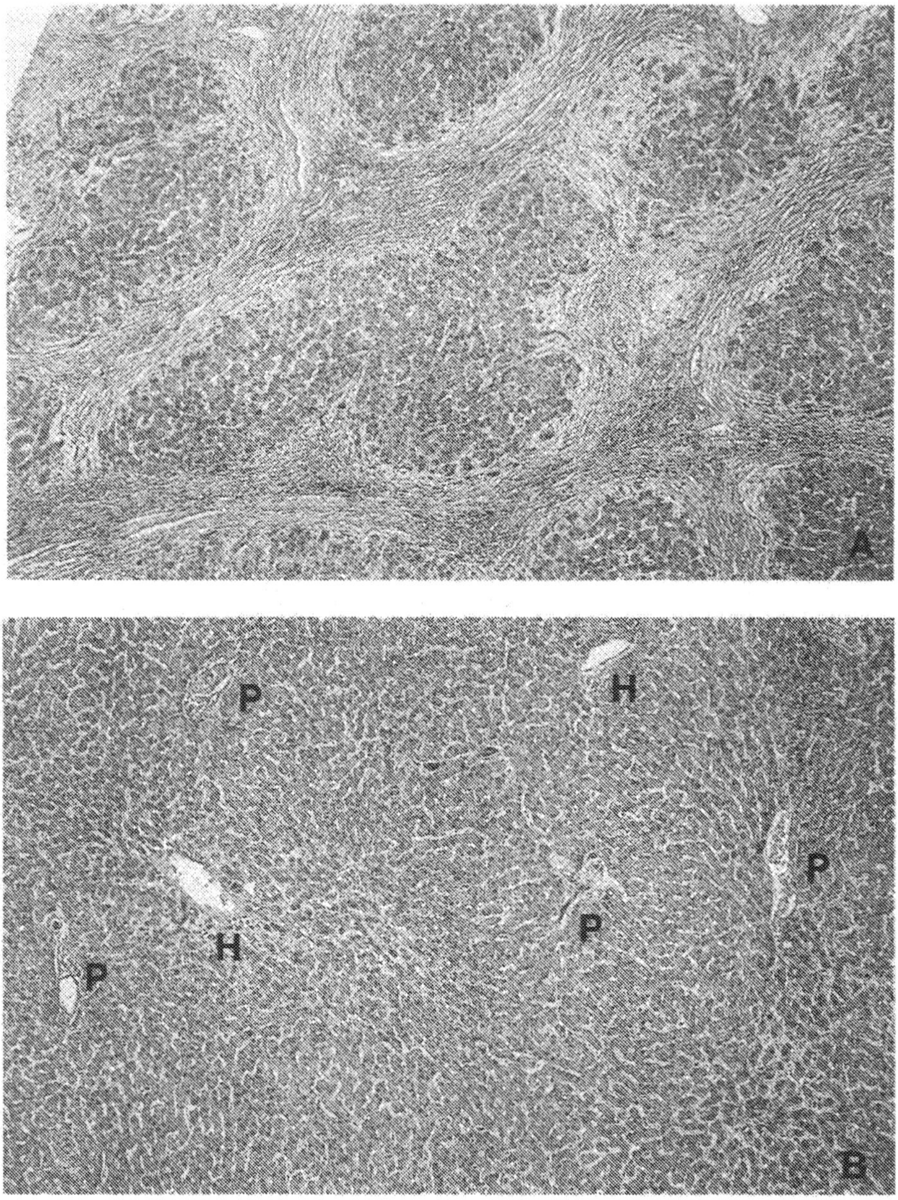


**Fig. 15** Sampling variation in severity of fibrosis in PBC. These two slides are both taken from a single block of liver obtained from a patient undergoing liver transplantation. In one area there is an established biliary cirrhosis (**A**). However, an adjacent field shows preservation of normal vascular relationships with no obvious fibrosis (**B**). P = portal tract, H = hepatic vein. Haematoxylin and eosin

**Table 5** Examples of two main forms of overlap syndrome which have been recognized in autoimmune liver disease

| | |
|---|---|
| 1. 'True' overlap syndrome (autoimmune hepatitis/primary biliary cirrhosis) | |
| Autoantibodies | ANA+, SMA+,AMA+ |
| Biochemistry | AST raised, alkaline phosphatase raised |
| Histology | Mixed hepatitic and biliary features |
| 2. 'Crossover' overlap syndrome ('autoimmune cholangitis') | |
| Autoantibodies | ANA+, SMA+, AMA- |
| Biochemistry | AST normal, alkaline phosphatase raised |
| Histology | PBC-like features |

Patient 1 has a 'true' overlap syndrome in which serological, biochemical and histological features of autoimmune hepatitis (AIH) and primary biliary cirrhosis (PBC) are present simultaneously. By contrast, patient 2 has the serological profile of AIH, with biochemical and histological features typical of PBC ('autoimmune cholangitis').

(35–54%) were found to have features of AIH, based on similar diagnostic criteria[58,59]. In most cases where overlapping features exist, the preferred diagnosis is one of autoimmune biliary disease (PBC or PSC) associated with prominent hepatitic features[60]. Nevertheless, the identification of a prominent hepatitic component, either histologically or by other methods, is clinically relevant as such patients appear to benefit from treatment with immunosuppression[57–61].

There has been much controversy regarding the precise nature of so-called 'autoimmune cholangitis'. Suggestions which have been made include AMA-negative PBC[62,64], a subtype of autoimmune hepatitis with prominent biliary features[56] or a distinctive syndrome which is neither PBC nor AIH[65]. However, it is now widely accepted that autoimmune cholangitis is best regarded as AMA-negative PBC. Evidence for this conclusion has included the results of several histological studies which have failed to identify any obvious differences between AMA-positive PBC and autoimmune cholangitis[62,63,65,66–68]. In the largest study, carried out by Goodman *et al.*[63], 200 patients with a histological diagnosis of PBC were divided into four serological groups based on their AMA and antinuclear antibody (ANA) status. Sixty-two patients were AMA-positive/ANA-negative ('typical' PBC), 74 patients were AMA-positive/ANA-positive (PBC/AIH overlap), 40 patients were AMA-negative/ANA-positive (autoimmune cholangitis) and the remaining 24 patients were AMA-negative and ANA-negative. A number of histological features were assessed including biliary features such as inflammatory bile duct lesions and bile duct loss and hepatitic features such as portal inflammation and interface hepatitis. No differences for any of the histological features assessed were found between the four serological groups identified. Immunohistochemical studies have also failed to demonstrate any differences between cases of AMA-positive PBC and autoimmune cholangitis in terms of the pattern of expression of the pyruvate dehyrogenase complex E2 subunit (PDC-E2) on the apical region of bile duct epithelial cells[69], or the phenotypic composition of portal inflammatory infiltrates[70]. On the basis of these observations it has been suggested that autoimmune cholangitis be used as an alternative term for PBC, to include both AMA-positive and AMA-negative cases[71,72] (Ishak KG *et al.*, in preparation).

## SUMMARY AND CONCLUSIONS

The final diagnosis of autoimmune cholestatic liver disease depends on a combination of biochemical, immunological, radiological and histological findings. In many cases (for example AMA-positive PBC or PSC associated with typical radiological changes) liver biopsy may not be required for diagnosis. In other cases (for example AMA-negative PBC or small duct PSC) liver histology is the main diagnostic investigation. Other indications for liver biopsy in autoimmune biliary disease include the identification and grading of necroinflammatory activity, which has potential therapeutic implications for the use of immunosuppressive agents; staging of fibrosis, which is most appropriate in a context of clinical trials; and exclusion of other intercurrent diseases. Finally liver biopsy material provides a valuable resource for studies investigating mechanisms of bile duct damage in PBC and PSC.

### Acknowledgements

I thank fellow members of the International Liver Group (Amelia Baptista, Leonardo Bianchi, Alastair Burt, Francesco Callea, Jan De Groote, Helmut Denk, Valeer Desmet, Kamal Ishak, Roderick MacSween, James Phillips, Bernard Portmann, Hemming Poulsen and Peter Scheuer) for helpful discussions relating to the histological diagnosis and classification of autoimmune biliary diseases, Miss TE Claridge who typed the manuscript, and Mrs R Smith who provided photographic assistance.

### References

1. Ludwig J. Idiopathic adulthood ductopenia: an update. Mayo Clin Proc. 1998;73:285–91.
2. Portmann B, MacSween RNM. Diseases of the intrahepatic bile ducts. In: MacSween RNM, Anthony PP, Scheuer PJ, Burt AD, Portmann BC, editors. Pathology of the Liver, 3rd edn. Edinburgh: Churchill Livingstone; 1994:477–512.
3. Van Den Oord JJV, Fevery J, de Groote J, Desmet VJ. Immunohistochemical characterization of inflammatory infiltrates in primary biliary cirrhosis. Liver. 1984;4:264–74.
4. Krams SM, Van de Water J, Coppel RL A *et al.* Analysis of hepatic T lymphocyte and immunoglobulin deposits in patients with primary biliary cirrhosis. Hepatology. 1990;12:306–313.
5. Nakanuma Y. Distribution of B lymphocytes in nonsuppurative cholangitis in primary biliary cirrhosis. Hepatology. 1993;18:570–5.
6. Terasaki S, Nakanuma Y, Yanazaki M, Unoura M. Eosinophilic infiltration of the liver in primary biliary cirrhosis: a morphological study. Hepatology. 1993;17:206–12.
7. Martinez OM, Villanueva JC, Gershwin ME, Sheri MK. Cytokine patterns and cytotoxic mediators in primary biliary cirrhosis. Hepatology. 1995;21:113–19.
8. Ishak KG. Sarcoidosis of the liver and bile ducts. Mayo Clin Proc. 1998;73:467–72.

9. Hoso M, Nakanuma Y, Kawano M *et al.* Granulomatous cholangitis in chronic hepatitis C: a new diagnostic problem in liver pathology. Pathol Int. 1996;46:301–5.
10. Chapman RW, Arborgh BMA, Rhodes JM, Summerfield JA, Dick R, Scheuer PJ. Primary sclerosing cholangitis: a review of its clinical features, cholangiography and hepatic histology. Gut. 1980;21:870–7.
11. Ludwig J, Colina F, Poterucha JJ. Granulomas in primary sclerosing cholangitis. Liver. 1995;15:307–12.
12. Ishak KG, Zimmerman HG. Drug induced and toxic granulomatous hepatitis. Baillière's Clin Gastroenterol. 1988;2:463–80.
13. Ferrell LD, Lee R, Brixko C *et al.* Hepatic granulomas following liver transplantation. Clinicopathologic features in 42 patients. Transplantation. 1995;60:926–33.
14. Kaplan KJ, Goodman ZD, Ishak KG. Liver involvement in Langerhans' cell histiocytosis: a study of nine cases. Mod Pathol. 1999;12:370–8.
15. Abt AB, Kirschner RH, Belliveau RE *et al.* Hepatic pathology associated with Hodgkin's disease. Cancer. 1974;33:1564–71.
16. Kadin ME, Donaldson SS, Dorfman RF. Isolated granulomas in Hodgkin's disease. N Engl J Med. 1970;283:859–61.
17. Harrison RF, Hübscher SG. The spectrum of bile duct lesions in end-stage primary sclerosing cholangitis. Histopathology. 1991;19:321–7.
18. Wee A, Ludwig J. Pericholangitis in chronic ulcerative cholitis: primary sclerosing cholangitis of the small bile ducts? Ann Intern Med. 1985;102:581–7.
19. Ludwig J. Small duct primary sclerosing cholangitis. Semin Liver Dis. 1991;11:1–17.
20. Angulo P, Lindor KD. Primary sclerosing cholangitis. Hepatology. 1999;30:325–32.
21. Boberg KM, Schrumpf E, Fausa O, Elgjo K, Kolmannskog F, Haaland T *et al.* Hepatobiliary disease in ulcerative colitis. An analysis of 18 patients with hepatobiliary lesions classified as small-duct primary sclerosing cholangitis. Scand J Gastroenterol. 1994;29:744–52.
22. Ludwig J, MacCarty RL, LaRusso NF, Krom RAF, Wiesner RH. Intrahepatic cholangiectases and large-duct obliteration in primary sclerosing cholangitis. Hepatology. 1986;6:560–8.
23. Oguma S, Belle S, Starzl TE, Demetris AJ. A histometric analysis of chronically rejected human liver allografts: insights into mechanisms of bile duct loss: direct immunological and ischaemic factors. Hepatology. 1989;9:204–9.
24. Wiesner RH, Ludwig J, van Hoek B, Krom RA. Current concepts in cell-mediated hepatic allograft rejection leading to ductopenia and liver failure. Hepatology. 1991;14:721–9.
25. Dilawari JB, Chawala YK. Pseudosclerosing cholangitis in extrahepatic portal venous obstruction. Gut. 1992;33:272–6.
26. Nakanuma Y, Hoso M, Sasaki M *et al.* Histopathology of the liver in non-cirrhotic portal hypertension of unkown aetiology. Histopathology. 1996;28:195–204.
27. Woolf GM, Vierling JM. Disappearing intrahepatic bile ducts: the syndromes and their mechanisms. Semin Liver Dis. 1993;13:261–75.
28. Forbes A, Blanshard C, Gazzard B. Natural history of AIDS related slcerosing cholangitis: a study of 20 cases. Gut. 1993;34:116–21.
29. Lucas SB. Other viral and infectious diseases and HIV-related liver disease. In: MacSween RNM, Anthony PP, Scheuer PJ, Burt AD, Portmann BC, editors. Pathology of the liver. 3rd Edition Edinburgh: Churchill Livingstone; 1994: pp 269–316.
30. Thompson HH, Pitt HA, Lewin KJ, Longmire WP. Sclerosing cholangitis and histiocytosis X. Gut 1984; 25: 526–530.
31. Baron TH, Koehler RE, Rodgers WH, Fallon MB, Ferguson SM. Mast cell cholangiopathy: another cause of sclerosing cholangitis. Gastroenterology. 1995;109:1677–81.
32. Terada T, Nakanuma Y. Intrahepatic cholangiographic appearance simulating primary sclerosing cholangitis in several hepatobiliary diseases. A post mortem cholangiographic and histopathological study in 154 livers at autopsy. Hepatology. 1995;22:75–81.
33. Wiesner RH, LaRusso NF, Ludwig J, Dickson ER. Comparison of the clinicopathologic features of primary sclerosing cholangitis and primary biliary cirrhosis. Gastroenterology. 1985;88:108–14.
34. Degott C, Zafrani ES, Callard P, Balkau B, Poupon RE, Poupon R. Histopathological study of primary biliary cirrhosis and the effect of ursodeoxycholic acid treatment on histology progression. Hepatology. 1999;29:1007–12.
35. Nakanuma Y. Necroinflammatory changes in hepatic lobules in primary biliary cirrhosis with less well defined cholestatic changes. Human Pathology. 1993;24:378–83.

36. Burt AD, MacSween RNM. Bile duct proliferation – its true significance. Histopathology. 1993;23:599–602.
37. Desmet V, Roskams T, Van Eyken P. Ductular reaction in the liver. Pathol Res Pract. 1995;191:513–24.
38. Nagore N, Howe S, Boxer L, Scheuer PJ. Liver cell rosettes: structural differences in cholestasis and hepatitis. Liver. 1989;9:43–51.
39. Crosby HA, Hübscher SG, Fabris L *et al.* Immunolocalization of putative human liver progenitor cells in livers from patients with end-stage primary biliary cirrhosis and sclerosing cholangitis using the monoclonal antibody OV-6. Am J Pathol. 1998;152:771–9.
40. Roskams T, De Vos R, Van Eyken P, Myazaki H, Van Damme B, Desmet V. Hepatic OV-6 expression in human liver disease and rat experiments: evidence for hepatic progenitor cells in man. J Hepatol. 1998;29:455–63.
41. Crosby HA, Hübscher SG, Joplin RE, Kelly DA, Strain AJ. Immunolocalization of OV-6, a putative progenitor cell marker in humal fetal and diseased pediatric liver. Hepatology. 1998;28:980–5.
42. Rubin E, Schaffner F, Popper H. Primary biliary cirrhosis. Chronic non-suppurative destructive cholangitis. Am J Pathol. 1965;46:387–407.
43. Scheuer PJ. Primary biliary cirrhosis. Proc R Soc Med. 1967;60:1257–60.
44. Popper H, Schaffner F. Non-suppurative destructive chronic cholangitis and chronic hepatitis. In: Popper H, Schaffner F, editors. Progress in Liver Diseases, vol. III. New York: Grune & Stratton; 1970:336–54.
45. Ludwig J, Dickson ER, McDonald GS. Staging of chronic non-suppurative cholangitis (syndrome of primary biliary cirrhosis). Virchows Arch (A). 1978;379: 103–12.
46. Ludwig J. Surgical pathology of the syndrome of primary sclerosing cholangitis. Am J Surg Pathol. 1989;33:43–49.
47. Hübscher SG. Histological grading and staging in chronic hepatitis: clinical applications and problems. Journal of Hepatology. 1998;29:1015–22.
48. Garrido MC, Hübscher SG. Accuracy of staging in primary biliary cirrhosis. J Clin Pathol. 1996;49:556–9.
49. Olsson R, Hagerstrand I, Broomé U *et al.* Sampling variability of percutaneous liver biopsy in primary sclerosing cholangitis. J Clin Pathol. 1995;48:933–5.
50. Horsmanns Y, Piret A, Brenard R, Rahier J, Geuvel AP. Autoimmune chronic active hepatitis responsive to immunosuppressive therapy evolving into a typical primary biliary cirrhosis syndrome: a case report. J Hepatol. 1994;21:194–8.
51. Colombato LA, Alvarez F, Cote J, Huet PM. Autoimmune cholangiopathy: the result of consecutive primary biliary cirrhosis and autoimmune hepatitis? Gastroenterology. 1994;107:1839–43.
52. Minuk GY, Sutherland LR, Pappas SC, Kelly JK, Martin SE. Autoimmune chronic active hepatitis (lupoid hepatitis) and primary sclerosing cholangitis in two young adult females. Canad J Gastroenterol. 1988;2:22–27.
53. Leggett BA, Hallam A, Powell EE, Powell LW. Autoimmune chronic active hepatitis evolving to primary sclerosing cholangitis: evidence for a common pathogenesis. Hepatology. 1992;16:191A.
54. Lawrence SP, Sherman KE, Lawson JM, Goodman ZY. A 38 year old man with chronic hepatitis. Semin Liver Dis. 1994;14:97–105.
55. Brunner G, Klinge O. A cholangitis with antinuclear antibodies (immunocholangitis) resembling chronic destructive non-suppurative cholangitis. Dtsch Med Wochenschr. 1987;112:1454–58.
56. Ben-Ari Z, Dhillon AP, Sherlock S. Autoimmune cholangiopathy: part of the spectrum of autoimmune chronic active hepatitis. Hepatology. 1993;18:10–15.
57. Chazouilleres O, Wendum D, Serfaty L, Montembault S, Rosmorduc O, Poupon R. Primary biliary cirrhosis–autoimmune hepatitis overlap syndrome: clinical features and response to therapy. Hepatology. 1998;28:296–301.
58. Czaja AJ. Frequency and nature of the variant syndrome of autoimmune liver disease. Hepatology. 1998;28:360–5.
59. Boberg KM, Fausa O, Haaland T *et al.* Features of autoimmune hepatitis in primary sclerosing cholangitis: an evaluation of 114 primary sclerosing cholangitis patients according to a scoring system for the diagnosis of autoimmune hepatitis. Hepatology. 1996;23:1369–76.

60. Lohse AW, Meyer zum Buschenfelde KH, Franz B, Kanzler S, Gerken G, Dienes HP. Characterisation of the overlap syndrome of primary biliary cirrhosis (PBC) and autoimmune hepatitis: evidence for it being a hepatitic form of PBC in genetically susceptible individuals. Hepatology. 1999;29:1078–84.
61. Czaja AJ. The variant forms of autoimmune hepatitis. Ann Intern Med. 1996;125:588–98.
62. Taylor SL, Dean PJ, Riely CA. Primary autoimmune cholangitis. An alternative to antimitochondrial antibody-negative primary biliary cirrhosis. Am J Surg Pathol. 1994;18:91–9.
63. Goodman ZD, McNally PR, Davis Dr, Ishak KG. Autoimmune cholangitis: a variant of primary biliary cirrhosis. Clinicopathologic and serologic correlations in 200 cases. Dig Dis Sci. 1995;40:1232–42.
64. Heathcote J. Autoimmune cholangitis. Gut. 1997;40:440–2.
65. Michieletti P, Wanless IR, Katz A *et al.* Antimitochondrial antibody negative primary biliary cirrhosis: a distinct syndrome of autoimmune cholangitis. Gut. 1994;35:260–5.
66. Sanchez-Pobre P, Castellano G, Colina F *et al.* Antimitochondrial antibody-negative chronic nonsuppurative destructive cholangitis. Atypical primary biliary cirrhosis or autoimmune cholangitis? J Clin Gastroenterol. 1996;23:191–8.
67. Kinoshita H, Omargi K, Whittingham S *et al.* Autoimmune cholangitis and primary biliary cirrhosis – an autoimmune enigma. Liver. 1999;19:122–8.
68. Lacerda MA, Ludwig J, Dickson ER, Jorgensen RA, Lindor KD. Antimitochondrial antibody-negative primary biliary cirrhosis. Am J Gastroenterol. 1995;90:247–9.
69. Tsuneyama K, Van de Water J, Van Thiel D *et al.* Abnormal expression of PDC-$E_2$ on the apical surface of biliary epithelial cells in patients with antimitochondrial antibody-negative primary biliary cirrhosis. Hepatology. 1995;22:1440–6.
70. Kaserer K, Exner M, Mosberger I, Penner E, Wrba F. Characterization of the inflammatory infiltrate in autoimmune cholangitis. A morphological and immunohistochemical study. Virchows Archiv. 1998;432:217–22.
71. Heathcote EJ. Autoimmune cholangitis. In: Lindor KD, Dickson ER, editors. Primary Biliary Cirrhosis, Primary Sclerosing Cholangitis and Adult Cholangiopathies. Philadelphia: WB Saunders; 1998:303–11.
72. Vierling JM. Autoimmune cholangiopathy. Clin Liver Dis. 1999;3:571–84.

# 21
# Clues to the aetiology of primary biliary cirrhosis

**A. TANAKA, P. S. C. LEUNG, J. VAN DE WATER, S. MUNOZ, R. L. COPPEL, A. ANSARI and M. E. GERSHWIN**

## INTRODUCTION

Primary biliary cirrhosis (PBC) is an organ-specific autoimmune disease, characterized by non-suppurative destructive cholangitis, involving small to interlobular biliary ducts. The presence of antimitochondrial antibodies (AMA) is one of the major diagnostic criteria. Although extensive research has resulted in defining the clinical, biochemical, histological and immunological manifestations of PBC, its aetiology remains obscure since the term PBC was coined in 1950[1]. As a result it is impossible to alter the clinical course of PBC by medical treatment, and currently no drug therapy can reverse the disease. Thus, at present, liver transplantation seems to be the only therapeutic regimen. However, donors for transplantation are not always available.

Recently, the application and advances of molecular and cellular biology have greatly facilitated our understanding of the immunological mechanism of PBC. In this chapter we will adress several major questions that are crucial in understanding the aetiology of PBC.

## WHAT ARE THE MAJOR MITOCHONDRIAL AUTOANTIGENS IN PBC?

Serologically, PBC is characterized by the presence of a high titre of AMA[2,3]. During the past decade a number of these antigens have been cloned and identified at the molecular level[4]. It is now well recognized that the targets of AMA are members of the 2-oxo-acid dehydrogenase complex (2-OADC), including the E2 subunit of the pyruvate dehydrogenase complex (PDC-E2), the E2 subunit of branched-chain 2-oxo-acid dehydrogenase complex (BCOADC-E2), the E2 subunit of the 2-oxoglutarate dehydrogenase complex (OGDC-E2), E1$\alpha$ subunit of PDC and dihydrolipoamide dehydrogenase-binding protein (E3BP), once termed protein X[4].

These molecules are located in the inner mitochondrial membrane. All of them, except for PDC-E1$\alpha$, have a lipoyl domain near the N-terminal, an E3 binding region in the middle and the catalytic site near the C-terminal which are interconnected by an alanine–proline-rich region (Figure 1). The number of lipoyl domains for each of these enzymes, however, differs. Thus, PDC-E2 has two lipoyl domains and both BCOADC-E2 and OGDC-E2 each have a single lipoyl domain (Figure 1).

Although the E3BP has been known to be recognized by AMA, it was only in 1997 that human E3BP was cloned and sequenced[5]. The protein has a multi-domain structure analogous to that of PDC-E2, with the exception that, similar to BCOADC-E2 and OGDC-E2, it contains only a single lipoyl domain (Figure 1).

## WHAT ARE THE B CELL EPITOPES OF THESE MITOCHONDRIAL AUTOANTIGENS?

The high structural similarity among the 2-OADC-E2 subunits and E3BP has prompted us to investigate whether there are any common epitope(s) among these antigens. The cloning and expression of recombinant human mitochondrial autoantigens in *Escherichia coli* has greatly facilitated the mapping of B cell epitopes of the 2-OADC enzymes. Several studies have shown that the predominant epitope of PDC-E2 is located within the inner lipoyl domain of PDC-E2[6,7]. AMA also react with the outer domain, but at a 100-fold lower dilution, and only 1/26 PBC sera react weakly to the E1/E3 binding region[7]. To map the B cell epitope more precisely, truncated constructs of PDC-E2 lipoyl domain were expressed in *E. coli*, and assayed for their immunoreactivity against sera from patients with PBC. The results suggest that anti-PDC-E2 autoantibodies recognize a conformational epitope encoded by the inner lipoyl domain of PDC-E2. These findings were further elegantly confirmed using similar truncated peptides of PDC-E2 and combinatorial human autoantibodies derived from an immunoglobulin library of patients with PBC[8]. Cloning recombinant full-length

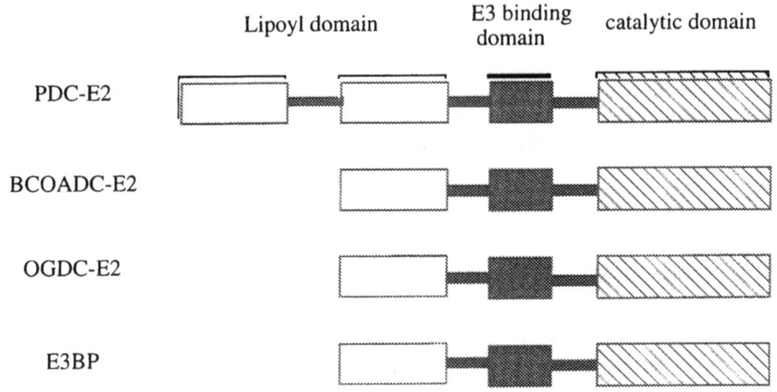


**Fig. 1** Diagrammatic representation of the structural and functional domains of 2-OADC E2 sub-units and E3 binding protein and their corresponding B-cell epitopes

and truncated BCOADC-E2, Leung *et al.*[9] defined the conformational epitope recognized by PBC sera and Moteki *et al.* mapped the AMA epitope of OGDC-E2 within an 81 amino acid polypeptide (residues 67–147) corresponding to the lipoyl domain of OGDC-E2[10]. Taken together, it appears that the reactive AMA to PDC-E2, BCOADC-E2 and OGDC-E2 each recognize conformational epitopes, and the lipoic acid domain is necessary for strong antibody binding.

The recent cloning and sequencing of human E3BP allowed us to analyse its epitope more precisely. Using full-length human E3BP cDNA, Dubel *et al.* revealed that 24 out of 45 PBC patients' sera (53%) reacted with the lipoyl domain of human E3BP (E3BP-LD)[11]. In addition, the reactivity against E3BP of beef heart mitochondria was completely abolished by pre-absorption of sera with E3BP-LD, suggesting that the lipoyl domain is the only epitope of the protein. Interestingly, the seroreactivity against beef heart mitochondria E3BP was also removed by pre-absorption with PDC-E2 protein, whereas beef heart mitochondria PDC-E2 was still recognized by PBC sera after pre-absorption with E3BP. These findings indicate that there are at least two autoepitopes on PDC-E2 lipoyl domain, one shared with E3BP and the other(s) not shared with E3BP. It is also of interest to note that most of the autoantibodies against E3BP were found to be of the IgG isotype (Table 1). Interestingly, except for PDC-E2 and E3BP, AMA do not crossreact. This is probably due to the high sequence homology between PDC-E2 and E3BP lipoyl domain (Table 2).

## WHAT IS THE NATURE OF T CELL RESPONSES TO MITOCHONDRIAL AUTOANTIGENS?

T cells play a central role in antigen-specific immune response, by helping B cells to produce specific antibodies and exerting cytotoxic activities. It is believed that mitochondrial autoantigens-specific T cell clones are present in patients with PBC, based on the assumption that the production of very specific autoantibodies, AMA, must require help from antigen-specific $CD4^+$ T cells. In 1995, autoreactive T cell clones specific for PDC-E2 were established from peripheral blood mononuclear cells (PBMC) of patients, and the T cell autoepitope of PDC-E2 was also identified[12,13]. The minimal autoepitopes recognized by these T-cell clones were all located within the same region of PDC-E2 peptide 163–176 (GDLLAEIETD-KATI), which corresponds to the inner lipoyl domain of human PDC-E2. Moreover, each of the six T-cell clones also reacted to the PDC-E2 peptide 36–49 (GDLIAEVETDKATD) of the outer lipoyl domain.

T-cell recognition of the peptide 163–176 can be affected by the tertiary structure of human PDC-E2. It was indicated that differential antigen processing in the APC could strongly influence the immunodominance pattern of the T-cell

**Table 1** Ig isotypes of AMA directed to E3BP-LD found in 24 PBC sera

| *Ig isotypes* | *No.* | *Percentage* |
|---|---|---|
| IgG | 23 | 95 |
| IgA | 4 | 16.6 |
| IgM | 3 | 12.5 |

**Table 2** Amino acid sequence of flanking lipoyl-lysine residues and comparison of each E2 subunit of human 2-OADC and human E3BP

| *Enzyme* | *Sequences* |
|---|---|
| PDC-E2 | **GDLLAEIETDKATI** |
| E3BP-LD | **GD**A**L**C**EIETDKA**VV |
| OGDC-E2 | DEVVL**EIETDK**TSV |
| BCOADC-E2 | F**D**SIC**E**VQS**DKA**SV |

Identical amino acids are shown in bold, and similar amino acids are underlined.

epitope of a given peptide, and that immunodominant epitopes correlate with nearby structurally unstable segments[14]. Despite the large molecular size of PDC, the inner lipoyl domain of human PDC-E2 is flexible and is preferentially cleaved by proteases. In addition, data from X-ray crystallography or two-dimensional nuclear magnetic resonance (NMR) of human PDC-E2 showed that peptide 163–176 is located at a structurally exposed region of the molecule[15–17], which partly explains the particular immunogenecity of this sequence. Thus the identification of the tertiary structure of other mitochondrial autoantigens, BCOADC-E2 or OGDC-E2, by X-ray crystallography or two-dimensional NMR will be helpful in the prediction and determination of T-cell autoepitopes of these molecules.

Recently we have also generated PDC-E2 specific T cell clones from livers and regional lymph nodes of patients with PBC[18]. PDC-E2 (peptide 163–176) specific T-cell precursor frequency was 100–150-fold higher in the hilar lymph nodes and liver than that of PBMC from patients with PBC. Interestingly, PDC-E2-specific T cell clones were also established from PBMC of normal individuals, and the precursor frequency in PBC patients was only 1.5–3.5-fold increased as compared with healthy controls. This result clearly demonstrates that PDC-E2-specific T cell clones are not eliminated from PBMC by negative thymic selection, and tolerance against PDC-E2 has to be established and maintained peripherally in healthy individuals. In addition, it was demonstrated that T cell clones reacted not only with PDC-E2 peptide 163–176, but also with PDC-E2 peptide 36–49 (GDLIAEVETDKATV) and OGDC peptide 100–113 (DEVVCEIETDKTSV), all of which share motifs with one another. This finding suggests the presence of crossreactivity among these three mitochondrial enzymes at the T-cell level. Since all these three peptides share ExETDK amino acid sequences, this could be a common T cell epitope 'motif'. Although it is likely that anti-PDC-E2 autoantibodies are produced by B cells through PDC-E2-specific T cells identified herein, whether the production of anti-OGDC autoantibodies can be achieved with help from OGDC-E2-specific T cells, or by crossreactivity of PDC-E2 specific T cells remains to be determined.

## ARE THERE ANY TISSUE-SPECIFIC ANTIGENS IN BILIARY EPITHELIAL CELLS IN PBC?

In PBC, tissue destruction in liver is mostly seen in biliary epithelial cells. It is difficult to explain this selectivity, since the 2-OADC enzymes are present in every mitochondrion in human tissues. Why would only biliary epithelial cells be chosen as a target of autoimmune reaction after T cell clones specific for human PDC-E2 are activated? Are there any specific antigens that are exclusively or preferentially expressed in human biliary epithelial cells?

We have taken advantage of a panel of PDC-E2-specific monoclonal antibodies to address these questions[19]. Among these there are eight murine monoclonal antibodies that have been mapped to four different regions of PDC-E2. In addition, we also used a PDC-E2-specific human Fab combinatorial antibody, derived from a PBC lymph node Fab combinatorial library. This Fab recombinant antibody reacts with the lipoyl domain of PDC-E2 and E3BP but not BCOADC-E2, OGDC-E2 or PDC-E1$\alpha$[20].

Using these antibodies we examined sections of liver from patients with PBC by indirect immunofluorescence and confocal microscopy and, for controls, several sections from patients with progressive sclerosing cholangitis (PSC) and hepatocarcinoma[21]. The PDC-E2-specific monoclonal antibodies gave typical mitochondrial immunofluorescence on biliary epithelium and on hepatocytes from patients with either PBC, PSC or hepatocarcinoma. However, one of the eight mouse monoclonal antibodies, C355.1, and a human combinatorial antibody, LC5, reacted with great intensity and specificity with the luminal region of biliary epithelial cells from patients with PBC. The selective reactivity of some anti-PDC-E2 monoclonal antibodies suggests the presence of tissue-specific autoantigens which are cross-reactive with PDC-E2 and the presence of a protein with PDC-E2 mimic peptide in the luminal region of biliary epithelial cells in PBC.

To further investigate this hypothesis we have generated other monoclonal antibodies against mitochondrial antigens[22]. By immunizing mice with a recombinant protein containing the lipoyl domains of PDC-E2, OGDC-E2, and BCOADC-E2[23], 35 new monoclonal antibodies which are specific for one or more mitochondrial antigens were obtained. By immunohistochemical staining and confocal microscopy, seven out of 35 monoclonal antibodies stained the apical region of biliary epithelial cells only in PBC, with a staining pattern similar to C355.1. Of these seven, one was reactive to PDC-E2, two were reactive to BCOADC-E2, three recognized OGDC-E2 and, interestingly, one monoclonal antibody was reactive to all three antigens. These results suggest that the tissue-specific autoantigens in the apical region of biliary epithelial cells contain epitopes or shared epitopes that are recognized by anti-BCOADC-E2, anti-OGDC monoclonal antibodies as well as C355.1 and anti-PDC-E2 monoclonals.

Recently, Sadamoto *et al.* reported that the expression of PDC-E2 and E3BP (or cross-reactive molecules) was induced by co-incubation of biliary epithelial cells from healthy individuals with lymph nodes from PBC patients[24]. They isolated lymph nodes from patients with PBC and co-cultured them with biliary epithelial cells from normal individuals for 7 days. After the incubation period, epithelial cell lysates were prepared and separated on SDS-PAGE gel and probed with anti-PDC antibodies. Quantitative analysis of the SDS-PAGE for expression of PDC-E2 and E3BP revealed an increase of 2.03- and 2.79-fold compared with the same cells incubated without lymph nodes, respectively.

Also, biliary epithelial cells from healthy subjects demonstrated a luminal staining pattern with antimitochondrial antibodies after co-incubation. Although their data suggest that PBC-specific antigens can be induced in biliary epithelial cells, further work is necessary to determine its exact molecular identity and whether it can be PDC-E2 and E3BP or cross-reactive molecules recognized by anti-PDC antibodies.

## IS THE BILIARY EPITHELIAL CELLS-SPECIFIC ANTIGEN PDC-E2 OR NOT?

What is the nature of the tissue-specific antigens in biliary epithelial cells recognized by these monoclonal antibodies? One hypothesis is that PDC-E2, normally located in mitochondrial inner membrane, is aberrantly expressed on the cell surface and recognized by autoantibodies or PDC-E2-specific monoclonal antibodies. This can be accounted for by the following: first, PDC-E2 may be overexpressed in biliary epithelial cells. *In-situ* hybridization of PDC-E2 mRNA, however, showed that there were no significant differences in the amount of PDC-E2 transcript between PBC and other liver diseases[25]. Second, mutant or tissue-specific variants of PDC-E2 may cause an abnormal turnover of the molecule, leading to the accumulation of PDC-E2 in the cells. Since biliary ducts are one of the routes by which toxic materials or metabolites are removed from the body, it may be possible that toxic substances accumulated in biliary epithelium alter the expression of PDC-E2 locally, leading to the production of tissue-specific variants of PDC-E2. Third, altered PDC-E2 mRNA would be produced by the abnormal transcription of PDC-E2. For example, if the leader sequence of PDC-E2 is modified, that could lead to aberrant subcellular distribution, from mitochondria to plasma membrane[26]. Alternatively, it is possible that abnormal splicing during synthesis of PDC-E2 mRNA would substitute an ER targeting signal instead of a mitochondrial targeting signal in PDC-E2. Thus, PDC-E2 are delivered into the endoplasmic reticulum (ER) and Golgi apparatus via a secretory route to be expressed on the cell surface of biliary ducts, instead of mitochondria. While these explanations are attractive, and can be possible, direct evidence supporting these mechanisms is lacking.

It remains possible that the molecule(s) on the ductular surface of biliary epithelial cells which are recognized by anti-PDC-E2 monoclonal antibodies may not be PDC-E2 itself, but are PDC-E2 mimics that cross-react with human PDC-E2 antibodies. Indeed, our data support the hypothesis that the recognition by monoclonal antibodies on the apical region is caused by the presence of the molecules which are cross-reactive with PDC-E2, because: (1) not all monoclonal antibodies specific for PDC-E2 display the luminal staining[21], and (2) OGDC- or BCOADC-specific monoclonal antibodies also stained the apical region[22], and (3) *in-situ* hybridization data do not show any overexpression in PDC-E2 mRNA in biliary epithelial cells[25]. Thus, based on these findings, it is postulated that the tissue-specific antigens are not PDC-E2, but share conformational epitope with mitochondrial antigens. The nature and identity of this molecule remain to be defined.

## DOES IgA-AMA BIND TO MITOCHONDRIAL ANTIGENS IN BILIARY EPITHELIAL CELLS?

Another hypothesis which explains the selective destruction of bile ducts in PBC is that IgA isotype might play an important role in the pathogenesis of PBC. IgA is the principal isotype of immunoglobulin in epithelial surfaces, including biliary epithelium. IgA is synthesized in plasma cells located in the lamina propria, and secreted IgA binds to a poly-Ig receptor which is present on the basolateral surfaces of biliary epithelial cells. Following internalization with the receptor, IgA is transported through the cytoplasm in a transport vesicle (transcytosis), and secreted into the bile ducts at the apical surface. If antimitochondrial IgA autoantibodies are responsible for the specific destruction of biliary epithelial cells in PBC, it is reasoned that this occurs by disruption of the metabolism of the cells whereby the IgA-AMA bind to the mitochondrial antigen and induce cellular dysfunction and hence the tissue specificity. Based on this hypothesis we purified serum IgA from patients with PBC and studied its localization and ability to penetrate cells using Madine–Darby canine kidney (MDCK) cells transfected with the human IgA receptor[27]. Interestingly, IgA from all PBC patients co-localized with PDC-E2 inside the cells, demonstrated by dual staining with anti-human IgA and anti-PDC-E2 mouse monoclonal antibody, whereas no co-localization was found when IgA from healthy controls were used. These results suggest that IgA-AMA can penetrate the epithelial cells, and that they recognize and bind to the mitochondria proteins. It is of note that the penetration of IgA was also observed, although to a lesser extent, in the MDCK cells which lack poly-Ig receptor, since in this situation IgA may be present in the cytoplasm without binding to the receptor and transport vesicle, and thus may be more accessible to cytoplasmic protein. However, whether these IgA antibodies recognize any of the mitochondrial 2-OADC subunits in PBC is unclear. Nevertheless, these data support the idea that the trafficking of IgA in biliary epithelial cells is a possible mechanism for selective damage of biliary epithelial cells, in which IgA-AMA can bind to mitochondrial antigens and result in cellular disruption in patients with PBC. However, the apical staining of anti-PDC-E2 monoclonal antibodies could also be accounted for by the presence of immune complex formed by secreted IgA and mitochondrial enzymes.

## DOES MICROBIAL INFECTION PLAY A ROLE IN THE AETIOLOGY OF PBC?

Several lines of evidence support the roles of infectious agents, especially bacteria, in the pathogenesis of PBC, and the mechanism called 'molecular mimicry' by microbes is one of the strong hypotheses being forwarded to account for breaking down of tolerance against mitochondrial antigens. It is reported that there is a high prevalence of bacteriuria with a very high recurrence rate in females with PBC compared to other forms of chronic liver disease[28]. Patients with recurrent urinary tract infections, all of whom have normal liver function, are reported to have weak AMA reactivity (69%)[29]. This (if true) suggests an association between *E. coli* or other bacteria causing urinary tract infection and the aetiology of PBC. In fact, cross-reactivity of AMA against prokaryotic antigens has been reported in a number of microbes, including *E. coli*, *Klebsiella pneumoniae*, *Proteus mirabilis*, *Staphylococcus aureus* and *Salmonella minnesota*, although the target components of AMA in these bacteria have not been fully determined[30]. Furthermore, the sera from patients with PBC have been shown to react with both human PDC-E2 and *E. coli* PDC-E2, and the epitope of *E. coli* PDC-E2 also maps to similar lipoyl domains[31]. Vilagut *et al.* demonstrated that the sera from patients with PBC reacted with extracts of *Mycobacterium gordonae*[32], and that antibodies to the *M. gordonae* 65 kDa heat-shock protein weakly cross-react with the mitochondrial autoantigens, PDC-E2 and BCOADC-E2[33], implicating the association of *M. gordonae* with the aetiology of PBC. In contrast, the presence of reactivity of patients' sera against *M. gordonae* was not supported by another report[34]. Klein *et al.* demonstrated that sera from 12 out of 28 patients (43%) with active pulmonary tuberculosis reacted to the PDC-E2 subunit, whereas only two of 82 patients with other bacterial and viral infections, including 25 patients with *E. coli* infections, reacted with the PBC-specific autoepitopes[35], also implicating mycobacterial infection in PBC.

These cross-reactivities are not surprising, because of the conserved structure of the PDC-E2 among many species. Evolutionarily, PDC-E2 is well conserved among various species, from eubacteria to mammals[36]. Although PDC-E2 is present in mitochondria, some evidence suggests that one component of the 2-OADC, dihydrolipoamide dehydrogenase, PDC, OGDC and BCOADC, is detectable in the membrane fraction of *E. coli*[37], *Neisseria meningitidis*[38] and *Trypanosoma brucei*[39]. It is also reported that the protein located in the membrane of *N. meningitidis* consists of 11 amino acid residues highly homologous with that of the lipoyl domain of the E2 component[38]. Since it is believed that the origin of mitochondria in mammalian cells is intracellular organisms, it is likely that mitochondrial components, usually located in the mitochondrial inner membrane, are detected in the membrane of the organisms. The presence of these displayed proteins on the cell surface of bacteria may contribute to tolerance breakdown.

It is important to realize that T-cell-mediated immune responses specific for the autoantigen are necessary to initiate the immune response by providing appropriate helper T cell function for the B cell to produce antibody response. Thus cross-reactivity at the T cell level is required to break self-tolerance. Previously we demonstrated cross-reactivity between human PDC-E2 and *E. coli* PDC-E2 at the T cell level[13]. One of the T cell clones was shown to cross-react with the exogenous peptide derived from the lipoic acid binding domain of *E. coli* PDC-E2 (EQSLITVEGDKASM). Moreover, the amino acids E, D and K, at positions 170, 172 and 173 respectively, of the human PDC-E2 are found to be essential amino acid residues for the T cell epitope. This sequence ExDK is also found in *E. coli* PDC-E2. In a recent study we found PDC-E2 163–176 specific T cell clones that cross-reacted with PDC-E2 peptide 36–49 and OGDC-E2 peptide 100–113, both of which have ExDK sequences[18]. These results indicate that molecular mimicry between human PDC-E2 and *E. coli* PDC-E2 is possible at the T cell level in PBC.

These results have prompted a search for the identity of the bacteria population in livers of patients with PBC. To date no-one has succeeded in identifying the bacteria by conventional culture techniques. By utilizing the more sensitive PCR technique, two groups, including ourselves, have attempted to detect bacterial genes in PBC livers. O'Donohue *et al.* searched the 16s rRNA gene by mycobacteria in 11 PBC liver specimens by polymerase chain reaction (PCR)[40] (Table 3). Although the PCR system is very sensitive, and is known to be sensitive for even 1 fg of *M. gordonae* DNA in 'spiked' samples, they failed to detect mycobacterial DNA in PBC livers. We also tried to detect mycobacterial DNA, as well as *Helicobacter* DNA, in PBC livers[41]. We used primers specific for groEL for detection of mycobacterial DNA, and primers for the 16s rRNA gene for the detection of *Helicobacter* DNA. Mycobacterial DNA was not found in any PBC livers, and *Helicobacter* DNA was found only in 1/29 PBC livers, which turned out to be *H. pylori* by sequencing. We also performed PCR using primers for another region of the 16s rRNA genes of *E. coli*, which is well conserved in all eubacteria, trying to clarify the profiles of all eubacteria in template DNA from livers. Although a number of bacteria were found in PBC liver, as well as control livers, we failed to define 'consensus' bacteria which were specifically detected only in PBC livers. Thus far, a clear association between microbes and the aetiology of PBC still remains to be defined.

## DOES VIRAL INFECTION HAVE ANY ROLE IN THE AETIOLOGY OF PBC?

Although viruses are often cited as possible causative factors in autoimmune diseases, including rheumatoid arthritis, Sjögren's syndrome-like disease, systemic lupus erythematosus (SLE), and multiple sclerosis, little is known about viral infection and pathogenesis of PBC. Recently, Mason *et al.* showed that antibodies against retroviral elements were detected in the sera of patients with PBC[42]. They investigated seroreactivity of HIV-1 p24 gag and human intracisternal A-type particle (HIAP) proteins using sera from patients with PBC and other liver diseases, as well as SLE and healthy controls. Twenty-seven out of 77 PBC sera (35%) reacted with HIV-1 p24 gag protein, and 37 (51%) reacted with HIAP proteins, whereas only one (4%) out of 25 healthy controls showed seroreactivity against either HIV-1 or HIAP. However, this reactivity is not disease-specific, since sera from 29% patients with SLE, 50% of the patients with chronic viral hepatitis and 39% of the patients with PSC or biliary atresia also reacted with HIV-1 protein. The reactivity against HIAP protein was also detected among patients with chronic liver diseases. Thus it is unlikely that mitochondrial antigens, which are disease-specific autoantigens in PBC, share

**Table 3** Summary of PCR for *Helicobacter* and *Mycobacterium*

| | *PBC (n = 29)* | *Controls (n = 26)* |
|---|---|---|
| *Helicobacter* | 1/29* | 0/26 |
| *Mycobacterium* | 0/29 | 0/26 |

*Sequence analysis revealed that *Helicobacter pylori* was detected in only one patient with PBC.

epitopes with the HIV-1 p24 and HIAP retroviral proteins. Nevertheless, the involvement of viral infection, or activation of human endogenous retroviruses, as a possible mechanism triggering the onset of PBC should not be underestimated. The activation of viral elements itself, or expression of specific proteins that may share a molecular mimic to the mitochondrial antigens in PBC, remains an unproven but attractive hypothesis. It should be noted that several lines of evidence suggest that viruses including Epstein–Barr virus, HIV, HTLV-1, and hepatitis virus C may be implicated in the pathogenesis of Sjögren's syndrome, which is also an autoimmune disease occurring in epithelial cells of exocrine glands and often present in patients with PBC[43,44].

## CAN PBC BE INITIATED AND DEVELOPED FROM MICROCHIMAERISM OF FETAL CELLS?

In addition to the presence of mitochondrial autoantigens there are several clinical and pathological features in PBC which could be clues to the aetiology of the disease. First PBC is predominant in women[45], with female to male ratios of up to 16: 1. Second, PBC often occurs in middle-aged individuals, and has not been found in children[3]. Third, the clinical features of PBC closely resemble that of chronic graft-versus-host disease (CGVHD)[46].

Interestingly, these characteristics are also shared with scleroderma, and recently a novel concept, *viz.* fetal microchimaerism for immunopathogenesis of scleroderma, was addressed. It is known that fetal cells migrate into maternal blood during and after pregnancy[47,48]. For example, fetal-derived DNA can be found in maternal blood as early as 4 weeks of gestation, and persists up to 27 or even 38 years after pregnancy. Although the physiological role of the migrating fetal cells in the maternal body is still unknown, they may persist to maintain tolerance against fetus, but also may play a role in the induction of autoimmunity. Nelson *et al.*, using quantitative PCR analysis on female patients with scleroderma who had previously given birth to at least one son, demonstrated that male DNA derived from the fetus was more frequently found in patients with scleroderma than in control patients[49]. Artlett *et al.* reported similar results[50]. These data suggest that persisting microchimaerism could be involved in the development of scleroderma, perhaps initiated by an allogeneic reaction.

These findings, and the common clinical features of PBC and scleroderma, prompted us to investigate the microchimaerism in PBC[51]. We obtained liver tissues from 37 female patients with PBC and 39 female control patients who have had at least one son. PBC was diagnosed after birth in all the 37 female PBC patients studied. Using PCR-assisted amplification of sequences unique to both the X and Y chromosome from liver tissues, and WAVE technology, a very sensitive technology based on an ion-pair reverse phase high-performance liquid chromatography (HPLC) system, data were analysed for the detection of the Y chromosome gene as well as the ratio of the yield of the Y chromosome PCR products to that of the X chromosome (Table 4). Surprisingly, the prevalence of Y chromosome was very high in both PBC and control livers, 26/37 (70%) in PBC and 28/39 (72%) in controls, and there was no significant difference between the two groups. The ratio of Y chromosome to X chromosome was also

**Table 4** The detection of Y-chromosome and Y/X ratio in patients with PBC and controls

| | *Y-chromosome* | | *Y/X ratio* |
|---|---|---|---|
| | *Positive* | *Negative* | |
| PBC ($n = 37$) | 26 (70%)* | 11 (30%) | 0.402 ± 0.143† |
| Controls ($n = 39$) | 28 (72%) | 11 (28%) | 0.271 ± 0.055 |

*PBC vs controls: $p = 1.000$, Fisher's exact test.
†PBC vs controls: $p = 0.923$, Mann–Whitney $U$-test.

similar between PBC and control groups, 0.402 ± 0.143 vs 0.271 ± 0.055, respectively, suggesting that microchimaerism by itself may not play a significant role in the development of PBC. Nevertheless, we cannot exclude the other possibilities such as select fetal MHC types which might contribute to disease susceptibility.

## CONCLUDING REMARKS

Whereas there have been great advances in the investigations of PBC in this decade, there are many questions, as reviewed in this chapter, which remain to be solved. The aetiology of PBC, like those of other autoimmune diseases, remains unknown. The use of clinical as well as epidemiological data, biochemistry, molecular biology and cellular biology, and frequent crosstalk among them, will provide clues to the aetiology of this enigmatic disease. We have shown examples of the clues in this chapter. We believe that a better therapeutic approach to patients with PBC based on further understanding of the disease will be acquired by continuous efforts, described herein, in the future.

### Acknowledgements

This work is supported in part by NIH grant DK 39588.

### References

1. Ahrens EH, Rayne MA, Kunkle HG, Eisenmenger WH, Blondeim SH. Primary biliary cirrhosis. Medicine. 1950;29:299–364.
2. Kaplan Marshall M. Primary biliary cirrhosis. N Engl J Med. 1996;335:1570–80.
3. Neuberger J. Primary biliary cirrhosis. Lancet. 1997;350:875–9.
4. Leung PS, Coppel RL, Ansari A, Munoz S, Gershwin ME. Antimitochondrial antibodies in primary biliary cirrhosis. Semin Liver Dis. 1997;17:61–69.
5. Harris RA, Bowker-Kinley MM, Wu P, Jeng J, Popov KM. Dihydrolipoamide dehydrogenase-binding protein of the human pyruvate dehydrogenase complex. DNA-derived amino acid sequence, expression, and reconstitution of the pyruvate dehydrogenase complex. J Biol Chem. 1997;272:6361–9.
6. Van de Water J, Gershwin ME, Leung P. The autoepitope of the 74-kD mitochondrial autoantigen of primary biliary cirrhosis corresponds to the functional site of dihydrolipoamide acetyltransferase. J Exp Med. 1988;167:1791–9.
7. Surh CD, Coppel R, Gershwin ME. Structural requirement for autoreactivity on human pyruvate dehydrogenase-E2, the major autoantigen of primary biliary cirrhosis. Implication for a conformational autoepitope. J Immunol. 1990;144:1321–8.

8. Cha S, Leung PSC, Coppel RL, Van de Water J, Ansari AA, Gershwin ME. Heterogeneity of combinatorial human autoantibodies against PDC-E2 and biliary epithelial cells in patients with primary biliary cirrhosis. Hepatology. 1994;20:574–83.
9. Leung PSC, Chuang DT, Wynn RM *et al.* Autoantibodies to BCOADC-E2 in patients with primary biliary cirrhosis recognize a conformational epitope. Hepatology. 1995;22:505–13.
10. Moteki S, Leung PS, Dickson ER *et al.* Epitope mapping and reactivity of autoantibodies to the E2 component of 2-oxoglutarate dehydrogenase complex in primary biliary cirrhosis using recombinant 2-oxoglutarate dehydrogenase complex. Hepatology. 1996;23:436–44.
11. Dubel L, Tanaka A, Leung PS *et al.* Autoepitope mapping and reactivity of autoantibodies to the dihydrolipoamide dehydrogenase-binding protein (E3BP) and the glycine cleavage proteins in primary biliary cirrhosis. Hepatology. 1999;29:1013–18.
12. Van de Water J, Ansari A, Prindiville T. Heterogeneity of autoreactive T cell clones specific for the E2 component of the pyruvate dehydrogenase complex in primary biliary cirrhosis. J Exp Med. 1995;181:723–33.
13. Shimoda S, Nakamura M, Ishibashi H. HLA DRB4 0101-restricted immunodominant T cell autoepitope of pyruvate dehydrogenase complex in primary biliary cirrhosis: evidence of molecular mimicry in human autoimmune disease. J Exp Med. 1995;181:1835–45.
14. Landry SJ. Local protein instability predictive of helper T-cell epitopes. Immunol Today. 1997;18:527–32.
15. Mattevi A, Obmolova G, Schulze E. Atomic structure of the cubic core of the pyruvate dehydrogenase multienzyme complex. Science. 1992;255:1544–50.
16. Davis AL, Laue ED, Perham RN. Three-dimensional structure of the lipoyl domain from *Baccilus stearothemophilus* pyruvate dehydrogenase multienzyme complex. J Mol Biol. 1995;229:1037–48.
17. Green JDF, Laue ED, Perham RN. Three-dimensional structure of a lipoyl domain from the dihydrolipoyl acetyltransferase component of the pyruvate dehydrogenase multienzyme complex of *Escherichia coli*. J Mol Biol. 1995;248:328–43.
18. Shimoda S, Van de Water J, Ansari A *et al.* Identification and precursor frequency analysis of a common T cell epitope motif in mitochondrial autoantigens in primary biliary cirrhosis. J Clin Invest. 1998;102:1831–40.
19. Surh CD, Coppel R, Gershwin ME. Comparative epitope mapping of murine monoclonal and human autoantibodies to human PDH-E2, the major mitochondrial autoantigen of primary biliary cirrhosis. J Immunol. 1990;144:2647–52.
20. Cha S, Leung PS, Gershwin ME, Fletcher MP, Ansari AA, Coppel RL. Combinatorial autoantibodies to dihydrolipoamide acetyltransferase, the major autoantigen of primary biliary cirrhosis. Proc Natl Acad Sci USA. 1993;90:2527–31.
21. Van de Water J, Turchany J, Leung PSC *et al.* Molecular mimicry in primary biliary cirrhosis: evidence for biliary epithelial expression of a molecule cross-reactive with pyruvate dehydrogenase complex-E2. J Clin Invest. 1993;91:2653–64.
22. Migliaccio C, Nishio A, Van de Water J *et al.* Monoclonal antibodies to mitochondrial E2 components define autoepitopes in primary biliary cirrhosis. J Immunol. 1998;161:5157–63.
23. Moteki S, Leung PS, Coppel RL *et al.* Use of a designer triple expression hybrid clone for three different lipoyl domains for the detection of antimitochondrial autoantibodies. Hepatology. 1996;24:97–103.
24. Sadamoto T, Joplin R, Keogh A, Mason A, Carman W, Neuberger J. Expression of pyruvate-dehydrogenase complex PDC-E2 on biliary epithelial cells induced by lymph nodes from primary biliary cirrhosis. Lancet. 1998;352:1595–6.
25. Harada K, Van de Water J, Leung PS, Coppel RL, Nakanuma Y, Gershwin ME. *In situ* nucleic acid hybridization of pyruvate dehydrogenase complex-E2 in primary biliary cirrhosis: pyruvate dehydrogenase complex-E2 messenger RNA is expressed in hepatocytes but not in biliary epithelium. Hepatology. 1997;25:27–32.
26. Kieber M, Becker K, Pfanner N, Neupert W. Mitochondrial protein import: specific recognition membrane translocation of preproteins. J Membrane Biol. 1993;135:191–207.
27. Malmborg AC, Shultz DB, Luton F *et al.* Penetration and co-localization in MDCK cell mitochondria of IgA derived from patients with primary biliary cirrhosis. J Autoimmun. 1998;11:573–80.
28. Burroughs AK, Rosenstein IJ, Epstein O, Hamilton-Miller JMT, Brumfitt W, Sherlock S. Bacteriuria and primary biliary cirrhosis. Gut. 1984;25:133–7.

29. Butler P, Valle F, Hamilton-Miller JMT, Brumfitt W, Baum H, Burroughs AK. M2 mitochondrial antibodies and urinary rough mutant bacteria in patients with primary biliary cirrhosis and in patients with recurrent bacteriuria. J Hepatol. 1993;17:408–14.
30. Baum H. Mitochondrial antigens, molecular mimcry and autoimmune disease. Biochem Biophys Acta. 1995;1271:111–21.
31. Fussey SP, Ali ST, Guest JR. Reactivity of primary biliary cirrhosis sera with *Escherichia coli* dihydrolipoamide acetyltransferase (E2p): characterization of the main immunogenic region. Proc Natl Acad Sci USA. 1990;87:3987–91.
32. Vilagut L, Vila J, Vinas O *et al. Mycobacterium gordonae* in primary biliary cirrhosis: possible aetiology for the disease. J Hepatol. 1993;18(Suppl. 1):S7.
33. Vilagut L, Pares A, Vinas O, Vila J, Jimenez de Anta T, Rodes J. Antibodies to mycobacterial 65-kD heat shock protein cross-react with the main mitochondrial antigens in patients with primary biliary cirrhosis. Eur J Clin Invest. 1997;27:667–72.
34. O'Donohue J, McFarlane B, Bomford A, Yates M, Williams R. Antibodies to atypical mycobacteria in primary biliary cirrhosis. J Hepatol. 1994;21:887–9.
35. Klein R, Wiebel M, Engelhart S, Berg PA. Sera from patients with tuberculosis recognize the M2a-epitope (E2-subunit of pyruvate dehydrogenase) specific for primary biliary cirrhosis. Clin Exp Immunol. 1993;92:308–16.
36. Yeaman SJ, Fussey SP, Danner DJ. Primary biliary cirrhosis: identification of two major M2 mitochondrial autoantigens. Lancet. 1988;1:1067–70.
37. Owen P, Kaback HR, Grame-Cook KA. Identification of antigen 19/27 as dihydrolipoyl dehydrogenase and its probable involvement in ubiquinone-mediated NADH-dependent transport phenomena in membrane vesicles of *Escherichia coli*. FEMS Microbiol. Lett. 1980;7:345–8.
38. de la Sierra IL, Pernot L, Prange T *et al.* Molecular structure of the lipoamide dehydrogenase domain of a surface antigen from *Neisseria meningitidis*. J Mol Biol. 1997;269:129–41.
39. Danson MJ, Conroy K, McQuattie A, Stevenson K. Dihydrolipoamide dehydrogenase from *Trypanosoma brucei*: characterization and cellular location. Biochem J. 1987;243:661–5.
40. O'Donohue J, Fidler H, Garcia-Barcelo M, Nouri-Aria K, Williams R, McFadden J. Mycobacterial DNA not detected in liver sections from patients with primary biliary cirrhosis. J Hepatol. 1998;28:433–8.
41. Tanaka A, Prindiville TP, Gish R *et al.* Are infectious agents involved in primary biliary cirrhosis?: a PCR approach. J Hepatol. 1999 (In press).
42. Mason AL, Xu L, Guo L *et al.* Detection of retroviral antibodies in primary biliary cirrhosis and other idiopathic biliary disorders. Lancet. 1998;351:1620–4.
43. Fox RI. Sjögren's syndrome. Curr Opin Rheumatol. 1995;7:409–16.
44. Koike K, Moriya K, Ishibashi K *et al.* Sialadenitis histologically resembling Sjögren syndrome in mice transgenic for hepatitis C virus envelope genes. Proc Natl Acad Sci USA. 1997;94:233–6.
45. Metcalf J, James O. The geoepidemiology of primary biliary cirrhosis. Semin Liver Dis. 1997;17:13–22.
46. Czaja AJ. Chronic graft-versus-host disease and primary biliary cirrhosis: sorting the puzzle pieces. Lab Invest. 1994;70:589–92.
47. Bianchi DW, Zickwolf GK, Weil GJ, Sylvester S, DeMaria MA. Male fetal progenitor cells persist in maternal blood for as long as 27 years postpartum. Proc Natl Acad Sci USA. 1996;93:705-8.
48. Evans PC, Lambert N, Maloney S, Furst DE, Moore JM, Nelson JL. Long-term fetal microchimerism in peripheral blood mononuclear cell subsets in healthy women and women with scleroderma. Blood. 1999;93:2033–7.
49. Nelson JL, Furst DE, Maloney S *et al.* Microchimerism and HLA-compatible relationships of pregnancy in scleroderma. Lancet. 1998;351:559–62.
50. Artlett CM, Smith JB, Jimenez SA. Identification of fetal DNA and cells in skin lesions from women with systemic sclerosis. N Engl J Med. 1998;338:1186–91.
51. Tanaka A, Lindor K, Gish R *et al.* Fetal microchimerisms alone do not contribute to the induction of primary biliary cirrhosis. (Submitted).

# 22 Nuclear protein antigens in primary biliary cirrhosis

H.J. WORMAN, B. TERJUNG and J.-C. COURVALIN

## INTRODUCTION

Antinuclear antibodies are frequently present in individuals with primary biliary cirrhosis (PBC). Although antinuclear antibodies of several different specificities can be present, those against two types of antigens appear to be highly specific for this disease. The first are integral proteins of the nuclear envelope membranes, with the most common antigen being nuclear pore membrane glycoprotein gp210. The second of the nuclear antigens recognized by specific autoantibodies from individuals with PBC are components of nuclear bodies, with the most common being Sp100.

## NUCLEAR ENVELOPE

The nuclear envelope is composed of the nuclear lamina, the nuclear pore complexes and the nuclear membranes. The nuclear lamina is a meshwork of intermediate (10 nm diameter) filaments associated with the inner nuclear membrane[1]. The protein building blocks of the lamina are called lamins and are similar in primary and secondary structure to cytoplasmic intermediate filament proteins[2, 3]. In human somatic cells at least four distinct nuclear lamin proteins, A, B1, B2 and C, polymerize in various ratios to form the lamina. Lamins A and C arise from the same gene on chromosome 1 by alternative RNA splicing and are identical for their first 566 amino acids but differ in their tail domain[4, 5]. Lamin B1 is encoded by a gene on chromosome 5[5, 6] and lamin B2 by another gene on chromosome 19[7]. Isoforms of lamin B2 and A/C arising by alternative RNA splicing are expressed in germ cells. Despite considerable study the precise functions of the nuclear lamina and lamins are not clear. Intriguingly, mutations in the gene encoding lamins A and C are associated with autosomal dominant Emery–Dreifuss muscular dystrophy[8].

The active transport of macromolecules and the passive diffusion of ions and small molecules between the nucleus and cytoplasm are mediated by the nuclear pore complexes. The nuclear pore complex consists of many different proteins. The non-membrane proteins of the pore complex have been termed nulceoporins, many of which contain repeat motifs of five (XFXFG), four (GLFG) and/or two (FG) amino acids[9]. In vertebrates some nucleoporins are modified by the post-translational addition of *O*-linked *N*-acetylglucosamine residues. Several integral membrane proteins have also been identified that are components of the nuclear pore complex[10–13]. Two or these which have been characterized in vertebrates, gp210 and POM121, have cytoplasmic carboxyl-terminal domains and amino-terminal domains located in the perinuclear space[11, 12, 14, 15].

The membranes of the nuclear envelope are divided into three distinct but connected domains. The outer nuclear membrane is associated with ribosomes on its outer surface and shares proteins with the contiguous rough endoplasmic reticulum[16]. The inner and outer nuclear membranes are connected by the pore membranes which are associated with the nuclear pore complexes. The inner nuclear membrane contains several unique integral proteins, some of which mediate the attachment of the lamina and chromatin. LBR, or lamin B receptor, is an inner nuclear membrane protein with a nucleoplasmic, aminoterminal domain followed by eight putative transmembrane segments[17–19].

The structure of the nuclear envelope is dramatically altered during cell division. When chromosomes condense during mitosis, the lamina and pore complexes disassemble into component polypeptides or smaller protein complexes. The nuclear membranes lose their differentiation and the distinct membrane domains appear to be 'resorbed' into a residual endoplasmic reticulum-like structure[20, 21]. Biochemically the mitotic nuclear membranes can be fractionated into distinct vesicles enriched in different integral membrane proteins[22, 23]. When cells enter anaphase, new nuclear envelopes reassemble in a stepwise process that proceeds through telophase with the integral proteins of the inner nuclear membrane targeted to decondensing chromosomes first[22, 23].

## NUCLEAR ENVELOPE ANTIGENS RECOGNIZED BY AUTOANTIBODIES IN PBC

### Gp210

Gp210 is an integral membrane glycoprotein of the nuclear pore complex localized to the nuclear pore membrane domain[10]. Gp210 is modified by N-linked glycosylation and has a molecular mass[11] of approximately 210 kDa. It has a carboxyl-terminal domain of 58 amino acids that faces the nuclear pore complex, a transmembrane segment of 20 amino acids and an amino-terminal domain of 1808 that resides in the perinuclear space (endoplasmic reticulum lumen) between the inner and outer nuclear membranes[11, 14]. A signal sequence is cleaved from the amino-terminal domain of the preprotein[11].

Ruffati *et al.*[24] reported in 1985 that 18 of 63 patients with PBC had autoantibodies that labelled the rim of the nucleus of fixed cells examined using immunofluorescence microscopy. Serum from only one of 431 control patients gave a similar pattern of nuclear fluorescence. Lassoued *et al.*[25] and Lozano *et al.*[26] then demonstrated in 1988 that autoantibodies from patients with PBC that labelled the nuclear rim reacted with a protein with an apparent molecular mass of 200 kDa. In 1990 Courvalin and collaborators[27] conclusively demonstrated that these autoantibodies recognized gp210. Subsequently, Nickowitz and Worman[28] showed that these autoantibodies recognized a linear stretch of only 15 amino acids near the protein's carboxyl-terminus that faces the nuclear pore complex. Two subsequent studies using enzyme-linked immunosorbent assays with either a recombinant fusion protein expressed in bacteria[29] or a chemically synthesized polypeptide[30] confirmed that the amino acid stretch near gp210's carboxyl-terminus is the predominant autoepitope(s). In a later study[31] using a portion of gp210 generated by protease digestion, autoantibodies from some patients with PBC were also shown to recognize a glycosylated fragment of the protein that is located in the perinuclear space.

The prevalence of gp210 autoantibodies in individuals with PBC has ranged from 9.5% to 41%, with a mean of approximately 25%, in various studies using different detection methods (Table 1). Gp210 autoantibodies have been reported in only 0–0.4% of hundreds of control subjects without PBC examined in several studies[25, 30–33]. Hence, the presence of gp210 autoantibodies appears to be more than 99% specific for the diagnosis of PBC. Of note, some patients with a diagnosis of PBC based upon clinical, biochemical and histological criteria but without detectable antimitochondrial antibodies have gp210 autoantibodies. Bandin *et al.*[30] identified seven of 285 such patients, Lassoued *et al.*[32] five of 150 and Nickowitz *et al.*[33] five of 159. Testing for gp210 autoantibodies may therefore be of clinical utility in diagnosing patients presumably with PBC but without detectable antimitochondrial antibodies.

Patients with PBC appear to have generally similar clinical characteristics whether or not they have gp210 autoantibodies. Of 150 patients with PBC studied by Lassoued *et al.*[32], however, those with gp210 autoantibodies had a lower incidence of several associated disorders including Raynaud's phenomenon and arthralgias. In contrast, Nickowitz *et al.*[33] found in a study of 159 subjects that those with gp210 autoantibodies had a higher incidence of associated arthritis. Both of these studies relied on retrospective reviews of medical records, and better clinical studies are needed to clarify these findings. There

**Table 1** Studies of the prevalence of gp210 autoantibodies in PBC

| *Study (ref.); number of subjects* | *Gp210 autoantibodies (%)* | *Detection method* |
|---|---|---|
| Lozano *et al.*, 1988[26]; $n = 38$ | 41.2 | Immunoblotting cellular protein |
| Lassoued *et al.*, 1990[32]; $n = 150$ | 26.7 | Immunoblotting cellular protein |
| Nickowitz *et al.*, 1994[33]; $n = 159$ | 9.4 | Immunoblotting fusion protein |
| Wesierska-Gadek *et al.*, 1995[31]; $n = 43$ | 27.9 | Immunoblotting cellular protein |
| Bandin *et al.*, 1996[30]; $n = 285$ | 25.6 | ELISA using synthetic polypeptide of predominant carboxyl-terminal epitope |

are no long-term follow-up studies examining whether the presence of detectable gp210 autoantibodies is a prognostic marker in PBC. Gp210 autoantibodies generally persist after orthotopic liver transplantation even though PBC is not apparent in the allograft[34, 35].

## LBR

LBR is an integral protein of the inner nuclear membrane[17–19]. It is encoded by a gene on chromosome 1[5, 36]. LBR is a member of a gene family that includes sterol reductases of the endoplasmic reticulum[37]. LBR differs from the other proteins in this family in that it has a basic amino-terminal domain of approximately 200 amino acids. It precedes the hydrophobic portion that is very similar to the sterol reductases of the endoplasmic reticulum. The amino-terminal domain of LBR faces the nucleoplasm and is involved in targeting to and/or retention in the inner nuclear membrane[21, 38, 39]. This domain of LBR also binds to B-type lamins[19] and HP1-type chromatin proteins[40, 41].

In 1990, two patients with PBC were identified who had autoantibodies that recognized LBR purified from avian erythrocytes[42]. These autoantibodies were later shown to be anti-idiotypic to some antibodies against B-type nuclear lamins, further suggesting that they recognized a lamin binding protein[43]. Subsequently, two additional patients with PBC were identified in a series of 159 that had autoantibodies that recognized the amino-terminal domain of LBR expressed in bacteria as a recombinant protein[33].

Recently, one additional patient with PBC and LBR autoantibodies has also been reported[30]. So far, antibodies against LBR have not been found in patients with any other diseases or in healthy controls. Examination of the four available serum samples from patients with PBC showed that LBR autoantibodies recognized the first 60 amino acids of the protein[44].

## Nuclear lamins

Autoantibodies against nuclear lamins are found in patients with several different autoimmune disease[45]. Patients with PBC also have lamin autoantibodies with a prevalence rate of about 2%[30, 32]. Autoantibodies against lamin B1 react with several different epitopes in the protein[46]. Hence, regarding their specificity and epitope recognition, lamin autoantibodies differ from autoantibodies against gp210 and LBR.

## Other nuclear envelope protein antigens

Two reports[47, 48] have been published in which p62, a nucleoporin that is modified by *O*-linked *N*-acetylglucosamine residues[49], was recognized by autoantibodies from some patients with PBC. Antibodies of this specificity, however, have not been reported in other large series that examined autoantibodies by immunoblotting of nuclear fraction[32, 33]. An apparently novel protein localized to the nuclear envelope of neutrophils and some myeloid cell lines is recognized by the so-called atypical-ANCA antibodies in individuals with primary sclerosing cholangitis and autoimmune hepatitis[50] (see also Chapter 13 in this volume). It is not known at this time whether this antigen is also recognized by autoantibodies from individuals with PBC. Autoantibodies against lamina-associated polypeptide 1A and lamina-associated polypeptide 2, integral proteins of the inner nuclear membrane, have been detected in patients with various rheumatic diseases but not PBC[51].

## NUCLEAR BODIES

Nuclear bodies appear as multiple 'dots' within the nucleus when cells are examined by immunofluorescence microscopy with appropriate antibodies. Most nuclei have five to 30 nuclear bodies per nucleus. The functions of the nuclear bodies are not clear but they may somehow be involved in cell growth suppression and differentiation based on studies of promyelocytic leukaemia cells. In most cases of acute promyelocytic leukaemia a protein known as promyelocytic leukaemia protein (PML) is fused to retinoic acid receptor alpha, usually as a result of a chromosomal t(15;17) translocation[52, 53]. In acute promyelocytic leukaemia cells, nuclear bodies are disrupted into a microparticulate pattern as a consequence of the expression of the PML–retinoic acid receptor alpha fusion protein and treatment with retinoic acid induces the formation of normal-appearing nuclear bodies[54, 55].

In addition to PML, several other proteins have been localized to nuclear bodies. In 1990 Szostecki *et al.* reported the cDNA cloning of Sp100 which is distributed in 'dots' throughout the nucleus and recognized by autoantibodies from patients with PBC. PML and Sp100 are both modified by the small ubiquitin-related protein, SUMO-1[57]. In 1996 Bloch *et al.*[58] reported the cDNA cloning of another nuclear body protein called Sp140, which is similar to Sp100 for part of its sequence. In 1997 Sternsdorf *et al.*[59] reported the identification of nuclear dot protein 52 (NDP52), a 52 kDa protein also localized to nuclear bodies. Recent results[60] suggest that different nuclear bodies are heterogeneous in their protein composition.

## NUCLEAR ENVELOPE ANTIGENS RECOGNIZED BY AUTOANTIBODIES IN PBC

### Sp100

The pattern of 'multiple nuclear dots' is readily distinguished from that generated by anti-centromere antibodies by using tissue culture cells for indirect immunofluorescence microscopy[61]. In 1987 Szostecki *et al.*[62] demonstrated that the predominant antigen recognized by autoantibodies from patients with PBC that produced the 'multiple nuclear dot' pattern recognized a protein with an apparent molecular mass of approximately 100 kDa, and called it Sp100. Subsequent studies[63, 64] confirmed that the predominant nuclear dot antigen in PBC had a molecular mass of approximately 100 kDa. In 1990 Szostecki *et al.*[56] reported the cDNA cloning of Sp100 which they accomplished by screening expression libraries with serum from a patient with PBC. Sp100 has sequence similarity to MHC class I domains and several trans-acting regulatory proteins, including HIV-1 nef proteins. Using recombinant fusion proteins, Szostecki *et al.*[65] identified at least three non-overlapping major autoantigenic domains of Sp100 that were recognized by the majority of sera. One domain, which has the sequence similarity with HIV nef proteins, contains multiple epitopes that were recognized by all anti-Sp100 examined by these investigators. Bluthner *et al.*[66] used phage-display technology to identify a stretch of 16 amino acids at position 296–311 as a major antigenic region on the Sp100 and a second antigenic region of 20 amino acids in length between amino acids 332 and 351. Hence, Sp100 appears to contain several different epitopes that are recognized by autoantibodies from patients with PBC.

The prevalence of Sp100 autoantibodies in individuals with PBC ranges from 18% to 44% in three studies using different detection methods (Table 2). Autoantibodies of this specificity have been reported in only a few individuals with other diseases or healthy controls[56, 64, 67, 68]. It therefore appears that the prevalence of Sp100 autoantibodies in PBC is between 20% and 40% and that they are rather specific for this disorder. The results of one study[67] suggest that their occurrence correlates with more frequent progression from early (I/II) to late (III/IV) histological stages of PBC within a 24-month observation period. Sp100 autoantibodies also appear to persist after orthotopic liver transplantation despite the absence of detectable disease in the allograft[34].

## Sp140

Using serum from a patient with PBC, Bloch *et al.*[58] identified a cDNA encoding a nuclear body protein they called Sp140. The amino-terminal portion of Sp140 is about 50% identical in sequence to the amino-terminal region of Sp100. The carboxyl-terminal domain of Sp140 is different and shows sequence similarity to a portion of the mouse transcription intermediate factor (TIF) 1-alpha[58]. The prevalence of Sp140 autoantibodies in patients with PBC is not presently clear.

## PML protein

Antibodies against PML are often seen together with Sp100 autoantibodies in individuals with PBC; however, they appear to be more difficult to detect[67, 69]. Sternsdorf *et al.*[69] used an immunoprecipitation assay with radiolabelled PML and an immunofluorescence microscopy assay with cells that overexpressed the protein to demonstrate that antibodies against PML are found in the majority of patients with PBC who had Sp100 autoantibodies. In contrast to Sp100, however, reactivity with recombinant PML in immunoblotting assays is only

**Table 2** Studies of the prevalence of Sp100 autoantibodies in PBC

| *Study (ref.); number of subjects* | *Sp100 autoantibodies (%)* | *Detection method* |
|---|---|---|
| Evans *et al.*, 1991[64]; $n = 50$ | 44 | 'Multiple nuclear dot' immunofluorescence |
| Zuchner *et al.*, 1997[67]; $n = 170$ | 21 | ELISA using recombinant polypeptide |
| Orth *et al.*, 1997[68]; $n = 33$ | 18 | 'Multiple nuclear dot' immunofluorescence |

weak. In a series of 170 patients with PBC, Zuchner *et al.*[67] reported the prevalence of PML autoantibodies to be 19% and Sp100 autoantibodies to be 21%.

## SPECULATION ON THE SIGNIFICANCE OF NUCLEAR ANTIGENS IN PBC

Although gp210, Sp100 or LBR autoantibodies are detectable in only a minority of patients with PBC, their high specificity suggests that they may be involved in the pathophysiology of this disease. Unfortunately, no studies have been able to link these specific autoantibodies or the proteins they recognize to the pathological lesion of PBC. In addition, no experimental data exist as to why or how these antibodies are generated in individuals with this disease. Molecular mimicry has been postulated as a mechanism of autoantibody generation in PBC[70]. The predominant autoepitope of gp210 is homologous to the *Escherichia coli mut Y* gene product, and this finding initially rekindled the question concerning the role of molecular mimicry in PBC[28]. However, we have not been able to show that the *mut Y* gene product is recognized by gp210 autoantibodies (Tartakovsky F, Worman H.J., unpublished observation). Cross-reactive bile duct proteins, which have been demonstrated for some antibodies against mitochondrial antigens[71–73], have not been reported with gp210, Spl00 or LBR autoantibodies. At this time molecular mimicry has not been shown to be a factor in the generation of antinuclear antibodies in individuals with PBC, and cross-reactive antigens have not been implicated in pathology.

Some LBR autoantibodies are anti-idiotypic to autoantibodies against B-type nuclear lamins[43]. As some patients with PBC also have antibodies against lamins, LBR antibodies may be generated by an idiotype–anti-idiotype network process in some instances. The hypothesis that an idiotype–anti-idiotype network mechanism is responsible for the production of nuclear envelope protein autoantibodies in all cases of PBC has not been formally tested. Some studies have suggested that antinuclear antibodies may arise as a result of antigenic presentation of proteolytic polypeptide fragments that arise during apoptotic cell death[74,75]. This mechanism is plausible for the generation of lamin autoantibodies, which are found in several diseases, as nuclear lamins are cleaved in apoptosis[76]. The high specificity of gp2l0, Spl00 and LBR autoantibodies for PBC, however, suggests that these autoantibodies do not simply arise as a result of generalized cell death and antigen presentation.

Despite speculation about the relationship of nuclear protein antigens to autoantibody generation and disease pathophysiology in PBC, nothing is really known. The high specificity of gp210, Spl00 and LBR autoantibodies for PBC as opposed to other diseases cries out for an explanation. Hopefully, future work will provide one.

### References

1. Aebi U, Cohn J, Buhle L, Gerace L. The nuclear lamina is meshwork of intermediate-type filaments. Nature. 1986;323:560–4.
2. McKeon FD, Kirschner MW, Caput D. Homologies in both primary and secondary structure between nuclear envelope and intermediate filament proteins. Nature. 1986;319:463–8.

3. Fisher DZ, Chaudhary N, Blobel G. cDNA sequencing of nuclear lamins A and C reveals primary and secondary structural homology to intermediate filament proteins. Proc Natl Acad Sci USA. 1986;83:6450–4.
4. Lin F, Worman HJ. Structural organization of the human gene encoding nuclear lamin A and nuclear lamin C. J Biol Chem. 1993;268:16321–6.
5. Wydner KL, McNeil JA, Lin F, Worman HJ, Lawrence JB. Chromosomal assignment of human nuclear envelope protein genes LMNA, LMNB1 and LBR by fluorescence *in situ* hybridization. Genomics. 1996;32:474–8.
6. Lin F, Worman HJ. Structural organization of the human gene (LMNB1) encoding nuclear lamin B1. Genomics. 1995;27:230–6.
7. Biamonti G, Giacca M, Perini G *et al.* The gene for a novel human lamin maps at a highly transcribed locus of chromosome 19 which replicates at the onset of S-phase. Mol Cell Biol. 1992;12:3499–506.
8. Bonne G, Di Barletta MR, Varnous S *et al.* Mutations in the gene encoding lamin A/C cause autosomal dominant Emery–Dreifuss muscular dystrophy. Nat Genet. 1999;21:285–8.
9. Rout MP, Wente SR. Pores for thought: nuclear pore complex proteins. Trends Cell Biol. 1994;4:357–65.
10. Gerace L, Ottaviano Y, Kondor-Koch C. Identification of a major polypeptide of the nuclear pore complex. J Cell Biol. 1982;95:826–37.
11. Wozniak RW, Bartnik E, Blobel G. Primary structure analysis of an integral membrane glycoprotein of the nuclear pore. J Cell Biol. 1989;108:2083–92.
12. Hallberg E, Wozniak RW, Blobel G. An integral membrane protein of the pore membrane domain of the nuclear envelope contains a nucleoporin-like region. J Cell Biol. 1992;122:513–21.
13. Wozniak RW, Blobel G, Rout MP. POM 152 is an integral protein of the pore membrane domain of the yeast nuclear envelope. J Cell Biol. 1994;125:31–42.
14. Greber UL, Senior A, Gerace L. A major glycoprotein of the nuclear pore complex is a membrane-spanning polypeptide with a large luminal domain and a small cytoplasmic tail. EMBO J. 1990;9:1495–502.
15. Söderqvist H, Hallberg E. The large C-terminal region of the integral pore membrane protein, POMl21, is facing the nuclear pore complex. Eur J Cell Biol. 1994;64:186–91.
16. Amar-Costesec A, Beaufay H, Wibo M *et al.* Analytical study of microsomes and isolated subcellular membranes from rat liver. II. Preparation and composition of the microsomal fraction. J Cell Biol. 1974;61:201–12.
17. Worman HJ, Yuan J, Blobel G, Georgatos SD. A lamin B receptor in the nuclear envelope. Proc Natl Acad Sci USA. 1988;85:8531–4.
18. Worman HJ, Evans, CD, Blobel G. The lamin B receptor of the nuclear envelope inner membrane: a polytopic protein with eight potential transmembrane domains. J Cell Biol. 1990;111:1534–42.
19. Ye Q, Worman HJ. Primary structure analysis and lamin B and DNA binding of human LBR, an integral protein of the nuclear envelope inner membrane. J Biol Chem. 1994;269:11306–11.
20. Yang L, Guan T, Gerace L. Integral membrane proteins of the nuclear envelope are dispersed throughout the endoplasmic reticulum during mitosis. J Cell Biol. 1997;137:1199–210.
21. Ellenberg J, Siggia ED, Moreira JE *et al.* Nuclear membrane dynamics and reassembly in living cells: targeting of an inner nuclear membrane protein in interphase and mitosis. J Cell Biol. 1997;138:1193–206.
22. Chaudhary N, Courvalin J-C. Stepwise reassembly of the nuclear envelope at the end of mitosis. J Cell Biol. 1993;122:295–306.
23. Buendia B, Courvalin J-C. Domain-specific disassembly and reassembly of nuclear membranes during mitosis. Exp Cell Res. 1997;230:133–44.
24. Ruffati A, Arslan P, Floreani A *et al.* Nuclear membrane-staining antinuclear antibody in patients with primary biliary cirrhosis. J Clin Immunol. 1985;5:357–61.
25. Lassoued K, Guilly M-N, André C *et al.* Autoantibodies to a 200 kD polypeptide(s) of the nuclear envelope: a new serological marker of primary biliary cirrhosis. Clin Exp Immunol. 1988;74:283–8.
26. Lozano F, Parés A, Borche L *et al.* Autoantibodies against nuclear envelope-associated proteins in primary biliary cirrhosis. Hepatology. 1988;8:930–8.

27. Courvalin J-C, Lassoued K, Bartnik E, Blobel G, Wozniak RW. The 210 kilodalton nuclear envelope polypeptide recognized by human autoantibodies in primary biliary cirrhosis is the major glycoprotein of the nuclear pore. J Clin Invest. 1990;86:279–85.
28. Nickowitz RE, Worman HJ. Autoantibodies from patients with primary biliary cirrhosis recognize a restricted region within the cytoplasmic tail of nuclear pore membrane glycoprotein gp210. J Exp Med. 1993;178:2237–42.
29. Tartakovsky F, Worman HJ. Detection of gp2l0 autoantibodies in primary biliary cirrhosis using a recombinant protein containing the predominant autoepitope. Hepatology. 1995;21:495–500.
30. Bandin O, Courvalin J-C, Poupon R, Dubel L, Homberg J-C, Johanet C. Specificity and sensitivity of gp2l0 autoantibodies detected using an ELISA and a synthetic polypeptide in the diagnosis of primary biliary cirrhosis. Hepatology. 1996;23:1020–4.
31. Wesierska-Gadek J, Hohenauer H, Hitchman E, Penner E. Autoantibodies from patients with primary biliary cirrhosis preferentially react with the amino-terminal domain of nuclear pore complex glycoprotein gp2l0. J Exp Med. 1995;182:1159–62.
32. Lassoued K, Brenard R, Degos F *et al.* Antinuclear antibodies directed to a 200 kD polypeptide of the nuclear envelope in primary biliary cirrhosis. A clinical and immunological study of a series of 150 patients with primary biliary cirrhosis. Gastroenterology. 1990;99:181–6.
33. Nickowitz RE, Wozniak RW, Schaffner F, Worman HJ. Autoantibodies against integral membrane proteins of the nuclear envelope in patients with primary biliary cirrhosis. Gastroenterology. 1994;106:193–9.
34. Luettig B, Boeker KH, Schoessler W. *et al.* The antinuclear autoantibodies Sp100 and gp2l0 persist after orthotopic liver transplantation in patients with primary biliary cirrhosis. J Hepatol. 1998;28:824–8.
35. Dubel L, Farges O, Courvalin J-C, Sebagh M, Johanet C. Persistence of gp2l0 and multiple nuclear dots antibodies does not correlate with recurrence of primary biliary cirrhosis 6 years after liver transplantation. J Hepatol. 1998;28:169–70.
36. Schuler E, Lin F, Worman HJ. Characterization of the human gene encoding LBR, an integral protein of the nuclear envelope inner membrane. J Biol Chem. 1994;269:11312–17.
37. Holmer L, Pezhman A, Worman HJ. The human LBR/sterol reductase multigene family. Genomics. 1998;54:469–76.
38. Soullam B, Worman, HJ. The amino-terminal domain of the lamin B receptor is a nuclear envelope targeting signal. J Cell Biol. 1993;120:1093–1100.
39. Soullam B, Worman HJ. Signals and structural features involved in integral membrane protein targeting to the inner nuclear membrane. J Cell Biol. 1995;130:15–27.
40. Ye Q, Worman HJ. Interaction between an integral protein of the nuclear envelope inner membrane and human chromodomain proteins homologous to *Drosophila* HP1. J Biol Chem. 1996;271:14653–6.
41. Ye Q, Callebaut I, Pezhman A, Courvalin J-C, Worman HJ. Domain-specific interactions of human HP 1-type chromodomain proteins and inner nuclear membrane protein LBR. J Biol Chem. 1997;272:14983–9.
42. Courvalin J-C, Lassoued K, Worman HJ, Blobel G. Identification and characterization of autoantibodies against the nuclear envelope lamin B receptor from patients with primary biliary cirrhosis. J Exp Med. 1990;172:961–7.
43. Lassoued K, Danon F, Brouet J-C. Human autoantibodies to lamin B receptor are also anti-idiotypic to certain anti-lamin B antibodies. Eur J Immunol. 1991;21:1959–62.
44. Lin F, Noyer CM, Ye Q, Courvalin J-C, Worman HJ. Autoantibodies from patients with primary biliary cirrhosis recognize a restricted region within the nucleoplasmic domain of inner nuclear membrane protein LBR. Hepatology. 1996;23:57–61.
45. Worman HJ, Courvalin J-C. Autoantibodies against nuclear envelope proteins in liver disease. Hepatology. 1991;14:1269–79.
46. Chou CH, Reeves WH. Recognition of multiple epitopes in the coiled-coil domain of lamin B by human autoantibodies. Mol Immunol. 1992;29:1055–64.
47. Wesierska-Gadek J, Hohenuer H, Hitchman E, Penner E. Autoantibodies against nucleoporin p62 constitute a novel marker of primary biliary cirrhosis. Gastroenterology. 1996;110:840–7.
48. Miyachi K, Shibata M, Onozuka Y, Kikuchi F, Imai N, Horigome T. Primary biliary cirrhosis sera recognize not only gp2l0 but also proteins of the p62 complex bearing N-acetylglucosamine residues from rat liver nuclear envelope. Anti-p62 complex antibody in PBC. Mol Biol Rep. 1996;23:227–34.

49. Davis LI, Blobel G. Nuclear pore complex contains a family of glycoproteins that includes p62: glycosylation through a previously unidentified cellular pathway. Proc Natl Acad Sci USA. 1987;84:7552–6.
50. Terjung B, Herzog V, Worman HJ *et al.* Atypical antineutrophil cytoplasmic antibodies with perinuclear fluorescence in chronic inflammatory bowel diseases and hepatobiliary disorders colocalize with nuclear lamina proteins. Hepatology. 1998;28:332–40.
51. Konstantinov K, Foisner R, Byrd D *et al.* Integral membrane proteins associated with the nuclear lamina are novel autoimmune antigens of the nuclear envelope. Clin Immunol Immunopathol. 1995;74:89–99.
52. Kakizuka A, Miller WH Jr, Umesono K *et al.* Chromosomal translocation t(15;17) in human acute promyelocytic leukemia fuses RAR alpha with a novel putative transcription factor, PML. Cell. 1991;66:663–74.
53. de The H, Lavau C, Marchio A, Chomienne C, Degos L, Dejean A. The PML-RAR alpha fusion mRNA generated by the t(15;17) translocation in acute promyelocytic leukemia encodes a functionally altered RAR. Cell. 1991;66:675–84.
54. Dyck JA, Maul GG, Miller WH Jr, Chen JD, Kakizuka A, Evans RM. A novel macromolecular structure is a target of the promyelocyte-retinoic acid receptor oncoprotein. Cell. 1994;76:333–43.
55. Weis K, Rambaud S, Lavau C *et al.* Retinoic acid regulates aberrant nuclear localization of PML-RAR alpha in acute promyelocytic leukemia cells. Cell. 1994;76:345–56.
56. Szostecki C, Guldner HH, Netter HJ, Will H. Isolation and characterization of cDNA encoding a human nuclear antigen predominantly recognized by autoantibodies from patients with primary biliary cirrhosis. J Immunol. 1990;145:4338–47.
57. Sternsdorf T, Jensen K, Will H. Evidence for covalent modification of the nuclear dot-associated proteins PML and Spl00 by PIC1/SUMO-1. J Cell Biol. 1997;139:1621–34.
58. Bloch DB, de la Monte SM, Guigaouri P, Filippov A, Bloch KD. Identification and characterization of a leukocyte-specific component of the nuclear body. J Biol Chem. 1996;271:29198–204.
59. Sterndorf T, Jensen K, Zuchner D, Will H. Cellular localization, expression, and structure of the nuclear dot protein 52. J Cell Biol. 1997; 138:435–48.
60. Bloch DB, Chiche J-D, Orth D, de la Monte S, Rosenzweig A, Bloch KD. Structural and functional heterogeneity of nuclear bodies. Mol Cell. 1999;19:4423–30.
61. Cassani F, Bianchi FB, Lenzi M, Volta U, Pisi E. Immunomorphological characterisation of antinuclear antibodies in chronic liver disease. J Clin Pathol. 1985;38:801–5.
62. Szostecki C, Krippner H, Penner E, Bautz FA. Autoimmune sera recognize a 100 kD nuclear protein antigen (sp-l00). Clin Exp Immunol. 1987;68:108–16.
63. Fusconi M, Cassani F, Govoni M *et al.* Anti-nuclear antibodies of primary biliary cirrhosis recognize 78-92-kD and 96-100-kD proteins of nuclear bodies. Clin Exp Immunol. 1991;83:291–7.
64. Evans J, Reuben A, Craft J. PBC 95k, a 95-kilodalton nuclear autoantigen in primary biliary cirrhosis. Arthritis Rheum. 1991;34:731–6.
65. Szostecki C, Will H, Netter HJ, Guldner HH. Autoantibodies to the nuclear Spl00 protein in primary biliary cirrhosis and associated diseases: epitope specificity and immunoglobulin class distribution. Scand J Immunol. 1992;36:555–64.
66. Bluthner M, Schafer C, Schneider C, Bautz FA. Identification of major linear epitopes on the sp100 nuclear PBC autoantigen by the gene-fragment phage-display technology. Autoimmunity. 1999;29:33–42.
67. Zuchner D, Sternsdorf T, Szostecki C, Heathcote EJ, Cauch-Dudek K, Will H. Prevalence, kinetics, and therapeutic modulation of autoantibodies against Spl00 and promyelocytic leukemia protein in a large cohort of patients with primary biliary cirrhosis. Hepatology. 1997;26:1123–30.
68. Orth T, Gerken G, Meyer Zum Buschenfelde KH, Mayet WJ. Antineutrophil nuclear antibodies (ANNA) in primary biliary cirrhosis: their prevalence and antigen specificity. Z Gastroenterol. 1997;35:113–21.
69. Sternsdorf T, Guldner HH, Szostecki C, Grotzinger T, Will H. Two nuclear dot-associated proteins, PML and Spl00, are often co-autoimmunogenic in patients with primary biliary cirrhosis. Scand J Immunol. 1995;42:257–68.
70. Burroughs AK, Butler P, Sternberg MJE, Baum H. Molecular mimicry in liver disease. Nature. 1992;358:377–8.

71. Cha S, Leung PS, Gershwin ME, Fletcher MP, Ansari AA, Coppel RL. Combinatorial autoantibodies to dihydrolipoamide acetyltransferase, the major autoantigen of primary biliary cirrhosis. Proc Natl Acad Sci USA. 1993;90:2527–31.
72. Van de Water J, Turchany J, Leung PS *et al.* Molecular mimicry in primary biliary cirrhosis. Evidence for biliary epithelial expression of a molecule cross-reactive with pyruvate dehydrogenase complex-E2. J Clin Invest. 1993;91:2653–64.
73. Cha S, Leung PS, Coppel RL, Van de Water J, Ansari AA, Gershwin ME. Heterogeneity of combinatorial human autoantibodies against PDC-E2 and biliary epithelial cells in patients with primary biliary cirrhosis. Hepatology. 1994;20:574–83.
74. Casciola-Rosen, LA, Anhalt G, Rosen A. Autoantigens targeted in systemic lupus erythematosus are clustered in two populations of surface structures on apoptotic keratinocytes. J Exp Med. 1994;179:1317–30.
75. Casciola-Rosen LA, Anhalt GJ, Rosen A. DNA-dependent protein kinase is one of a subset of autoantigens specifically cleaved early during apoptosis. J Exp Med. 1995;182:1625–34.
76. Lazebnik YA, Takahashi A, Moir RD *et al.* Studies on the lamin proteinase reveal multiple parallel biochemical pathways during apoptotic execution. Proc Natl Acad Sci USA. 1995;92:9042–6.

# 23
# Thoughts on the infectious aetiology of primary biliary cirrhosis

R. JOPLIN

## INTRODUCTION

Primary biliary cirrhosis (PBC) is characterized by features consistent with autoimmune aetiological mechanisms. However, the initiating events in autoimmunity, by which tolerance to self-antigens is broken, are still poorly understood. Indeed, as will be considered, characteristic features of infection and autoimmunity are not mutually exclusive. Recent reports increasingly lend support to earlier speculation and hypotheses that proposed involvement of infectious agents in aetiological mechanisms in autoimmunity. Conversely, autoimmune phenomena are associated with certain infections. It has long been suggested that some features of PBC may have more in common with a response to infection than an autoimmune reaction. Evidence for involvement of an infectious agent in the aetiology of PBC will be considered in this chapter.

## CIRCUMSTANTIAL EVIDENCE SUGGESTIVE THAT AN INFECTIOUS AGENT MAY BE INVOLVED IN THE AETIOLOGY OF PBC

It has been noted for many years that not all features of PBC have correlates in other autoimmune conditions. Some paradoxical features are included in Table 1. An increasing body of circumstantial evidence, which could be interpreted as favouring involvement of an infectious agent, includes: geographical/environmental variation, weak MHC associations, sequence homology between autoantigens and known infectious agents, Th1/Th2 balance, poor response to immunosuppressive therapies, recurrence of PBC following liver transplantation, evidence of transmissibility.

### Geographical/environmental associations

Epidemiological studies demonstrate geographical clustering. The highest incidence is in northern Europe followed by southern Europe, North America and

**Table 1** Comparison between PBC and other organ-specific autoimmune diseases

| | *PBC* | *Other conditions* |
|---|---|---|
| **Autoantibody/antigen** | | |
| Autoantibody frequency in patients | >95% | Variable |
| Tissue distribution of autoantigen | Ubiquitous | Restricted |
| Antibody specificity | Single epitope | Multiple epitopes |
| Antibody disease restricted | Yes | No |
| Antibody inhibitory of enzyme activity | Yes | Yes |
| **Animal model** | No | Yes |
| **Childhood incidence** | No | Yes |
| **HLA linkage** | Weak | Strong |
| **Female dominance** | 90% female | Variable |
| **Response to immunosuppressive therapy** | Poor | Good |
| **Familial occurrence** | Rare | Common |
| **Recurrence after transplantation** | Yes | Yes |
| **Environmental/geographical factors** | Yes | Yes |
| **Th1 dominance** | Yes | Yes |
| **HLA-DR on targets** | Yes | Yes |
| **Association with other autoimmune conditions** | Yes | Yes |

Australasia (including Japan) with extremely low incidence in Africa and the Indian sub-continent[1]. It is of interest that patients of Asian extraction develop PBC when translocated to an area of high incidence[2]. One study demonstrated association between PBC patients resident in the Sheffield region of North East England and their water supply[3]. Approaching 90% of patients with PBC in the Sheffield area received their water supply from just one of five different reservoirs. No factor unique to the water supplied by that resevoir was ever identified.

## MHC association

Serotyping studies demonstrate an association of HLA DR8 with development of PBC, but the association is weak and HLA DR8 is neither an essential element in developing PBC nor alone sufficient to precipitate it[4], suggesting a relatively greater importance for environmental factors.

## Autoantigens

More than 95% of patients with PBC have detectable antibodies to one or more components of the mitochondrial oxo-acid dehydrogenase complexes[5–7]. These antigens are highly conserved. Strong sequence homology exists between the major human mitochondrial antigens, pyruvate dehydrogenase dihydrolipoamide acetyltransferase (PDC-E2) and pyruvate dehydrogenase E3 binding protein (PDC-E3bp) and prokaryotic PDC-E2. The similarity between prokaryotic and eukaryotic PDC-E2 and E3bp has led to speculation that molecular mimicry for an extrinsic protein of a bacterial agent may be the basis of breakdown in immune tolerance of self-PDC-E2 (see below for specific examples).

The major immune target in PBC appears to be the biliary epithelium. Studies of the distribution of PDC-E2/E3bp in human tissues show that in PBC liver, but not controls, high-intensity, diffuse distribution of PDC-E2/E3bp is present in the biliary epithelium[8–9]. Van de Water *et al.* suggested that biliary epithelial cells (BEC) contain a mimicking antigen which cross-reacts with antibodies to PDC-E2[10]. However, no direct evidence has been found for any foreign or altered antigen which might explain the high-intensity or atypical distribution of PDC-E2/E3bp in BEC in PBC[11].

## Th1/Th2 balance

The reason for increased presence of PDC-E2/E3bp (or other cross-reactive protein) in BEC in PBC is unknown. Expression of a number of antigens important in lymphocyte recognition can be up-regulated or induced *de novo* on BEC by a range of proinflammatory cytokines including interferons alpha and gamma (IFN$\alpha$ and IFN$\gamma$), interleukin-1 (IL-1) and tumour necrosis factor alpha (TNF$\alpha$)[12,13]. The balance of cytokines in the local environment of the portal tract may thus influence the immunogenicity of target cells, and specific cytokines have also been shown to influence expression of certain autoantigens. The size and number of SP100 protein containing nuclear dots increased in HEp2 cells exposed to IFN-$\alpha$, $\beta$ and $\gamma$ but not TNF-$\alpha$. Thus, in common with ICAM and MHC, sp100 is a cytokine-inducible protein[14]. IFN-$\gamma$ is produced by the Th1 subset of helper T cells, and several studies have demonstrated that Th1 cytokines predominate in the liver of patients with PBC[15–16]. Increase in IFN-$\gamma$ is also observed in the liver of patients with hepatitis C infection[17]. The possibility of involvement of a viral factor in PBC is discussed further below. Increased IFN-$\gamma$ in the vicinity of bile ducts could be involved in induction of MHC class II and ICAM on target cells. However, neither IFN-$\gamma$ nor IFN-$\alpha$ up-regulated PDC-E2/E3bp on BEC *in vitro*, suggesting that other mechanisms of induction of PDC-E2/E3bp exist *in vivo*[18].

## Immunosuppressive therapy

In contrast to most classic autoimmune conditions, patients with PBC appear to respond poorly to immunosuppressive therapy; evidence which may be consistent with the hypothesis that an infectious element may be important in PBC. However, immune response to bile ducts is considered to be dominant during the early inflammatory stage of disease; diagnosis of PBC usually occurs only when bile duct damage is advanced. At this time secondary bile duct pathology may have become established as a result of biliary obstruction and cholestasis. Thus, coexistence of both immune and cholestatic mechanisms at the time of diagnosis leads to difficulties in reversing the effect of any damage using a monotherapeutic approach. In early studies the lack of efficacy of immunosuppressive agents may have been a direct result of the administration of a monotherapeutic agent at a stage in the disease when both immunological mechanisms and bile acid toxicity probably contributed to the inflammatory damage. Combination of the anticholestatic agent, ursodeoxycholic acid and immunosuppressive therapies appears more effective than corticosteroids administered alone[19]. Nonetheless, no drug is capable of inducing remission or arresting the progression of PBC and ultimately patients develop end-stage disease for which liver transplantation is the only effective therapeutic option.

## Recurrence of PBC following liver transplantation

Despite difficulties in confidently identifying recurrent PBC in the allograft, several studies have now reported independently that PBC may recur in a small proportion of patients[20]. One possible mechanism for apparent recurrence of PBC is that as BEC are immune targets in PBC, the patients' lymphocytes will already be sensitized to biliary antigens which then become targets in the allograft. Recurrence of PBC may be influenced by the specific immunosuppressive protocol to which patients are subjected following transplantation. Patients receiving tacrolimus (FK-506)-based immunosuppression were reported as more likely to develop recurrence earlier and more aggressively than those receiving cyclosporin-based treatment[21]. In one study, atypical distribution of the major autoantigen, PDC-E2 was observed on BEC in the allografts of patients whose original disease was PBC irrespective of evidence for disease recurrence[22], suggesting that a transmissible factor retained in an extrahepatic reservoir in the host has the capability to induce PBC 'changes' in the allograft.

## Transmissibility

Examples of PBC in genetically and non-genetically linked individuals are described infrequently. In genetically linked individuals presentation in the second generation appears to occur earlier (higher prevalence between mother and daughter than between siblings[23]), suggesting greater importance of environmental factors relative to genetic linkages. A few reports suggest transmissibility between genetically non-linked individuals[24].

The concept of transmissibility of PBC between patients and normal subjects has been investigated using an *in vitro* experimental approach. BEC purified from normal liver were incubated with homogenates of lymph nodes harvested from the hilum of explanted livers of patients with PBC. The atypical pattern of PDC-E2 seen previously only on PBC BEC was induced on normal BEC, indicating that some transmissible factor present in the lymph nodes of patients with PBC (but not controls) can induce up-regulation of PDC-E2 in normal BEC[25]. To date the factor in PBC lymph nodes which is responsible for inducing PDC-E2 in normal BEC has not been identified.

# EVIDENCE FOR INVOLVEMENT OF SPECIFIC INFECTIOUS AGENTS

## A role for chronic bacterial infection in PBC?

Connections have been proposed between several bacterial species and PBC.

### *Mycobacteria*

Granulomatous lesions are frequently observed in the liver of patients with PBC, and the hypothesis that mycobacterial infection may be involved in the pathogenesis of PBC investigated. Sera from 43% of patients with active pulmonary tuberculosis were reported to recognize PDC-E2 compared with < 2% of sera from patients with other bacterial or viral infections[26]. Vilagut *et al.* reported sera from patients with PBC (and not controls) reacted with extracts of *Mycobacterium gordonae*[27]. The authors suggested *M. gordonae* might play a pathogenic role in PBC. However, O'Donohue *et al.* failed to find significant differences between PBC and control groups with respect to prevalence of mycobacteria[28].

### *Escherichia coli*

Hopf *et al.* reported a high incidence of rough form mutants of *Escherichia coli* in faecal samples from patients with PBC[29]. Butler *et al.* reported weak reactivity of sera with PDC-E2 in 69% of patients with recurrent urinary tract infection but normal liver function, and rough forms of *E. coli* were identified in the urine of patients with bacteriuria[30]. These reports failed to be substantiated by others[31].

### *Salmonella*

Antibodies to the nuclear antigen gp210 (found in up to 50% of patients with PBC) from 25 patients with PBC reacted with a homologous protein in *Salmonella typhimurium* (exact identity with six consecutive amino acids). Molecular mimicry was suggested with bacterial antigenic determinants[32]. No further follow-up references could be found for the relevance of this observation.

Apart from the lack of forthcoming data to support clinical correlation between specific bacterial infections and PBC many experimental data also fail to support the hypothesis of bacterial infection as a plausible mechanism of induction of PBC. First, the sequence homology between epitopes of human and bacterial E2 is relatively weak[33]. Secondly, absorption of PBC sera with bacterial lysates failed to remove all antibody reactivity against mammalian antigen, suggesting that the major immune response is directed against mammalian (human) PDC-E2 rather than bacterial enzyme. Thirdly, PBC sera are highly inhibitory of mammalian PDC (99% inhibition of enzyme activity) but are less inhibitory of the activity of yeast or bacterial PDC (70% and 26% inhibition, respectively), again suggesting reaction directed against mammalian PDC-E2[34]. Furthermore, immunization of a wide range of laboratory animals with PDC-E2 resulted in production of antibodies to PDC-E2 but not biliary tract damage, indicating that AMA are not pathogenetic; conversely, use of suspensions of bacterial antigen as the immunogen produced biliary tract damage but not anti-mitochondrial antibodies (AMA)[35]. Thus, despite speculation about the possible significance of similarity between pro and eukaryotic PDC-E2, there is very little evidence currently to support the hypothesis that such homology is important in pathogenetic mechanisms in PBC.

### *A viral aetiology for PBC?*

Viral infection has often been proposed as important in precipitating autoimmune conditions. Hypothetically, the immune system could inadvertently attack autologous antigens if immune processing of viral proteins resulted in generation of cross-reactive antibodies/lymphocytes capable of binding to host tissues. Candidate viral agents for induction of autoimmune conditions have included cytomegalovirus, Epstein–Barr virus and a range of enteroviruses. Parallels can be drawn between PBC and insulin-dependent diabetes mellitus (IDDM). Both are characterized by an extended subclinical period and by immune-mediated destruction of a minor population of cells. Coxsackie B4 virus has been implicated in IDDM. Viral antigen has sequence similarity with the islet cell autoantigen glutamic acid decarboxylase and viral RNA was detected in the peripheral blood of 35.7% of patients with newly diagnosed IDDM compared with only 8% later in the course; data interpreted as evidence for an initiating role of Coxsackie B infection in IDDM[36–37]. No such viral associations have been described in PBC.

Retroviruses have been implicated in the aetiology of various autoimmune disorders, for example as a triggering mechanism in systemic lupus erythematosus[38]. Furthermore the ability of exogenous retroviruses (ExRV) to induce conditions that resemble autoimmuity is well documented. Mason *et al.* used Western blotting to test patients with PBC and controls for human immunodeficiency virus (HIV-1) and human intracisternal A-type particle (HIAP, found in a high proportion of patients with Sjögren's syndrome). Significant seroreactivity was found for HIV-1 p24 gag and HIAP in 35% of patients with PBC and also in a number of other biliary and non-biliary controls and viral and autoimmune conditions[39]. The significance of this study is unclear.

Endogenous retroviruses (EndRV) are estimated to constitute up to 1% of human DNA and have been implicated as aetiological agents in autoimmunity because of their structural and sequence similarities to exogenous retroviruses known to be associated with immune dysregulation. Their tissue-specific or differentiation-dependent expression could account for localization of autoimmune reactions to anatomically restricted sites. The long terminal repeat sequences of integrated retroviruses contain promoters which could induce expression of specific host antigens in response to environmental or endogenous factors. For example activation of certain retroviruses is regulated by endogenous oestrogen, a mechanism of interest in view of the female predominance in many autoimmune conditions. In one preliminary report, evidence was presented in support of the suggestion that autoimmune recognition is triggered in PBC by a virus which either mimics PDC-E2 or activates and up-regulates native PDC-E2[40]. Representational difference analysis was undertaken between PBC liver and skin. The products were cloned, sequenced and used to screen a cDNA library constructed from BEC from the livers of patients with PBC. Significant viral homology could be demonstrated in eight of 28 clones, two of which resembled PBC autoantigens. Furthermore, one had 95% homology for the endogenous retrovirus Erv-9. In BEC from three out of four patients with PBC, retrovirus-like particles were observed while similar structures were observed in only one out of four normal controls. The results of this small study have yet to be substantiated.

## THE T-CELL RESPONSE TO AUTOANTIGEN

### Activation of T-cells

The endpoint of immune recognition of antigen is destruction of 'infected' targets. Destruction of BEC in PBC could be mediated through a number of mechanisms which may or may not include direct T-cell interaction with BEC[41].

The initiating event for recognition of antigen is constant, however: naive T-cells that survived deletion during development and entered peripheral circulation become primed through a complex reaction between many different molecules including intercellular adhesion molecules, T-cell receptor and MHC molecules complexed with antigen and suitable co-stimulatory signals. This process is achieved most efficiently in localized secondary lymphatic organs (lymph nodes) where antigens encountered by dendritic cells in the tissues are presented to T cells. In the case of the liver, dendritic cells activated by antigen in the liver migrate to lymph nodes in the porta hepatis. T cells activated by interaction with dendritic cells in the portal nodes then migrate back to the original site of dendritic cell activation by a poorly understood tissue-specific homing mechanism, and are sequestered at the original site of dendritic cell activation[42]. In the presence of persisting antigen, T cells are retained and inflammation established. In the absence of persistent antigen some activated T cells return to the circulation as memory cells which have the ability to respond directly to antigen on targets without the requirement for co-stimulatory factors such as CD80 or CD86. Memory T cells (CD45RO) are abundant in portal infiltrates in PBC[43] and immunohistochemistry indicates that numerous cells in the draining lymph nodes of patients with PBC contain material that is recognized by antibodies to PDC-E2/E3bp[44]. Thus, although BEC are thought not to express the co-stimulatory molecules required to activate naive class II restricted T cells[45], high intensity of PDC-E2/E3bp in BEC of patients with PBC could perpetuate inflammation in the liver if T cells had become sensitized to this or other cross-reactive antigen in the regional lymph nodes.

## T cell cross-reactivity

T cells derived from liver and peripheral blood of patients with PBC react with epitopes of both native and recombinant PDC-E2 and T cell cross-reactivity with *E. coli* PDC-E2 has been demonstrated[10,46–48]. T-cell cross-reactivity with an infectious agent could break T-cell tolerance of self-antigen if T-cells specific for PDC-E2/E3bp survived deletion in the thymus. Mechanisms of induction of tolerance to self-antigens during development are still only partially understood. It is clear that, during development, recognition of antigen by developing thymocytes in the thymic environment leads to apoptosis of these cells[49]. Theoretically only those thymocytes expressing receptors for non-self antigens will mature and persist as naive T cells in the peripheral circulation. However, several problems exist with this concept. First, every thymocyte would have to sample every self-antigen to ensure deletion of all autoreactive T cells. Secondly, thymocytes specific for antigens not available in the thymic environment would not be deleted. Thirdly, intracellular antigens (mitochondrial antigens, for example), do not enter the exogenous pathway for antigen presentation. Therefore, unless specialized cells exist in the thymus to secrete the full range of autologous proteins and some mechanism exists to ensure sampling of all these antigens by every thymocyte, the potential exists for autoreactive cells to escape deletion in the thymus and enter the peripheral circulation. Jones *et al.* demonstrated that T-cells from patients with PBC react with PDC-E2/E3-bp but also found that T cells from normal subjects react with intact pyruvate dehydrogenase complex, although not specifically the E2 and E3bp, components[45]. These data suggest that T cells with specificity for mitochondrial enzymes can escape deletion in the thymus, and the potential exists for cross-reaction with homologous foreign antigens, thereby breaking T-cell tolerance to self-antigen.

## EVIDENCE FOR INVOLVEMENT OF AN INFECTIOUS AGENT IN PBC: SUMMARY, CONCLUSIONS AND FUTURE PERSPECTIVES

Specific infectious agents have been implicated in a range of autoimmune disorders. Patients with PBC display autoimmune abnormalities including specific circulating autoantibodies and autoreactive T cells. Other features of PBC are inconsistent with autoimmune mechanisms. Unlike patients with other autoimmune conditions, patients with PBC appear to respond poorly to immunosuppression, and immunosuppressive therapy has been reported to exacerbate recurrence of PBC after liver transplantation. In most autoimmune conditions specific MHC associations can be demonstrated, but no clear-cut MHC association has been described in PBC, and associations which have been reported (HLA DR8) are relatively weak. Unlike most autoimmune conditions, familial occurrence of PBC is rare, but, when it does occur, individuals of different generations tend to present at the same chronological time-point rather than at the same age, suggesting a relatively more important role for environmental factors compared to genetic constitution. Although patients with PBC have well-defined autoantibodies these differ from autoantibodies in other autoimmune conditions in that reactivity is directed against a single dominant epitope, whereas in most autoimmune conditions multiple epitopes are recognized. Some of these apparent paradoxes could be interpreted as circumstantial evidence for involvement of an infectious agent in PBC. Extensive analysis of B-cell epitopes of the mitochondrial autoantigens in PBC demonstrated molecular mimicry between human and bacterial antigens at both B- and T-cell levels, and a number of bacterial species have been implicated in PBC. However, no report of bacterial involvement in PBC has been substantiated and the significance of studies reporting an association of PBC with specific bacterial species remains unclear. The possible involvement of a viral agent is also an attractive hypothesis, but likewise lacks supporting data. The basic conflict between whether the initiating event in PBC is infectious or autoimmune remains unresolved, and important questions relating to early events in PBC remain unanswered. Success in relating features observed at diagnosis to the temporally far-removed initiating events may depend critically on well-designed prospective studies. Improved studies to define the BEC antigens recognized by patients' T cells and characterization of the repertoire of T cells that survive thymic deletion and enter the peripheral circulation may also improve the potential for devising hypotheses about how tolerance of such cells for autoantigens might be broken.

### Acknowledgements

I am grateful to Professor James Neuberger and Professor Eric Jenkinson for constructive suggestions regarding the preparation of this chapter.

## References


1. James OFW. Definition and epidemiology of primary biliary cirrhosis. In: Neuberger JM, editor. Primary Biliary Cirrhosis. Eastbourne, UK: West End Studios; 1999:53–9.
2. Anand AC, Elias E, Neuberger JM. End-stage primary biliary cirrhosis in a first generation migrant South Asian population. Eur J Gastroenterol Hepatol. 1996;7:663–6.
3. Triger DR. Primary biliary cirrhosis: an epidemiological study. Br Med J. 1984;281:772–5.
4. Agarwal K, Jones DEJ, Bassendine MF. Genetic susceptibility to primary biliary cirrhosis. Eur J Gastroenterol Hepatol. 1999;11:603–6.
5. Fussey SPM, Guest JR, James OFW *et al.* Identification and analysis of the major M2 autoantigens in PBC. Proc Natl Acad Sci USA. 1988;85:8654–8.
6. Coppell RL, McNeilage J, Surh CD *et al.* Primary structure of the human M2 mitochondrial autoantigen of PBC: dihydrolipoamide acteyltransferase. Proc Natl Acad Sci USA. 1988;85:7317–21.
7. Leung PSC, Van de Water J, Coppel RL *et al.* Molecular characterisation of the mitochondrial autoantigens in primary biliary cirrhosis. Immunol Res 1991;10:518–43.
8. Joplin R, Johnson GD, Matthews JB *et al.* Distribution of pyruvate dehydrogenase dihydrolipoamide acetyltransferase (PDC-E2) and another mitochondrial marker in salivary gland and biliary epithelium from patients with primary biliary cirrhosis. Hepatol. 1994;19:1375–80.
9. Joplin R, Wallace LL, Johnson GD *et al.* Subcellular localisation of pyruvate dheydrogenase dihydrolipoamide acetyltransferase in human intrahepatic biliary epithelial cells. J Pathol. 1995;176:381–90.
10. Van de Water J, Ansari AA, Surh CD *et al.* Evidence for the targeting by 2-oxo-dehydrogenase enzymes in the T-cell response of primary biliary cirrhosis. J Immunol. 1991;146:89–94.
11. Joplin R, Wallace LL, Lindsay JG *et al.* The human biliary epithelial cell plasma membrane antigen in primary biliary cirrhosis: pyruvate dehydrogenase X? Gastroenterology. 1997;113:1727–33.
12. Ayres RCS, Neuberger JM, Shaw J *et al.* Intercellular-adhesion molecule and MHC antigens on human intrahepatic bile-duct cells – effect of pro-inflammatory cytokines. Gut. 1993;9:1245–9.
13. Saidman S, Duquesnoy RJ, Zeevi A *et al.* Recognition of major histocompatibility complex antigens on cultured human biliary epithelial cells by alloreactive lymphocytes. Hepatology. 1991;13:239–46.
14. Grotzinger T, Sternsdorf T, Jensen K, Will H. Interferon-modulated expression of genes encoding the nuclear-dot-associated proteins Sp100 and promyelocytic leukemia protein (PML). Eur J Biochem. 1996;238:554–60.
15. Harada K, Van de Water J, Leung PSC *et al. In situ* nucleic acid hybridization of cytokines in primary biliary cirrhosis: predominance of the Th1 subset. Hepatology. 1997;25:791–6.
16. Shindo M, Mullin G, Braun-Elwert L *et al.* Cytokine mRNA expression in the liver of patients with primary biliary cirrhosis (PBC) and chronic hepatitis B (CHB). Clin Exp Immunol. 1996;105:254–9.
17. Ascher NL. The role of the host immune state in recurrent hepatitis C. Liver Transplant Surg. 1997;3:179–80.
18. Sadamoto T, Neuberger JM, Joplin R. Effect of pro-inflammatory cytokines on human biliary epithelial cells (BEC): interleukin-1 up-regulates pyruvate dehydrogenase E2/X (PDC-E2/X). Hepatology. 1997;26:1264 (abstract).
19. Leuschner U. Medical treatment of vanishing bile duct syndrome. In: Alvaro D, Benedetti A, Strazzabosco M. editors. Vanishing Bile Duct Syndrome. Pathophysiology and Treatment. Lancaster: Kluwer; 1997;213–23.
20. Neuberger JM. Primary biliary cirrhosis transplantation and recurrent disease. In: Lindor KD, Heathcote JE, Poupon R, editors. Primary Biliary Cirrhosis: from Pathogenesis to Clinical Treatment. Lancaster: Kluwer; 1998:155–61.
21. Dmetrewski J, Mayer AD, Hubscher SG *et al.* Histological recurrence of primary biliary cirrhosis after liver transplantation: effect of immunosuppresssion. J Hepatol. 1996;24:253–7.
22. Van de Water J, Gerson LB, Ferrell LD *et al.* Immunohistochemical evidence of disease recurrence after liver transplantation for primary biliary cirrhosis. Hepatology. 1996;24:1079–84.
23. Jones DEJ, Watt FE, Metcalf JV *et al.* Familial primary biliary cirrhosis reassessed: a geographically-based population study. J Hepatol. 1999;30:402–407.

24. Delpre G, Niv Y. Primary biliary cirrhosis occurring in a married couple. J Hepatol. 1998;28:232 (abstract).
25. Sadomoto T, Joplin R, Keogh A *et al.* Expression of pyruvate dehydrogenase complex E2 on normal biliary epithelial cells induced by lymph nodes from primary biliary cirrhosis. Lancet. 1998;352:1595–6.
26. Klein R, Wiebel M, Engelhart S *et al.* Sera from patients with tuberculosis recognise the M2a-epitope (E2-subunit of pyruvate dehydrogenase) specific for primary biliary cirrhosis. Clin Exp Immunol. 1993;92:308–16.
27. Vilagut L, Vila J, Pares A *et al.* Cross-reactivity of anti-mycobacterium gordonae antibodies with the major mitochondrial autoantigens in primary biliary cirrhosis. J Hepatol. 1994;21:673–7.
28. O'Donohue J, Fiddler H, Garcia-Barcelo M *et al.* Mycobacterial DNA not detected in liver sections from patients with primary biliary cirrhosis. J Hepatol. 1998;28:433–8.
29. Hopf U, Stemerowicz R, Rodloff A *et al.* Relation between *Escherichia coli* R (rough)-forms in gut, lipid A and primary biliary cirrhosis. Lancet. 1989;2:1421–2.
30. Butler P, Valle F, Hamilton-Miller J *et al.* M2 mitochondrial antibodies and urinary rough mutant bacteria in patients with primary biliary cirrhosis and recurrent bacteriuria. J Hepatol. 1993;17:408–14.
31. O'Donohue J, Workman MR, Rolando N *et al.* Urinary tract infections in primary biliary cirrhosis and other chronic liver diseases. Eur J Clin Microbiol Infect Dis. 1997;16:743–6.
32. Nickowitz RE, Worman HJ. Autoantibodies from patients with primary biliary cirrhosis recognise a restricted region within the cytoplasmic tail of nuclear-pore membrane glycoprotein gp210. J Exp Med. 1993;6:2237–42.
33. Fussey SPM, Lindsay JG, Fuller C *et al.* Autoantibodies in primary biliary cirrhosis – analysis of reactivity against eukaryotic and prokaryotic 2-oxo acid dehydrogenase complexes. Hepatology. 1991;13:467–74.
34. Teoh KL, Mackay IR, Rowley MJ *et al.* Enzyme inhibitory autoantibodies to pyruvate dehydrogenase complex in primary biliary cirrhosis differ for mammalian, yeast and bacterial enzymes: implications for molecular mimicry. Hepatology. 1994;19:1029–33.
35. Howell CD, Li J, Chen W. Animal models of primary biliary cirrhosis. In: Lindor KD, Heathcote JE, Poupon R, editors. Primary Biliary Cirrhosis: from Pathogenesis to Clinical Treatment. Lancaster: Kluwer; 1998;53–63.
36. Hyoty H, Hilttunen M, Lonnrot M. Enterovirus infections and insulin dependent diabetes mellitus – evidence for causality. Clin Diagnostic Virol. 1998;9:77–84.
37. Andreoletti L, Hober D, Heber-Vandenberghe C *et al.* Coxsackie B virus infection and beta cell autoantibodies in newly diagnosed IDDM adult patients. Clin Diagnostic Virol. 1998; 9:125–33.
38. Sekigawa I, Kaneko H, Hishikawa T *et al.* HIV infection and SLE: their pathogenic relationship. Clin Exp Rheumatol. 1998;6:175–80.
39. Mason AL, Xu LZ, Guo LS *et al.* Detection of retroviral antibodies in primary biliary cirrhosis and other idiopathic biliary disorders. Lancet. 1998;351:1620–4.
40. Xu L, Guo L, Joplin R *et al.* A viral etiology of primary biliary cirrhosis. Hepatology. 1997;26:1250 (abstract).
41. Joplin R, Neuberger JM. Immunopathology of primary biliary cirrhosis. Eur J Gastroenterol Hepatol. 1999;11:587–93.
42. Picker LJ, Treer JR, Ferguson-Darnell B *et al.* Control of lymphocyte recirculation in man. Differential regulation of peripheral lymph node homing receptor L-selectin on T-cells during virgin to memory transition. J Immunol. 1993;150:1105–21.
43. Leon MP, Spickett G, Jones DEJ *et al.* CD4+ T-cell subsets defined by isoforms of CD45 in primary biliary cirrhosis. Clin Exp Immunol. 1995;99:233–9.
44. Joplin R, Lindsay JG, Hubscher SG *et al.* Distribution of dihydrolipoamide acetyltransferase (E2) in the liver and portal lymph nodes of patients with primary biliary cirrhosis: an immunohistochemical study. Hepatology. 1991;14:442–7.
45. Leon MP, Bassendine MF, Wilson JL *et al.* Immunogenicity of biliary epithelium: investigation of antigen presentation to CD4+ T-cells. Hepatology. 1996;24:561–7.
46. Jones DEJ, Palmer JM, Yeaman SJ *et al.* T-cell responses to native human proteins in primary biliary cirrhosis. Clin Exp Immunol. 1997;107:562–8.

47. Van de Water J, Ansari A, Prindiville T *et al.* Heterogeneity of autoreactive T-cell clones specific for the E2 component of the pyruvate dehydrogenase complex in primary biliary cirrhosis. J Exp Med. 1995;181:723–33.
48. Shimoda S, Nakamura M, Ishibishi H *et al.* HLA DRB4 0101-restricted immunodominant T-cell autoepitope of pyruvate dehydrogenase complex in primary biliary cirrhosis: evidence of molecular mimicry in human autoimmune disease. J Exp Med. 1995;181:1835–45.
49. Anderson KL, Anderson G, Michell RH *et al.* Intracellular signalling pathways involved in the induction of apoptosis in immature thymic T-lymphocytes. J Immunol. 1996;11:4083–91.

# 24
# Primary sclerosing cholangitis as an autoimmune disease: pros and cons

R.W. CHAPMAN

## INTRODUCTION

Primary sclerosing cholangitis (PSC) is a disease of the intrahepatic and/or extrahepatic bile ducts which is characterized by concentric obliterative fibrosis and bile duct strictures eventually leading to biliary cirrhosis.

It is clear that any proposed hypothesis will have to take account of the close association between PSC and inflammatory bowel disease. The prevalence of inflammatory bowel disease in patients with PSC varies from 21–98% and the prevalence of PSC in patients with inflammatory bowel disease from 2.4–7.5%. These variations may reflect genuine differences in study populations as the reported prevalence of PSC in UC in Northern European populations is around 80%[2,3], whereas in Southern Europe the prevalence is between 40 and 50%[4,5]. It is possible, however, that different screening methods (sigmoidoscopy versus colonoscopy) may lead to an underestimation of inflammatory bowel disease in some studies. Approximately, 1–14% of patients with PSC have Crohn's disease, usually a Crohn's colitis[1,2]. Interestingly, there is a male predominance of 2 : 1 which is not observed in inflammatory bowel disease and is in contrast with the female predominance seen in classical autoimmune diseases, such as primary biliary cirrhosis and autoimmune hepatitis[1,2]. It is also intriguing that the increased risk of developing ulcerative colitis which is associated with non-smoking is also observed in primary sclerosing cholangitis[6,7]. This effect is seen, even in patients who do not have associated inflammatory bowel disease. The mechanism for this is not clear but may be due to the effects of smoking on the immune system along with other factors, such as altered blood flow or different mucous production.

In the light of the close association with inflammatory bowel disease and biliary tract fibrosis, a number of possible causes have been suggested, including ascending portal bacteraemia, abnormal bile acid metabolism, viral infections, and copper toxicity (Table 1). There has been little data to support these hypotheses.

**Table 1** Possible causes of primary sclerosing cholangitis

| |
|---|
| Non-immune |
| Portal bacteraemia |
| Portal endotoxaemia |
| Absorbed colonic toxins |
| Copper accumulation and toxicity |
| Viral infections |
| Ischaemic damage |
| Immune mediated |

## SECONDARY SCLEROSING CHOLANGITIS

A number of different aetiological factors can give rise to histological and cholangiographic features which are similar to those seen in primary sclerosing cholangitis. These are listed in Table 2. It is clear that essentially diverse causes of bile duct obstruction can initiate a disease process which results in sclerosing-like lesions of the intra- and extrahepatic bile ducts. This article will deal with primary or idiopathic sclerosing cholangitis of the type associated with inflammatory bowel disease.

## BILE DUCT PATHOLOGY

As well as having to accommodate the clinical features described above, any proposed pathogenetic mechanism in PSC must account for the diverse, and

**Table 2** Possible causes of secondary sclerosing cholangitis

| |
|---|
| Biliary calculi and recurrent cholangitis |
| Biliary stricture |
| Benign/iatrogenic |
| Chronic pancreatitis |
| Carcinoma of head of pancreas |
| Cholangiocarcinoma |
| Cystic fibrosis |
| Biliary atresia |
| Biliary duct malformations |
| Choledochal cysts |
| Biliary infections |
| Cytomegalovirus AIDS |
| Cryptosporidium cholangiopathy |
| Ascariasis |
| Liver flukes |
| Bacterial (recurrent ascending cholangitis) |
| Chemotherapy e.g. following FUDR infusion |
| Formalin treatment for hydatid cysts |
| Post-surgical complications after bile duct surgery |

often focal, pathology which can affect the biliary system at a number of different sites.

Firstly, small ducts alone may be involved, which are only detectable on microscopic liver histology. The characteristic histology is periductular inflammation and concentric fibrosis resulting in epithelial atrophy and progressive ductopenia[8]. Secondly, the small, median and large intrahepatic ducts can be affected and lastly the extrahepatic ducts, either alone or along with the intrahepatic bile ducts. Apart from a few cases of small duct PSC, the diagnosis is established in the majority of cases by endoscopic retrograde cholangiography (ERCP). Moreover, pancreatic duct involvement can be seen on pancreatography in 10–50% of cases and suggests that derivatives of the embryonic fore gut are potential targets in PSC.

The pancreatic changes are identical to bile duct changes with stricturing and dilation of first and second order ducts.

## IMMUNE MEDIATED HYPOTHESIS

The finding of strong HLA associations, the detection of autoantibodies, and alterations in T cell function, together with the association of other autoimmune-mediated diseases, have led to the suggestion that PSC is immune mediated (Table 3). However, whether PSC is an autoimmune disease remains controversial. The evidence will be reviewed below (Table 4).

## IMMUNOGENETICS

Early studies of HLA and PSC reported an increased frequency of HLA-B8 and -DR3 in PSC patients. The first large series from King's College Hospital in London confirmed these associations[9] and reported a strong negative association with the HLA-B44-DR4 haplotype. In addition, once DR3-positive PSC patients are excluded, a secondary positive association with DR2 emerged. The HLA-A1-B8-DR3 haplotype was present in 40% of PSC patients compared with only 12% of the controls[9]. As this extended haplotype HLA-A1-B8-DR3-DQ2 is associated with susceptibility to a number of organ-specific autoimmune dis-

**Table 3** The features of primary sclerosing cholangitis compared with classical autoimmune diseases

| *Characteristic* | *Classical autoimmune disease* | *Primary sclerosing cholangitis* |
|---|---|---|
| Age | Children and adults | Children and adults |
| Sex | Female predominance | Male predominance |
| Associated autoimmune disease | Yes | Yes (particularly strong) association with IBD) |
| HLA associations (Classes I and II) | Yes | Yes |
| Response to immunosuppression | Usually good | Good in children<br>Poor in adults |

**Table 4** Immune mechanisms in primary sclerosing cholangitis

| | |
|---|---|
| Humoral immunity | Increased circulating immune complexes<br>Elevated immunology levels (IgM IgG)<br>Low titres non-organic<br>autoantibodies ANA/SMA<br>High titres anti-neutrophil<br>cytoplasmic antibody (ANCA) |
| Cell-mediated immunity | Reduction in circulating peripheral<br>CD8 T cells<br>Portal T cell infiltrate<br>Selective increase in δ8 T cells in liver/blood<br>Increased activated and memory T cells<br>Restricted T-cell receptor repertoire<br>Aberrant expression of HLA-DR on BEC<br>Increased adhesion molecules on BEC |
| Immune effector mechanisms | Enhanced cytokine expression in the liver |
| Immunogenetic mechanisms | HLA associations |

eases, such as autoimmune hepatitis, insulin-dependent diabetes mellitus, myasthenia gravis and thyrotoxicosis, the association of PSC with this haplotype provided circumstantial evidence that there may be a possible autoimmune basis for this disease also.

These early studies relied on serotyping for antigen assignment where subsequent studies have employed more specific genotyping molecular techniques. More recently, three major studies of HLA Class II associations with PSC have assessed the validity of the earlier serological studies[10–12]. A detailed discussion of these studies and their possible interpretation may be found elsewhere. To summarize, these studies broadly agree that there is a possible association with DR3 (DRB1*0301) and a negative association with DR4 (DRB1*04). These studies identified two susceptibility haplotypes A1-B8-DRB3*0101 DRB1*0301-DQA1*0501-DQB1*0201 and DRB3*0101-DRB1*1301-DQA1*0103-DQB1*0603. The two studies from the UK[10,12] found a secondary association with DR2 (DRB1*501) not confirmed in the Scandinavian study. As the alleles, BR3*0101(DR52a) and DRB5*101 (included in DR1*501 haplotypes, DR2), both encode a leucine residue at position 38 of the DR beta chains, Farrant *et al.* proposed that hydrophobicity of the leucine at position 38 confers susceptibility to PSC whereas alanine (usually encoded by DRB1*04, DR4) in this position confers protection[10]. Although leucine homozygocity was more frequent in the PSC group in both the King's[10] and Swedish studies[11] compared with the controls, given that only 28% and 24% of PSC patients were homozygous, respectively, this amino acid substitution cannot be crucial for the development of PSC. The most recent study, which included 256 patients from five European countries confirmed that PSC is positively associated within the three HLA Class II haplotypes, DR3/DQ2-DR2/DQ6 and DR6. In addition, those studies confirmed the negative association with the haplotype DR4[13]. These HLA associations would appear to be also true for Southern European patients from Spain and Italy who have a lower prevalence of colitis[4,5]. A study from Oxford and Birmingham[12] and one from the Mayo Clinic[14] both suggested that the presence of DR4, whilst protective when present, is associated with a poor prognosis, although other studies have failed to confirm this[15]. In a recent study analysis of 124 Norwegian patients, the DR3/DQ2 haplotype was significantly associated with poor prognosis, while the DR2 haplotype was an indicator of a more favourable disease course. DR4 was not associated with a poor prognosis, but a further analysis has revealed that it may be associated with cholangiocarcinoma (Spurkland A., personal communication). The finding that patients with DR3 have a poorer prognosis and DR2 a more favourable course are in keeping with the results reported in autoimmune hepatitis.

Recent studies have revealed strong HLA Class I and Class III associations with PSC. In one study, the greatest risk of disease was associated with the inheritance of the Cw*0701-B8-DRB1*0301 haplotype[16]. Cw*0701 may be inherited as part of the extended B8-DRB1*0301 haplotype and the C locus may mark the telemeric limit of the HLA encoded susceptibility to PSC[16]. PSC was associated with the TNF-$\alpha$-308A2 (TNF2 allele lying in the Class III region) an association which is stronger than that for DR3 and slightly greater than that for B8[17]. Whilst the authors argue that these data suggest that the primary susceptibility allele in PSC may lie closer to B8 than a DR3 locus, it is not possible from the current data to identify the prime susceptibility allele with any certainty. One explanation for these results would be that the susceptibility to PSC is mediated by more than one gene on the short arm of chromosome 6[17]. Whether the HLA associations are playing a major pathogenic role, for example in enhancing antigen presentation or whether they are markers by linkage disequilibrium of other genes conferring susceptibility such as TNF-$\alpha$ remain unclear.

In recent years, a number of studies have considered the immunogenetic associations of inflammatory bowel disease and have found the immunogenetic background to be different from that of PSC. It has been recently proposed that the immunogenetic associations with PSC and IBD differ from those with PSC alone. From these observations, they suggest that two types of PSC may have a different immunopathogenesis and whilst it is intriguing to speculate that colitis-associated PSC may be different from non-colitis-associated PSC, further studies are required to confirm this. Unpublished data from the PSC European Study group would not support this suggestion (Spurkland A., personal communication).

## HUMORAL IMMUNE FACTORS

In PSC, a number of humoral immune abnormalities have been described but many of these do not specifically relate to the disease. For example, low titres of antinuclear antibodies and smooth muscle antibodies were detected in 32% and 16% of PSC patients, respectively[2].

### Antineutrophil cytoplasmic antibody (ANCA)

Perinuclear ANCA (pANCA) have been detected in the sera of 26–85% of patients with PSC, with or without ulcerative colitis and up to 68% with ulcerative colitis alone[18,19]. The prevalence of ANCA in patients with Crohn's colitis is much lower 0–25% and it usually occurs in lower titres than in ulcerative colitis[18,19]. The difference in reported prevalence is probably a reflection of differences between ethnic groups and also possibly due to different techniques used to detect the antibody. High ANCA titres are seen in PSC and also in Type I autoimmune hepatitis although they are not consistently in other forms of liver disease. The target antigen or antigens, to which ANCA are directed in circulating mature neutrophils in patients with PSC and UC, have been elusive despite intensive investigation by a number of laboratories. They are not directed against proteinase-3 or myloperoxidase, the antigens responsible for cytoplasmic cANCA and perinuclear pANCA, respectively, in Wegener's granulomatosis. A recent study has suggested that the antigen may reside in the nuclear envelope although this interesting finding remains to be confirmed[20].

Although ANCA is a diagnostic marker of disease in both UC and PSC it does not appear to play an important part in the pathogenesis of either disease. Circulating ANCA from patients with UC and/or PSC have not been shown to modulate neutrophil function either *in vitro* or *in vivo*. Furthermore, a significant proportion of patients with UC and PSC are ANCA-negative, and the titre of ANCA does not correlate with disease activity, nor does it fall following colectomy or liver transplantation[21]. ANCA positivity is associated with the presence of both intra- and extrahepatic disease in PSC. It is to be hoped that if the identification of the antigen site is confirmed as nuclear envelope protein, this will allow further assessment of the role of the antibody as genetic marker, and also as a participant in the pathogenesis of PSC. Current evidence would suggest, however, that the circulating ANCA seen in the majority of patients with PSC is an epiphenomenon.

### Cellular immune abnormalities in PSC

A number of immune mechanisms have been shown to be present and activated in PSC. These are shown in Table 4[5]. However, their particular role in pathogenesis remains unproven. Recent studies have suggested that there may be oligoclonal restriction of the T cell repertoire. Studies by Broomé *et al.*[22] indicated that the hepatic T cells in PSC preferentially have V beta 3 T cell repertoires, which is not seen in T cells isolated from peripheral blood. Interestingly, in an English study, oligoclonal T cell receptors were noticed in PSC patients and, when cell lines were established, the cell lines proliferated when exposed to culture with enterocytes, and were indeed cytotoxic for enterocyte cell lines[23]. These studies provide limited support for the hypothesis that T cells found in hepatobiliary infiltrates may react against epithelial cells of gut derivation, raising the possibility that there may be shared antigens between cholangiocytes and enterocytes.

## POSSIBLE TARGETS OF IMMUNE ATTACK

It is unclear whether biliary epithelial cells (BEC) can act as antigen-presenting cells and are the targets of the immune response in PSC. In common with primary biliary cirrhosis, BEC in PSC aberrantly express Class II HLADR[24] and ICAM-1[25] which are both required for presentation of antigens to the CD4 T cell.

However, there is conflicting data as to whether other costimulatory molecules B7.1/B7.2 are also expressed on BEC[26] and the costimulatory molecules may not be expressed concomitantly[27]. The histological findings rarely show CD4 cells in the proximity of BEC and peribiliary CD8 T cells are uncommon in the early stages of PSC[28].

## ALTERNATIVE HYPOTHESIS

Vierling has suggested an alternative hypothesis in which the initial event is the reaction of an immunogenetically susceptible host to bacterial cell wall products[28]. This reaction results in the hepatic macrophages producing TNF-$\alpha$ and endotoxin. The exposure to bacterial components and increased gut permeability would be increased by the presence of inflammatory bowel disease but could also, in theory, occur during episodes of gut infection. The resulting increase in peribiliary cytokine secretion and chemokine would attract activated neutrophils, monocytes, macrophages, T cells and fibroblasts. He further postulated that the deposition of concentric fibrosis could result in atrophy of the BEC secondary to ischaemia[28]. The resulting bile duct loss would lead to progressive cholestasis, fibrosis and secondary biliary cirrhosis. This hypothesis does not explain the relative scarcity of patients with Crohn's colitis and does not take into account the strong circumstantial evidence of immune mediation and autoimmunity, previously described.

## CONCLUSION – PSC, AN AUTOIMMUNE DISEASE OR NOT?

One of the cardinal properties of the immune system is its ability to discriminate between self and non-self antigens. An important consequence of the need and ability to generate diversity in antigen specificity is that the generation of B and T cells showing receptor specificity for self, rather than non-self, antigens will inevitably occur. The majority of individuals, however, do not develop autoimmune diseases, demonstrating that there are effective mechanisms in place to maintain self-tolerance. Autoimmunity may be defined as immune reactivity against self molecules to an extent that is sufficient to cause pathogenesis and organ damage.

There is no doubt that immune mechanisms play an essential role in the pathogenesis of PSC. The question is whether they are the cause or consequence of the tissue injury. As previously stated, susceptibility to PSC is strongly associated with MHC Class II loci, particularly the HLA1-B8-DR3 haplotype and other associated alleles which are, in turn, associated with other autoimmune diseases and may mediate a T-cell specificity. In the portal tracts, there is an organ-specific T cell infiltrate which contains activated and memory T cells in close proximity to the possible target cells (the biliary epithelial cells). There is a disease-specific autoantibody ANCA which serves as a diagnostic marker but does not, on current evidence, appear to be a driving force in the pathogenetic process. Cytokine expression is enhanced in the liver and there is conflicting evidence to suggest that the epithelial cells in PSC express the necessary costimulatory signals to allow them to act as antigen-presenting cells. However, it is still unclear as to whether PSC is an organ-specific autoimmune disease. It is probable that multiple interacting genetic and environmental factors contribute to the development of autoimmunity in general, and possible PSC in particular. For the present, the question of whether PSC is an autoimmune disease or not must therefore remain unanswered.

## References


1. Wiesner RH, LaRusso NF. Clinicopathologic features of the syndrome of primary sclerosing cholangitis. Gastroenterology. 1980;1980:200–6.
2. Chapman RWG, Arborgh BAM, Rhodes JM *et al.* Primary sclerosing cholangitis; a review of its clinical features, cholangiography and hepatic histology. Gut. 1980;21:870–7.
3. Broomé U, Olsson R, Lööf L *et al.* Natural history and prognostic factors in 305 Swedish patients with primary sclerosing cholangitis. Gut. 1996;38:610–15.
4. Escorsell A, Pares A, Rodés J, Soli-Herruzo J, Miras M, de la Morena E. Epidemiology of primary sclerosing cholangitis in Spain. J Hepatol. 1994;21:787–91.
5. Okolicsanyi L, Fabris L, Viaggi S *et al.* Primary sclerosing cholangitis: clinical presentation, natural history and prognostic variables. An Italian multicenter study. Eur J Gastroenterol Hepatol. 1996;8:686–91.
6. van Erpecum KM, Smits SJ, van de Meeberg PC *et al.* Risk of primary sclerosing cholangitis is associated with nonsmoking behaviour (see comments). Gastroenterology. 1996;110(5):1503–6.
7. Loftus EVJ, Sandborn WJ, Mahoney DW, Zinsmeister AR, Offord KP, Melton LJ. Primary sclerosing is associated with nonsmoking a case-control study (see comments). Gastroenterology. 1996;110(5):1496–502.
8. Ludwig J, Barham SS, La Russo NF, Elveback LR, Wiesner RH, McCall JT. Morphologic features of chronic hepatitis associated with primary sclerosing cholangitis and chronic ulcerative colitis. Hepatology. 1981;1:632–40.
9. Donaldson PT, Farrant JM, Wilkinson ML, Hayllar K, Portmann BC, Williams R. Dual association of HLA DR2 and DR3 with primary sclerosing cholangitis. Hepatology. 1991;129–33.
10. Farrant JM, Doherty DG, Donaldson PT *et al.* Amino acid substitutions at position 38 of the DR beta polypeptide confer susceptibility to and protection from primary sclerosing cholangitis. Hepatology. 1992;16(2):390–5.
11. Olerup O, Olsson R, Hultcrantz R, Broome U. HLA-DR and HLA-DQ are not markers for rapid disease progression in primary sclerosing cholangitis. Gastroenterology. 1995;108(3):870–8.
12. Mehal WZ, Lo YM, Wordsworth BP *et al.* HLA DR4 is a marker for rapid disease progression in primary sclerosing cholangitis. Gastroenterology. 1994;106(1):160–7.
13. Spurkland A, Saarinen S, Bopberg KM *et al.* HLA Class II haplotypes in primary sclerosing cholangitis patients from five European populations. Tissue Antigens. 1999;53(5):459–69.
14. Aguilar HI, Nuako K, Krom RAF, Wiesner RH. Do primary sclerosing cholangitis (PSC) patients who express HLA-DR4 haplotype have a more rapidly progressive disease? (abstract). Hepatology. 1994;20:154A.
15. Moloney MM, Donaldson PT, Thomson LJ, Williams R. HLA-DR4 and DR4 subtypes confer resistance to primary sclerosing cholangitis and are not associated with poor prognosis (abstract). Hepatology. 1996;24:169A.
16. Bernal W, Maloney M, Underhill J, Donaldson PT. Association of tumor necrosis factor polymorphism with primary sclerosing cholangitis. J Hepatol. 1999;30:237–41.
17. Mitchell SA, Grove J, Spurkland A *et al.* Association of the TNF A-308 but not the interleukin 10, 592 promoter polymorphism with genetic susceptibility to primary sclerosing cholangitis. Gut. 2000;(in press).
18. Duerr RH, Targan SR, Landers CJ *et al.* Neutrophil cytoplasmic antibodies: a link between primary sclerosing cholangitis and ulcerative colitis. Gastroenterology. 1991;100(5 pt 1):1385–91.
19. Lo SK, Fleming KA, Chapman RW. Prevalence of anti-neutrophil antibodies in primary sclerosing cholangitis and ulcerative colitis using an alkaline phosphatase technique. Gut. 1992;33(10):1370–5.

20. Terjung B, Herzog V, Worman HJ *et al.* Atypical antineutrophil antibodies with perinuclear fluorescence in chronic inflammatory bowel disease and the hepatobiliary disorders colocalize with nuclear envelope lamina proteins. Hepatology. 1998;28:332–40.
21. Lo SK, Fleming KA, Chapman RW. A 2-year follow-up study of anti-neutrophil antibody in primary sclerosing cholangitis: relationship to clinical activity, liver biochemistry and ursodeoxycholic acid treatment. J Hepatol. 1994;21(6):974–8.
22. Broomé U, Grunwald J, Scheynius A *et al.* Preferential V beta3 usage by hepatic T lymphocytes in patients with primary sclerosing cholangitis. J Hepatol. 1997;26:527–34.
23. Probert CS, Christ AD, Saubermann LJ *et al.* Analysis of human common bile duct-associated T cells: evidence of oligoclonality, T cell clonal persistence, and epithelial cell recognition. J Immunol. 1997;158:1941–8.
24. Chapman RW, Kelly PM, Heryet A, Jewell DP, Fleming KA. Expression of HLA-DR antigens on bile duct epithelium in primary sclerosing cholangitis. Gut. 1988;29(4):422–7.
25. Bloom S, Fleming K, Chapman R. Adhesion molecule expression in primary sclerosing cholangitis and primary biliary cirrhosis. Gut. 1995;36(4):604–9.
26. Spengler U, Leifeld L, Braunschweigeer I *et al.* Anomalous expression of costimulatory molecules B7-1, B7-2 and CD28 in primary biliary cirrhosis. J Hepatol. 1997;26:31–6.
27. Broomé U, Hultcrantz R, Scheynius A. Lack of concomitant expression of ICAM-1 and HLA-DR on bile duct cells from patients with primary sclerosing cholangitis and primary biliary cirrhosis. Scand J Gastroenterol. 1993;28(2):126–30.
28. Vierling J. Aetiopathogenesis of primary sclerosing cholangitis. In: Manns M, Chapman RW, Stiehl A, Wiesner R, Eds. Primary Sclerosing Cholangitis. London: Kluwer Academic Publishers, 1998:37–45.

# 25
# Overlap syndromes and changing diagnoses

J. HEATHCOTE

## INTRODUCTION

What is meant by the term 'overlap' syndrome? There has never been a clear definition; rather it is the opinion of the particular author describing the syndrome. Hence the term might mean two autoimmune liver diseases being present at the same time in one patient, or a patient who at one time appears to have all the typical features of one autoimmune disease, later losing those features and developing the clinical, biochemical, serological and histological features of another autoimmune disease. These two situations are in fact very rare and for the most part 'overlap syndrome' appears to refer to patients who have all the typical features of autoimmune liver disease albeit autoimmune hepatitis (AIH) or primary biliary cirrhosis (PBC) or primary sclerosing cholangitis (PSC), but who in addition have some features of one or other of these well-recognized autoimmune liver diseases.

There are other conditions which have been thought by some to be 'overlap syndromes', for instance, patients who have all the features of PBC but lack antimitochondrial antibodies (AMA) even by the most specific tests but do test positive for antinuclear antibodies (ANA) and/or smooth muscle antibodies (SMA). It is probably more correct to call such patients AMA-negative PBC, there being no true overlap except for the serological pattern[1]. Such patients have been referred to as 'outliers'; so too has cryptogenic cirrhosis which responds to corticosteroid therapy, i.e. cirrhosis lacking any obvious aetiology but hypergammaglobulinaemia is present, in the absence of the common non-organ specific autoantibodies, although testing for antisoluble liver antigens is positive in a few[2].

## IMPLICATIONS OF A DIAGNOSIS OF AN OVERLAP SYNDROME

### Aetiological

The causes of all autoimmune liver diseases remain unknown. It is unlikely that any of the autoantibodies are themselves directly responsible for the pathogenesis of disease, although there are now some preliminary animal data which support the concept that AMA may cause a non-supportive destructive cholangitis[3]. The fact that several different autoantibodies may be found in one or other of the autoimmune liver diseases suggests that they are more likely epiphenomena, or that there could be a common aetiological agent but a different response to the inciting agent, possibly in part due to the specific HLA configurations of the patient.

### Therapeutic

To the clinician the crucial questions to be answered are whether subjects thought to have an overlap syndrome have a different prognosis from those subjects who seem to have a single autoimmune disease, and whether or not a patient with an 'overlap syndrome' needs an additional or a different therapeutic regimen.

## PITFALLS IN THE DIAGNOSIS OF AN 'OVERLAP SYNDROME'

Before making a diagnosis of an autoimmune 'overlap syndrome' it is particularly important to exclude other possible aetiological factors which may initiate certain autoimmune phenomena, e.g.: the non-organ, non-species specific antibodies such as ANA, SMA, AMA, anti-LKM1. Both ANA and/or ASMA may be detected in a third of patients with Wilson disease[4]. Such antibodies may also be detected in the serum of a few patients with alcohol-induced liver disease[5]. Similarly these same autoantibodies are frequently found in the serum of patients with ongoing chronic viral hepatitis B or C[6]. It is rare although quite possible for a patient, particularly someone who comes from a high prevalence area for viral hepatitis, to be both a hepatitis carrier and in addition to have an autoimmune liver disease[7]. It is probably inappropriate to classify such patients as having an overlap syndrome, as one is due to a virus and the other is clearly autoimmune. Initial features obtained at the time of the history and physical examination may suggest autoimmune disease, e.g. the presence of non-hepatic autoimmune conditions, vitiligo, thyroiditis, diabetes, coeliac disease, glomerolonephritis, Sicca syndrome, scleroderma, etc.

It is particularly important to include the possibility of a drug-induced liver disease with autoimmune features. For many years it was not appreciated that alphamethyldopa, nitrofuratoin and minocyclin[8], to name but a few, could all cause typical features of autoimmune hepatitis including an excellent response to immunosuppressive therapy!

## 'OVERLAP' SYNDROMES OF AUTOIMMUNE LIVER DISEASE

Many physicians make a diagnosis of an 'overlap syndrome' based predominantly on the serological and biochemical laboratory findings. This is likely erroneous as all biochemical, serological and immunological findings should be interpreted only in the light of the complete clinical history and well-reviewed liver histology. Some have suggested that the response to a specific therapy, e.g.

prednisone or ursodeoxycholic acid, can be used to determine the specific and/or dominant autoimmune liver disease present in an 'overlap syndrome'. This too is erroneous as abnormal liver biochemical tests tend to improve, at least in the short term, in most patients given either of these two drugs.

It is clear that specific criteria for the diagnosis of overlap syndromes need to be established. This can be achieved only by careful scrutiny of the data, preferably pooled from a team of international collaborators. Until then the definition of autoimmune overlap syndromes will continue to be diverse.

## THE PRESENCE OF TWO AUTOIMMUNE LIVER DISEASES SIMULTANEOUSLY

If such a situation ever truly exists it is best described in the paediatric literature. There are reports of children who present with all the clinical, biochemical, serological, immunological and histological findings of AIH but who are found to have PSC when their biliary tree is outlined either by using endoscopic retrograde cholangio pancreatography (ERCP) or magnetic resonance cholangiography (MRC). Often the only hint of biliary pathology is an elevation in serum gammaglutamyl transpeptidase (GGT)[10]. The typical changes of stricturing and beeding, i.e. the hallmark of PSC, are relatively late manifestations of this disease. Hence it may take many years to prove that a patient with all the features of AIH except for perhaps a more than usually elevated GGT does in fact have PSC. In adults who truly have PSC a biochemical response to corticosteroids is rarely observed, but this is not the case in paediatric patients; hence it may very well be that in children AIH and PSC can present simultaneously. As no child has yet been seen to develop PBC, possible overlap of AIH with this diagnostic dilemma is not a problem in the paediatric population.

## ONE DOMINANT AUTOIMMUNE LIVER DISEASE WITH ADDITIONAL FEATURES OF ANOTHER

It is appropriate to review only current literature, as our understanding of the different patterns of autoimmune liver disease has changed markedly since the mid-1950s when they were first recognized. There have been substantial changes in both conduct and interpretation of laboratory tests, radiological examination and histopathology. Testing for hepatitis B was introduced in the 1970s and for hepatitis C in the 1990s, but only recently have we had techniques available that detect virus in the absence of marker antibodies[11]. All these co-founding factors need to be accounted for before making a diagnosis of an autoimmune 'overlap' syndrome.

## FROM THE PERSPECTIVE OF AIH

It has long been noted that some patients with otherwise obvious type 1 AIH tested positive for the hallmark of PBC, namely AMA[12]. Further testing with the more specific ELISA or immunoblotting methods shows some AMA in these circumstances (especially when in low titre), are false-positive, but in others AMA testing is still positive by immunoblot, which employs the specific substrates for AMA. In the absence of other features of PBC, such patients respond well to immunosuppressive therapy. There has long been an argument as to whether bile duct lesions on liver histology can be a feature of AIH. In the older literature this was considered acceptable, but it is now recognized that bile duct changes are more likely but not always secondary to hepatitis C[13]. The recently modified international criteria for AIH now give the presence of bile duct lesions a mark against the diagnosis of AIH[14].

In subjects with AIH and ulcerative colitis it has been noted that duct lesions on histology are not uncommon (even in the absence of hepatitis C) despite negative ERCP findings. It may be that such patients have an 'overlap' of AIH and PSC (confined to the intrahepatic bile ducts). The rate of disease progression in such patients is noted to be faster than in subjects with AIH and no ulcerative colitis[15]. Long-term follow-up of such patients with repeat examinations of the biliary tree has not been reported to date, i.e. perhaps the typical changes on ERCP develop later. Copper retention in the liver is seen in any patient with cholestasis, as copper is normally excreted via the biliary system. A positive copper stain in AIH has been said to indicate an 'overlap' – generally with PBC and such patients often test positive for AMA.

The clinical relevance to the clinician of discerning whether or not a patient has AIH ± biliary tract disease is that the therapy may differ. Patients with cholestatic liver disease have a much higher rate of osteoporosis (regardless of gender) and treatment with long-term corticosteroid is likely to worsen their bone disease. Hence it may be preferable in patients with AIH who have cholestatic features and who require immunosuppressive therapy, to wean them off corticosteroid therapy and maintain them on azathioprine as soon as possible.

A recent large review of 162 patients with AIH suggested that 5% of such patients had overlapping features of PBC[16] (Table 1). All these patients with AIH had scored positive for AIH using the original international AIH scoring system. The authors noted that if patients tested AMA positive their AIH score tended to be in the probable range, i.e. between 10 and 15. These authors also noted that their patients with AIH with features of PBC had lower IgG and higher IgM values than those with pure AIH, in addition fewer tested positive for SMA. This observation has recently been confirmed.

**Table 1** Frequencies of the variant syndromes in autoimmune chronic liver disease[16]

| | *Clinical diagnoses* | | | |
|---|---|---|---|---|
| *Variant types* | *AIH (n = 162)* | *PBC (n = 37)* | *PSC (n = 26)* | *Total patients (n = 225)* |
| AIH + PBC | 8 (5) | 7 (19) | 0 (0) | 15 (7) |
| AIH + PSC | 0 (0) | 0 (0) | 14 (54) | 14 (6) |
| Autoimmune cholangitis | 11 (7) | 0 (0) | 0 (0) | 11 (5) |
| Total variants | 19 (12)* | 7 (19)† | 14 (54)*† | 40 (18) |

Numbers in parentheses are percentages.
*$p = 0.000004$; †$p = 0.006$.

## FROM THE PERSPECTIVE OF PBC

A large group (130) of patients with AMA-positive, biopsy-proven PBC have been assessed for features of AIH[17] (Table 2). In this study the International Immune Hepatitis (IAIH) scoring system was not used; rather the definition of AIH features made by the authors were: patients who had two of the following three criteria: (1) serum alanine transaminase (ALT) levels $\geqslant$ 5-fold elevated, (2) serum IgG levels at least twice the upper limit of normal or an SMA positive to a titre of $\geqslant$ 1:80 and (3) a liver biopsy showing moderate or severe periportal or periseptal lymphocytic piecemeal necrosis. Twelve of these 130 (9.2%) patients also had features of AIH. The authors did not comment on whether other non-hepatic autoimmune features were more or less common in those PBC patients with apparent AIH overlap. They did report that standard treatment with ursodeoxycholic acid (UDCA) given to five patients caused the biochemical cholestatic features to improve, but the liver histology worsened in three of these five over a 2-year period. A further six patients were treated only with corticosteroids and both the cholestatic and hepatitic features improved over a median duration of therapy of 4 months. Some patients were given a combination of UDCA and immunosuppressive therapy (including azathioprine) for 18 months and a sustained biochemical response of alkaline phosphate and GGT as well as ALT was noted, with little change in the immunoglobulin pattern. There was no mention of any changes in serum bilirubin measurements. A recent paper suggests that PBC patients with features of AIH have an HLA profile more in keeping with AIH than PBC; these authors also suggest combination therapy with UDCA plus prednisone may be beneficial in such cases[18].

Review of a larger (222) PBC cohort using the same criteria to identify AIH features showed a prevalence of PBC/AIH overlap (5%) less, and 2 years of treatment with UDCA led to an equal improvement in both the cholestatic and hepatitic biochemical features as well as immunoglobulin (IgG and IgM) both in the patients with PBC alone and in those with the overlapping features with AIH (Joshi S, personal communication). Hence it remains unclear as to whether treatment of PBC patients with features of AIH should be any different from treatment of patients with PBC alone. Clearly further studies are warranted. UDCA has now been shown both *in vitro* and *in vivo* to have several immunoregulatory effects, and has been used with benefit in patients with mild AIH without the addition of corticosteroid therapy[19].

Bile acids are said to be immunosuppressive, and it was suggested that it could be the effectiveness of UDCA treatment in reducing intracellular hydrophobic bile acid levels that permits autoimmune features to appear! This is an interesting concept, but the same authors have shown that long-term (10

**Table 2** PBC–AIH overlap[16]

Definition of AIH if one or more:
1. ALT > 5 × ULN
2. SMA-positive and/or IgG > 2 ULN
3. Liver biopsy with piecemeal necrosis (moderate/severe)

130 PBC patients assessed,
12 (9.2%) AIH criteria present

years) of UDCA given to patients with PBC without cirrhosis normalizes their survival, and they suggest that it is unlikely that UDCA initiates further autoimmune disease[20].

## FROM THE PERSPECTIVE OF PSC

The IAIH scoring system was applied to a large group of 114 patients with PSC (proven by ERCP)[21]. Two had a score of greater than 15, i.e. definite AIH, and 38 had a score of 10 or more, suggesting probable AIH! Patients who appear to have features of AIH and PSC have more concurrent autoimmune diseases (38%) than those who appear to have uncomplicated PSC (7%) (Table 3). Czaja *et al.*, using the IAIH scoring system in 26 patients, with ERCP-proven PSC, showed 54% to have a positive score, i.e. > 10![16]. Because of the complications of steroid therapy in patients at high risk for biliary sepsis in addition to osteoporosis, corticosteroid therapy in such patients is generally not recommended, but when tried it has rarely been shown to give rise to any clinical benefit.

## CHANGING DIAGNOSES

Although apparently extremely rare, there are case reports of patients who have all the hallmarks of PBC, namely a high serum alkaline phosphatase, a positive AMA test and typical liver histology, who have responded well to UDCA therapy and who then quite suddenly have an elevation in serum transaminase levels, loss of AMA with the appearance of ANA and a change in liver histology, to a pattern more typical of AIH (Figure 1).

Introduction of corticosteroid therapy has been shown to lead to resolution of disease[22]. Such cases are rare but do indicate what we already know, i.e. that a person with one autoimmune disease is at higher risk of another (albeit both hepatic) than someone with no autoimmune disease. A flare-up in serum transaminase levels in a patient with PBC is not unusual. This may be iatrogenic, i.e. secondary to the introduction of an hepatoxic drug, e.g. non-steroidal anti-inflammatories or a concurrent viral hepatitis. It is only when there is a

**Table 3** Aggregate scores in 114 PSC patients according to a scoring table for the diagnosis of AIH[22]

| *Classification* | *Score* | *No. of patients (%)* |
|---|---|---|
| Definite AIH | > 15 | 2 (2) |
| Probable AIH | 15 | 0 (0) |
| | 14 | 2 (2) |
| | 13 | 7 (6) |
| | 12 | 7 (6) |
| | 11 | 10 (9) |
| | 10 | 12 (11) |
| Not AIH | 5–9 | 55 (48) |
| | < 5 | 19 (17) |

Scores represent values before evaluation of response to therapy.

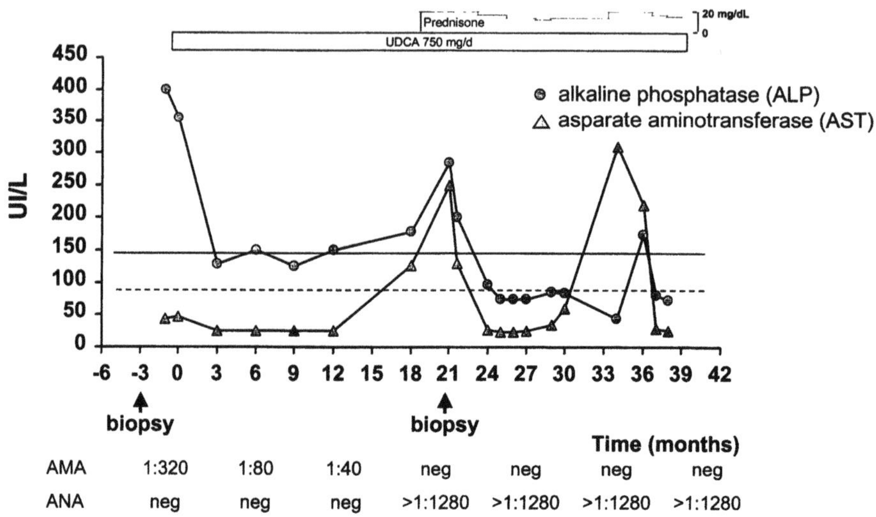


**Fig. 1** Consecutive PBC and AIH[22]

change in liver histology and a simultaneous change in serum autoantibodies that true dynamic change in the patient's autoimmune liver disease can be certain. Other cases have been described where AMA was not lost but other autoantibodies appeared[17], although a marked change in the biochemical pattern, i.e. from cholestasis to hepatitis, with a rise in ALT values, was observed. This change may be autoimmune; alternatively an exogenous insult such as a drug reaction could cause this pattern of disease.

## SUMMARY

It is clear that currently there is insufficient data to be confident about the definition/diagnosis of autoimmune liver disease 'overlap' syndromes. It is important that these syndromes be carefully delineated and defined so that studies of appropriate therapies can be instituted. There are those who advocate immunosuppressive therapy for all autoimmune liver disease, those who advocate UDCA for patients with cholestatic features and others who advocate a combination of corticosteroid therapy and UDCA for those with combined features of cholestasis and hepatitis. The consequences of choosing the wrong treatment are grave. If immunosuppressive therapy is withheld from subjects with an AIH mortality significantly increases, whereas immunosuppressive therapy (corticosteroids) given to patients with a cholestatic pattern liver disease will increase morbidity (osteroporosis) and possibly mortality. In order to ascertain the appropriate therapy in these circumstances a much greater understanding of the pathogenesis of overlap syndromes is required.

## References

1. Micheletti P, Wanless IR, Katz A *et al.* Antimitochondrial antibody negative primary biliary cirrhosis: a distinct syndrome of autoimmune cholangitis. Gut. 1994;35:260–5.
2. Czaja A. Variant forms of autoimmune hepatitis. Current Gastroenterol Rep. 1999;1:63–70.
3. Bassendine MF, Palmer JM, Decruz D *et al.* Approaches to a murine model of AMA positive non-supportive destructive cholangitis (NSDC). J Hepatol. 1998;28:59 (abstract).
4. Gregorio GV, Pensati P, Iorio R *et al.* Autoantibody prevalence in children with liver disease due to chronic hepatitis C virus (HCV) infection. Clin Exp Immunol. 1998;112:471–6.
5. Laskin C, Vidins E, Blendis L *et al.* Autoantibodies in alcoholic liver disease. Am J Med. 1990;89:129–33.
6. Clifford BD, Donahue D, Smith L *et al.* High prevalence of serological markers of autoimmunity in patients with chronic hepatitis C. Hepatology. 1995;21:613–19.
7. Somashekhar B, Schiano T, Hartman G, Black M. Chronic hepatitis with combined features of autoimmune chronic hepatitis and chronic hepatitis C: favorable response to prednisone and azathioprine. Ann Intern Med 1995;123:32–4.
8. Gough A, Chapman S, Wagstaff K *et al.* Minocycline induced autoimmune hepatitis and systemic lupus erythematosus-like syndrome. Br Med J. 1996;312:169–72.
9. Laskin C, Vidins E, Blendis L *et al.* Autoantibodies in alcoholic liver disease. Am J Med. 1990;89:129–33.
10. Wilschanski M, Chait P, Wade JA *et al.* Primary sclerosing cholangitis in 32 children: clinical, laboratory and radiographic features, with survival analysis. Hepatology. 1995;22:1411–20.
11. Cacciola I, Pollicino T, Squadrito G *et al.* Occult hepatitis B virus infection in patients with chronic hepatitis C liver disease. N Engl J Med. 1999;341:22–6.
12. Czaja A, Carpenter HA, Manns M. Antibodies to soluble liver antigen, P45011D6, and mitochondrial complexes in chronic hepatitis. Gastroenterology. 1993;105:1522–8.
13. Bach N, Thung SN, Schaffner F. The histological features of chronic hepatitis C and autoimmune chronic hepatitis: a comparative analysis. Hepatology. 1992;15:572–7.
14. Meeting Report. International autoimmune hepatitis group. J Hepatol. (In press).
15. Czaja A. The variant forms of autoimmune hepatitis. Ann Intern Med. 1996;125:588–98.
16. Czaja A. Frequency and nature of the variant syndromes of autoimmune liver disease. Hepatology. 1998;28:360–5.
17. Chazouilleres O, Wendum D, Serfaty L *et al.* Primary biliary cirrhosis – autoimmune hepatitis overlap syndrome: clinical features and response to therapy. Hepatology. 1998;28:296–301.
18. Lohse AW, Meyer zum Buschenfelde KH, Franz B *et al.* Characterization of the overlap syndrome of primary biliary cirrhosis (PBC) and autoimmune hepatitis: evidence for it being a hepatitis form of PBC in genetically susceptible individuals. Hepatology. 1999;29:1078–84.
19. Nakamura K, Yoneda M, Yokohama S *et al.* Efficacy of UDCA in Japanese patients with type 1 autoimmune hepatitis. J Gastroenterol Hepatol. 1998;13:457–9.
20. Poupon RE, Bonnand AM, Chretien Y *et al.* Ten year survival in ursodeoxycholic acid-treated patients with primary biliary cirrhosis. Hepatology. 1999;29:1668–71.
21. Boberg KM, Fausa O, Haaland T *et al.* Features of autoimmune hepatitis in primary sclerosing cholangitis: an evaluation of 114 primary sclerosing cholangitis patients according to a scoring system for the diagnosis of autoimmune hepatitis. Hepatology. 1996;23:1369–76.
22. Colombato LA, Alvarez F, Cote J, Huet MP. Autoimmune cholangiography: the result of consecutive primary biliary cirrhosis and autoimmune hepatitis. Gastroenterology. 1994;107:1839–43.

# 26
# Autoimmune liver disease and malignancy

U. BROOMÉ and A. BERGQUIST

## INTRODUCTION

Primary biliary cirrhosis (PBC), primary sclerosing cholangitis (PSC), and chronic autoimmune hepatitis represent the vast majority of autoimmune liver diseases. An increased prevalence of extrahepatic autoimmune manifestations, such as Raynaud's phenomenon, Sjögren's syndrome, autoimmune thyroiditis and inflammatory bowel disease (IBD), are present in all these disorders.

The risk for carcinoma of the liver in autoimmune liver disease varies considerably between the different diagnoses and is the main topic of this chapter. In other systemic autoimmune disorders, such as rheumatoid arthritis and systemic lupus erythematosus, an excess risk of developing both lymphatic and solid malignancies has been noted[1,2]. Therefore, the risk of acquiring extrahepatic malignancies in autoimmune liver diseases will also be discussed. The underlying mechanisms for the increased incidence of malignancies among patients with autoimmune disorders are unknown, but disturbances of the immune system are likely to be involved. Treatment with immunosuppressive drugs may further increase the risk of malignancy occurring. Moreover, a closer medical surveillance of patients with chronic disorders may lead to an increased overall identification of malignancy and overestimation of the cancer risk.

## PRIMARY BILIARY CIRRHOSIS (PBC)

### PBC and hepatocellular carcinoma

Male sex and cirrhosis (regardless of its aetiology) are well-documented risk factors for the development of hepatocellular carcinoma (HCC)[3]. The risk of acquiring HCC is estimated to be 3% per year in well-compensated cirrhosis, though variations are seen depending on its underlying cause[4]. It has been suggested that PBC is a relatively rare precursor of HCC[5,6]. The first observations of cases of HCC with an underlying PBC were published in 1979[7]; three female patients with stage IV PBC were described. Since then, several reports on HCC in PBC have been published[8–12]. The results concerning the risk of developing HCC in PBC are conflicting. An increased risk of developing HCC in patients with PBC has been reported by some authors[7,9,13–15], but others were unable to confirm this finding[12,16]. Circumstances influencing the incidence of HCC in PBC are related to several factors such as the stage of the liver disease, other concomitant hepatic disorders such as hepatitis B and C, female predominance, and the autopsy rate. These factors will be discussed below.

HCC seems to develop almost exclusively in stage IV (or cirrhotic) PBC. However, a few cases with early-stage PBC and concomitant HCC have been reported[10,17,18]. In a large cohort study including 667 PBC patients from one hospital in England, 16 HCCs were diagnosed[9]. A total of 273 of the patients had histologically confirmed fibrosis of stage III–IV. All patients with HCC had stage III–IV PBC. The overall annual incidence of HCC was 2.4% and the incidence of HCC in the group with histological advanced disease was 5.9% per year. In a recent study from Italy, Floreani and co-workers presented an overall prevalence of HCC of 2.3% among 175 patients with PBC[19]. All HCC patients had cirrhosis and the prevalence of HCC for PBC patients with stage IV disease was 10.8%. However, 11.5% of all the PBC patients had an associated hepatitis C infection, and 50% (two out of four) of the HCC patients had hepatitis C. The relatively high rate of HCV-infected patients in this study complicates the evaluation of the cancer risk of PBC itself. A logistic regression analysis indicated that a history of cigarette smoking and presence of hepatitis C infection were independent variables for the development of HCC in PBC[19].

In a Swedish study including 559 PBC patients, only two HCC were found[12]. This figure was not significantly higher than the expected number. Altogether 148 patients died during the follow-up period; since autopsies were made in only 39% of the cases, some patients with HCC may have gone undetected. A Japanese autopsy study demonstrated HCC as an incidental finding in as many as four out of six PBC patients with HCC[11]. Melia and co-workers showed – with isotopic and/or ultrasound investigations – that three out of five PBC patients with HCC lacked evidence of HCC. Since these patients had increased alpha-fetoprotein levels autopsies were made showing the presence of HCC[8].

The low overall HCC risk in PBC has been suggested as being explained by the female predominance in PBC, since male sex acts as an independent risk factor for the development of HCC. However, Farinati *et al.* found no difference between the incidence of HCC in women with stage IV PBC and those females with cirrhosis from other causes[20]. In the study by Jones and co-workers 89.4% of the stage III–IV patients were females[9]. The incidence of HCC was significantly higher in male stage III–IV patients than in female patients ($p < 0.005$). In the studies by Nakanuma and Floreani, however, no male dominance of HCC in PBC was found[11,14]. The development of HCC in PBC has been shown to influence survival, especially in male patients[8,9]. Since the presence of HCC affects the timing of liver transplantation, it is of importance to define HCC early in the course of PBC. It seems justified to screen for HCC in cirrhotic PBC patients, although the cost-effectiveness of screening for HCC in cirrhosis has not yet been demonstrated in a large-scale study. In summary, patients with stage IV PBC run an increased risk of developing HCC. The risk seems higher in men, and HCC in PBC seems to have an impact on survival. The largest studies on HCC in PBC are summarized in Table 1.

Cholangiocarcinomas (CC) are not overrepresented in patients with PBC. There is one case on record with a patient with underlying PBC presenting with both carcinoma in the common bile duct and a HCC[21].

## PBC and extrahepatic carcinoma

The possible increase in the risk of developing breast cancer in PBC was first suggested in 1983. Wolke *et al.* presented a study including 208 patients (187 female) with PBC[22]. During the follow-up period – ranging between 1 month and almost 16 years, six of the patients developed breast cancer. The relative risk in this group was 4.4, compared to an age-matched cohort in the normal population. Such an increased risk for developing breast cancer has, however, not been confirmed in a far larger study, including 559 patients, by Lööf *et al.*[12]. In a recent study from Italy, including 175 PBC patients, extrahepatic malignancies developed in eight cases (4.5%)[19]. Breast cancer was found in only two patients, giving a proportional incidence ratio of 0.43 and indicating a lower incidence of breast cancer than in the general population. These data should be viewed in the light of the relatively low risk of breast cancer in rheumatoid arthritis, the most common systemic autoimmune disorder mostly affecting females[2]. Today there is no convincing evidence of an increased risk of developing cancer of the breast in PBC; consequently these patients do not need an intensified screening for breast cancer.

The majority of the PBC patients also suffer from Sjögren's syndrome[23]. Moreover, PBC is known to induce lymphoid hyperplasia[24]. Results of several studies show that patients with Sjögren's syndrome run an increased risk of developing lymphoma[25]. In this context it is therefore of interest to emphasize that PBC patients do not seem to run an increased risk of developing either non-Hodgkin or Hodgkin lymphoma. One case report of a PBC patient with lymphoma has been presented, but in studies including larger groups of PBC patients no increased risk of developing lymphoma has been found[12,19].

# PRIMARY SCLEROSING CHOLANGITIS (PSC)

## Hepatic malignancies in PSC

An association between ulcerative colitis (UC) and CC was first described in 1954[26]. Later, in 1971, Converse *et al.* found that bile duct carcinoma in UC most commonly occurs in patients with pre-existing PSC[27]. Today we know that PSC can be complicated by CC, gall bladder carcinoma and HCC. The increased risk for CC in PSC is well established, the prevalence of CC varying in different studies between 5% and 20%[28,29]. The main reasons for variations in the number of PSC patients found to have CC are probably differences in selection of patients and diagnostic ambitions. This is well reflected in a Swedish study including 305 PSC patients[28]. The overall prevalence of CC in this study was 8%. However, among PSC patients with a follow-up of more than 5 years, 16% developed CC. Seventy-nine patients in the study died or underwent liver

**Table 1** Hepatocellular carcinoma in patients with PBC; results from nine different studies

| *Author, country year* | *Type of study* | *Follow-up time* | *Number of PBC patients (female)* | *HCC (%)* | *Number of dead patients (autopsy)* | *Comments* |
|---|---|---|---|---|---|---|
| Melia, England, 1984 | Cohort study, one centre | 1978–83 | 130 (112) | 5 (3.8) | 52 (17%) | All HCC cirrhosis; 16.7% of males developed HCC |
| Wolke, USA, 1984 | Cohort study, one centre | 45 months | 208 (187) | 1 (0.5) | n.s. | No increased risk for HCC vs Connecticut population |
| Nakanuma, Japan, 1990 | Autopsy study | 1977–87 | 319 (283) | 13 (4.1) | All | None |
| Lööf, Sweden, 1994 | Population cohort study | 108 (64.8 months) | 559 (ns) | 2 (0.3) | 148 (39%) | No increased risk for HCC vs Swedish population |
| Farinati, Italy, 1994 | Cohort study, one centre, comparison with other females with cirrhosis | 57 months | 89 (89) | 2 (2.2) | n.s. | Same risk of HCC in PBC females as for women with cirrhosis of other causes |
| Turissini, USA, 1997 | Cohort study, one hospital | 60 months | 614 | 4 (0.65) | 49 (33%) | No increased risk for HCC vs normal population |
| Jones, England, 1997 | Cohort study, one centre | 87.7 (55.3 months) | 667 | 16 (2.4) | 147 (32 OLT) | All HCC stage III–IV, 20% of males with stage III–IV developed HCC |
| van Dam, Netherlands, 1997 | Register study of death certificates | 1979–92 | 596 | ns | All | Increased risk of HCC vs normal population; SMR 25.5 |
| Floreani, Italy, 1999 | Multicentre study | 6.8 years | 175 (166) | 4 (2.3) | n.s. | HCV in 50% of HCC patients; all HCC cirrhosis, PIR 26.3 |

n.s.: not stated

**Table 2** Diagnostic tools for cholangiocarcinoma in PSC

| *Method* | *Sensitivity* | *Specificity* |
|---|---|---|
| Clinical features/rapid disease progression[31] | Poor | Poor |
| Mayo Model Risk Score > 4.4[37] | Good | Good |
| Ultrasound/computer tomography[39] | Moderate | Moderate |
| ERCP[31] | Poor | Poor |
| Tumour markers (CA 19-9, CEA)[45] | Moderate | Moderate |
| PET[47] | Excellent (?) | Excellent (?) |
| Brush cytology[42] | Poor | Excellent |

transplantation and 30% of these patients were found to have CC. In the group of PSC patients who died, only 69% underwent autopsy. It has been recognized in several studies that CC in some PSC patients will be revealed only by autopsy[30].

CC in PSC develops when patients are in their 40s, i.e. about 20 years earlier than CC in patients without PSC[29,31,32]. Liver transplantation is a well-established treatment in end-stage PSC, with excellent survival rates[33]. If CC is fully developed, liver transplantation is not recommended, since tumour recurrence is frequent. However, in a recent study it was shown that incidentally detected CC less than 1 cm in diameter discovered at the time of gross examination of the explanted liver did not influence chances of survival[34]. Gallbladder carcinoma is of rare occurrence in PSC[31,35].

## Diagnosis of CC in PSC

CC in the setting of PSC is difficult to diagnose and is often diagnosed at an advanced stage of tumour growth and spread, or accidentally at liver transplantation in end-stage PSC[29,36–38]. Clinically, biliary malignancy is often suspected when a PSC patient shows rapid, progressive liver disease with increasing bilirubin levels, weight loss and abdominal pain. However, end-stage PSC without CC can also present with rapid disease progression, and it is not possible to distinguish clinically between end-stage PSC and PSC complicated by CC[31]. Moreover, it is very difficult to differentiate between malignant and non-neoplastic strictures cholangiographically[31] since fibrotic strictures of the bile ducts are already present at the onset of the disease in PSC. In a retrospective study only encompassing PSC patients with CC, the benefit of computer tomography (CT), cholangiography, ultrasound (US) and magnetic resonance (MR) imaging in demonstrating CC in PSC was evaluated[39]. Polypoid bile duct masses on cholangiography were seen in only two patients. The most sensitive method was MR imaging, although this was done in only a minority of the patients. It was possible to detect CC in PSC in 80% of the patients with a combination of radiological methods. However, in studies in which PSC patients, both with and without CC, were included, lesions highly suspicious of being malignant were noted also in PSC patients not suffering from CC[31].

The tumours in PSC are often scirrous in nature, and even if a change suspected of being malignant is found at CT or US, it is still difficult to obtain a representative biopsy specimen. Moreover, even if representative material is gathered, it can still sometimes be difficult to differentiate between non-neoplastic and malignant bile duct changes in needle biopsies from patients with PSC. Rizzi and co-workers noted that 78.5% of all CC in PSC patients had an overexpression of the p53 protein; this was not seen in bile ducts with benign proliferation[40]. Inactivation of the p53 tumour suppressor gene is a frequently occurring step in the progression of cellular changes to cancer. In another study no overexpression of p53 was found in areas of bile duct dysplasia[41]. It would therefore seem that p53 mutation is a late event in tumour development in PSC; should overexpression of p53 be found, the change speaks in favour of bile duct malignancy.

Brush cytology from strictures obtained at ERCP have a good specificity, but a relatively low sensitivity[42,43]. DNA measurements by image cytometry on cytology specimens from strictures in PSC and CC are another means with increased sensitivity of detecting malignant transformation of bile duct epithelium[44]. Rising titres of the tumour markers carcinoembryonic antigen (CEA) or carbohydrate antigen 19-9 (CA 19-9) in the blood may be taken to support a suspicion of CC. However, increased tumour marker figures are not specific for CC since they are also seen in bacterial cholangitis. In a study published in 1995 by Ramage *et al.* a combination of the two tumour markers of CA 19-9 and CEA was evaluated, showing that (CA 19-9 + (CEA × 40)) > 400 give an 86% sensitivity in diagnosing CC in the setting of PSC[45]. This formula is recommended when using tumour markers. In a recent prospective study four different tumour markers (CEA, CA 50, CA 19-9 and CA 242) were assayed in order to try to find CC at an early phase of development in 74 PSC patients. However, it was concluded that all these tumour markers were lacking both in sensitivity and specificity[46].

In a study by Nashan *et al.*[37], the Mayo Model risk score was evaluated in 48 PSC patients undergoing liver transplantation. Ten patients suffered from CC, the cancer being incidentally found in nine of these. The Mayo PSC Natural History Model is based on a formula including bilirubin level, histological stage, age of the patient and presence of splenomegaly. A marked increase in the incidence of biliary malignancy was shown at a score above 4.4. However, patients with biliary malignancy did not differ from non-cancer patients in their clinical course, the year before transplantation. Therefore, Mayo Model scoring may be helpful in evaluating the probability of CC in PSC patients before liver transplantation. Interestingly, in a recent report from Keiding *et al.*, positron emission tomography with a radiolabelled glucose analogue accumulating in malignancies has been evaluated as a means of detecting CC in PSC[47]. The study shows very promising results regarding the possibility of revealing small CC in PSC. There is currently a need for spotting PSC patients before manifest cancer occurs, and identifying patients at increased risk of developing CC.

## PSC patients at increased risk for CC

The factors responsible for the malignant bile duct change in PSC are not known. The fact that patients with chronic *Clonorchis sinensis* infection run an increased risk of developing CC may be taken to suggest that long-standing inflammation of the bile ducts enhances the risk of the development of CC. When the cholangiocytes are continuously exposed to the concerted actions of chronic inflammatory change and hydrophobic bile acids, the cells may become predisposed to oncogenic mutations and further progression to the malignant state. This may partly be caused by a failure to activate apoptosis and delete cells with genetic damage from the epithelial lining[48]. It is important to be aware that CC in PSC occurs in patients both with and without cirrhosis[31]. PSC patients who are previous or current smokers appear to be at increased risk of developing CC[31]. In another recent study, investigating risk factors for gallbladder carcinoma in patients without PSC, cigarette smoking was also found to be an independent risk factor[49]. Smoking has been considered a risk factor for HCC both in HBsAg chronic carriers and in patients with PBC[19,50].

Presence of colorectal dysplasia/cancer in patients with concomitant ulcerative colitis seems to be another risk factor for the occurrence of CC in PSC[51,52]. In a case–control study comparing 40 PSC patients with 80 age- and sex-matched controls with UC without PSC, 10 PSC patients developed CC. Among the 10 PSC patients with CC, nine had a concomitant inflammatory bowel disease. Seven of the patients with CC also had colorectal dysplasia/cancer. Thus, CC was significantly more common among UC patients with PSC and colorectal neoplasia than among patients with UC and PSC lacking evidence of colorectal dysplasia/carcinoma ($p < 0.02$).

Biliary duct dysplasia in liver biopsies has previously – by the Oxford group – been suggested to precede CC in PSC[53]. This is a controversial proposal, as Ludwig *et al.* found only one patient with bile duct dysplasia among 60 cases who underwent liver transplantation[54]. However, none of the patients included in the study by Ludwig suffered from CC. If premalignant changes could be detected in PSC, patients at increased risk could be treated with liver transplantation before the occurrence of manifest cancer. An evaluation of biliary duct dysplasia in PSC has recently been made, and it seems that with the adoption of strict definitions of this change, an acceptable agreement can be achieved among liver pathologists on the criteria for diagnosis. Moreover, the findings suggested that bile duct dysplasia mostly occurred in PSC patients with CC and in patients who later will develop this feared complication[55]. Presence of biliary duct dysplasia in a liver biopsy should increase the suspicion of the presence of CC in another part of the liver[41]. Dysplasia is sometimes difficult to distinguish from reactive changes in biliary epithelia. In brush cytology from bile ducts, architectural relationships between the cells cannot be assessed. DNA aneuploidy is presumed to be an early sign of malignant transformation of the colonic mucosa and is sometimes seen prior to the development of colorectal dysplasia in patients with UC. The parallel to PSC is obvious, and this makes it tempting to hypothesize that DNA aneuploidy could precede malignant transformation in bile duct cells in PSC as in the colorectal mucosae in UC. DNA measurements of bile duct cells from brush samples may be a more objective way than evaluation of dysplasia in the estimation of premalignancy. We are currently – prospectively – evaluating this technique, and it seems very promising.

## PSC and HCC

There have been several case reports on HCC in PSC[31,56]. In a study from the Mayo Clinic, including 134 PSC patients with cirrhosis undergoing liver transplantation, HCC was found in three patients (2%). There was no evidence of hepatitis B or C infection in the PSC patients with HCC, nor any other risk factors for the development of HCC. No significant differences in clinical characteristics in PSC patients with or without HCC were noted. Consequently, HCC can occur in end-stage PSC[57].

Case reports have also described the association of PSC with fibrolamellar carcinoma[58].

## PSC and the risk of colorectal carcinoma

UC is a well-known risk factor for the development of colorectal carcinoma. The two most important conditions responsible for this complication are long duration of the disease and extensive colitis. The cause of the neoplastic change in UC remains unexplained; 80–90% of all patients with PSC suffer from a concomitant inflammatory bowel disease (IBD). The majority of the patients with PSC who have an associated IBD have UC with pancolitis. Lately the presence of PSC has been shown to increase the risk of colorectal cancer of dysplasia in patients with UC[51,52,59–61]. In a study from Sweden the absolute cumulative risk of developing colorectal dysplasia/cancer in the PSC/UC group was 9%, 31% and 50%, respectively, after 10, 20 and 25 years of disease duration (Figure 1). In the group with UC only, the corresponding risk was 2%, 5% and 10%, respectively[52]. Almost identical cumulative incidence rates of colorectal neoplasia were found both in a recent case–control study from Finland including 45 patients with UC and concomitant PSC and 45 pair-matched control patients

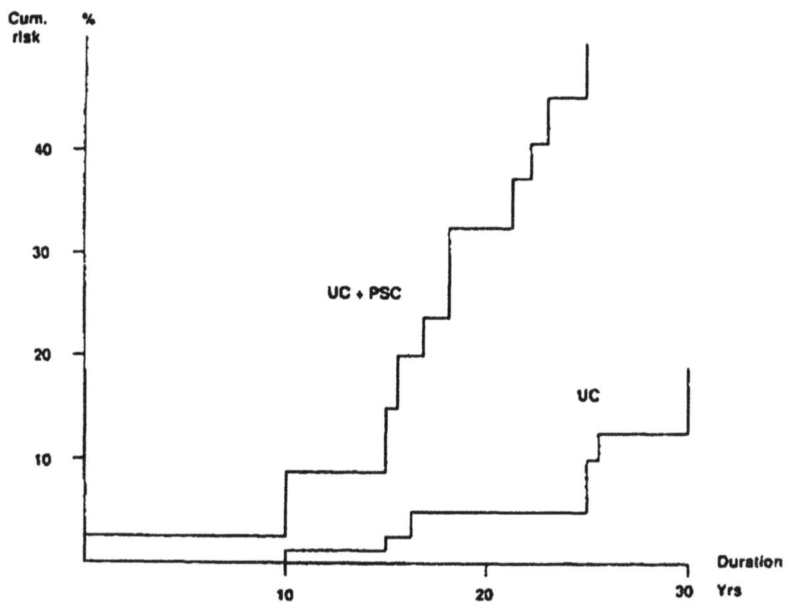


**Fig. 1** Absolute cumulative risk of developing colorectal neoplasia in patients with ulcerative colitis with primary sclerosing cholangitis compared with patients with ulcerative colitis without primary sclerosing cholangitis ($p < 0.001$)[52].

with UC only, and in a population-based study from Sweden including 125 PSC patients[61,62]. The reason for this is not clear. However, it should be kept in mind that other studies have failed to show an increased risk for UC patients with PSC to develop colorectal dysplasia/cancer[63,64]. The disagreement between the results may be explained by differences in study designs. Patients with cholestatic liver disease have a decreased bile acid excretion and a relatively high proportion of secondary bile acids[65]. It has been speculated that secondary bile acids play a role as carcinogenic agents in the colorectal mucosa in PSC. This theory is supported by the observation that right-sided cancers seem to be more common in patients with PSC than in patients with UC alone[60]. The colitis in PSC often runs a quiescent course; this is not the case with UC patients without PSC[66]. This difference may lead to an underestimate of the presence and duration of UC. Colonoscopy with multiple biopsies should therefore always be performed in PSC patients; if UC is found, colonoscopic cancer surveillance should be considered. PSC patients with UC remain at an increased risk of developing colon cancer/dysplasia even after they have undergone liver transplantation[67]. Therefore, an annual colonoscopy of these patients is warranted also after transplantation.

### Extrahepatic malignancies in PSC

Knowledge of the risk of developing extrahepatic malignancies, outside the colon in PSC, is poor. We are currently evaluating the risk of extrahepatic malignancies in a large Swedish cohort including 613 well-defined PSC patients. All cancers occurring in the cohort are traced via files from the Swedish Cancer Registry. Preliminary data show that the total number of cancers in the cohort was 160. The previously known high prevalence of cholangiocarcinoma and colorectal carcinoma was confirmed.

## AUTOIMMUNE HEPATITIS (AIH)

The development of HCC in patients with AIH is a rare event[68]. In an English study including 217 patients with AIH seen in one hospital between 1985 and 1993, eight patients developed HCC. The mean duration of AIH before occurrence of HCC was 17.1 years. Cirrhosis was present at the time of AIH diagnosis in all patients with AIH and HCC. All had steroid-responsive autoimmune hepatitis. Six of the eight patients had HCV RNA in the liver but only four had HCV RNA in the serum. Moreover, only two out of six HCV patients developed detectable antibodies to the hepatitis C virus. Thus, among 217 AIH patients, two developed HCC without an association to hepatitis C infection. Both virus-free AIH patients with HCC were males. These results support the notion that HCC is an uncommon complication to AIH.

## References

1. Mellmkjaer L, Andersen V, Linet M, Gridley G, Hoover R, Olsen J. Non-Hodgkin lymphoma and other cancers among a cohort of patients with systemic lupus erythematosus. Arthritis Rheum. 1997;40:761–8.

2. Mellemkjar L, Linet M, Gridley G, Frisch M, Mööler H, Olsen J. Rheumatoid arthritis and cancer risk. Eur J Cancer. 1996;32A:1753–7.
3. Bassendine M. Aetiological factors in hepatocellular carcinoma. Ballières Clin Gastroenterol. 1987;1:1–16.
4. Colombo M, De Franchis R, Ninno D *et al.* Hepatocellular carcinoma in Italian patients with cirrhosis. N Engl J Med. 1991;325:675–80.
5. De Bac C, Stroffolini T, Gaeta G, Taliani G, Giusti G. Pathogenic factors in cirrhosis with and without hepatocellular carcinoma. Hepatology. 1994;201:1225–30.
6. Kaczynski J, Hansson G, Hermodsson S, Olsson R, Wallerstedt S. Minor role of hepatitis B and C infection in the etiology of hepatocellular carcinoma in low-endemic area. Scand J Gastroenterol. 1996;31:809–13.
7. Krasner N, Johnson P, Portmann B, Watkinson G, Macsween R, Williams R. Hepatocellular carcinoma in primary biliary cirrhosis: report of four cases. Gut. 1979;20:255–8.
8. Melia W, Johnson P, Neuberger J, Zaman S, Portmann B, Williams R. Hepatocellular carcinoma in primary biliary cirrhosis: detection by alpha-fetoprotein estimation. Gastroenterology. 1984;87:660–3.
9. Jones D, Metcalf J, Collier J, Bassendine M, James O. Hepatocellular carcinoma in primary biliary cirrhosis and its impact on outcomes. Hepatology. 1997;26:1148–52.
10. Gluskin L, Guariglia P, Payne J, Banner B, Economou P. Hepatocellular carcinoma in a patient with precirrhotic primary biliary cirrhosis. J Clin Gastroenterol. 1985;7:441–4.
11. Nakanuma Y, Terada T, Doishita K, Miwa A. Hepatocellular carcinoma in primary biliary cirrhosis: an autopsy study. Hepatology. 1990;11:1010–16.
12. Lööf, Adami H-O, Sparén P-O *et al.* Cancer risk in primary biliary cirrhosis: a population-based study from Sweden. Hepatology. 1994;20:101–4.
13. Johnson P, Krasner N, Portmann B, Eddlestone A, Williams R. Hepatocellular carcinoma in Great Britain: influence of age, sex, HBsAg status and aetiology of underlying cirrhosis. Gut. 1978;198:1022–6.
14. Floreani A, Biagini M, Chiaramonte M, Milani S, Naccarato R, Surrenti C. Incidence of hepatic and extra-hepatic malignancies in primary biliary cirrhosis. Ital J Gastroenterol. 1991;23:523–4.
15. van Dam G, Gips C. Primary biliary cirrhosis in the Netherlands. Scand J Gastroenterol. 1997;32:77–83.
16. Turissini S, Kaplan M. Hepatocellular carcinoma in primary biliary cirrhosis. Am J Gastroenterol. 1997;92:676–8.
17. Terris G, Lande P, Vaury P. Carcinome hépatocellulaire et cirrhosis biliaire primitive: une nouvelle observation. Gastroenterol Clin Biol. 1982;6:593–4.
18. Wakai T, Shirai T, Tsukada K, Aono T, Kurosaki I. Hepatocellular carcinoma associated with precirrhotic primary biliary cirrhosis successfully treated by a right hepatic lobectomy: report of a case. Surg Today. 1996;26:723–6.
19. Floreani A, Baragiotta A, Baldo V, Menegon T, Farinati F, Naccarato R. Hepatic and extrahepatic malignancies in primary biliary cirrhosis. Hepatology. 1999 (In press).
20. Farinati F, Floreani A, De Maria N, Fagiouli S, Naccarato R, Chiaramonte M. Hepatocellular carcinoma in primary biliary cirrhosis. J Hepatol. 1994;21:315–16.
21. Imada J, Hoshino H, Nishimura D *et al.* Case report: Multiple cancers: hepatocellular carcinoma and adenocarcinomas of the common bile duct and the gall bladder in a woman with primary biliary cirrhosis. J Gastroenterol Hepatol. 1996;11:546–50.
22. Wolke A, Schaffner A, Kapelman B, Sacks H. Malignancy in primary biliary cirrhosis: high incidence of breast cancer in affected women. Am J Med. 1084;76:1075–8.
23. Sherlock S, Heathcote J. Primary Biliary Cirrhosis, (2nd edn.) Oxford: Oxford University Press, 1999. (Bircher J, ed. Oxford Textbook of Clinical Hepatology, vol. 2).
24. Kaplan M. Primary biliary cirrhosis. N Engl J Med. 1996;335:1570–80.
25. Kruize A, Hené R, van der Heide A *et al.* Long term follow-up of patients with Sjögren's syndrome. Arthritis Rheum. 1996;39:297–303.
26. Parker R, Kendall E. The liver in ulcerative colitis. Br Med J. 1954;2:1030–2.
27. Converse C, Reagan J, DeCosse J. Ulcerative colitis and carcinoma of the bile ducts. Am J Surg. 1971;121:39–45.
28. Broomé U, Olsson R, Lööf L *et al.* Natural history and prognostic factors in 305 Swedish patients with primary sclerosing cholangitis. Gut. 1996;38:610–15.
29. Rosen C, Nagorney D, Wiesner R, Coffey R, LaRusso L. Cholangiocarcinoma complicating primary sclerosing cholangitis. Ann Surg. 1991;213:21–5.

30. La Russo N, Wiesner R, Ludwig J. Sclerosing Cholangitis, (2nd edn.) Oxford: Oxford University Press, 1999. (Bircher J, ed. Oxford Textbook of Clinical Hepatology, vol. 2).
31. Bergquist A, Glaumann H, Persson B, Broomé U. Risk factors and clinical presentation of hepatobiliary carcinoma in patients with primary sclerosing cholangitis – a case control study. Hepatology. 1998;27:311–16.
32. Kaczynski J, Hansson G, Wallerstedt S. Incidence, etiologic aspects and clinicopathologic features in intrahepatic cholangiocellular carcinoma. Acta Oncol. 1998;37:77–83.
33. Wiesner R, Poryako M, LaRusso N, Steers J, Krom R, Dickson E. Liver transplantation for primary sclerosing cholangitis: impact of risk factors and outcome. Liver Transplant Surg. 1996;2:99–108.
34. Goss J, Shackleton C, Farmer D *et al.* Orthotopic liver transplantation for primary sclerosing cholangitis. A 12-year single experience. Ann Surg. 1997;225:472–83.
35. Dorudi S, Chapman R, Kettlewell M. Carcinoma of the gallbladder in ulcerative colitis and primary sclerosing cholangitis. Report of two cases. Dis Colon Rectum. 1991;34:827–8.
36. Miros M, Kerlin P, Walker N, Harper J, Lynch S, Strong R. Predicting cholangiocarcinoma in patients with primary sclerosing cholangitis before transplantation. Gut. 1991;32:1369–73.
37. Nashan B, Schlitt H, Tusch G *et al.* Biliary malignancies in primary sclerosing cholangitis: timing for liver transplantation. Hepatology. 1996;23:1105–11.
38. Farley D, Weaver A, Nagourney D. 'Natural history' of unresected cholangiocarcinoma: patient outcome after noncurative resection. Mayo Clin Proc. 1995;70:425–9.
39. Campbell W, Ferris J, Holbert B, Thaete F, Baron R. Biliary tract carcinoma complicating primary sclerosing cholangitis: evaluation with CT, cholangiography, US and MR imaging. Radiology. 1998;207:41–50.
40. Rizzi P, Ryder S, Portmann B, Ramage J, Naoumov N, Williams R. p53 Protein overexpression in cholangiocarcinoma arising in primary sclerosing cholangitis. Gut. 1996;38:265–8.
41. Bergquist A, Glaumann H, Stål P, Wang G-S, Broomé U. Apoptosis and bile duct cell dysplasia in patients with primary sclerosing cholangitis with and without cholangiocarcinoma. J Hepatol. 1998;28: abstract P/C07/001.
42. Mansfield J, Griffin S, Wadehra V, Matthewson K. A prospective evaluation of cytology from biliary strictures. Gut. 1997;40:671–7.
43. Rabinovitz M, Zajko A, Hassanein T *et al.* Diagnostic value of brush cytology in the diagnosis of bile duct carcinoma; a study in 65 patients with bile duct strictures. Hepatology. 1990;12:747–52.
44. Sears R, Duckworth C, Decaestecker C *et al.* Image cytometry as a discriminatory tool for cytologic specimens obtained by endoscopic retrograde cholangiopancreatography. Cancer Cytopathol. 1998;84:119–26.
45. Ramage J, Donaghy A, Farrant J, Iorns R, Williams R. Serum tumor markers for the diagnosis of cholangiocarcinoma in primary sclerosing cholangitis. Gastroenterology. 1995;108:865–9.
46. Hultcrantz R, Olsson R, Danielsson Å *et al.* A 3-year prospective study on serum tumor markers used for detecting cholangiocarcinoma in patients with primary sclerosing cholangitis. J Hepatol. 1999;30:669–73.
47. Keiding S, Hansen S, Rasmussen H *et al.* Detection of cholangiocarcinoma in primary sclerosing cholangitis by positron emission tomography. Hepatology. 1998;28:700–6.
48. Celli A, Que F. Dysregulation of apoptosis in the cholangiopathies and cholangiocarcinoma. Sem Liver Dis. 1998;18:177–85.
49. Khan Z, Neugut A, Ahsan H, Chabot JA. Risk factors for biliary tract cancers. Am J Gastroenterol. 1999;94:149–52.
50. Yu M, Hsu F, Sheen I *et al.* Prospective study of hepatocellular carcinoma and liver cirrhosis in asymptomatic chronic hepatitis B virus carriers. Am J Epidemiol. 1997;145:1039–47.
51. Brentnall T, Hagitt R, Rabinovitch P *et al.* Risk and natural history of colonic neoplasia in patients with primary sclerosing cholangitis and ulcerative colitis. Gastroenterology.1996;110:331–8.
52. Broomé U, Löfberg R, Veress B, Eriksson S. Primary sclerosing cholangitis and ulcerative colitis: evidence for increased neoplastic potential. Hepatology. 1995;22:1404–8.
53. Martins E, Fleming K, Garrido M, Hine K, Chapman R. Superficial thrombophlebitis, dysplasia, and cholangiocarcinoma in primary sclerosing cholangitis. Gastroenterology. 1994;107:537–42.
54. Ludwig J, Wahlström H, Batts K, Wiesner R. Papillary bile duct dysplasia in primary sclerosing cholangitis. Gastroenterology. 1992;102:2134–8.

55. Fleming K, Clausen O, Glaumann H, Bergquist A, Smith D. Biliary dysplasia in primary sclerosing cholangitis as a marker of increased risk of cholangiocarcinoma. Hepatology. 1998;28:A1136.
56. Ismail T, Angrisani L, Hübscher S, McMaster P. Hepatocellular carcinoma complicating primary sclerosing cholangitis. Br J Surg. 1991;78:360–1.
57. Harnois D, Gores G, Ludwig J, Steers J, LaRusso N, Wiesner R. Are patients with cirrhotic stage primary sclerosing cholangitis at risk for the development of hepatocellular cancer? J Hepatol. 1997;27:512–16.
58. Snook J, Kelly P, Chapman R. Fibrolamellar hepatocellular carcinoma complicating ulcerative colitis with primary sclerosing cholangitis. Gut. 1989;30:243–5.
59. Bansal P, Sonnenberg A. Risk factors of colorectal cancer in inflammatory bowel disease. Am J Gastroenterol. 1996;91:44–8.
60. Marchesa P, Lashner BA, Lavery I *et al.* The risk of cancer and dysplasia among ulcerative colitis patients with primary sclerosing cholangitis. Am J Gastroenterol. 1997;92:1285–8.
61. Kornfelt D, Ekbom A, Ihre T. Is there an excess risk for colorectal cancer in ulcerative colitis patients with primary sclerosing cholangitis? A population-based study. Gut. 1997;41:518–21.
62. Leidenius M, Farkkila M, Karkkainen P *et al.* Colorectal dysplasia and carcinoma in patients with ulcerative colitis and primary sclerosing cholangitis. Scand J Gastroenterol. 1997;32:706.
63. Loftus E, Sandborn W, Tremaine W *et al.* Risk of colorectal neoplasia in patients with primary sclerosing cholangitis. Gastroenterology. 1996;110:432–40.
64. Nuako K, Ahlqvist D, Sandborn W *et al.* Primary sclerosing cholangitis and colorectal carcinoma in patients with chronic ulcerative colitis: a case control study. Cancer. 1998;82:822–6.
65. Nagengast F, Grubben M, vanMunster I. Role of bile acids in colorectal carcinogenesis. Eur J Cancer. 1995;31:1067–70.
66. Lundqvist K, Broomé U. Differences in colonic disease activity in patients with ulcerative colitis with and without primary sclerosing cholangitis. Dis Colon Rectum. 1997;40:541–6.
67. Bleday R, Lee E, Jessurun J *et al.* Increased risk of early colorectal neoplasms after hepatic transplant in patients with inflammatory bowel disease. Dis Colon Rectum. 1993;36:908.
68. Burroughs A, Bassendine M, Thomas H, Sherlock S. Primary liver cell cancer in autoimmune chronic liver disease. Br Med J. 1981;282:2–73.

# Section VI
# Therapy of autoimmune liver diseases – state of the art

# 27
# Therapy of autoimmune diseases – state of the art

A.J. CZAJA

## INTRODUCTION

Prednisone alone or in combination with azathioprine is the established treatment of autoimmune hepatitis[1–5]. Remission occurs in 65% of treated patients within 2 years[6,7] and immediate survival is improved[8]. The 10-year life expectancy of treated patients is 93% and is similar to that of an age- and sex-matched normal population[9]. Patients with histological cirrhosis at presentation have the same 10-year survival expectation as those without this finding (89% and 90%, respectively) and they respond similarly to initial therapy[9]. In contrast, untreated patients with disease of comparable severity have a 3-year survival of 50% and a 10-year life expectancy of 10%[10]. Prospective studies describe a mortality as high as 40% within 6 months[8].

Currently available treatment regimens are not ideal. Relapse after drug withdrawal occurs in from 20% to 87% of patients within 1 year[6,7,11,12]; 13% develop drug-related complications that prematurely terminate therapy[1]; 9% deteriorate despite compliance with the appropriate treatment schedule (treatment failure)[1,13]; 13% improve but not to a degree to satisfy remission criteria (incomplete response)[1,2]; and 40% progress to histological cirrhosis within 10 years of presentation[14]. Indeed, only 17% of treated patients experience a complete and sustained resolution of their disease for at least 5 years[15]. Furthermore, codification of criteria for the diagnosis of autoimmune hepatitis has identified many patients with inconsistent or unusual findings[16–18] and these variant syndromes lack uniform diagnostic criteria and established treatment algorithms[18,19]. Successful therapy, as defined by a high benefit–risk ratio, requires accurate diagnosis, proper indications for treatment, adherence to established drug protocols, therapy until an optimal endpoint, early recognition of an adverse result, and alternative management schemes for the unsatisfactory outcome.

## TREATMENT INDICATIONS

Absolute indications for treatment are sustained severe laboratory abnormalities, bridging necrosis or multilobular necrosis on liver biopsy examination, and/or the presence of incapacitating symptoms (Table 1)[1–5]. An acute onset of severe illness (duration less than 6 months) or fulminant presentation warrants an immediate treatment trial with predisone alone or in combination with azthioprine[20]. Patients with a fulminant presentation who fail to improve at least one biochemical abnormality after 2 weeks of corticosteroid therapy are candidates for liver transplantation[20].

Lesser degrees of clinical, biochemical or histological change are associated with better prognoses and the treatment decision must be individualized to balance the benefits and risks of the medication (Table 1)[1–5]. The presence of interface hepatitis alone is insufficient to compel therapy[21,22]. This histological lesion has been associated with a low frequency of cirrhosis (≤ 7% within 5 years) and normal 5-year life expectancy if untreated[21,22].

Patients with inactive or minimally active cirrhosis and those with mild serum aminotransferase (AST) abnormalities (less than three-fold normal) and few or no symptoms do not require corticosteroid therapy (Table 1)[1–5]. Similarly, patients with features of liver failure and mild or no inflammatory activity are better candidates for liver transplantation than a regimen of corticosteroids (Table 1)[1–5]. The diagnosis of autoimmune hepatitis *per se* does not compel corticosteroid treatment.

## INITIAL TREATMENT SCHEDULES

The preferred initial treatment strategy is prednisone in combination with azathioprine (Table 2). The combination schedule is as effective as a higher dose of prednisone alone and it is associated with fewer side-effects[23]. Ideal candidates for the combination protocol are postmenopausal women and individuals with

**Table 1** Indications for treatment of autoimmune hepatitis

| *Absolute indications* | *Relative indications* | *No indications* |
|---|---|---|
| Aspartate aminotransferase level ≥ 10-fold normal | Aspartate aminotransferase level < 10-fold normal | Minimal aspartate aminotransferase elevation |
| Aspartate aminotransferase level ≥ 5-fold normal and γ-globulin level ≥ 2-fold normal | Aspartate aminotransferase level < 5-fold normal and γ-globulin level < 2-fold normal | Minimal γ-globulin elevation |
| Bridging necrosis | Interface hepatitis | Inactive cirrhosis |
| Multilobular necrosis | Disease progression | Liver failure with mild or no inflammatory component |
| Incapacitating symptoms | Mild–moderate symptoms | Serious co-morbidities |
| Acute onset fulminant disease | | |

**Table 2** Conventional treatment schedules for autoimmune hepatitis

| *Treatment type* | *Daily doses* | | *Ideal patient attributes* |
|---|---|---|---|
| Combination | Prednisone | Azathioprine | Postmenopausal |
| | 30 mg × 1 week | 50 mg × 1 week | Osteoporosis |
| | 20 mg × 1 week | 50 mg × 1 week | Diabetes |
| | 15 mg × 2 weeks | 50 mg × 1 week | Hypertension |
| | 10 mg until endpoint | 50 mg until endpoint | Obesity |
| | | | Emotional lability |
| Prednisone | Prednisone | | Cytopenia |
| | 60 mg × 1 week | | Pregnancy |
| | 40 mg × 1 week | | Malignancy |
| | 30 mg × 2 weeks | | Short-term trial |
| | 20 mg until endpoint | | (3–6 months) |
| Adjunctive | Calcium 1–1.5 g/day | | Postmenopausal |
| | Vitamin D 50 000 units/week | | |
| | Female hormone replacement if postmenopausal | | |
| | Diphosphonates (alendronate 10 mg daily or etidronate 400 mg/day × 2 weeks every 3 months) | | |
| | Multivitamins daily | | |
| | Regular exercise | | |
| | Weight control general diet | | |

osteoporosis, brittle diabetes, obesity, labile hypertension or emotional lability (Table 2)[1–5]. Prednisone alone in higher dose than when combined with azathioprine is warranted in patients with pre-existent severe cytopenia, pregnancy or contemplation of pregnancy, or active malignancy (Table 2)[1–5]. The straight prednisone regimen is also justified in patients in whom only a short treatment period (≤ 6 months) is anticipated. The advantages of the combination schedule in reducing the overall frequency of side-effects do not become apparent for at least 1 year[23]. Controlled clinical trials have established efficacy only in type 1 autoimmune hepatitis but the same treatment schedules are generally applied to all forms.

Adjunctive therapies should include a regular exercise programme that is tailored to individual tolerance (walking, swimming or biking); vitamin supplementation, especially vitamin K as indicated (10 mg daily); calcium supplementation (1–1.5 g daily); and vitamin D (50 000 units once each week). Postmenopausal women should be considered for hormonal replacement therapy, and symptomatic osteoporosis in any patient should be treated with physical therapy and bisphosphonates, such as alendronate, 10 mg daily[24], or etidronate, 400 mg daily for 2 weeks every 3 months[25, 26]. Recent studies have indicated that etidronate may have limited efficacy in cholestatic chronic liver disease but similar deficiencies have not yet been described in hepatocellular disease[27]. Asymptomatic patients on long-term corticosteroid treatment should be monitored for bone disease by annual bone mineral densitometry of the lumbar spine and femur. Manifestations of osteopenia warrant therapeutic interventions identical to those used in patients with symptomatic osteoporosis[24–26].

## TREATMENT ENDPOINTS

Treatment is continued until remission, drug toxicity, incomplete response, or treatment failure (Table 3)[1–5]. Alternative strategies are instituted if the response to conventional therapy is inadequate or if the risks of protracted or repeated treatment are substantial. *Remission* connotes absence of symptoms, resolution of laboratory abnormalities except for a less than two-fold elevation of the serum AST level, and histological improvement to normal, portal hepatitis or inactive cirrhosis (Table 3)[1,2]. *Drug toxicity* connotes intolerance to prednisone and/or azathioprine that compels discontinuation of treatment or reduction in the dose of medication (Table 3)[1,2]. Cytopenia, nausea, emotional lability, hypertension, cosmetic changes and diabetes are typically dose-related and these side-effects can improve with dose reduction. Severe reactions, including psychosis, extreme cytopenia and symptomatic osteopenia with or without vertebral compression, justify immediate discontinuation of the offending agent. *Treatment failure* connotes clinical, biochemical and/or histological deterioration despite compliance

**Table 3** Treatment endpoints and courses of action

| | *Remission* | *Treatment failure* | *Drug toxicity* | *Incomplete response* |
|---|---|---|---|---|
| Definition | Asymptomatic. Tests normal (AST ≤ 2-fold normal). Normal or near-normal biopsy. | Clinical and/or laboratory deterioration. Ascites. Encephalopathy. Worse biopsy. | Vertebral compression. Severe obesity. Psychosis. Cytopenia. Brittle diabetes. | None or some improvement. No remission after 3 years. No deterioration. |
| Action | Gradual drug withdrawal over 6 weeks. Monitor at 3-weeks intervals for relapse. Repeat original therapy if relapse. | High-dose prednisone (60 mg daily) or prednisone (30 mg daily) and azathioprine (150 mg daily) for ≥ 1 month. | Immediate dose reduction (by 50%) if mild effect. Complete withdrawal if serious effect or no better on lower dose. Control disease with single tolerated agent. | Empirical therapy with indefinite prednisone at lowest dose possible. Empirical therapy with indefinite azathioprine (2 mg per kg daily). |
| Outcome | Relapse, 50% within 6 months. 'Cure', 17%. | Clinical and test improvement, 75%. Histological remission, 20%. Liver failure possible. | Side-effects improve. Disease suboptimally treated. | Disease controlled. Transplantation if liver failure (usually ascites) after 4 years of treatment. |
| Other therapies – empirical or investigational | | Transplantation Mercaptopurine. Cyclosporin. Tacrolimus. | Mercaptopurine. Cyclosporin Tacrolimus. Budesonide. | Mercaptopurine. Budesonide. Ursodiol. |

AST = serum aspartate aminotransferase level.

with conventional treatment strategies and *incomplete response* connotes improvement that is insufficient to satisfy criteria for remission after protracted therapy (Table 3)[1,2]. The probability of entering remission during initial therapy increases at a constant rate during the first 3 years of treatment and 87% of patients who enter remission do so during this interval[1–5]. Therapy extended beyond 3 years has a decreasing probability of inducing remission (7% per annum of therapy) and an increasing likelihood of producing side-effects (7% per annum of therapy)[1–5]. Inability to achieve remission after 3 years of standard treatment is associated with diminishing benefit–risk ratio and this compels alternative therapeutic actions. The appropriate courses of action for each treatment endpoint are shown in Table 3.

## ADVERSE OUTCOMES

*Relapse* after drug withdrawal is the most common management problem and is characterized by recrudescence of symptoms (usually easy fatigability, myalgia, arthralgia and/or anorexia), increase in the serum AST level to at least three-fold normal and/or histological changes of moderate to severe interface hepatitis[6,7]. Reinstitution of the original treatment programme invariably induces another remission, but relapse after drug withdrawal typically recurs[6]. The frequency of relapse is 50% within 6 months after drug withdrawal and 70% within 3 years[6]. Patients who relapse and require re-treatment progress to cirrhosis, develop oesophageal varices and die of liver failure more commonly than those who sustain remission after treatment[6,7]. The most common consequence of relapse and repeated therapy, however, is the development of drug-related complications (54% versus 26%). Indeed, the frequency of side-effects after two relapses is 70%[7]. This high occurrence of complication erodes the net benefit–risk ratio of conventional therapy and justifies alternative management strategies.

The best method of managing relapse is to prevent its occurrence. The bases for relapse may relate to premature discontinuation of the medication and/or inability to permanently disrupt the pathogenic mechanisms of the disease. Histological improvement lags behind clinical and laboratory improvement by 3–6 months[1–5] and therapy should be extended for at least this interval before tissue sampling and treatment withdrawal[1–5]. Active histological disease is found in 55% of patients with normal serum AST and $\gamma$-globulin levels during therapy, and these patients invariably relapse after cessation of treatment[27]. Indeed, the degree of histological improvement prior to drug withdrawal influences the probability of relapse and the ideal histological endpoint is reversion of the hepatic architecture to normal[15]. Such patients have only a 20% frequency of subsequent relapse[15]. In contrast, patients with portal hepatitis at termination of therapy have a 50% frequency of relapse within 6 months[15] and those who progress to cirrhosis during treatment or who have interface hepatitis at drug withdrawal have a 100% frequency of relapse[15]. Not all patients are able to achieve histological normality and pursuit of this ideal treatment endpoint must be balanced against the risks associated with the continued administration of maintenance therapy. Liver biopsy assessment is the only method of establishing histological remission and pursuit of an ideal treatment endpoint requires this evaluation[15,28].

Patients who have relapsed multiply, despite compliance with the treatment protocol and demonstration of histological remission, are treated with a low-dose prednisone regimen that is tailored to control symptoms and maintain serum AST levels below five-fold normal (Table 4)[29]. An alternative strategy is to administer azathioprine indefinitely at a dose of 2 mg/kg per day (Table 4)[30]. The regimens have not been compared head-to-head and there is no objective basis for preference.

*Treatment failure* justifies institution of higher than conventional doses of prednisone alone (60 mg daily) or prednisone (30 mg daily) in conjunction with azathioprine (150 mg daily) (Table 3)[13]. Treatment is continued at this dose for at least 1 month. The dose of medication is then reduced each month of clinical and laboratory improvement until standard maintenance levels are achieved. Clinical and biochemical improvement can be anticipated in 75% of patients within 2 years but histological remission is achievable in only 20% (Table 3)[13]. These patients are commonly on long-term variable-dose therapy and they are at risk for drug toxicity as well as disease progression. Many may become candidates for liver transplantation.

*Drug toxicity* justifies reduction in dose of the offending agent by 50% or termination of its use depending on the severity of the side-effect (Table 3). Usually

**Table 4** Treatment strategies after multiple relapses

| *Features* | *Low-dose prednisone* | *Indefinite azathioprine* |
|---|---|---|
| Objectives | Control clinical and laboratory features of liver inflammation on the lowest dose of prednisone possible. | Maintain clinical, biochemical and histological remission using corticosteroid-sparing agent. |
| Method | Induce clinical and laboratory remission on conventional therapy. Decrease prednisone dose by 2.5 mg each month until symptoms and/or serum AST levels ≥ 5-fold normal. Maintain indefinitely on low-dose prednisone with or without azathioprine (depending on original treatment schedule). | Induce clinical and laboratory remission on conventional therapy. Increase dose of azathioprine to 2 mg/kg per day and withdraw prednisone in gradual fashion. Maintain indefinitely on fixed daily dose of azathioprine. |
| Results | Median prednisone dose, 7.5 mg. Improvement of pre-existent steroid-related complications, 85%. Stable survival No new side-effects. | 10-year sustained remission, 80%. Stable survival |
| Complications | Theoretical risk of corticosteroid-related complications | Withdrawal arthralgias, 53%. Withdrawal myalgias, 14%. Myelosuppression, 6%. Neoplasm, 7%. Dose reduction, 32%. Theoretical risk of teratogenicity and oncogenicity. |

some form of therapy can be maintained with the alternative tolerated medication in adjusted dose (prednisone or azathioprine). Azathioprine-induced myelosuppression can be anticipated by testing for thiopurine methyltransferase activity prior to its institution[31,32]. 6-Mercaptopurine is the active form of azathioprine and it may have differences in intestinal absorption and/or metabolism that favour its use as a substitute in individuals who are intolerant of azathiopurine. The dose is usually started at 25 mg/day and increased to 100 mg/day or 1.5 mg/kg body weight[33]. Other non-steroidal immunosuppressive agents can also be considered, including cyclosporin and tacrolimus (Table 3). These treatments, however are best administered in the context of a clinical trial as they have increased expense, toxicity, unestablished efficacy and no likely endpoint.

*Incomplete response* warrants empirical or investigational therapy. The most common treatment strategy is to maintain control of the inflammatory process on the lowest doses of medication possible (Table 3).The dose of prednisone is reduced by 2.5 mg each month until symptoms recur (typically easy fatigability) and/or the serum AST level increases to five-fold the upper limit of normal or higher. Azathioprine can be used as a corticosteroid-sparing agent and its dose can be increased to 2 mg/kg daily as the dose of prednisone is decreased.

## LIVER TRANSPLANTATION

Liver transplantation should be considered in all patients with decompensated autoimmune hepatitis. There are no findings prior to therapy that predict immediate and long-term prognosis and the transplantation decision should be deferred, if possible, until after a treatment trial with corticosteroids[20]. Some patients with advanced liver disease, ascites and/or endogenous encephalopathy at presentation can be salvaged with such treatment and immediate liver transplantation can be avoided[20].

The likelihood of a significant response to corticosteroid treatment can usually be determined within 2 weeks and it is presaged by the resolution of at least one pretreatment laboratory abnormality, improvement in a pretreatment hyperbilirubinaemia and/or failure of any test to worsen during the treatment period[20]. Death invariably occurs in patients with multilobular necrosis and an unimproved hyperbilirubinaemia, and these patients must be evaluated expeditiously for transplantation[20].

Long-term survival and the ultimate need for liver transplantation also depend on the response to corticosteroid therapy[34]. Inability to induce remission after 4 years of continuous effort identifies a subgroup of patients at risk for liver failure. These patients have a high mortality unless activated at the first sign of decompensation (usually the development of ascites)[34].

The 5-year survival after transplantation is 92% and this is comparable to that of untransplanted patients who enter remission during conventional corticosteroid therapy[34–36]. Autoantibodies and hypergammaglobulinaemia disappear[34] or reduce in level[35] within 2 years, and recurrent disease is rare ($\leq$ 30%)[34–37]. Inadequate immunosuppression[38,39] and the mismatching of an HLA DR3-negative donor organ with an HLA DR3-positive recipient[40] (unconfirmed) have been associated with disease recurrence. Adjustments in the immunosuppressive regimen are usually sufficient to control these manifestations[34–36,39]. Recurrent disease can be severe and result in graft failure or cirrhosis[35]. Recurrence may also complicate retransplantation[35].

Importantly, patients with autoimmune hepatitis may have other manifestations of heightened immunoreactivity after transplantation, including higher frequencies of acute rejection (81% vs 47%, $p < 0.001$), steroid-resistant rejection (38% vs 13%, $p = 0.003$) and chronic rejection (11% vs 2%) than disease-control patients with alcoholic liver disease[41]. Patients with autoimmune hepatitis who undergo liver transplantation require close monitoring and conservative adjustments in their immunosuppressive regimens[39].

## EMPIRICAL INVESTIGATIONAL THERAPIES

*Tacrolimus (FK-506)* is a macrolide antibiotic with 10–200 times the immunosuppressive activity of cyclosporin[42, 43]. Preliminary, open-label studies using 3 mg twice daily followed by dose adjustments according to the trough serum level (mean daily dose 7.2 ± 0.8 mg) have demonstrated laboratory improvements in 21 patients treated for 1 year (Table 5)[43]. Modest reductions in leukocyte and platelet counts have been observed, as have increases in serum creatinine and blood urea nitrogen levels. These drug-related consequences have been well tolerated and the net benefit–risk ratio of therapy has been satisfactory[43]. Accordingly, tacrolimus remains a drug of promise that warrants additional study.

*Ursodeoxycholic acid* has putative choleretic, cytoprotective and immunomodulatory actions that may be of advantage in the treatment of autoimmune hepatitis[44]. The drug may preserve or enhance hepatocyte membrane integrity by replacing noxious hydrophobic bile acids in the liver tissue[44] and/or altering the expression of HLA class I antigens on the hepatocyte surface[45]. It may also suppress immunoglobulin production by peripheral blood mononuclear cells[46], inhibit interleukin-2, interleukin-4 and interferon-γ production[46], improve lymphocyte function[47] and inhibit apoptosis. Ursodeoxycholic acid may also inhibit nitric oxide production and in turn improve mitochondrial function and immune responsiveness[48]. Preliminary studies in patients with chronic hepatitis of various or

**Table 5** Novel treatments of autoimmune hepatitis

| *Promising empirical or investigational therapies* | | *Theoretical therapies* | *Anecdotal therapies* |
|---|---|---|---|
| Tacrolimus | 3 mg twice daily | T cell vaccination | Cyclophosphamide (1–1.5 mg/kg daily) |
| Ursodeoxycholic acid | 13–15 mg/kg daily | Cytotoxic T lymphocyte antigen 4 | Leukocytaphoresis |
| Budesonide | 6–9 mg daily | Gene therapy | Bilirubin adsorption |
| Cyclosporin | 5–6 mg/kg daily | FcRn blockade to enhance IgG depletion | Myeloablation and stem cell transplant. Intravenous IgG (400 mg/kg 5 days/month × 5 months) |

uncertain aetiologies have shown biochemical improvements using 250 mg, 500 mg and 750 mg daily for 2 months[49,50]. Limited uncontrolled studies in autoimmune hepatitis have demonstrated clinical and biochemical improvement in eight patients treated with ursodeoxycholic acid, 600 mg daily, for 2 years, and reduction in the histological features of inflammation but not fibrosis in four patients who underwent successive liver biopsies[51]. Other studies in patients with type 1 autoimmune hepatitis who were selected by their recalcitrance to conventional corticosteroid therapy found no advantage to the adjunctive use of ursodeoxycholic acid (13–15 mg/kg per day) (Table 5)[52]. The precise role of ursodeoxycholic acid in the management of autoimmune hepatitis remains unknown and additional studies are necessary to define its place.

*Budesonide* is a second-generation corticosteroid that has a high first-pass clearance by the liver, low systemic availability, and metabolites that lack glucocorticoid activity[53]. It has been used safely and effectively in patients with asthma, allergic rhinitis, nasal polyposis, and inflammatory bowel disease[53]. Importantly, budesonide also has promise as a potent yet safe corticosteroid for immune-mediated chronic liver disease and a small open-label study involving 13 patients with autoimmune hepatitis has justified this expectation[54]. Patients treated with varying doses of budesonide (usually 6–8 mg daily) for 9 months have shown improvement in the laboratory indices of liver inflammation and tolerance for the drug (Table 5)[54]. Controlled treatment trials are necessary to establish its advantages over conventional therapy.

*Cyclosporin* is a potent immunosuppressive agent that impairs clonal expansion of cytotoxic T cells, blocks release of cytokines such as interleukin 2, and decreases antibody production by B cells[55]. In doses of 5–6 mg/kg daily it can induce rapid clinical and biochemical improvement in patients recalcitrant to or intolerant of conventional corticosteroid therapy and the medication is well tolerated at least in the short term (Table 5)[56–60]. Recent experiences in corticosteroid-resistant disease have also demonstrated histological improvement using doses of 2–3 mg/kg daily[61]. Unfortunately, treated patients become dependent on the medication and successful termination of therapy after induction of remission has not been reported. Tacrolimus has greater immunomodulatory effects and less toxicity than cyclosporin and it may supplant this agent in future clinical trials.

## PROMISING THEORETICAL TREATMENTS

*T cell vaccination* is an experimental therapy that stimulates a regulatory T cell network in the peripheral circulation and induces tolerance to autoreactive pathogenic T lymphocytes[62]. A T cell vaccine has been prepared from splenocytes taken from mice with experimental autoimmune hepatitis (Table 5). When these irradiated T cells are injected as a suspension into the peritoneum of naive mice they protect the animals from severe experimental autoimmune hepatitis induced by an infusion of freshly prepared syngeneic liver antigen[62]. Indeed, the histological scores, indicative of disease severity, are significantly reduced in the vaccinated group compared to a control group that have received irradiated Con-A activated splenocytes from naive animals and solvent alone[62]. Furthermore, vaccination of animals already afflicted with the experimental hepatitis has a therapeutic effect that is comparable to that achieved by prednisone alone or in combination with azathioprine[62]. The mechanisms by which T cell vaccination induces tolerance include anti-idiotype recognition, which confers specificity; anti-ergotype recognition, which confers efficacy; and humoral anti-lymphocyte effects, which confer potency. The mediators of the experimental liver disease and the targets of successful T cell vaccination were the CD4 cells[62]. Ideally, the antigen-specific T cell clone responsible for autoimmune hepatitis will be defined and a clone-specific vaccine can be developed not only for the prevention of the disease but for its treatment.

*Cytotoxic T lymphocyte antigen 4 (CTLA-4)* appears on the surface of helper T lymphocytes after they become activated and blocks the generation of co-stimulatory signals necessary to activate helper T lymphocytes[63]. Activated lymphocytes thereby stop proliferating and they become anergic despite ligation of the sensitizing antigen to the immunoreceptors. Soluble CTLA-4 can be used therapeutically as an immunosuppressant allowing animals[64] and humans[65] to accept foreign grafts. Furthermore, CTLA-4 polymorphisms have been described in various autoimmune diseases[66–69]. These polymorphisms probably impair self-tolerance by altering the natural inhibitory effects of CTLA-4 on helper T cell activation[70]. CTLA-4 has a theoretical application in the treatment of autoimmune hepatitis but there have been no reported clinical experiences (Table 5).

*Gene therapy* offers the advantage of delivering a gene product that is either missing or functionally insufficient. Gene delivery of CTLA-4 using a non-replicative vector has been more efficient than injections of CTLA-4 protein in treating experimental allergic encephalomyelitis[71]. A similar experimental approach might be considered in the treatment of autoimmune hepatitis if a single perturbation in normal immunoregulation can be defined (i.e. CTLA-4 polymorphism) and linked to perpetuation of the disease.

*Intravenous immunoglobulin (IgG)* has long been recognized as a mechanism of attenuating diseases that are mediated by pathogenic autoantibodies or immune complexes[72], presumably by increasing degradation of pathogenic IgG. Such treatment has also been effective anecdotally in the management of autoimmune hepatitis complicated by corticosteroid-related aseptic necrosis of the femoral head[73]. Intravenous immunoglobulin administered as 400 mg/kg body weight daily for 5 days each month for 5 months and then 400 mg/kg for 1 day each month thereafter has been associated with clinical, biochemical, and histological improvement[73]. A transporter receptor for IgG, named FcRn (Fc receptor for the neonate), has been identified and it prevents IgG catabolism by lysosomes[72]. Therapies that alter or interfere with FcRn function might facilitate depletion of pathogenic IgG[72]. Such novel strategies might include neutralizing monoclonal antibodies that alter FcRn, synthetic ligands with higher affinity for FcRn than IgG that can saturate the receptor, and anti-sense nucleotides that can down-regulate FcRn expression[72]. None of these hypothetical approaches has been tested in an experimental fashion.

## ANECDOTAL THERAPIES

Leukocytaphoresis and bilirubin absorption therapy[74], cyclophosphamide (1–1.5 mg/kg body weight per day)[75], and acute myeloablative immunosuppression followed by syngeneic stem cell transplantation[76] have all been reported to be effective in isolated cases. Pentoxifylline, as an inhibitor of nuclear factor *k*B (NF-*k*B) and tumour necrosis factor-$\alpha$ (TNF-$\alpha$), blocks hepatic stellate cell activation and has theoretical value as an antifibrogenic agent[77]. Its use as an adjunct to corticosteroid treatment has yet to be evaluated in autoimmune hepatitis. Similarly, efforts to manipulate the cytokine network are just now being implemented.

## References

1. Czaja AJ. Diagnosis, prognosis, and treatment of classical autoimmune chronic active hepatitis. In: Krawitt EL, Wiesner RH, editors. Autoimmune Liver Disease. New York: Raven Press; 1991:143–66.
2. Czaja AJ. Autoimmune hepatitis. Current therapeutic concepts. Clin Immunother. 1994;1:413–29.
3. Czaja AJ. Diagnosis and therapy of autoimmune liver disease. Med Clin N Am. 1996;80:973–94.
4. Czaja AJ. Autoimmune liver disease. In: Krawitt EL, Wiesner RH, editors. Treatment of Autoimmune Hepatitis. Amsterdam: Elsevier; 1998:499–515.
5. Czaja AJ. Drug therapy in the management of type 1 autoimmune hepatitis. Drugs. 1999;57:49–68.
6. Czaja AJ, Ammon HV, Summerskill WHJ. Clinical features and prognosis of severe chronic active liver disease (CALD) after corticosteroid-induced remission. Gastroenterology. 1980;78:518–23.
7. Czaja AJ, Beaver SJ, Shiels MT. Sustained remission following corticosteroid therapy of severe HBsAg-negative chronic active hepatitis. Gastroenterology. 1987;92:215–19.
8. Soloway RD, Summerskill WHJ, Baggenstoss AH *et al.* Clinical biochemical, and histological remission of severe chronic active liver disease: a controlled study of treatments and early prognosis. Gastroenterology. 1972;63:820–33.
9. Roberts SK, Therneau TM, Czaja AJ. Prognosis of histological cirrhosis in type 1 autoimmune hepatitis. Gastroenterology. 1996;110:848–57.
10. Geall MG, Schoenfield LJ, Summerskill WHJ. Classification and treatment of chronic active liver disease. Gastroenterology. 1972;63:458–65.
11. Hegarty JE, Nouri-Aria KT, Portmann B, Eddleston ALWF, Williams R. Relapse following treatment withdrawal in patients with autoimmune chronic active hepatitis. Hepatology. 1983;3:685–9.
12. Czaja AJ, Ludwig J, Baggenstoss AH, Wolf A. Corticosteroid-treated chronic active hepatitis in remission. Uncertain prognosis of chronic persistent hepatitis. N Engl J Med. 1981;304:5–9.
13. Schalm SW, Ammon HV, Summerskill WHJ. Failure of customary treatment in chronic active liver disease: causes and management. Ann Clin Res. 1976;8:221–7.
14. Davis GL, Czaja AJ, Ludwig J. Development and prognosis of histologic cirrhosis in corticosteroid-treated HBsAG-negative chronic active hepatitis. Gastroenterology. 1984;87:1222–7.
15. Czaja AJ, Davis GL, Ludwig J, Taswell HF. Complete resolution of inflammatory activity following corticosteroid treatment of HBsAg-negative chronic active hepatitis. Hepatology. 1984;4:622–7.
16. Czaja AJ. Chronic active hepatitis: the challenge for a new nomenclature. Ann Intern Med. 1993;119:510–17.
17. Czaja AJ. The variant forms of autoimmune hepatitis. Ann Intern Med. 1996;125:588–98.
18. Czaja AJ. Frequency and nature of the variant syndromes of autoimmune liver disease. Hepatology. 1998;28:360–5.
19. Czaja AJ. Variant forms of autoimmune hepatitis. Curr Gastroenterol Rep. 1999;1:63–70.
20. Czaja AJ, Rakela J, Ludwig J. Features reflective of early prognosis in corticosteroid-treated severe autoimmune active hepatitis. Gastroenterology. 1988;95:448–53.
21. Schalm SW, Korman MG, Summerskill WHJ, Czaja AJ, Baggenstoss AH. Severe chronic active liver disease. Prognostic significance of initial morphologic patterns. Am J Dig Dis. 1977;22:973–80.
22. Cooksley WGE, Bradbear RA, Robinson W *et al.* The prognosis of chronic active hepatitis without cirrhosis in relation to bridging necrosis. Hepatology. 1986;6:345–8.

23. Summerskill WHJ, Korman MG, Ammon HV, Baggenstoss AH. Prednisone for chronic active liver disease: dose titration, standard dose, and combination with azathioprine compared. Gut. 1975;16:876–83.
24. Liberman UA, Weiss SR, Broll J *et al.* Effect of oral alendronate on bone mineral density and the incidence of fractures in portmenopausal osteoporosis. N Engl J Med. 1995;333:1437–43.
25. Guanabens N, Pares A, Monegal A *et al.* Etidronate versus fluoride for treatment of osteopenia in primary biliary cirrhosis: preliminary results after 2 years. Gastroenterology. 1997;113:219–24.
26. Wolfhagen FHJ, van Buuren HR, den Ouden JW *et al.* Cyclical etidronate in the prevention of bone loss in corticosteroid-treated primary biliary cirrhosis. A prospective, controlled pilot study. J Hepatol. 1997;26:325–30.
27. Lindor KD, Jorgenson RA, Petz JL, Dickson ER. Etidronate for cholestasis induced osteoporosis: a randomized trial. Gastroenterology. 1999;116:A1239 (abstract).
28. Czaja AJ, Wolf AM, Baggenstoss AH. Laboratory assessment of severe chronic active liver disease (CALD): correlation of serum transaminase and gamma globulin levels with histologic features. Gastroenterology. 1981;80:687–92.
29. Czaja AJ. Low dose corticosteroid therapy after multiple relapses of severe HBsAg-negative chronic active hepatitis. Hepatology. 1990;11:1044–9.
30. Johnson PJ, McFarlane IG, Williams R. Azathioprine for long-term maintenance of remission in autoimmune hepatitis. N Engl J Med. 1995;333:958–63.
31. Ben Ari Z, Mehta A, Lennard L, Burroughs AK. Azathioprine-induced myelosuppression due to thiopurine methyltransferase deficiency in a patient with autoimmune hepatitis. J Hepatol. 1995;23:351–4.
32. Yates CR, Krynetski EY, Loennechen T *et al.* Molecular diagnosis of thiopurine *S*-methyltransferase deficiency: genetic basis for azathioprine and mercaptopurine intolerance. Ann Intern Med. 1997;126:608–14.
33. Pratt DS, Flavin DP, Kaplan MM. The successful treatment of autoimmune hepatitis with 6-mercaptopurine after failure with azathioprine. Gastroenterology. 1996;110:271–4.
34. Sanchez-Urdazpal L, Czaja AJ, van Hoek B, Krom RAF, Wiesner RH. Prognostic features and role of liver transplantation in severe corticosteroid-treated autoimmune chronic active hepatitis. Hepatology. 1992;15:215–21.
35. Ratziu V, Samuel D, Sebagh M *et al.* Long-term follow-up after liver transplantation for autoimmune hepatitis: evidence of recurrence of primary disease. J Hepatol. 1999;30:131–41.
36. Gonzalez-Koch AR, Czaja AJ, Carpenter HA *et al.* Orthotopic liver transplantation for autoimmune hepatitis: long-term outcome and incidence of disease recurrence. Hepatology. 1999;30:427A.
37. Sempoux C, Horsmans Y, Lerut J, Rahier J, Geubel A. Acute lobular hepatitis as the first manifestation of recurrent autoimmune hepatitis after orthotopic liver transplantation. Liver. 1997;17:311–15.
38. Neuberger J, Portmann B, Calne R, Williams R. Recurrence of autoimmune chronic active hepatitis following orthotopic liver grafting. Transplantation. 1984;37:363–5.
39. Devlin J, Donaldson P, Portmann B, Heaton N, Tan K-C, Williams R. Recurrence of autoimmune hepatitis following liver transplantation. Liver Transplant Surg. 1995;1:162–5.
40. Wright HL, Bou-Abboud CF, Hassanein T *et al.* Disease recurrence and rejection following liver transplantation for autoimmune chronic active liver disease. Transplantation. 1992;53:136–9.
41. Hayashi M, Keefe EB, Krams SM *et al.* Allograft rejection after liver transplantation for autoimmune liver disease. Liver Transplant Surg. 1998;4:208–14.
42. Thomson AW, Carroll PB, McCauley J *et al.* FK 506: a novel immunosuppressant for treatment of autoimmune disease. Rationale and preliminary clinical experience at the University of Pittsburgh. Springer Semin Immunopathol. 1993;14:323–44.
43. Van Thiel DH, Wright H, Carroll P *et al.* Tacrolimus: a potential new treatment for autoimmune chronic active hepatitis: results of an open-label preliminary trial. Am J Gastroenterol. 1995;90:771–6.
44. James OFW. Ursodeoxycholic acid treatment for chronic cholestatic liver disease. J Hepatol. 1990;11:5–8.
45. Calmus Y, Gane P, Rouger P, Poupon R. Hepatic expression of class I and class II major histocompatibility complex molecules in primary biliary cirrhosis: effect of ursodeoxycholic acid. Hepatology. 1990;11:12–15.

46. Yoshikawa M, Tsujii T, Matsumura K *et al.* Immunostimulatory effects of ursodeoxycholic acid on immune responses. Hepatology. 1992;16:358–64.
47. Gianni L, Di Padova F, Zuin M, Podda M. Bile acid-induced inhibition of the lymphoproliferative response to phytohemagglutinin and pokeweed mitogen: an *in vitro* study. Gastroenterology. 1980;78:231–5.
48. Hattori Y, Murakami Y, Hattori S, Kuroda H, Kasai K, Shimoda SI. Ursodeoxycholic acid inhibits the induction of nitric oxide synthetase. Eur J Pharmacol. 1996;300:147–50.
49. Bateson MC. Ursodeoxycholic acid therapy in chronic active hepatitis. Postgrad Med J. 1990;66:781–3.
50. Crosignani A, Batterzzati PM, Setchell KDR *et al.* Effects of ursodeoxycholic acid on serum liver enzymes and bile metabolism in chronic active hepatitis: a dose–response study. Hepatology. 1991;13:339–44.
51. Nakamura K, Yoneda M, Yokohama S *et al.* Efficacy of ursodeoxycholic acid in Japanese patients with type 1 autoimmune hepatitis. J Gastroenterol Hepatol. 1998;13:490–5.
52. Czaja AJ, Carpenter HA, Lindor KD. Ursodeoxycholic acid as adjunctive therapy for problematic type 1 autoimmune hepatitis: a randomized placebo-controlled treatment trial. Hepatology. 1999;30:1381–6.
53. Clissold SP, Heel RC. Budesonide: a preliminary review of its pharmacodynamic properties and therapeutic efficacy in asthma and rhinitis. Drugs. 1984;28:485–518.
54. Danielsson A, Prytz H. Oral budesonide for treatment of autoimmune chronic active hepatitis. Aliment Pharmacol Ther. 1994;8:585–90.
55. Canafax DM, Ascher NL. Cyclosporine immunosuppression. Clin Pharmacol. 1983;2:515–24.
56. Mistilis SP, Vickers CR, Darroch MH, McCarthy SW. Cyclosporin, a new treatment for autoimmune chronic active hepatitis. Med J Australia. 1985;143:463–5.
57. Hyams JS, Ballow M, Leichtner AM. Cyclosporine treatment of autoimmune chronic active hepatitis. Gastroenterology. 1987;93:890–3.
58. Minuk GH. Cyclosporin A in nontransplant-related liver disease. Am J Gastroenterol. 1989;84:1345–50.
59. Jackson LD, Song E. Cyclosporin in the treatment of corticosteroid resistant autoimmune chronic active hepatitis. Gut. 1995;36:459–61.
60. Sherman KE, Narkewicz M, Pinto PC. Cyclosporine in the management of corticosteroid-resistant type 1 autoimmune chronic active hepatitis. J Hepatol. 1994; 21:1040–7.
61. Fernandes NF, Redeker AG, Vierling JM, Villamil FG, Fong T-L. Cyclosporine therapy in patients with steroid resistant autoimmune hepatitis. Am J Gastroenterol. 1999;94:241–8.
62. Lohse AW, Dienes HP, Meyer zum Buschenfelde K-H. Suppression of murine experimental autoimmune hepatitis by T-cell vaccination or immunosuppression. Hepatology. 1998;27:1536–43.
63. Schwartz RS. The new immunology – the end of immunosuppressive drug therapy? N Engl J Med. 1999;340:1754–6.
64. Lin H, Bolling SF, Linsley PS *et al.* Long-term acceptance of major histocompatibility complex mismatched cardiac allografts induced by CTLA4Ig plus donor-specific transfusion. J Exp Med. 1993;178:1801–6.
65. Guinan EC, Boussiotis VA, Neuberg D *et al.* Transplantation of anergic histoincompatible bone marrow allografts. N Engl J Med. 1999;340:1704–14.
66. Djilali-Saiah I, Schmitz J, Harfouch-Hammond E, Mougenot JF, Bach JF, Caillat-Zucman S. CTLA-4 gene polymorphism is associated with predisposition to coeliac disease. Gut. 1998;43:187–9.
67. Krokowski M, Bodalski J, Bratek A, Machejko P, Caillat-Zucman S. CTLA-4 gene polymorphism is associated with predisposition to IDDM in a population from central Poland. Diabetes Metab. 1998;24:241–3.
68. Gonzalez-Escribano MF, Rodriguez R, Valenzuela A, Garcia A, Garcia-Lozano JR, Nunez-Roldan A. CTLA4 polymorphisms in Spanish patients with rheumatoid arthritis. Tissue Antigens. 1999;53:296–300.
69. Kemp EH, Ajjan RA, Husebye ES *et al.* A cytotoxic T lymphocyte antigen 4 (CTLA-4) gene polymorphism is associated with autoimmune Addison's disease in English patients. Clin Endocrinol. 1998;49:609–13.
70. McCoy KD, Le Gros G. The role of CTLA-4 in the regulation of T cell immune response. Immunol Cell Biol. 1999;77:1–10.

71. Croxford JL, O'Neill JK, Ali RR *et al.* Local gene therapy with CTLA4-immunoglobulin fusion protein in experimental allergic encephalomyelitis. Eur J Immunol. 1998;28:3904–16.
72. Yu Z, Lennon VA. Mechanism of intravenous immune globulin therapy in antibody-mediated autoimmune diseases. N Engl J Med. 1999;340:227–8.
73. Carmassi F, Morale R, Puccetti R *et al.* Efficacy of intravenous immunoglobulin therapy in a case of autoimmune-mediated chronic active hepatitis. Clin Exp Rheumatol. 1992;10:13–17.
74. Sawada K, Ohnishi K, Kosaka T *et al.* Exacerbated autoimmune hepatitis successfully treated with leukocytapheresis and bilirubin adsorption therapy. J Gastroenterol. 1997;32:689–95.
75. Kanzler S, Gerken G, Dienes HP, Meyer zum Buschenfelde KH, Lohse AW. Cyclophosphamide as alternative immunosuppressive therapy for autoimmune hepatitis. Gastroenterology. 1996;110:1228 (abstract).
76. Slavin S. Treatment of life-threatening autoimmune diseases with myeloablative doses of immunosuppressive agents: experimental background and rationale for ABMT. Bone Marrow Transplant. 1993;12:85–8.
77. Lee KS, Cottam HB, Houglum K, Wasson DB, Carson D, Chojkier M. Pentoxifylline blocks hepatic stellate cell activation independently of phosphodiesterase inhibitory activity. Am J Physiol. 1997;36:G1094–G1100.

# 28
# Therapy of primary biliary cirrhosis

**R. POUPON, C. CORPECHOT and R. E. POUPON**

## INTRODUCTION

Non-suppurative destructive cholangitis, more commonly known as primary biliary cirrhosis (PBC), is an uncommon progressive, destructive liver disease that leads to end-stage liver failure and premature death over decades. Although liver transplantation is life-saving, there continues to be great need for effective pharmacological treatments. The only drug currently approved specifically for the treatment of PBC is ursodeoxycholic acid (UDCA). Concurrently, increasing experimental evidence supports the use of UDCA in cholestatic diseases [1–3].

## UDCA AS THE FIRST-LINE THERAPY

The increasing use of UDCA as first-line therapy is based on a body of evidence showing that this bile acid slows the progression of the disease towards its irreversible terminal phase.

### Effect of UDCA therapy on survival

Long-term UDCA treatment improves survival free of orthotopic liver transplant (OLT). This has been demonstrated by the analysis of the combined raw data from three clinical trials involving 548 patients followed for up to 4 years and treated with the optimal dose regimen of UDCA (13–15 mg/kg per day) (see below)[4].

Other evidence comes from long-term observational studies. Survival of UDCA-treated patients is better than that predicted by the Mayo model for PBC[5]. However, it should be emphasized that 10-year survival of UDCA-treated patients with PBC remains slightly lower than that of an age- and sex-matched general population, the difference being mainly explained by the mortality among patients with cirrhosis at the outset of treatment[5,6].

## Controversy or misleading conclusions about UDCA efficacy?

The problem of the design of a clinical trial and the choice of the endpoints in a disease with a slow progression is a difficult task. Because of the increased use of OLT in the most severe patients, the combined endpoint OLT or death may be considered as the most relevant hard endpoint. Using this endpoint, large numbers of patients, and a sufficient length of follow-up are obviously needed to test the efficacy of UDCA. A tempting alternative is to perform meta-analysis of published trials. Two groups recently reported systematic review and meta-analysis of randomized controlled trials of UDCA in PBC[7, 8]. The meta-analysis by Goulis *et al.*[7] showed no difference between UDCA and placebo in the incidence of death, liver-related death, OLT, death or OLT (eight studies on 1114 patients). This work raises several methodological issues. One of the main concerns is the analysis of time-related endpoints, i.e. survival or survival without OLT, given that the length of follow-up was quite different in the selected trials. Most of the studies lasted 2 years or less. Given the patient selection and the slow progression of the disease, it is highly unlikely that an effect of UDCA on survival without OLT, or on survival, could be shown in this period. This meta-analysis also included trials in which patients were treated with what is now demonstrated as insufficient doses of UDCA[9, 10]. A major criticism is that the heterogeneity in the trials makes it unlikely that the meta-analysis might lead to reliable conclusions. The paper by Goulis *et al.*[7] is misleading in that the conclusions of the authors are based only on the meta-analysis of the 2-year randomized controlled trials, whereas they only review one by one the five studies with extended follow-up. In a meta-analysis performed on these five studies using the data summarized in this paper, we found that the risk of OLT or death is lower in the UDCA group than in the group originally assigned to placebo (OR: 0.68 [95% CI 0.48–0.95]). In other words this means a 32% reduction in the risk of dying or being transplanted. This is in agreement with the results of a combined analysis of the individual data from three larger trials[4].

The second meta-analysis, performed by Gluud *et al.* and published in abstract form[8], also concludes that UDCA has no efficacy on survival without OLT, survival, or liver histology.

Because of the limitations of the meta-analysis it is unlikely that these results are strong enough to contradict the results of our combined analysis[4]. It is well established that meta-analysis is inferior to actual data obtained from larger trials[11]. Summarizing all the information contained in a group of trials into a single odds ratio may considerably oversimplify a very complex issue.

## Effect on histology

UDCA treatment slows the histological progression and delays the onset of cirrhosis[12]. No significant changes in histological stages of the disease have been found in any trial of 2 years' duration. In contrast, a long-term clinical trial (median follow-up 3.4 years) has provided evidence that the rate of progression to cirrhosis is lower in the UDCA group than in the placebo group (10% vs 42%)[13]. In addition to short duration of therapy, lack of power of classical statistical methods may also account for the apparent absence of effect of UDCA therapy on histological progression. To test this hypothesis we used a multistage continuous-time Markov model to analyse the histological progression rate in 103 patients with PBC who were enrolled in a double-blind, placebo-controlled trial. UDCA therapy was associated with lower yearly transition rates from early stages to cirrhosis ($p < 0.001$). The median times of remaining free of stage IV (cirrhosis) starting from stages I and II were: (a) for UDCA-treated patients 20.6 years (95% CI 13–48) and 12 years (95% CI 8–33), respectively; (b) for placebo-treated patients 6.6 years (95% CI 5.3–9.9) and 4.7 years (95% CI 4–7), respectively[14].

Thus recent studies seem to indicate: (a) that long-term treatment, about 4 years, is needed to induce a clear benefit on liver histology; (b) UDCA treatment might be efficient when given to patients at the early stages of the disease but less or no more efficient in patients with advanced stages. These preliminary results need to be confirmed. One possible approach would be to analyse combined individual histological data of the larger trials.

### Other effects

UDCA therapy consistently ameliorates serum liver tests including serum bilirubin that keeps its potent prognostic value in patients receiving UDCA treatment[15]. UDCA therapy delays the onset and severity of portal hypertension. The risk of newly developing endoscopically confirmed varices was 16% for the UDCA-treated patients compared with 58% for the placebo-treated patients after 4 years of follow-up[16].

### Optimal dose of UDCA

Among all the published clinical trials only three used the initially proposed dose, namely 13–15 mg/kg per day. Two recent clinical trials were conducted to address the issue of the optimal daily dose[9, 10]. These two studies show that doses ranging from 13 to 20 mg/kg per day afford the optimal enrichment in biliary UDCA, as well as the most significant changes of liver tests. Doses equal to 10 mg/kg per day or less should be considered as suboptimal for treating PBC.

However, it should be emphasized that the dose regimen must be adapted to patient status. In particular, in patients having pruritus, hyperbilirubinaemia, severe ductopenia or cirrhosis, we recommend: (a) starting with a low dose, i.e. 200 mg/day, to avoid side-effects; (b) checking serum bile acid and bilirubin levels every month. The optimal daily dose may only be reached 6–8 months after the outset of treatment. Ideally, serum UDCA and endogenous bile acid levels should be assessed to determine the optimal dose, which in fact may vary from one patient to another because of differences in absorption, metabolism of bile acids and liver metabolic activity.

## SECOND-LINE THERAPY FOR PBC

Efforts at developing effective medical therapy for PBC should focus on improving the efficacy of UDCA. To achieve this goal we need better information on pathogenesis, natural history of subsets of patients with this syndrome, and causes of resistance to UDCA therapy. Ideally, well-designed randomized trials should assess the efficacy of potent and safe anti-inflammatory or immunosuppressive drugs in combination with UDCA.

So far three classes of drug have been tested in combination with UDCA in pilot trials: colchicine, methotrexate and corticosteroids (prednisone, budesonide)[17]. In patients with early stages of the disease the combination of UDCA with budesonide shows further improvement in biochemistries and liver histology compared with UDCA alone[18]. In contrast, the results of a pilot study indicate that budesonide does not provide additional benefit to UDCA[19]. However, it must be emphasized that in this latter study the selected patients had a suboptimal response to UDCA, while in the previous one they were naive. These results are encouraging and suggest that appropriate long-term trials should be designed to evaluate the risk – benefit of this combination in appropriate selected patients.

In this regard, we aimed at defining subsets of patients at risk of rapid histological progression under UDCA therapy. We studied the histological progression by assessing 480 biopsy specimens over 712 patient-years. After 5 years of UDCA therapy the probabilities of developing cirrhosis from stages I, II and III were 4%, 12% and 59%, respectively. Serum bilirubin level and lymphocytic piecemeal necrosis were identified as independent risk factors of rapid progression. For example, after 5 years of UDCA therapy the risk of developing cirrhosis is about 10% in a patient having stage II PBC, serum bilirubin within the normal range (< 17$\mu$mol/L) and moderate lymphocytic piecemeal necrosis, whereas it reaches 26% in a patient having the same characteristics but with severe lymphocytic piecemeal necrosis.

In conclusion, the only medical treatment for PBC that should be used outside clinical trials is UDCA. Clinical trials should be conducted to assess the risk – benefit of corticosteroids, colchicine or methotrexate in combination with UDCA in highly selected subsets of patients.

## References


1. Rodrigues CM, Fan G, Ma X, Kren BT, Steer CJ. A novel role for ursodeoxycholic acid in inhibiting apoptosis by modulating mitochondrial membrane perturbation. J Clin Invest. 1998;101:2790–9.
2. Van Nieuwkerk CMJ, Oude Elferink RPJ, Groen AK *et al.* Effects of ursodeoxycholate and cholate feeding on liver disease in FVB mice with disrupted mdr2 P-glycoprotein gene. Gastroenterology. 1996;111:165–71.
3. Beuers U, Boyer JL, Paumgartner G. Ursodeoxycholic acid in cholestasis: potential mechanisms of action and therapeutic applications. Hepatology. 1998;28:1449–53.
4. Poupon RE, Lindor KD, Cauch-Dudek K, Dickson ER, Poupon R, Heathcote EJ. Combined analysis of randomized controlled trials of ursodeoxycholic acid in primary biliary cirrhosis. Gastroenterology. 1997;113:884–90.
5. Poupon RE, Bonnand A-M, Chrétien Y, Poupon R and the UDCA – PBC Study Group. Ten-year survival in ursodeoxycholic acid-treated patients with primary biliary cirrhosis. Hepatology. 1999;29:1668–71.
6. Bateson MC, Gedming P. Ursodeoxycholic acid therapy for primary biliary cirrhosis. A 10-year British single-centre population-based audit of efficacy and survival. Postgrad Med J. 1998;74:482–5.
7. Goulis J, Leandro G, Burroughs AK. Randomised controlled trials of ursodeoxycholic-acid therapy for primary biliary cirrhosis: a meta-analysis. Lancet. 1999;354:1053–60.
8. Gluud C, Christensen E. Ursodeoxycholic acid (UDCA) in primary biliary cirrhosis (PBC) – a Cochrane hepato-biliary systemic review. J Hepatol. 1999;30(Suppl. 1):83 (abstract).

9. van Hoogstraten HJF, de Smet MBM, Renooij W *et al.* A randomized trial in primary biliary cirrhosis comparing ursodeoxycholic acid in daily doses of either 10/mg/kg or 20 mg/kg. Aliment Pharmacol Ther. 1998;12:965–71.
10. Angulo P, Dickson ER, Therneau TM *et al.* Comparison of three doses of ursodeoxycholic acid in the treatment of primary biliary cirrhosis: a randomized trial. J Hepatol. 1999;30:830–5.
11. LeLorier J, Grégoire G, Benhaddad A, Lapierre J, Derderian F. Discrepancies between meta-analyses and subsequent large randomized, controlled trials. N Engl J Med. 1997;337:536–42.
12. Angulo P, Batts KP, Therneau TM, Jorgensen RA, Dickson ER, Lindor KD. Long-term ursodeoxycholic acid delays histological progression in primary biliary cirrhosis. Hepatology. 1999;29:644–7.
13. Parés A, Caballeria L, Rodés J *et al.* Long-term effects of ursodeoxycholic acid in primary biliary cirrhosis: results of a double-blind controlled multicentric trial. J Hepatol. 2000;32:561–6.
14. Corpechot C, Carrat F, Bonnand A-M, Poupon RE, Poupon R. A Markov model for assessment of histological progression in PBC provides evidence that UDCA is effective in early stages. Hepatology. 1999;30:474 (abstract).
15. Bonnand A-M, Heathcote EJ, Lindor KD, Poupon RE. Clinical significance of serum bilirubin levels under ursodeoxycholic acid therapy in patients with primary biliary cirrhosis. Hepatology. 1999;29:39–43.
16. Lindor KD, Jorgensen RA, Therneau TM, Malinchoc M, Dickson ER. Ursodeoxycholic acid delays the onset of esophageal varices in primary biliary cirrhosis. Mayo Clin Proc. 1997;72:1137–40.
17. Poupon RE, Poupon R. Ursodeoxycholic acid for primary biliary cirrhosis. In: Boyer JL, Jansen PLM, Manns MP, Reichen J, editors. Cholestatic Liver Diseases. Dordrecht: Kluwer; 1998:271–7.
18. Leuschner M, Maier K-M, Schlichting J *et al.* Oral budesonide and ursodeoxycholic acid for treatment of primary biliary cirrhosis: results of a prospective double-blind trial. Gastroenterology. 1999;117:918–25.
19. Angulo P, Smith C, Jorgensen RA, Keach JC, Dickson ER, Lindor KD. Budesonide in the treatment of patients with primary biliary cirrhosis with suboptimal response to ursodeoxycholic acid. Hepatology 1999;20:471 (abstract).

# 29 Therapy of primary sclerosing cholangitis

U. BEUERS and G. PAUMGARTNER

## INTRODUCTION

Primary sclerosing cholangitis (PSC) is a chronic progressive fibrosing disease of the intrahepatic and/or extrahepatic bile ducts. Men are more often affected than women (2:1), and an accompanying chronic inflammatory bowel disease, most frequently ulcerative colitis, is seen in 70–80% of patients. The main age of manifestation is 25–40 years, but PSC has been diagnosed between the ages of 2 and 80 years[1–3]. In most untreated patients PSC progresses to liver cirrhosis. Mean life expectancy after diagnosis for patients with untreated PSC was 10–12 years in follow-up studies with large interindividual variations[1–3]. Among the major risks are complications of cirrhosis, liver failure, and cholangiocarcinoma, which develops at a frequency of about 8% during an observation period of one decade[3].

The aetiopathogenesis of PSC is unclear at present, but the recent gain in knowledge has allowed the formation of a plausible hypothetical model of PSC[4]. This model indicates that PSC is an immune-mediated disease caused by an agent/toxin of putatively intestinal origin which affects immunogenetically susceptible subjects by initiating complex cytokine- and chemokine-mediated processes at the level of the bile ducts[4].

A careful look at a typical histological specimen of a patient with PSC mirrors the problems a clinician is confronted with when he or she considers adequate treatment for the patient who suffers from PSC. On the one hand, there is a chronic inflammatory process in the (peri-)portal areas of the liver of unknown cause, which may call for some kind of anti-inflammatory treatment. On the other hand, progressive onion-skin-like fibrosis around the intrahepatic and extrahepatic bile ducts may be observed (although only in a minority of liver biopsies due to their small size) which might increasingly deprive the cholangiocytes of nutritional and oxygen support[4] and may lead to mechanical obstruction of the bile duct lumen. Mechanical obstruction of larger bile ducts may call for interventional treatment measures.

No specific curative treatment, either for the inflammatory process or for progressive fibrosis around the bile ducts, is so far available for patients with PSC. This chapter summarizes data on medical and interventional treatment of PSC. Indication, timing and outcome of liver transplantation as the treatment of choice in late-stage disease of the patient with PSC-related liver cirrhosis will be discussed by Professor Neuberger in another chapter of these proceedings.

## MEDICAL TREATMENT

### Anti-inflammatory/immunosuppressive agents (Table 1)

In clinical practice, patients with PSC sometimes need treatment with immunosuppressive drugs such as corticosteroids or azathioprine for their accompanying inflammatory bowel disease. No clear benefit of immunosuppressive treatment for bile duct disease has been described under these conditions. For treatment of PSC only two randomized, placebo-controlled trials of immunosuppression were performed.

Cyclosporin administered at doses of 3 mg/kg per day did not improve symptoms, serum liver tests, or survival when compared to placebo[5] in 34 patients with PSC during a 2-year treatment period. A trend towards delay of histological progression was observed[5].

Methotrexate administered at doses of 15 mg/week for 2 years did not improve symptoms, serum liver tests (other than alkaline phosphatase), histological and cholangiographic findings or survival when compared to placebo in 24 patients with PSC[6]. This study was weakened by inclusion of 12 patients (50%) with stage 4 disease (cirrhosis). An uncontrolled pilot study had shown some improvement of serum liver tests and of inflammatory activity in liver of patients with early-stage disease[7].

In a series of uncontrolled studies a number of drugs have been tested in small groups of patients. Neither budesonide[8] nor nicotine[9], pentoxifylline[10] or prednisone combined with colchicine[11] showed any beneficial effect on serum liver tests. Treatment with tacrolimus for 12 months led to some improvement of serum liver tests[12]. These data, however, await approval in a randomized, placebo-controlled trial.

In summary, these studies do not admit recommendation of any of the anti-inflammatory/immunosuppressive drugs evaluated so far for the long-term treatment of patients with PSC.

### Antifibrotic treatment

Two drugs with antifibrotic activity, colchicine and penicillamine, have been evaluated in well-designed randomized, placebo-controlled trials. Colchicine, administered at a dose of 1 mg/day for 3 years, was completely ineffective with regard to symptoms, serum liver tests, histological features or survival when compared to placebo treatment in 84 patients[13].

**Table 1** Medical treatment of PSC as evaluated in randomized, placebo-controlled trials (RCT) or in pilot studies (P) which included eight or more patients with PSC

| *Agent* | *Study design* | *Patients (n)* | *Reference* | *Recommendation for treatment (November 1999)* |
|---|---|---|---|---|
| *Anti-inflammatory/immunosuppressive agents* | | | | |
| Cyclosporin | RCT | 34 | 5 | No |
| Methotrexate | RCT | 24 | 6 | No |
| | P | 10 | 7 | |
| Budesonide | P | 21 | (8) | (No) |
| Nicotine | P | 8 | 9 | No |
| Pentoxifylline | P | 20 | (10) | (No) |
| Prednisone/ colchicine | P | 12 | 11 | No |
| Tacrolimus | P | 10 | 12 | No |
| *Antifibrotic agents* | | | | |
| Colchicine | RCT | 84 | 13 | No |
| Penicillamine | RCT | 70 | 14 | No |
| *Anticholestatic agents* | | | | |
| Ursodeoxycholic acid (≥ 10 mg/kg/per day) | | | | Yes |
| | RCT | 14 | 17 | |
| | P/RCT | 20 | 18 | |
| | RCT | 105 | 19 | |
| | RCT | 24 | (20) | |
| | RCT | 18 | (21) | |
| | P | 15 | 15 | |
| | P | 12 | 16 | |

Pencillamine at a dose of 750 mg/day was not only ineffective with regard to symptoms, serum liver tests, histological progression or survival, but caused major side-effects in 21% of patients[14].

Thus, antifibrotic treatment using the above-mentioned drugs is not justified in patients with PSC.

## Anticholestatic treatment

Improvement of serum liver tests in patients with PSC treated with ursodeoxycholic acid (UDCA) was reported in pilot studies 10 years ago[15,16]. In a small, randomized, placebo-controlled trial which included 14 patients for a treatment period of 1 year, significant improvement of serum liver tests including bilirubin, gammaglutamyltransferase (GGT), alkaline phosphatase and serum aminotransferases was observed in patients treated with UDCA at a dose of 13–15 mg/kg a day as compared to placebo-treated patients. In addition, a multiparametric score revealed significant improvement of histological features in patients treated with UDCA mainly due to decrease of inflammatory activity[17]. A 3-year pilot study with a placebo-controlled study period which included 20 patients showed significant improvement of serum activities of alkaline phosphatase, GGT and aminotransferases during UDCA treatment as compared to placebo. Portal inflammation improved significantly in comparison to pretreatment conditions[18]. The largest trial published so far ($n$ = 105 patients) also revealed significant improvement of serum bilirubin levels and other serum liver tests in patients treated with UDCA as compared to placebo-treated patients. An analysis of liver histology was not reported, and a difference in survival free of liver transplantation during a median follow-up of 2.2 years was not observed[19]. Finally, improvement of serum liver tests and liver inflammatory activity was reported in a preliminary publication from Oxford, UK, when UDCA was administered at a daily dose of 20 mg/kg[20] ($n$ = 24), but not at 10 mg/kg[21] ($n$ = 18). Thus, the adequate dose may play a role when patients with PSC are treated with UDCA, and 15 mg/kg may today be regarded as the minimum recommended daily dose in the treatment of PSC.

None of the controlled studies showed significant effects on symptoms or survival free of liver transplantation. However, it must be kept in mind that more than 500 patients with primary biliary cirrhosis (PBC) had to be observed for a period of 4 years before a significant survival benefit of UDCA treatment was detected[22]. In addition, significant improvement of serum bilirubin in two of the studies[17,19] is remarkable as serum bilirubin levels are a strong prognostic marker in PSC[23] and the prognostic value is not affected by UDCA treatment in patients with PBC[24].

As no major side-effects were reported during UDCA long-term treatment, UDCA can be recommended for treatment of PSC at daily doses of at least 15 mg/kg, although its efficacy with regard to transplant-free survival has not been proven in this disease.

Experimental evidence indicates that UDCA may exert its anticholestatic effect at different levels[25]: at the level of the bile ducts, UDCA (at millimolar concentrations) reduces bile duct injury caused by hydrophobic bile acids[26,27]; at the level of the liver cells, UDCA (at micromolar concentrations) improves the impaired hepatobiliary secretion of hepatocytes[28,29]. This effect may at least in part be explained by UDCA-induced stimulation of hepatobiliary exocytosis and, thereby, insertion of transport proteins into the canalicular membranes of cholestatic hepatocytes[25,30,31]. In addition to these anticholestatic effects, UDCA has recently been shown to exert antiapoptotic effects[32,33].

## ENDOSCOPIC TREATMENT

Medical treatment alone insufficiently affects the natural course of PSC. In an 8-year follow-up study, patients treated continuously with UDCA developed strictures of the large bile ducts over time[34]. The more advanced the disease, the higher was the percentage of patients with strictures of large bile ducts[34].

Although no data from controlled trials are available for endoscopic treatment, a number of studies showed that dilation and/or stenting of major strictures led to an overall clinical and/or biochemical improvement in 60–80% of patients[35–39]. As long-term stenting may increase the risk of ascending bacterial cholangitis, short-term stenting was proposed for patients with PSC. The most recent publication on short-term stenting in PSC reported a 4-year experience with this technique[40]. In 32 patients with dominant strictures, 10-Fr stents were placed for a mean period of 11 days. Cholestatic symptoms improved after 2 months in 83% of patients, 80% were re-intervention-free after 1 year and 60% after 3 years; 24-hour antibiotic prophylaxis was always administered[40].

Do these measures affect the prognosis of patients with PSC? An 8-year follow-up study provided an excellent prognosis for patients with PSC under combined treatment with UDCA and endoscopic measures. When the prognosis of these patients was compared to their estimated survival as evaluated by the Mayo model for PSC, transplant-free survival was significantly improved[34].

Thus, endoscopic treatment of dominant strictures by dilation and/or short-term stenting should be part of the treatment in patients with PSC. Prophylactic administration of antibiotics during and after endoscopic retrograde cholangiography (ERC) (e.g. 1 day) is highly recommended[41].

## SURGICAL TREATMENT

In most centres bile duct surgery – with the exception of cholecystectomy – is avoided in PSC and has been largely replaced by endoscopic interventions because prior abdominal surgery may increase mortality after liver transplantation[42]. Liver transplantation is the recommended treatment in cirrhotic patients with late-stage disease. One-year survival has been reported to be above 85% in experienced centres[43].

## SUMMARY AND OUTLOOK

At present no specific curative treatment of PSC exists. Available data indicate that the natural course of PSC may be beneficially affected by medical treatment

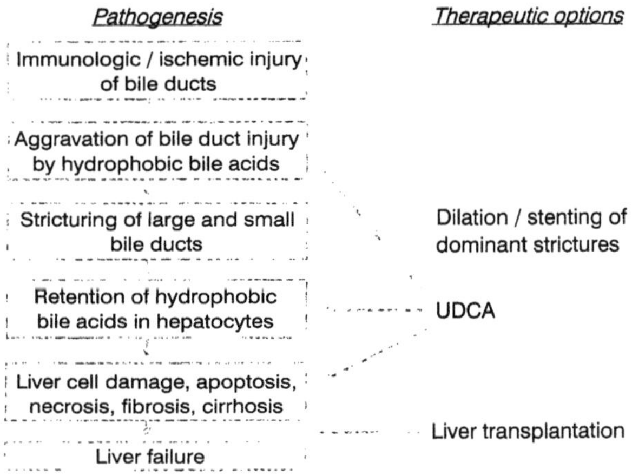


**Fig. 1** Pathogenetic mechanisms putatively involved in the progression of primary sclerosing cholangitis. Detailed considerations on the aetiopathogenesis of PSC ('immunological/ischaemic bile duct injury') have recently been published[4]. Therapeutic options are discussed in the text

with UDCA at adequate doses, endoscopic measures for dilation of dominant bile duct strictures, and liver transplantation in end-stage disease.

Future efforts should be directed towards the elucidation of the pathomechanisms leading to portal inflammation and bile duct fibrosis in early stages of PSC and therapeutic agents will probably be specifically targeted against cytokines and chemokines involved in the initiation of bile duct injury.

## References

1. Lee Y-M, Kaplan MM. Primary sclerosing cholangitis. N Engl J Med. 1995;332:924–33.
2. Angulo P, Lindor KD. Primary sclerosing cholangitis. Hepatology. 1999;7:325–32.
3. Broomé U, Olsson R, Lööf L *et al.* Natural history and prognostic factors in 305 Swedish patients with primary sclerosing cholangitis. Gut. 1996;38:610–15.
4. Vierling JM. Aetiopathogenesis of primary sclerosing cholangitis. In: Manns MP, Chapman RW, Stiehl A, Wiesner R, editors. Primary Sclerosing Cholangitis. Lancaster: Kluwer; 1998:37–45.
5. Wiesner R, Steiner B, LaRusso N, Lindor K, Baldus W. A controlled clinical trial evaluating cyclosporin in the treatment of primary sclerosing cholangitis. Hepatology. 1991;14:63A (abstract).
6. Knox TA, Kaplan MM. A double-blind controlled trial of oral-pulse methotrexate therapy in the treatment of primary sclerosing cholangitis. Gastroenterology. 1994;106:494–9.
7. Knox TA, Kaplan MM. Treatment of primary sclerosing cholangitis with oral methotrexate. Am J Gastroenterol. 1991;86:546–52.
8. Angulo P, Batts KP, Jorgensen RA, Keach JC, LaRusso NF, Lindor KD. Budesonide in the treatment of primary sclerosing cholangitis: a pilot study. Hepatology. 1999;30:477A (Abstract).
9. Angulo P, Bharucha AE, Jorgensen RA *et al.* Oral nicotine in treatment of primary sclerosing cholangitis: a pilot study. Dig Dis Sci. 1997;44:602–7.
10. Bharucha AE, Jorgensen RA, Lichtman SN *et al.* A pilot study evaluating pentoxifylline in the treatment of primary sclerosing cholangitis. Hepatology. 1997;26:402A (abstract).
11. Lindor KD, Wiesner RH, Colwell LJ, Steiner B, Beaver S, LaRusso NF. The combination of prednisone and colchicine in patients with primary sclerosing cholangitis. Am J Gastroenterol. 1991;86:57–61.
12. Van Thiel DH, Carroll P, Abu-Elmagd K *et al.* Tacrolimus (FK 506), a treatment for primary sclerosing cholangitis: results of an open-label preliminary trial. Am J Gastroenterol. 1995;90:455–9.

13. Olsson R, Broomé U, Danielsson A *et al.* Colchicine treatment of primary sclerosing cholangitis. Gastroenterology. 1995;108:1199–203.
14. LaRusso NF, Wiesner RH, Ludwig J, MacCarty RL, Beaver SJ, Zinsmeister AR. Prospective trial of penicillamine in primary sclerosing cholangitis. Gastroenterology. 1988;95:1036–42.
15. Chazouilleres O, Poupon R, Capron J-P *et al.* Ursodeoxycholic acid for primary sclerosing cholangitis. J Hepatol. 1990;11:120–3.
16. O'Brien CB, Senior JR, Arora-Mirchandani R, Batta AK, Salen G. Ursodeoxycholic acid for the treatment of primary sclerosing cholangitis: a 30-month pilot study. Hepatology. 1991;14:838–47.
17. Beuers U, Spengler U, Kruis W *et al.* Ursodeoxycholic acid for treatment of primary sclerosing cholangitis: a placebo controlled trial. Hepatology. 1992;16:707–14.
18. Stiehl A, Walker S, Stiehl L *et al.* Effects of ursodeoxycholic acid on liver and bile duct disease in primary sclerosing cholangitis. A 3 years' pilot study with a placebo-controlled study period. J Hepatol. 1994;20:57–64.
19. Lindor KD and the Mayo PSC/UDCA Study Group. Ursodiol for the treatment of primary sclerosing cholangitis. N Engl J Med. 1997;336:691–5.
20. Mitchell SA, Bansi D, Hunt N *et al.* High dose ursodeoxycholic acid (UDCA) in primary sclerosing cholangitis (PSC): results after two years of a randomized double-blind, placebo-controlled trial. Gut. 1997;40(Suppl.1):TH 115 (abstract).
21. Lo SK, Herrmann R, Chapman RW *et al.* Ursodeoxycholic acid in primary sclerosing cholangitis: a double-blind placebo-controlled trial. Hepatology. 1992;16:92A (abstract).
22. Poupon RE, Lindor KD, Cauch-Dudek K, Dickson ER, Poupon R, Heathcote EJ. Combined analysis of randomized controlled trials of ursodeoxycholic acid in primary biliary cirrhosis. Gastroenterology. 1997;113:884–90.
23. Wiesner RH, Grambsch PM, Dickson ER *et al.* Primary sclerosing cholangitis: natural history, prognostic factors and survival analysis. Hepatology. 1989;10:430–6.
24. Bonnand AM, Heathcote EJ, Lindor KD, Poupon RE. Clinical significance of serum bilirubin level under ursodeoxycholic acid therapy in patients with primary biliary cirrhosis. Hepatology. 1999;29:39–43.
25. Beuers U, Boyer JL, Paumgartner G. Ursodeoxycholic acid in cholestasis: potential mechanisms of action and therapeutic applications. Hepatology. 1998;28:1449–53.
26. Heuman DM, Bajaj RS, Lin Q. Adsorption of mixtures of bile salt taurine conjugates to lecithin –cholesterol membranes: implications for bile salt toxicity and cytoprotection. J Lipid Res. 1996;37:562–73.
27. Van Nieuwkerk CM, Oude Elferink RP, Groen AK *et al.* Effects of ursodeoxycholate and cholate feeding on liver disease in FVB mice with a disrupted mdr2 P-glycoprotein gene. Gastroenterology. 1996;111:165–71.
28. Jazrawi RP, de Caestecker JS, Goggin PM *et al.* Kinetics of hepatic bile acid handling in cholestatic liver disease: effect of ursodeoxycholic acid. Gastroenterology. 1994;106:134–42.
29. Stiehl A, Rudolph G, Sauer P, Theilmann L. Biliary secretion of bile acids and lipids in primary sclerosing cholangitis. Influence of cholestasis and effect of ursodeoxycholic acid treatment. J Hepatol. 1995;23:283–9.
30. Beuers U, Nathanson MH, Isales CM, Boyer JL. Tauroursodeoxycholic acid stimulates hepatocellular exocytosis and mobilizes extracellular $Ca^{++}$ mechanisms defective in cholestasis. J Clin Invest. 1993;92:2984–93.
31. Beuers U, Bilzer M, Chittattu A *et al.* Inhibition of bile flow, hepatobiliary exocytosis, and mrp2-insertion into the canalicular membrane by taurolithocholic acid is reversed by tauroursodeoxycholic acid in the perfused rat liver. Hepatology. 1999;30:463A (abstract).
32. Benz C, Angermüller S, Töx U *et al.* Effect of tauroursodeoxycholic acid on bile-acid-induced apoptosis and cytolysis in rat hepatocytes. J Hepatol. 1998;28:99–106.
33. Rodriguez CMP, Fan G, Ma X, Kren BT, Steer CJ. A novel role for ursodeoxycholic acid in inhibiting apoptosis by modulating mitochondrial membrane perturbation. J Clin Invest. 1998;101:2790–9.
34. Stiehl A, Rudolph G, Sauer P *et al.* Efficacy of ursodeoxycholic acid and endoscopic dilation of major duct stenoses in primary sclerosing cholangitis. An 8-year prospective study. J Hepatol. 1997;26:560–6.
35. Johnson GK, Geenen JE, Venu RP, Hogan WJ. Endoscopic treatment of biliary duct strictures in sclerosing cholangitis: follow up assessment of a new therapeutic approach. Gastrointest Endosc. 1987;33:9–12.

36. Gaing AA, Geders JM, Cohen SA, Siegel JH. Endoscopic management of primary sclerosing cholangitis: review and report of an open series. Am J Gastroenterol. 1993;88: 2000–8.
37. van Milligen AWM, van Bracht J, Rauws EAJ *et al.* Endoscopic stent therapy for dominant extrahepatic bile duct strictures in primary sclerosing cholangitis. Gastrointest Endosc. 1996;44:293–9.
38. Lee JG, Schutz SM, England RE, Leung JW, Cotton PB. Endoscopic therapy of sclerosing cholangitis. Hepatology. 1995;21:661–7.
39. Wagner S, Gebel M, Meier P *et al.* Endoscopic management of biliary tract strictures in primary sclerosing cholangitis. Endoscopy. 1996;28:546–51.
40. Ponsioen CY, Lam K, van Milligen de Wit AWM, Huibregtse K, Tygat GNJ. Four years' experience with short term stenting in primary sclerosing cholangitis. Am J Gastroenterol. 1999;94:2403–7.
41. Olsson R, Björnsson E, Bäckman L *et al.* Bile duct bacterial isolates in primary sclerosing cholangitis: a study of explanted livers. J Hepatol. 1998;28:426–32.
42. Farges O, Malassagne B, Sebagh M, Bismuth H. Primary sclerosing cholangitis: liver transplantation or biliary surgery. Surgery. 1995;117:146–55.
43. Neuberger J. Liver transplantation in autoimmune liver diseases. In: Manns MP, Paumgartner G, Leuschner U, editors. Immunology and Liver. Lancaster: Kluwer; 2000.

# 30
# New steroids and new immunosuppressive drugs in autoimmune liver disease

U. LEUSCHNER

## INTRODUCTION

Immunosuppressive drugs have been used for 40 years for the treatment of autoimmune chronic active hepatitis. The best-known substances are hydrocortisone, prednisone and prednisolone. Prednisolone is a metabolite of prednisone and its effect on autoimmune hepatitis does not differ from that of prednisone. To reduce corticoid-related side-effects, glucocorticoids were combined with the antimetabolite azathioprine. Combination therapy with glucocorticoids and azathioprine is now the standard treatment of autoimmune chronic active hepatitis.

Because of severe side-effects, an intolerance of standard therapy, and because in some patients combination therapy with glucocorticoids and azathioprine is contraindicated, alternative immunosuppressive agents were necessary having a maximal efficacy and minimal adverse effects. Further, since liver transplantation has become one of the most important options for treatment of final-stage chronic liver disease, stronger immunosuppressive substances with considerably fewer side-effects were needed in order to prevent allograft rejection.

## NEW IMMUNOSUPPRESSIVE DRUGS

Cyclosporin A (CsA) was isolated from a fungus (*Tolypocladium inflatum*) and introduced into therapy in 1978. It quickly became established as the predominant drug after liver transplantation when used in combination with prednisone (or prednisolone) and azathioprine. One-year patient survival improved from 40% to 74%, although there are no controlled studies comparing the two treatment regimens[1].

Later more powerful immunosuppressants have been developed, such as tacrolimus (the former FK506) and mycophenolate-mofetil, for treatment of allograft recipients. CsA was compared to FK506 in two liver transplantation studies in 1994[2,3]. Tacrolimus reduced the rejection episodes compared to CsA but was not superior concerning graft or patient survival. Therefore the use of FK506 has been proposed in the early post-transplantation period when the risk of rejection is greater, and the less potent CsA in lower doses after a treatment period of 3–4 years[4]. At that time withdrawal, or at least reduction, of steroids is obviously possible in about 20% of the patients, as shown in several studies[5–7].

The new immunosuppressants have not been used exclusively after liver transplantation, but they have been used in other autoimmune liver diseases, e.g. chronic active autoimmune hepatitis, primary biliary cirrhosis (PBC) and primary sclerosing cholangitis (PSC) (Table 1). In addition, cytostatics, the bile acid ursodeoxycholic acid (UDCA) and the leukotriene antagonist Pranlukast have been used. Anti-interleukin-2 receptor antibodies, anti-CD3 antibodies and the very interesting CD154 antibody (hu5C8) are still experimental, although promising[8–12]. CD154 is the ligand for the receptor CD40. The CD154-specific monoclonal antibody allowed renal allotransplantation in outbred MHC-mismatched rhesus monkeys without acute rejection[13] and the effect persisted for more than 10 months after treatment end. No further drugs were required and the animals remained healthy during and after therapy. Although the CD154 antibody was used after renal transplantation in non-human primates, the promising agent or a similar antibody could possibly also be beneficial in liver transplant recipients and in humans.

## TREATMENT OF AUTOIMMUNE LIVER DISEASES

### Budesonide

The topical steroid budesonide (Table 1) has been used in patients with chronic autoimmune hepatitis, primary biliary cirrhosis[14,15] and after liver transplantation

**Table 1** 'New' immunosuppressive drugs in autoimmune liver diseases

| | | |
|---|---|---|
| Topical steroid | Budesonide | Autoimmune hepatitis, PBC, liver rejection in rats |
| Drugs used after liver transplant | Cyclosporin A | Autoimmune hepatitis, PBC, liver rejection, chronic hepatitis C |
| | Tacrolimus | Autoimmune hepatitis, liver rejection |
| | Mycophenolate | Liver rejection |
| Cytostatics | Cyclophosphamide | Autoimmune hepatitis |
| | Chlorambucil | Autoimmune hepatitis |
| | Fludarabine | Autoimmune hepatitis |
| Other substances | Ursodeoxycholic acid | PBC, PSC, acute hepatitis, chronic hepatitis, liver rejection |
| | Methotrexate | PBC, autoimmune hepatitis |
| | Pranlukast | PBC |
| Experimental | Anti-IL-2 | |
| | FTY720, CTLA4 Ig, anti-CD80/86 | |
| | Anti-Fas L | |
| | CD154 antibody (hu5C8): kidney | |
| | Others | |

in rats. Budesonide is a non-halogenated glucocorticoid which is rapidly absorbed in the small intestine. Its relative receptor binding affinity to glucocorticoid receptors is 100 times higher than that of hydrocortisone, 50 times higher than that of prednisolone and 20 times higher than that of methylprednisolone (Table 2). Systemic bioavailability of budesonide is 10–15% compared to 55% of hydrocortisone, and 76% and 70% of methylprednisolone and prednisone, respectively[16]. Budesonide is metabolized to 16$\alpha$-hydroxy-prednisolone and 6$\beta$-hydroxy-budesonide. The glucocorticoid activity of these two metabolites is about one-tenth to one-hundredth of budesonide.

In an open study 13 patients with chronic autoimmune hepatitis were treated with 6–8 mg budesonide per day over a period of 6–10 weeks[14]. Thereafter the dose was individualized (2–6 mg/day) according to laboratory data. The total treatment time was 9 months. During therapy the improvement in liver function tests was statistically significant ($p < 0.01$). The frequency of side-effects was low. There was a marginal reduction of serum cortisol concentrations. When patients were stratified into groups with and without liver cirrhosis the decrease in the cirrhosis group was statistically significant due to portosystemic shunts ($p < 0.01$).

In a randomized double-blind trial with 40 patients with PBC, 3 × 3 mg budesonide plus UDCA (10–15 mg/kg per day) improved liver function tests significantly ($p < 0.05$–$0.001$) compared to a group treated with UDCA and placebo. Liver histology also improved. Plasma cortisol concentrations decreased but did not reach abnormally low concentrations. After 2 years' total treatment time adrenocorticotrophic hormone (ACTH)-stimulated cortisol secretion was regular in both treatment groups. Bone mineral density measured by DEXA decreased slightly but not significantly in both groups[15].

In the rat budesonide has been given after liver transplantation using an acute rejection model[17]. In the study groups treated with three different doses of budesonide the dosage of 1 mg/kg per day prevented histomorphological alterations which correlated with alanine aminotransferase (ALT) and aspartate transaminase (AST) and alkaline phosphatase levels in the serum. Lower doses were not as effective. The authors conclude that the topical glucocorticoid budesonide has a beneficial effect on liver allograft rejection.

## Cyclosporin A, tacrolimus

Cyclosporin A, tacrolimus and mycophenolate mofetil (MMF) have been used in patients with autoimmune hepatitis. Most studies report on very small patient numbers in corticosteroid-resistant type I hepatitis.

**Table 2** Relative receptor binding affinity (RBA) of different glucocorticoids in humans

| | |
|---|---|
| Hydrocortisone | 8 |
| Prednisolone | 16 |
| Methylprednisolone | 42 |
| Betamethasone | 58 |
| Budesonide | 845 |
| Beclomethasone monopropionate | 1022 |
| Fluticasone propionate | 1800 |

Dexamethasone RBA = 100.

In a 51-year-old man with type I autoimmune hepatitis refractory to corticosteroids, CsA dramatically reduced systemic symptoms and inflammation. This patient initially responded to corticosteroids but later became resistant[18]. In a 14-year-old boy with chronic autoimmune hepatitis and growth failure due to glucocorticoid therapy, CsA improved ALT and normalized growth[19]. In 1994 six patients with corticoid- or corticoid–azathioprine-resistant type I autoimmune hepatitis and considerable side-effects were treated with CsA administered orally twice per day in doses ranging from 3 to 6 mg/kg[20]. Five of the six patients nearly normalized ALT within 10 weeks. Remission was sustained for up to 1 year, as long as therapeutic CsA levels were maintained. Histology improved in all three patients in whom liver biopsies were taken. According to these three studies CsA appears to have a beneficial effect on liver function tests, symptoms and liver histology in those patients who do not fully respond to glucocorticoids alone or in combination with azathioprine.

In a pilot study CsA was given to 10 patients with chronic hepatitis C (genotype 1b) not responding to interferon therapy. Oral CsA was given for 3 months in increasing doses from 1.5–2.0 to 3.0–4.0 mg/kg per day. Serum ALT, AST and *g*-glutamyl transpeptidase gradually decreased in all but one patients, while HCV-RNA titres determined by reverse transcription polymerase chain reaction (RT-PCR) did not change. Whether this a positive effect on the course of the disease is unknown[21].

There are two placebo-controlled double-blind studies with patients with PBC[22,23]. In one study with 29 patients CsA was administered in a dose of 4 mg/kg per day. Fatigue and itching stabilized, bilirubin, ALT, alkaline phosphatase, $\gamma$-globulins and antimitochondrial antibody (AMA) decreased significantly[22]. Liver histology deteriorated in 1/13 patients in the CsA group and in 5/7 in the placebo group. In the second study, with 349 patients who were followed up for 6 years, CsA was administered in a dose of 3 mg/kg per day[23]. In the CsA-treated group albumin, alkaline phosphatase, bilirubin and ALT improved modestly, but serum creatinine deteriorated significantly. Survival was not prolonged. Fatigue and liver histology did not improve. Considering the toxicity of CsA the results of this long-lasting study with a large number of patients were disappointing.

The first report on tacrolimus in patients with autoimmune hepatitis was published in 1995[24]. The immunosuppressive activity of FK506 is 10–200 times greater than that of cyclosporin. Twenty-one patients were treated with an oral dose of 3 mg twice per day over a period of 12 months. Tacrolimus was successful, the response to therapy was rapid and sustained, but a minor increase of serum blood urea nitrogen (BUN) and creatinine levels occurred. The authors anticipated that with continued therapy hepatic failure and the necessity of liver transplantation may be averted.

## Cytostatics

Cytostatics, such as cyclophosphamide, fludarabine and chlorambucil, have been used for treatment of autoimmune hepatitis and PBC[25–28]. The number of patients treated is small. In 1997 three patients with severe autoimmune hepatitis who received cyclophosphamide in a dose of 1–1.5 mg/kg were treated with a tapering dose of corticosteroids beginning with 1 mg/kg per day. The authors observed neither relapse of the disease nor severe side-effects in a cumulative observation period of more than 12 years[26]. The dose of 3 mg/kg used previously was toxic and cannot be recommended for treatment of autoimmune hepatitis. The long-term toxicity of cyclophosphamide has been demonstrated in patients with rheumatoid arthritis and other diseases. With compounds such as cyclophosphamide, but also with CsA, FK506 and azathioprine, there seems to be an increased risk of developing malignancies (especially when the CD4/CD8 ratio is low)[29–31]. Chlorambucil has been used in only one study[28]. The results were dubious; depression of bone marrow occurred in 30% of the patients treated. Fludarabine has been used in one patient with steroid-resistant autoimmune hepatitis. The results were favourable.

## Ursodeoxycholic acid, methotrexate, Pranlukast

There are many studies in which the tertiary bile acid UCDA has been administered to patients with autoimmune hepatitis, PBC and PSC. Because UDCA seems to have only immunomodulatory but not immunosuppressive properties, it will not be discussed here but can be looked up in the literature[32].

Although methotrexate (MTX) is not a new drug it will be discussed briefly because recently the first placebo-controlled double-blind trial has been published[33], showing that low-dose MTX (7.5 mg/week) is not useful in PBC. Liver function parameters such as bilirubin, albumin, prothrombin time and the Mayo Score deteriorated in both groups; deterioration tended to be greater in the MTX group. The group with patients randomized to MTX also showed a trend towards a more frequent and earlier death or transplantation. This may be different in patients who responded incompletely to UDCA, and when treated with a higher dosage of 12–15 mg/kg[34].

In 1998 the first report on MTX being successful in the treatment of type I autoimmune hepatitis not responding to standard therapy with glucocorticoids and azathioprine was published[35]. MTX dosage was 7.5 mg/week, which resulted in normalisation of liver enzymes and improvement of histology.

Pranlukast is a leukotriene antagonist. It inhibits the infiltration of pulmonary alveoli by inflammatory cells in asthma patients and inhibits the release of leukotrienes by eosinophils[36]. When Pranlukast was administered in a dose of 450 mg/day to 12 patients with PBC stage I and II according to the Scheuer classification, in all patients alkaline phosphatase, $\gamma$-glutamyl transpeptidase, IgG and IgM decreased significantly ($p < 0.05$). The absolute eosinophil count improved 6 months after onset of therapy.

## Mode of action of immunosuppressants

Immunosuppressive drugs influence $Th_1$-related, $Th_2$-related and monocyte-related cytokine expression. The $Th_1$-related cytokines interleukin 2 and interferon gamma (IFN-$\gamma$) have proinflammatory properties. The expression is reduced by CsA and FK506. The monocyte-related tumour necrosis factor alpha (TNF-$\alpha$) perpetuates an existing inflammation and is inhibited by glucocorticoids, CsA and FK506. The $Th_2$-related cytokines IL-4 and IL-10 have anti-inflammatory properties. Fludarabine, for example, increases IL-4 and decreases

**Table 3** Major effects of modern immunosuppressants

| *Drug* | *T-cell proliferation/differentiation* | *B-cell proliferation/differentiation* | *Cytotoxicity* | *Cytokine production* |
| --- | --- | --- | --- | --- |
| Steroids | + | + | +<br>Prostaglandins–phospholipase A2 | IL-1, 2, 6, 8; TNF-$\alpha$ |
| Azathioprine → | 6-mercaptopurine<br>+ | +<br>| | |
| Cyclosporin A | +, $CD_4$ | (+) | +<br>Antibody-dependent cell toxicity | IL-2, 3, 4; IFN-$\gamma$; TNF-$\alpha$ |
| Tacrolimus | + | (+) | +<br>Free radicals, $NO_2/NO_3$ | IL-2, 3, 4; IFN-$\gamma$; TNF-$\alpha$ |
| Mycophenolate | + | + | Inhibits purine metabolism | |
| Pranlukast | Leukotriene antagonist suppressing eosinophil infiltration | | | |

+ = Suppresses.

the proinflammatory cytokine IL-2. Further, glucocorticoids, azathioprine, CsA, FK506 and MMF decrease differentiation and proliferation of T cells, while B cells are mainly influenced by glucocorticoids, azathioprine and MMF, to a lesser extent by the modern compounds CsA and FK506. Pranlukast prevents eosinophil infiltration of the liver (Table 3). The experimental FTY720 is synergistic with CsA but non-toxic and influences apoptosis[9]. Anti-Fas L, together with CTLA4 Ig or antiCD80/86, prolongs hepatocyte survival[12], while treatment with the humanized monoclonal antibody against CD154, which is a ligand of the CD40 receptor, mediates endothelial and antigen-presenting cell activation and facilitates their interaction with T cells and platelets[13]. Although CD154 has been used only after kidney transplantation, similiar agents could be of greatest interest also for liver recipients. Anti-IL-2 receptor antibodies (BT563) have already been used after liver transplantation in patients. They constitute a safe and efficient addition to the immunosuppressive regimen after liver transplant[8,10].

### Side-effects

Side-effects of immunosuppressants are listed in Table 4. Hyperglycaemia, nephrotoxicity, neurotoxicity, osteoporosis and the development of neoplasias are best known. Therefore one of the aims of the development of modern immunosuppressants needs to be the reduction of adverse reactions.

## SUMMARY

New immunosuppressive drugs have been used after liver transplantation, in chronic autoimmune hepatitis, in primary biliary cirrhosis and primary sclerosing cholangitis. Most of the modern drugs improved liver function tests, some of them liver histology, and they are less toxic compared to older compounds. New immunosuppressants influence $Th_1$-related, $Th_2$-related and monocyte-related cytokines, T- and B-cell differentiation and proliferation. Cytokine antibodies are still experimental, although first studies with IL-2 antibodies in humans have already been published.

**Table 4** Side-effects of immunosuppressants

| *Side-effects* | *Steroids* | *Azathioprine* | *CsA* | *FK506* | *MMF* |
|---|---|---|---|---|---|
| Nephrotoxicity | | | ++ | ++ | |
| Hypertension | + | | +++ | ++ | |
| Diabetes | +++ | | + | + | |
| Neurotoxicity | | | ++ | ++ | |
| Psychological complications | + | | + | + | |
| Hepatotoxicity | | + | + | + | |
| Myelotoxicity | | ++ | (+) | (+) | |
| Hyperlipidaemia | ++ | | | (+) | |
| Hirsutism | ++ | | + | | |
| Gingival hyperplasia | | | + | | |
| Malignancies | | (?) | + | (+) | |
| Intestinal bleeding | | | | | ++ |
| Infections | + | | + | + | + |

## References


1. Iwatsuki S, Starzl TE, Todd S *et al.* Experience in 1000 liver transplants and cyclosporin-steroid therapy: a survival report. Transplant Proc. 1988;20:498–504.
2. European FK506 Multicenter Liver Study Group. A randomized trial comparing tacrolimus (FK506) and cyclosporin in prevention of liver allograft rejection. Lancet. 1994;344:423–8.
3. The US Multicenter FK506 Liver Study Group. A comparison of tacrolimus (FK506) and cyclosporin for immunosuppression in liver transplantation. N Engl J Med. 1993;331:1110–15.
4. Lucey MR. Immunosuppression after liver transplantation. J Hepatol. 1996;24:503–5.
5. MacDiarmid SV, Farmer DA, Goldstein L *et al.* A prospective randomized trial of steroid withdrawal in orthotopic liver transplant recipients. Presented to the ASTP 14th Annual Meeting, Chicago, 1995.
6. Stegall MD, Wachs ME, Everson G *et al.* Prednisone withdrawal 14 days after liver transplantation with mycophenolate – a prospective trial of cyclosporin and tacrolimus. Transplantation. 1997;64:1755–60.
7. Gómez-Sanz R, Moreno E, Colina F *et al.* Steroid withdrawal is safe and beneficial in stable cyclosporin-treated liver transplant patients. J Hepatol. 1998;28:150–6.
8. Neuhaus P, Bechstein WO, Blumhardt G *et al.* Comparison of quadruple immunosuppression after liver transplantation with ATG or IL-2 receptor antibody. Transplantation. 1993;55:1320–7.
9. Suzuki S, Enosawa S, Kakefuda T *et al.* A novel immunosuppressant, FTY720, with a unique mechanism of action, induces long-term graft acceptance in rat and dog allotransplantation. Transplantation. 1996;61:200–5.
10. Langrehr JM, Glanemann M, Guckelberger O *et al.* A randomized, placebo-controlled trial with anti-interleukin-2 receptor antibody for immunosuppressive induction therapy after liver transplantation. Clin Transplant. 1998;12:303–12.
11. Reding R, Vraux H, de Ville de Goyet J *et al.* Monoclonal antibodies in prophylactic immunosuppression after liver transplantation. A randomized controlled trial comparing OKT3 and anti-IL-2 receptor monoclonal antibody LO-Tact-1. Transplantation. 1993;55:534–41.
12. Kawahara T, Yagita H, Kasai S *et al.* Allogenic hepatocyte transplantation: contribution of Fas–Fas ligand interaction to allogenic hepatocyte rejection. J Gastroenterol Hepatol. 1998;13(Suppl.):S119–23.
13. Kirk AD, Burkly LC, Batty DS *et al.* Treatment with humanized monoclonal antibody against CD154 prevents acute renal allograft rejection in nonhuman primates. Nat Med. 1999;5:686–93.
14. Danielson A, Prytz H. Oral budesonide for treatment of autoimmune chronic active hepatitis. Aliment Pharmacol Ther. 1994;8:585–90.
15. Leuschner M, Maier K-P, Schlichting J *et al.* Oral budesonide and ursodeoxycholic acid for treatment of primary biliary cirrhosis: results of a prospective double-blind trial. Gastroenterology. 1999;117:918–25.
16. Brattsand R. Overview of newer glucocorticoid preparations for inflammatory bowel disease. Can J Gastroenterol. 1990;4:407–14.
17. Weber T, Kalbhenn T, Herrmann G *et al.* Local immunosuppression with budesonide after liver transplantation in the rat. A preliminary histomorphological analysis. Transplantation. 1997;64:705–8.
18. Mistilis SP, Vickers CR, Dessoch MH *et al.* Cyclosporin, a new treatment for autoimmune chronic active hepatitis. Med J Aust. 1985;143:463–5.
19. Hyams JS, Ballow M, Leichther AM. Cyclosporin treatment of autoimmune chronic active hepatitis. Gastroenterology. 1987;93:890–3.
20. Sherman KE, Narkewicz M, Pinto PC. Cyclosporine in the management of corticosteroid-resistant type I autoimmune chronic active hepatitis. J Hepatol. 1994;21:1040–7.
21. Kakumu S, Takayanagi M, Iwata K *et al.* Cyclosporine therapy affects aminotransferase activity but not hepatitis C virus RNA levels in chronic hepatitis C. J Gastroenterol Hepatol. 1997;12:62–6.
22. Wiesner RH, Ludwig J, Lindor KD *et al.* A controlled trial of cyclosporine in the treatment of primary biliary cirrhosis. N Engl J Med. 1990;322:1419–24.
23. Lombard M, Portmann BP, Neuberger J *et al.* Cyclosporine A treatment in primary biliary cirrhosis: results of a long-term placebo controlled trial and effect on survival. Gastroenterology. 1993;104:519–26.

24. Van Thiel DH, Wright H, Carroll P *et al.* Tacrolimus: a potential new treatment of autoimmune chronic active hepatitis: results of an open-label preliminary trial. Am J Gastroenterol. 1995;90:771–6.
25. Gilmore IT, Cowan RE, Axon ATR *et al.* Controlled trial of cyclophosphamide in active chronic hepatitis. Br Med J. 1979;6171:1120–1.
26. Kanzler S, Gerken C, Dienes HP *et al.* Cyclophosphamide as alternative immunosuppressive therapy for autoimmune hepatitis – report of three cases. Z Gastroenterol. 1997;35:571–8.
27. Tassiulas IO, Davis JC, Fessler BJ *et al.* Fludarabine in nonmalignant disorders. In: Cheson BD, Keating MJ, Plunkett W, (editors). Nucleoside Analogs in Cancer Therapy. New York: Marcel Dekker; 1997:383–413.
28. Hoofnagle JH, Davis GL, Schafer DF *et al.* Randomized trial of chlorambucil for primary biliary cirrhosis. Gastroenterology. 1986;91:1327–34.
29. Silman AJ, Petrie J, Hazleman B *et al.* Lymphoproliferative cancer and other malignancy in patients with rheumatoid arthritis treated with azathioprine: a 20 year follow-up study. Ann Rheum Dis. 1988:47:988–92.
30. Nalesnik MA, Jaffe A, Starzl TE *et al.* The pathology of posttransplant lymphoproliferative disorders occurring in the setting of cyclosporine A–prednisolone immunosuppression. Am J Pathol. 1988;133:173–92.
31. Puri CP, Campbell RA. Cyclophosphamide and malignancy. Lancet. 1977;1:1306.
32. Berg PA, Leuschner U, (editors). Bile Acids and Immunology. Dordrecht: Kluwer; 1996.
33. Hendrickse MT, Rigney E, Giaffer MH *et al.* Low-dose methotrexate is ineffective in primary biliary cirrhosis: long-term results of a placebo-controlled trial. Gastroenterology. 1999;117:400–7.
34. Bonis PAL, Kaplan M. Methotrexate improves biochemical tests in patients with primary biliary cirrhosis who respond incompletely to ursodiol. Gastroenterology. 1999;117:395–9.
35. Burak KW, Urbanski SJ, Swain MG. Successful treatment of refractory type 1 autoimmune hepatitis with methotrexate. J Hepatol. 1998;29:990–3.
36. Kobayashi S, Yoshida K, Mori A *et al.* Inhibitory effect of ONO-1078, a novel leukotriene receptor antagonist, on human peripheral blood eosinophils. Jpn J Allergol. 1996;45:1166–71.

# 31 Transplantation for autoimmune liver disease

J. NEUBERGER

## INTRODUCTION

The three major autoimmune liver diseases are primary biliary cirrhosis (PBC), primary sclerosing cholangitis (PSC) and autoimmune hepatitis (AIH). Despite the widespread use of ursodeoxycholic acid (UDCA) for the treatment of PBC and PSC, and corticosteroids and azathioprine for AIH, many patients progress to end-stage liver disease or develop symptoms making life intolerable. For these patients liver transplantation may be indicated. In this chapter the indications and contraindications for liver transplantation will be discussed, together with the outcomes, postoperative complications and evidence for disease recurrence.

Although the number of patients transplanted in Europe for autoimmune liver diseases has remained roughly constant, these represent a reduction in the proportion of transplants because viral hepatitis and alcoholic liver disease are becoming increasingly common indications. Thus, data from the European Liver Transplant Registry[1] show that of the 13 676 primary liver transplants done in Europe between January 1988 and December 1997 for patients with cirrhosis, 2125 (16%) were for patients with PBC, 1032 (8%) were for PSC and only 584 (4%) were for AIH. In 1989 PBC was the primary indication in 40% of those grafted for cirrhosis; in 1995, it accounted for less than 20%. Although it might appear that the 1- and 5-year survival figure of 81% and 76% represent a cause for congratulation, these figures show a significant mortality and do not reflect morbidity. The long-term consequences of immunosuppressive therapy (such as renal failure and malignancy) emphasize the need for increasing efforts to find safe and effective remedies for the underlying condition, so that liver replacement becomes a therapy no longer required.

## INDICATIONS FOR TRANSPLANTATION

Liver transplantation is indicated for patients with liver disease either because of quality of life, because of the liver disease, that is unacceptable to the patient, or because the anticipated survival in the absence of transplantation is estimated to be less than 1 year.

### *Quality of life*

Assessing the quality of life for an individual patient is difficult and the clinician has to distinguish poor quality of life as a consequence of liver disease from other causes of poor quality, such as depression, side-effects of treatment and other treatable conditions. Since autoimmune liver diseases are associated with other autoimmune diseases, it is important to exclude diseases such as thyroid disease, Addison's disease and gluten-sensitive enteropathy.

### *Length of life*

Although most transplant centres consider transplantation when the anticipated length of life is less than 1 year, this figure is arbitrary and more detailed analysis of the risks and benefits of transplantation and surgical non-intervention is required to refine the process. In practice, however, the indications for transplantation are relatively well defined and these are summarized in Table 1. Once hepatic decompensation occurs, the short-term mortality starts to increase. The decision to place a patient on the transplant list will depend on many factors, summarized in a recent consensus document[2].

### *Contraindications to transplantation*

In general, these can be divided into those conditions which preclude good survival after surgery or those conditions which make it unlikely the patient will survive surgery, and for these the patients are referred to recent reviews. A summary is given in Table 2. It is important that these contraindications are regularly reviewed: for example, the advent of effective anti-retroviral agents may mean that transplantation of HIV-infected patients will become possible.

**Table 1** General indications for transplantation for chronic parenchymal disease

| |
|---|
| Serum bilirubin > 180 μmol/L for >6 months in cholestatic liver disease; > 50 μmol/L for non-cholestatic liver disease |
| Serum albumin < 30 g/L |
| Ascites resistant to treatment |
| Spontaneous bacterial peritonitis |
| Hepatic encephalopathy |
| Progressive muscle wasting |
| Recurrent variceal bleeding |
| Development of primary liver cell cancer* |
| Intractable pruritus/lethargy |
| Progressive osteopenia* |
| Hepatopulmonary syndrome* |

*These may also, paradoxically, be contraindications to liver replacement.

**Table 2** Contraindications for liver transplantation (although these will vary to some extent between centres and few are absolute)

| |
|---|
| Advanced age |
| Extensive portal and mesenteric vein thrombosis |
| Active bacterial/fungal/viral infection |
| HIV infection |
| Extrahepatic primary malignancy |
| Primary liver cell cancer extending outside the liver |
| Cholangiocarcinoma |
| Severe extrahepatic disease (cardiac, respiratory, neurological) preventing successful transplantation or rehabilitation) |

## TIMING OF TRANSPLANTATION AND USE OF PROGNOSTIC MODELS

The timing of transplantation is one of the more difficult areas in transplantation practice: transplantation too late in the course of the disease may increase the risk of the patient dying from the procedure, whereas transplantation too early may reduce the patient's life because of the small but finite risk of the patient dying from the surgery. Thus choosing the optimal time of transplantation depends on understanding the risks and benefits of surgery or no surgery at any time during the course of the patient's illness.

The development of prognostic models has given the clinician some guidance for selecting the optimal time for surgery. These models have been well developed for PBC[3–9] and less so for PSC[10–12]. There are very few prognostic models for patients with AIH, and indications for transplantation follow those for general parenchymal liver disease. These models compare well with each other[13]. In these models the risks of surviving in the absence of transplantation and the probability of surviving after transplantation can be estimated for an individual patient at any time during the course of the illness. Although these models have given considerable insight into the natural history of PBC, the use of these models remains limited. The models are developed from follow-up of patients: data collected at entry into the study are usually assessed using a Cox regression model[14]; those factors which correlate with death/survival are weighted and, using a simple formula, a prognostic index calculated. The prognostic index can be used to give an estimate of either the probability of surviving for a given period of time or the median survival probability. Extrapolation to the individual must be done with caution: the confidence interval may be wide. The validity of the model may be affected by changes in treatment. With the exception of the time-dependent model of Christensen *et al.*[15], these models are static: this means that for valid use the models can only be used once, when the patient presents.

### Prognostic models for PBC

Shapiro and colleagues[16] first emphasized the importance of serum bilirubin as a prognostic marker for PBC; subsequently others have developed prognostic markers and there are now several models that have been described (Table 3). While serum bilirubin remains the major prognostic factor, the presence of cirrhosis, age and serum albumin are also important prognostic factors. Ursodeoxycholic acid is used extensively for the treatment of patients with PBC; even though there is uncertainty whether the use of the drug affects the prognosis, there is overall agreement that the use of UDCA is associated with an improvement in liver tests. The Mayo Clinic model, when applied to patients with PBC treated with UDCA for 6 months, still accurately predicts outcome[17].

Other prognostic variables have been described: these include serum hyaluronic acid[18], procollagen peptide type III[19] and dynamic liver function tests such as the lignocaine metabolism (MEGX) test, indocyanine green clearance, caffeine clearance and galactose elimination capacity[20,21]. Although many of these markers and tests have been shown to correlate well with survival, none has yet achieved widespread use in clinical practice.

## Prognostic models for PSC

Fewer models for PSC have been described, and prognostic variables are defined in Table 4[22]. In contrast to PBC, the natural history of PSC is more variable, with a more fluctuating course which may in part depend on the presence of coincidental cholangitis.

### *Additional problems associated with PSC*

Selection and timing of transplantation in patients with PSC are associated with two additional problems: the presence of inflammatory bowel disease and the probability of cholangiocarcinoma.

In many patients with PSC there is coexisting inflammatory bowel disease, usually ulcerative colitis. In many patients the ulcerative colitis is often mild and may indeed be subclinical. There remains controversy in the literature to whether patients with PSC who have ulcerative colitis do have an increased risk of colonic neoplasia[23,24]. It is inappropriate to transplant patients with active colitis although, once this is treated, transplantation can be undertaken. Although some have suggested that patients with PSC and ulcerative colitis have a worse prognosis than those without clinical colitis[25], our own data do not support this (see below). In general, non-transplant surgical intervention in patients with PSC is unhelpful and may indeed increase the morbidity of transplantation[26,27], although in the rare cases of a single dominant extra-hepatic stricture in the patient without advanced cirrhosis, stenting, dilatation or biliary resection may be useful.

### *Cholangiocarcinoma*

The major diagnostic problem in patients with PSC is the increased risk of cholangiocarcinoma. Many studies have shown convincingly that the presence of cholangiocarcinoma has a significant adverse effect on survival after transplantation[22,28]. Smoking seems to be a risk factor for hepatobiliary malignancy[29]. In most cases the cholangiocarcinoma develops insidiously and it is often very difficult to diagnose this condition pretransplant[29]. Serum markers for cholangiocarcinoma, such as CEA and CA19–9, lack the necessary sensitivity and specificity required for a certain diagnosis of cholangiocarcinoma[30,31]. These

**Table 3** Prognostic factors in different models for prognosis PBC

| | *Age* | *Varical bleeding* | *Ascites* | *Bilirubin* | *PT* | *Hepatomegaly* | *Fibrosis* | *Cholestasis* | *Mallory's hyaline* | *Albumin* |
|---|---|---|---|---|---|---|---|---|---|---|
| European | + | | | + | | | + | + | | + |
| Mayo | + | | (+) | + | + | | | | | + |
| Yale | + | | | + | | + | + | | | |
| Australia | + | | | + | | | | | | + |
| Glasgow | + | + | + | + | | | + | + | + | |
| Oslo | | + | | + | | | | | | |
| Royal Free | + | | + | + | | | | | | + |

(+) = Oedema; PT = prothrombin time; fibrosis = fibrosis/cirrhosis.

**Table 4** Prognostic factors in different models for prognosis in PSC

| | *Age* | *Bilirubin* | *IBD* | *Hepatomegaly* | *Splenomegaly* | *Alkaline phosphatase* | *Stage* | *Haemoglobin* |
|---|---|---|---|---|---|---|---|---|
| Mayo | + | + | + | | | | + | + |
| King's | + | | | + | + | + | + | |
| Multicentre | + | + | | | + | | + | |

IBD = inflammatory bowel disease; stage = histological stage.

tumours are often difficult to visualize on imaging, whether by ERCP, PTC, ultrasound, CT scanning or MRI scanning[32,33]. We have found that biopsy of any possible stricture is highly specific but not very sensitive. Although brushings or bile cytology may be of value in this instance, it is often difficult to obtain satisfactory brushings of hilar lesions in those with extensive extrahepatic sclerosing cholangitis[34,35]. Furthermore, there is a significant risk of inducing biliary sepsis, which may be fatal. A high clinical suspicion and, where appropriate, frozen section histology during the laparotomy preceding hepatectomy, will reduce the number of liver replacements in this condition.

### *Survival after transplantation*

Comparison of outcome between centres is usually difficult because of differences in case-mix. Indeed, one centre with a patient 5-year survival of 85% may actually be doing worse than another with a 5-year survival of only 70% if the former are operating on less sick and lower-risk patients.

### *Prediction of survival after transplantation*

To predict survival after transplantation is of value for several reasons: not only does this allow for identification of the risk factors predicting survival but also, by comparing prognosis with and without transplantation, it allows the optimal timing of transplantation to be determined. Those factors which predict survival after transplantation are not necessarily those that predict survival without transplantation. Wiesner *et al.*[22] recently compared the predictive accuracy of the Child–Pugh score (developed to predict survival after shunt surgery) with the Mayo Risk score for PSC (developed to predict survival in the absence of transplantation) for survival and resource utilization after transplantation. They concluded that the Child–Pugh was a better overall predictor of outcome and resource utilization after transplantation. Of course, there are limitations with such an approach; nevertheless, useful clinical additional information can be gained.

*PSC* Univariate analysis of 118 patients grafted at the Liver Unit, Birmingham and followed for up to 9 years identified seven variables associated with a poor outcome after surgery[37]: high serum creatinine, high serum bilirubin, biliary tree malignancy, previous upper abdominal surgery, hepatic encephalopathy, ascites and coexisting Crohn's disease. In contrast, coexisting ulcerative colitis had a beneficial association with outcome. The final Cox model included inflammatory bowel disease, ascites, previous upper abdominal surgery, high serum creatinine and biliary tree malignancy. The model, validated in another group of patients with PSC, grafted in another centre, may help in understanding the timing of the procedure, and suggests that upper abdominal surgery pretransplant should, if possible, be avoided. The reasons for the discordant association of ulcerative colitis and Crohn's disease are uncertain.

*PBC* Assessment of those variables associated with a poor short-term survival after transplantation for PBC identified earlier year of transplant, ascites (with or without diuretic treatment), low serum albumin, high serum bilirubin, high serum urea and high serum creatinine, low serum sodium and rhesus negativity as significant factors[38]. In the final Cox regression model, year of transplant, albumin/age ratio, plasma bilirubin and ascites or diuretic treatment were the only factors included. Several of these factors also predict outcome in the absence of transplantation, although the prognostic value differs in the two models. By assessing the 6-month survival probability with and without transplantation, it can be clearly shown that there is a benefit of transplantation when the 6-month survival probability in the absence of transplantation falls below 0.85. However, it must be noted that patients may be grafted for conditions other than end-stage disease, and that patients should be listed at a time which will also reflect the likely length of wait for a liver to become available.

### *Survival after transplantation for PBC*

Between 1982 and 1995, in the Birmingham Liver Transplant Unit, 312 patients have been grafted for PBC. The overall 1-, 2- and 5-year survival values are 82.5%, 81.7% and 76%, respectively. As may be hoped for, results have improved during the lifetime of the unit with 1-, 2- and 5-year survival figures of 72.5%, 70.5% and 69.6% in patients grafted during the 1980s compared with the respective figures in patients grafted in the 1990s of 87.4%, 86.8% and 77.2%. This improvement in outcome may reflect a number of factors, including better selection, as well as improved immunosuppression, and better surgical, anaesthetic and microbiological techniques. Several studies have confirmed that the actual observed survival after transplantation is superior to the length of life predicted from prognostic models[39–42].

### *Survival after transplantation for PSC*

The number of patients transplanted for PSC is lower than for PBC, with 101 grafted between 1986 and 1995 in our unit. The overall 1-, 2- and 5-year survival figures are currently 79%, 75% and 68%; as with patients with PBC there has been an improvement in survival in patients grafted during the 1980s and the 1990s – with 1-, 2- and 5-year survival figures of 60%, 55% and 50% before 1990 compared with 84%, 80% and 73%. Seven patients had a cholangiocarcinoma, and in these patients 1-year survival was 29%. These figures compare with the European Liver Transplant Registry Data in which survival of 1032 patients grafted for PSC between 1988 and December 1997 was 81%, 71% and 67% at 1, 5 and 9 years respectively. Of the 101 patients with PSC, 65% had ulcerative colitis. The 1-, 2- and 5-year survival figures in these patients are, if anything, higher than in those without colitis, at 83%, 79% and 69%.

### *Survival after transplantation for AIH*

Survival after transplantation for patients with AIH is broadly similar to that seen after transplantation for other autoimmune liver diseases: in our own unit the overall survival rates for the 86 adult patients at 1, 3, 5 and 10 years are 83%, 74%, 72% and 69%; for those grafted after 1990 the 1-, 3- and 5-year survival figures are 89%, 80% and 78% respectively.

## Rejection post-transplant

Several studies have shown that patients with autoimmune liver disease are at greater risk of both acute and chronic allograft rejection[43–46]. For example, in our own series the incidence of severe acute allograft rejection at 7 days in patients grafted for PBC was 63%, for AIH 61% and for PSC 50%. In contrast, for patients grafted for liver disease where immune mechanisms were not implicated in the pathophysiology, acute rejection was found in 42% of those with alcoholic liver disease and in 37% of those with alcohol-related liver disease[43]. However, there is no difference in graft survival in patients with and without early acute graft rejection.

In contrast, ductopenic rejection is associated with graft loss: although there are many factors which are associated with ductopenic rejection, it does seem that all three autoimmune diseases are risk factors for graft loss from chronic rejection[42,47–48]. It remains unclear whether the immunosuppressive protocol used should be different according to the indication for transplant.

It also remains unclear why there is a higher incidence of acute and chronic rejection in patients grafted for autoimmune diseases. Farges *et al.*[44] suggested this may be due to pretransplant immunoglobulin protecting the patient from rejection, but this could not be confirmed in our series and does not explain why those with a toxic cause of acute liver failure have a lower risk than those with autoimmune disease.

## Quality of life after transplantation

Now that many of the technical problems of transplantation have been overcome, clinicians are starting to assess the quality of life after transplantation. While this can never be stated to be normal, it is better than no life at all[49,50,51].

### *Inflammatory bowel disease (IBD) after transplantation*

PSC is associated with IBD: the course of IBD in patients with PSC after transplantation is variable. Riley *et al.*[52] described the development of IBD in 14 of 6800 liver and kidney allograft recipients; all but two had received a liver graft, but of these 12 only two were grafted for PSC, the remainder for a variety of indications including four with autoimmune hepatitis. In a study of 30 patients, Papatheodoridis *et al.*[53] found that in half the colitis remained the same after transplantation, and in the other half the colitis deteriorated. Colitis developed *de novo* in three patients and none had developed colonic cancer. It is unknown why IBD will develop in patients already receiving immunosuppressive drugs which, in the ungrafted patient, are effective therapies.

## RECURRENCE OF AUTOIMMUNE LIVER DISEASE AFTER TRANSPLANTATION

If autoimmune disease is defined in the most simplistic way as an immune response against self-antigens, then in patients following transplantation the immune response will be against the donor alloantigen, on bile duct cells or hepatocytes which retain the donor phenotype. Thus, a more appropriate term may be 'alloimmune disease'.

Recurrent autoimmune disease has been suggested after transplantation of other organs, such as recurrent sarcoidosis in the lung[54] and autoimmune diabetes after pancreas transplantation[55]. The diagnosis of recurrent autoimmune disease in the allograft is often difficult, since there will be several confounding factors which may render invalid those diagnostic criteria which apply to the native liver.

*Immunosuppression* After transplantation, patients are maintained on immunosuppressive therapy using drugs which may also be used for the treatment of autoimmune disease. This may mask or modify the features of recurrent disease.

*Rejection* The graft remains at risk of rejection and it is unusual for an allograft biopsy to be devoid of infiltrating leukocytes. There may be overlap between the histological features of rejection from recurrent disease.

*Other causes of graft damage* The allograft may be affected by factors which are not found in the native liver, and may mimic features of recurrent disease. Such factors include infections (bacterial, viral or protozoan), ischaemia, preservation damage, reperfusion damage and drug toxicity.

*De novo autoimmunity* *de novo* autoimmune features may occur after transplantation. For example, Kerkar and colleagues[56] have reported that seven of 200 paediatric liver allograft recipients have, after transplantation, developed autoimmune liver disease associated with elevated titres of autoantibodies, elevated serum immunoglobulin G and histological features of chronic active hepatitis. The indications for transplantation were not those in which autoimmunity is believed to be implicated (such as extrahepatic biliary atresia or Alagille's syndrome). These autoimmune features, which became apparent at a median of 24 months after transplantation, responded well to increased immunosuppression. Heneghan and colleagues identified three adult liver allograft recipients who developed features of *de novo* autoimmune hepatitis after transplantation for Ecstasy overdose, HCV cirrhosis and PSC: in all three cases there was a significant transaminitis, liver/kidney microsomal antibodies at a titre greater than 1 in 640 and portal and periportal hepatitis on liver histology. Markers of inflammation resolved on treatment with high-dose corticosteroids[57]. In these cases the antigen may be the donor cytochrome P450 rather than the asialoglycoprotein receptor, the autoantigen in AIH.

## Primary sclerosing cholangitis

In the native liver the diagnosis of PSC is made on a combination of clinical, serological, pathological and radiological features. The clinical, biochemical and immunological findings (including the antineutrophil cytoplasmic antibody (ANCA)) are not specific for PSC. Although the histological features of fibrous cholangitis and fibro-obliterative lesions are characteristic of the condition, these are found in less than half the cases of PSC on needle biopsies and may be found in other conditions affecting the biliary tree. The definitive diagnosis of sclerosing cholangitis is made by imaging the biliary tree showing the characteristic dilatation and strictures affecting intrahepatic and/or extrahepatic biliary tree. Imaging will not, however, differentiate primary from secondary biliary cirrhosis, so the confirmation of primary sclerosing cholangitis is made by excluding the secondary causes. Many of the causes of secondary biliary cirrhosis will be present in the allograft. For example, most liver allograft recipients have Roux-en-Y loops fashioned at the time of surgery, which is associated with cholangitis and thus sclerosing cholangitis.

Sebagh and colleagues[58] studied 24 patients who developed non-anastomotic strictures after transplantation. The histological diagnosis of sclerosing cholangitis was made on the basis of periductal fibrosis and large-duct obstruction, and were present in 23 of the 24 cases. In all instances there were histological features present in the first postoperative year; cholangiographic features of sclerosing cholangitis were detected in all but two in the first year (median 3.5 months). Of these, 10 patients had ABO-incompatible grafts; 12 patients having hepatic artery thrombosis, three focal fibrointimal hyperplasia, four preservation-related ischaemia and three arteriopathic chronic ductopenia rejection (some patients had more than one possible risk factor). Thus, after transplantation, cholangitis may be attributed to several causes. Patel *et al.*[59] analysed 10 patients who underwent regrafting for non-anastomotic biliary strictures. Recurrence of biliary strictures requiring intervention was significantly more common in those regrafted for biliary strictures than those regrafted for other indications (50% compared with 11%, respectively).

It remains uncertain whether ANCA are markers of PSC or are implicated in the pathogenesis of the disease. Haagsma and colleagues[60] showed that titres of pANCA fall in the first few months after transplantation but thereafter rise, so that after 1 year the titres are similar to those found prior to surgery. In the nine patients studied between 3 and 48 months after transplantation there was no histological evidence of PSC recurrence. Our own studies have reached broadly similar conclusions, although in two ANCA became negative after transplantation.

In Birmingham, until recently, annual review protocol biopsies have been undertaken. We therefore assessed the histological features of PSC in 22 patients grafted for PSC who had survived more than 1 year compared with 22 patients who had been grafted for other indications but had a Roux-loop[61].

Although the latter group is useful for comparison, these patients clearly cannot be regarded as a true control. None of the patients had an ABO-incompatible graft, hepatic artery thrombosis or evidence (at the time of biopsy or subsequently) of arteriopathic or ductopenic rejection. The timing of the biopsies excluded the possibility of preservation damage. Features of biliary obstruction were seen in 10–32% of patients. Periductal fibrosis was observed more commonly in those grafted for PSC than either the Roux-control group or the general allograft population. The more characteristic fibro-obliterative lesions were found in only three of the patients grafted for PSC but in none of the other patients. Thus, in our experience, the histological features associated with PSO are seen more commonly in those grafted for PSC than in those grafted for other conditions. A recent study from the Mayo Clinic[62] reported findings in 150 patients transplanted for PSC, with a median follow-up of 55 months. Features suggestive of recurrent PSC were found in 20% of the 120 eligible patients. In 11 of these 24 patients, histological features compatible with recurrent PSC were reported. The median time to the diagnosis of recurrent disease was 421 days if the diagnosis was based on cholangiography and 42 months if based on histology. Five patients with recurrent PSC died and two underwent regrafting. In the control group only one of 464 had histological features of recurrent PSC. More recently, in an analysis of 380 patients grafted for PSC in Pittsburgh and followed for a median of 6 years follow-up, Abu-Elmagd and colleagues[63] reported recurrence of PSC in 52 grafts (13.7%) at a mean onset of 4 years after transplantation. The diagnosis of recurrence was made either on imaging the biliary tree or on histology. The probability of recurrence increased with time: 3.6% at 1 year, 12% at 5 years, 25% at 10 years. Factors associated with recurrence included older recipient age and the presence of inflammatory bowel disease.

Not all studies have confirmed these observations. Haagsma *et al.* found no histological features of recurrent PSC in the allograft in nine patients[60]. However, in a larger study, Sheng *et al.*[64] analysed the cholangiograms of 643 liver allograft recipients with a choledochojejunostomy. Overall, in those transplanted for conditions other than PSC, 13% had intrahepatic biliary strictures whereas 27% of those grafted for PSC had such strictures. When those with hepatic artery thrombosis were excluded, intrahepatic strictures were found in 18% of those grafted for PSC compared with 9% in the comparison group. That there was no statistically significant difference between the two groups (20 of 112 and 53 of 575 respectively) may be a consequence of small numbers rather than a true difference. Others have reported a greater incidence of biliary complications in patients grafted for PSC than for other indications[65,66], but in both series the numbers of patients were relatively small.

Thus, in conclusion, it therefore remains uncertain whether PSC recurs in the allograft. The uncertainty arises as a consequence of the difficulties in differentiating primary recurrent sclerosing cholangitis from secondary sclerosing cholangitis. Nonetheless, nearly all studies have shown that, when known causes of biliary strictures are excluded, those grafted for PSC have a greater probability of having both histological and radiological features compatible with the possibility of PSC than those grafted for other indications.

## Primary biliary cirrhosis (PBC)

As with PSC, the diagnosis of PBC in the native liver is made on the basis of the clinical, biochemical, immunological and histological features. The presence of antimitochondrial antibodies reacting with the components of the pyruvate dehydrogenase complex is virtually diagnostic of the condition[67]. However, in the allograft, demonstration of these antibodies may not imply disease recurrence, merely persistence of the immune or other abnormalities which allow development of the disease. After transplantation there is a small and transient fall in the titre of antimitochondrial antibody which is followed by a persistence of the AMA with a similar but not always identical antigen recognition[70]. Others[71] have shown that other PBC-specific autoantibodies, Sp100 and gp210, also persist after transplantation but do not correlate with histological evidence of disease recurrence. The persistence or *de-novo* development of the autoimmune conditions associated with PBC (such as thyroid disease or sicca syndrome) does not necessarily imply disease recurrence.

The possibility of disease recurrence has generated much controversy since the initial report of three patients with clinical and histological features of PBC in the allograft[67]. There is, however, consensus that the diagnosis of PBC recurrence can be made only on the basis of histology, which in the native liver is best described as a non-suppurative destructive cholangitis or a granulomatous cholangitis.

The bile ducts in the allograft may be affected in a variety of situations including acute and chronic rejection, graft versus host disease, ischaemia, drug toxicity and infections, notably hepatitis C virus. In most cases these possible diagnoses can be excluded by appropriate clinical or serological investigations. Granulomas around the bile ducts are strongly suggestive of recurrent PBC but granulomatous infiltration may be associated with a variety of causes including infection (viral, especially recurrent HCV, microbial, especially tuberculosis, foreign-body reaction) but granulomas occurring after 1 year are most commonly associated with recurrent PBC[68].

The initial report[67] suggesting recurrence of PBC was followed by a subsequent study in which three more patients with histological features of recurrent PBC were described. These histological features included bile duct damage, a predominantly lymphoid cell infiltrate around the portal tract, occasional granuloma formation, deposition of orcein-positive granules in the absence of cholestasis and bile duct proliferation[69]. One of these patients subsequently developed features of chronic ductopenic rejection and underwent regrafting. Examination of the explanted liver, however, failed to show any evidence of features suggestive of recurrent PBC.

Our own studies in Birmingham also suggest recurrence of PBC. In a prospective analysis of protocol biopsies, of 83 patients grafted for PBC who had survived for more than 1 year, histological features of recurrent PBC were found in 13 of 83 patients[70]. The histological features leading to the diagnosis of PBC in the allograft included a mononuclear cell portal tract infiltrate, portal granulomas, bile duct damage and disappearance, and bile ductular proliferation. Of the 13 patients, the disease was at histological stage 1/2 apart from one patient who had developed a cirrhosis. The features were patchy and were not always seen in subsequent biopsies. None of these features was seen in biopsies from 100 patients grafted for other conditions, followed for a similar period and treated with a similar immunosuppressive protocol.

Some studies have shown similar results. For instance, Balan and colleagues[72] evaluated 60 patients who had survived for more than 1 year after liver transplantation for PBC at a median period of 3.3 years. At the time of the analysis, 55 had normal liver tests and a normal liver histology. Five patients, assessed between 2 and 6 years after transplantation, had features suggestive of recurrent PBC, with the florid bile duct lesion, bile duct damage and portal granulomas. Patients were asymptomatic and liver tests were normal. All but one of the patients had AMA detectable in the serum. Four patients were treated with cyclosporin-based immunosuppression and one with tacrolimus. Of potential interest was the observation that all five patients had at least one HLA match with the donor liver at either the class I or II loci. Other centres have also reported that PBC may recur in the allograft[73,74].

Not all studies, however, have confirmed these findings. In early studies looking at failed allografts, Fennel *et al.*[75] and Demetris *et al.*[76] were unable to find any convincing histological evidence of PBC recurrence in the allograft. Features of early recurrence may have been masked by features of rejection or other complications. The study by Gouw *et al.*[77] involved careful prospective histological evaluation of 19 patients grafted for PBC for a period of up to 11 years (median 5). Although the AMA were positive, the authors were unable to find any convincing evidence of recurrent PBC and could find no other serological or histological differences between patients grafted for PBC and those grafted for other indications. Hart *et al.*[78] reached similar conclusions.

Some centres (including our own in Birmingham), which reported in preliminary studies that there was no evidence for recurrent PBC, have later reached different conclusions[70,79,80]. There are several explanations which may account for these revisions:

*Numbers and duration of follow-up* Our preliminary study from Birmingham on 19 patients grafted for PBC, and who had survived for more than 1 year, led us to conclude that there was no evidence for PBC recurrence[79]; however, when more patients were evaluated over a longer period, these conclusions were reversed.

*Immunosuppression* Some patients grafted for PBC were included in a prospective, randomized study comparing cyclosporin-based immunosuppression with tacrolimus-based immunosuppression. When the 1- and 2-year post-transplant biopsies were studied, it was found that those receiving tacrolimus-based immunosuppression had histological evidence of PBC recurrence not only earlier but more severely[81]. Those given tacrolimus in the study had less rejection, suggesting that those patients had a greater degree of immunosuppression; thus, as with recurrence of HBV infection, the degree of immunosuppression may affect the extent of disease recurrence. In a study from Pittsburgh[82] which, contrary to previous reports, found evidence of recurrent

PBC; histological features of PBC were found in 7.9% of patients at 5 years after liver transplantation and in 21.6% at 10 years. Risk factors for recurrence included recipient age, cold ischaemia age and immunosuppression.

## Implications of PBC recurrence

The possibility of disease recurrence has important implications for the pathogenesis of the disease: AMA and other PBC-specific autoantibodies persist after transplantation but have not been shown to be pathogenic. Biliary epithelial cells from the native livers of patients with PBC, but not with other conditions, have plasma membrane expression of the antigen recognized by AMA. We studied the grafts of patients with and without histological evidence of recurrent PBC with an affinity-purified antibody to the E2 component of pyruvate dehydrogenase[83] and were unable to find any evidence of aberrant antigen expression in any of the groups studied. However, Van der Water *et al.*[84] used a different antibody (a monoclonal antibody which reacts with the inner lipoyl domain of PDC-E2) and found that all sections from patients grafted for PBC showed a pattern of staining identical to that seen in the native PBC liver, whether or not there was evidence of disease recurrence.

These results raise the possibility that there is some factor (possibly infective or toxic) which is associated with the development of aberrant antigen expression on biliary epithelial cells and sets the scene for cell damage. The other implications are that immunosuppressive therapy may be of limited value in prevention or possibly progression of the disease process.

### *Autoimmune hepatitis*

The diagnosis of autoimmune hepatitis (AIH) is made in the patient with a native liver on the basis of internationally agreed criteria which include clinical, biochemical and histological features. The combination of elevated serum immunoglobulins (especially IgG), high titres of autoantibodies, interface hepatitis and a prompt response to corticosteroids, in the absence of known risk factors, such as drug ingestion or HCV infection, is virtually pathognomonic of the disease. Following liver transplantation, lymphocytic infiltration around the portal tracts is found in allograft rejection and autoantibodies may be present in low titre.

The first report of recurrence of autoimmune hepatitis after transplantation was a single case study in which the diagnosis was suggested by the development of spider naevi in a woman 18 months after transplantation[85]. The diagnosis was suggested by the development of raised IgG and antibodies to actin and liver-specific lipoprotein. The biopsy showed typical histological features of AIH. The reintroduction of corticosteroids was associated with a prompt resolution of all these abnormalities. The recipient was HLA-B8-DR3 positive, whereas the donor had neither of these antigens.

In 1992, Wright and colleagues from Pittsburgh published a retrospective analysis of 43 patients grafted for putative AIH[86]. Disease recurrence occurred in 11 (26%). All patients had hyperglobulinaemia and elevated levels of autoantibodies. The authors suggested that recurrence was most likely in HLA-DR3-

positive recipients of DR3-negative grafts. These findings must be interpreted with caution since molecular confirmation of HLA assignments was not available at the time. The Mayo Clinic[87] described recurrence of AIH in four (11%) of their series at a mean interval of 72 months. Serum anti-SMA or anti-ANA were present in two. Two of the four patients were mismatched at the DR3 locus. Remission, induced by increased immunosuppression, occurred in all but one. Devlin *et al.*[88] described severe AIH occurring 10 years after transplantation in a woman; there was a prompt response to the introduction of corticosteroids. The recipient was HLA $Al_1$ B8 DR3 and the donor was negative for all three antigens. Prados *et al.*[89] estimated the risk of AIH recurrence at 8% in the first year and 68% at 5 years. Interestingly, in that series from Madrid, none of those with liver–kidney microsomal antibodies developed recurrence.

Birnbaum and colleagues[90] reported recurrence of autoimmune hepatitis in five of six children at a mean time of 11 months after transplantation. They suggest that the recurrence is more severe in children, since in three patients, retransplantation was required. The recurrence was both in cyclosporin- and tacrolimus-treated patients. Others[91] have also described graft loss from recurrent AIH.

Overall, the diagnosis of recurrent autoimmune hepatitis is readily made on serological and histological evidence. There is usually a prompt response to increased immunosuppression, and recurrence has little adverse impact on the graft. The data do suggest that HLA mismatching may play a role in the development of recurrent AIH, although the mechanism is unclear. The recurrence of AIH suggests that the defect leading to AIH lies in the lymphocytes rather than the liver, an observation supported by the recent case report of remission of AIH in a patient following successful bone marrow transplantation[92].

## CONCLUSIONS

For the three major autoimmune liver conditions treated by transplantation, it is clear that in both PBC and AIH there is evidence for recurrent disease affecting the graft. Recurrent AIH responds well to increased immunosuppression, and donor/recipient HLA matching may be implicated, although the factors which determine which patients experience recurrence have not been identified. Risk factors for recurrence have not been identified either, but the type or degree of immunosuppression may affect the rate and severity of recurrence. PSC recurrence is difficult to define because of the inherent problems in distinguishing primary and secondary sclerosing cholangitis in the graft. Histological and radiological studies do suggest that the condition recurs, although further and longer-term studies are required.

### References


1. Registry of the European Liver Transplant Registry. Hôpital Paul Brousse, 1999.
2. Lucey M, Brown KA, Everson GT *et al.* Minimal listing criteria for placement of adults on the liver transplant waiting list. Transplantation. 1998;66:956–62.
3. Roll J, Boyer JL, Barry D, Klatskin G. The prognostic importance of clinical and histologic features in asymptomatic and symptomatic primary biliary cirrhosis. Nw Engl J Med. 1983;308:1–8.

4. Christensen E, Neuberger J, Crowe J, *et al.* Beneficial effect of azathioprine and prediction of prognosis in primary biliary cirrhosis: final result of an international trial. Gastroenterology. 1985;89:1084–91.
5. Dickson E, Grambsch P, Fleming T, Fisher L, Langworthy A. Prognosis in primary biliary cirrhosis: model for decision making. Hepatology. 1989;10:1–7.
6. Rydning A, Schrumpf E, Abdel-noor M, Elgio K, Jenssen E. Factors of prognostic importance in primary biliary cirrhosis. Scand J Gastroenterol.1990;25:119–26.
7. Goudie B, Burt AD, Macfarlane G *et al.* Risk factors and prognosis in primary biliary cirrhosis. Am J Gastroenterol. 1989;84:713–16.
8. Jeffrey G, Reed W, Shilkin K. Natural history and prognostic variables in primary biliary cirrhosis. Hepatology. 1990;12:955.
9. Hughes M, Raskino C, Pocock S, Biagini M, Burroughs A. Prediction of short-term survival with an application in primary biliary cirrhosis. Stat Med. 1992;11:1371–1745.
10. Wiesner R, Grambsch P, Dickson ER *et al.* Primary sclerosing cholangitis: natural history, prognostic factors and survival analysis. Hepatology. 1989;10:430–6.
11. Farrant M, Hayllar K, Wilkinson M *et al.* Natural history and prognostic variables in primary sclerosing cholangitis. Gastroenterology. 1991;100:1710–17.
12. Dickson ER, Murtaugh P, Wiesner R *et al.* Primary sclerosing cholangitis: refinement and validation of survival models. Gastroenterology. 1992;103:1893–901.
13. Klion F, Fabry T, Palmer M, Schaffner F. Prediction of survival of patients with primary biliary cirrhosis: examination of the Mayo Clinic model on a group of patients with known end-point. Gastroenterology. 1992;102:310–13.
14. Christensen E. Multivariate survival analysis using Cox's regression model. Hepatology. 1987;7:1346–50.
15. Christensen E, Altman D, Neuberger J, de Stavola B, Tygstrup N, Williams R. Updating prognosis in primary biliary cirrhosis using a time dependent Cox regression model. Gastroenterology. 1993;105:1865–76.
16. Shapiro J, Smith H, Schaffner F. Serum bilirubin: a prognostic factor in primary biliary cirrhosis. Gut. 1979;20:137–40.
17. Poupon R, Balkau B, Guechot J, Heintzman F. Predictive factors in ursodeoxycholic acid treated patients with primary biliary cirrhosis. Hepatology. 1994;19:635–40.
18. Nyberg A, Engstrom-Laurent A, Lööf L. Serum hyaluronate in primary biliary cirrhosis: a biochemical marker for progressive liver damage. Hepatology. 1988;8:142–6.
19. Eriksson E, Zettervall O. The N-terminal propeptide of collagen type III in serum as a prognostic indicator in primary biliary cirrhosis. J Hepatol. 1982;2:370–8.
20. Clements D, Elias E, McMaster P. Preliminary study of indocyanine green clearance in primary biliary cirrhosis. Scand J Gastroenterol. 1991;26:119–23.
21. Reichen J, Widmer T, Cutting J. Accurate prediction of death by serial determination of galactose elimination capacity in primary biliary cirrhosis: a comparison with the Mayo model. Hepatology. 1991;14:504–10.
22. Wiesner R, Grambsch P, Dickson E *et al.* Primary sclerosing cholangitis: natural history, prognostic factors and survival analysis. Hepatology. 1989;10:430–6.
23. Brentali T, Haggitt R, Rabonivitch P *et al.* Risk and natural history of colonic neoplasia in patients with primary sclerosing cholangitis and ulcerative colitis. Gastroenterology. 1996;110:331–8.
24. Loftus E, Sandborn W, Tremaine W *et al.* Risk of colorectal neoplasia in patients with primary sclerosing cholangitis. Gastroenterology. 1996;110:432–44.
25. Shaked A, Colonna J, Goldstein L, Busuttil R. The interrelationship between sclerosing cholangitis and ulcerative colitis in patients undergoing liver transplantation. Ann Surg. 1992;215:598–605.
26. Ismail T, Angrisani L, Powell J *et al.* Primary sclerosing cholangitis: surgical options, prognostic variables and outcome. Br J Surg. 1991;78:564–7.
27. Thompson J, Wood P, Burnett D, Shae B, Rikkers L. The role of non-transplant procedures for sclerosing cholangitis. Am J Surg .1988;156:506–8.
28. Rosen C, Nagorney D, Wiesner R, Coffey R, LaRusso N. Cholangiocarcinoma complicating primary sclerosing cholangitis. Ann Surg. 1991;213:21–5.
29. Bergquist A, Glaumann H, Persson B, Broome U. Risk factors and clinical presentation of hepatobiliary carcinoma in patients with primary sclerosing cholangitis: a case–control study. Hepatology. 1998;27:311–16.

30. Fisher A, Thiese N, Min A *et al.* CA19-9 does not predict cholangiocarcinoma in patients with primary sclerosing cholangitis undergoing liver transplantation. Liver Transplant Surg. 1995;1:94–8.
31. Ramage J, Farrant JM, Iorns R, Williams R. Serum tumour markers for diagnosis of cholangiocarcinoma in patients with primary sclerosing cholangitis. Gut. 1992;33:S1.
32. Takayasu K, Ikeya S, Mukai K, Muramatsu Y, Makuuchi M, Hasegawa H. CT of hilar cholangiocarcinoma: late contrast enhancement in six patients. Am J Roentgenol. 1990;154:1203–6.
33. Shulte S, Baron R, Teefey S *et al.* CT of the extrahepatic bile ducts: wall thickness and contrast enhancement in normal and abnormal ducts. Am J Roentgenol. 1990;154:79–85.
34. Cobb C, Floyd W. Usefulness of bile cytology in the diagnostic management of patients with biliary tract obstruction. Acta Cytol. 1985;29:93–100.
35. Davidson B, Varsamidakis N, Dooley J *et al.* Value of exfoliative cytology for investigating bile duct strictures. Gut. 1992;33:1408–11.
36. Wiesner RH, Seaberg EC, Kim WR *et al.* Predicting outcomes of liver transplantation in patients with primary sclerosing cholangitis (PSC) using the Mayo PSC model and the Child-Pugh score. Transplantation. 1999;67:S244 (abstract).
37. Neuberger J, Gunson B, Komolit P, Davies MH, Christensen E. Pretransplant prediction of prognosis after liver transplantation in primary sclerosing cholangitis using a Cox regression model. Hepatology 1999;29:1375–9.
38. Christensen E, Gunson B, Neuberger J. Optimal timing of liver transplantation for patients with primary biliary cirrhosis: use of prognostic models. J Hepatol. 1999;30:285–92.
39. Keiding S, Ericzon B, Eriksson *et al.* Survival after liver transplantation of patients with PBC in the Nordic countries. Scand J Gastroenterol. 1990;25:11–18.
40. Markus B, Dickson ER, Grambsch P *et al.* Efficacy of liver transplantation in patients with primary biliary cirrhosis. N Engl J Med 1989;320:1709–13.
41. Bonsel G, Klompmaker I, van de Veer F, Habbema J, Slooff M. Use of prognostic models for assessment of value of liver transplantation in primary biliary cirrhosis. Lancet. 1990;335:493–7.
42. Neuberger J, Gunson B, Buckels JAC, Elias E, MacMaster P. Referral of patients with primary biliary cirrhosis for liver transplantation. Gut. 1990;31:1069–72.
43. Neuberger J. Incidence, timing and risk factors for acute and chronic rejection. Liver Transplant Surg.1999;5 (Suppl 1):530–6.
44. Farges O, Saliba F, Fahramant H *et al.* Incidence of rejection and infection after liver transplantation as a factor of the primary disease: possible influence of alcohol and polyclonal immunoglobulins. Hepatology. 1996;23:240–8.
45. Wiesner RH, Demetris AJ, Belle SH *et al.* Acute hepatic allograft rejection: incidence, risk factors and impact on outcome. Hepatology. 1998;28:638–45.
46. Hayashi M, Keefe EB, Krams SM *et al.* Allograft rejection after liver transplantation for autoimmune liver diseases. Liver Transplant Surg. 1998;4:208–14.
47. Candinas D, Gunson B, Nightingale P, Hubscher S, MacMaster P, Neuberger J. Sex mismatch as a risk factor for chronic rejection of liver grafts. Lancet. 1995;346:1117–21.
48. Wiesner RH, Ludwig J, van Hoek B, Krom RAF. Current concepts in cell-mediated hepatic allograft rejection leading to ductopenia and liver failure. Hepatology. 1991;14:721–9.
49. Hunt C, Tart J, Dowdy E, Bute B, Williams D, Clasen P. Effect of orthotopic liver transplantation on employment and health status. Liver Transplant Surg. 1996;2:148–53.
50. Jeyarajah DR, Netto GJ, Lee SP *et al.* Recurrent primary sclerosing cholangitis after orthotopic liver transplantation. Transplantation. 1998;66:1300–6.
51. Adams PC, Ghent C, Grant D, Wall W. Employment after liver transplantation. Hepatology. 1995;21:140–4.
52. Riley TR, Schoen RE, Lee RG, Rakela J. A case series of transplant recipients who despite immunosuppression developed inflammatory bowel disease. Am J Gastroenterol. 1997;92:279–82.
53. Papatheodoridis GV, Hamilton M, Mistry PK, Davidson B, Rolles K, Burroughs AK. Ulcerative colitis has an aggressive course after orthotopic liver transplantation for primary sclerosing cholangitis. Gut. 1998;43:639–44.
54. Muller C, Briegel J, Haller M *et al.* Sarcoidosis recurrence following lung transplantation. Transplantation. 1996;61:1117–19.

55. Stegall M, Lafferty K, Kam I, Gill R. Evidence of recurrent autoimmunity in human allogeneic islet transplantation. Transplantation. 1996;61:1272–4.
56. Kerkar N, Hadzic N, Davies E *et al.* Graft dysfunction associated with autoimmunity in paediatric liver transplantation. Hepatology. 1996;24:235A (abstract).
57. Heneghan MA, Portmann B, Rela M, Heaton ND, O'Grady JG. Autoimmune hepatitis occurring de-novo following orthotopic liver transplantation in adults. Transplantation. 1999;67:S199 (abstract).
58. Sebagh M, Farges O, Kalil A *et al.* Sclerosing cholangitis following human orthotopic liver transplantation. Am Surg Pathol. 1995;19:81–90.
59. Patel T, Reddy S, Gores G, Wiesner R, Krom R. Recurrence following retransplantation for biliary strictures. Hepatology. 1996;24:243A (abstract).
60. Haagsma E, Mulder A, Gouw A *et al.* Neutrophil cytoplasmic autoantibodies after liver transplantation in patients with primary sclerosing cholangitis. J Hepatol. 1993;19:8–14.
61. Harrison RF, Davies MH, Neuberger JM *et al.* Fibrous and obliterative cholangitis in liver allografts: evidence of recurrent primary sclerosing cholangitis. Hepatology. 1994;20:356–61.
62. Graziadei I, Wiesner R, Marotta P *et al.* Strong evidence for recurrence of primary sclerosing cholangitis after liver transplantation. Hepatology. 1997;26:176A (abstract).
63. Abu-Elmagd K, Demetris AJ, Rakela J *et al.* Recurrence of primary sclerosing cholangitis (PSC) after hepatic transplantation: single center experience with 380 grafts. Transplantation. 1999;67:S236 (abstract).
64. Sheng R, Zajko AB, Campbell WL *et al.* Biliary structures in hepatic transplants:prevalence and types in patients with primary sclerosing cholangitis vs those with other liver diseases. Am J Radiol. 1993;161:297–300.
65. Letourneau JG, Day DL, Hunter OW *et al.* Biliary complications after liver transplantation in patients with primary sclerosing cholangitis. Radiology.1988;167:349–51.
66. McEntee G, Wiesner RH, Rosen C *et al.* A comparative study of patients undergoing liver transplantation for primary sclerosing cholangitis and primary biliary cirrhosis. Transplant Proc. 1991;23:1563–4.
67. Neuberger J, Portmann B, MacDougall B, Calne RY, Williams R. Recurrence of primary biliary cirrhosis after liver transplantation. N Engl J Med. 1982;306:1–4.
68. Ferrell L, Lee R, Brixko C *et al.* Hepatic granulomas following liver transplantation. Hepatology. 1995;60:926–44.
69. Polson R, Portmann B, Neuberger J *et al.* Evidence for disease recurrence after liver transplantation for primary biliary cirrhosis. Gastroenterology. 1989;97:715–25.
70. Hubscher S, Elias E, Buckels J *et al.* Primary biliary cirrhosis. Histological evidence of disease recurrence after liver transplantation. J Hepatol. 1993:18;173–84.
71. Luettig B, Boeker KH, Schoessler W *et al.* The antinuclear autoantibodies Sp100 and gp210 persist after orthotopic liver transplantation in patients with primary biliary cirrhosis. J Hepatol. 1998;28:824–8.
72. Balan V, Bans Bm Porayko Metal. Histological evidence for recurrence of primary biliary cirrhosis after liver transplantation. Hepatology. 1993:18;1392–8.
73. Pappo O, Ramos H, Starzl TE, Fung Ji, Demetris AJ. Structural integrity and identification of causes of liver allograft dysfunction occurring greater than 5 years after transplantation. Am J Pathol. 1995:19;192–206.
74. Samuel O, Gugenheim J, Mehta G *et al.* Liver transplantation for primary biliary cirrhosis. Transplant Proc. 1990;22:497–8.
75. Fennell RH, Shikes G, Vierling J. Relationship of pre-transplant hepatobiliary disease to bile duct damage occurring in liver allograft. Hepatology. 1983;3:84–9.
76. Demetris AJ, Markus BH, Esquivel C *et al.* Pathologic analysis of liver transplantation for primary biliary cirrhosis. Hepatology. 1988:6;937–47.
77. Gouw A, Haagsma E, Manns M *et al.* Is there recurrence of primary biliary cirrhosis after liver transplantation. J Hepatol. 1994;20:500–6.
78. Hart J, Busuttil R, Lewin KJ. Disease recurrence following liver transplantation. Am J Sung Pathol. 1990:14;79–91.
79. Buist L, Hubscher S, Vickers C, Neuberger J, McMaster P. Does transplantation cure primary biliary cirrhosis? Transplant Proc. 1989;21:2402.
80. Sebagh M, Farges O, Dubel L, Samuel D, Bismuth H, Reynes M. Recurrence of primary biliary cirrhosis (PBC) after liver transplantation: the risk is real. J Hepatol. 1996; (suppl. 1):25;125 (abstract).

81. Dmetrewski J, Mayer AD, Hubscher S, Neuberger JM. Histopathological recurrence of primary biliary cirrhosis after liver transplantation. J Hepatol. 1996;24:253–7.
82. Abu-Elmagd K, Demetris J *et al.* Transplantation for primary biliary cirrhosis: recurrence and outcome in 421 patients. Hepatology. 1997;26:176A (abstract).
83. Neuberger J, Wallace L, Joplin R, Babbs C, Hubscher S. Hepatic distribution of E2 component of pyruvate dehydrogenase complex after transplantation. Hepatology. 1995;22:798–801.
84. Van de Water J, Gerson LB, Ferrell L *et al.* Immunohistochemical evidence of disease recurrence after liver transplantation for primary biliary cirrhosis. Hepatology. 1996;74:1079–84.
85. Neuberger J, Portmann B, Calne R, Williams R. Recurrence of autoimmune chronic active hepatitis following orthotopic liver grafting. Transplantation. 1984;37:363–6.
86. Wright HL, Ben-Abboud C, Hussapein T *et al.* Disease recurrence and rejection following liver transplantation for autoimmune chronic active liver disease. Transplantation. 1992;53:136–9.
87. Roberts S, Czaja A, Chariton M *et al.* Recurrent autoimmune hepatitis following orthotopic liver transplantation. Hepatology. 1995;72:215A (abstract).
88. Devlin J, Donaldson P, Portmann B, Heaton N, Tan K-C, Williams R. Recurrence of autoimmune hepatitis following liver transplantation. Liver Transplant Surg. 1995;1:162–5.
89. Prados E, Cuervas-Mons V, de la Mata M *et al.* Outcome of autoimmune hepatitis after liver transplantation. Transplantation. 1998;66:1645–50.
90. Birnbaum AH, Benkov KJ, Pittman NS, McFarlane-Ferreira Y, Rosh JR, LeLeiko NS. Recurrence of autoimmune hepatitis in children after liver transplantation. J Pediatr Gastroenterol Nutr. 1997;25:20–5.
91. Ratziu V, Samuel D, Sebagh M *et al.* Long-term follow-up after liver transplantation for autoimmune hepatitis: evidence of recurrent disease. J Hepatol. 1999:30:131–41.
92. Vento S, Cainelli S, Renzini C, Ghironzi G, Concia E. Resolution of autoimmune hepatitis after bone marrow transplantation. Lancet. 1996;348:544–5.

# Section VII
# Therapy of autoimmune liver diseases – the future

# 32
# T cell vaccination as potential therapy for autoimmune hepatitis

A.W. LOHSE

## INTRODUCTION: ROLE OF AUTOREACTIVE CD4 LYMPHOCYTES IN MEDIATING AUTOIMMUNE DISEASE

Autoimmune diseases are mediated by lymphocytes reactive with self-antigens. While autoantibody-producing B cells are an important component of many autoimmune diseases, including autoimmune hepatitis, it is thought that autoreactive T lymphocytes play the key role in the aetiopathogenesis of most if not all autoimmune diseases, be it as helper cells allowing and supporting maturation of autoreactive B cells, or more importantly as critical mediators of autoreactive cell damage directly. Within the T cell compartment the CD4-positive cells seem to play the most important role in autoimmune diseases. While in human autoimmune diseases the evidence for CD4 cells as key mediator is only indirect, various experimental animal models have shown convincingly that CD4 cells induce and transfer the autoimmune disease process.

The experimental autoimmune disease model studied best is experimental autoimmune encephalomyelitis (EAE), the animal model for multiple sclerosis. This model can be induced in various animal species and strains, most reliably in Lewis rats, by immunization with myelin basic protein (MBP) in complete Freund's adjuvant (CFA)[1]. About 10 days later the animals develop ascending paralysis that can easily be scored clinically. If the animals survive they start recovering within 5 days. More than 10 years ago it was shown that this disease is entirely mediated by CD4-positive T cells reacting specifically with MBP[2]. Anti-MBP specific T cell lines and clones were able to transfer the disease effectively to naive syngeneic animals[2].

Experimental autoimmune hepatitis (EAH) as an animal model autoimmune hepatitis is induced by immunization of crude liver antigens in CFA intraperitoneally[3]. This disease also appears to be mediated by CD4-positive T cells as shown both by *in-vitro* responses and by passive transfer experiments[3].

## PRINCIPLES OF T CELL VACCINATION

Autoimmunity is not the result of unopposed proliferation of 'forbidden clones' of autoreactive T cells that have somehow escaped negative selection in the thymus, as was previously believed. On the contrary, autoreactive T cells are a physiological component of the normal immune repertoire, and this natural autoreactivity seems to be tightly regulated in order to prevent development of autoimmune disease under normal conditions[4,5]. This phenomenon can best be explained in the above-mentioned model of EAE: after induction of EAE in susceptible Lewis rats these animals recover, and this recovery is associated with a regulatory immune response against the disease-causing anti-MBP specific CD4 cells. Furthermore, the animals not only manage to recover by down-regulating the aberrant, artificially induced autoreactivity, but upon recovery these animals are protected from further bouts of the same disease process[5]. In other words, a second immunization with MBP in CFA fails to induce EAE in these recovered animals, nor can passive transfer of MBP-specific T cells reinduce disease.

These experiments demonstrate the ability of the immune system to regulate autoreactive T cells, and they also demonstrate that this regulatory capacity can be learned or augmented. T cell vaccination is based on this observation as it attempts to augment this natural regulatory capacity by challenging the immune system with autoreactive T cells which have been rendered harmless by prior attenuation[6,7]. The easiest way to achieve attenuation experimentally is by irradiation. Thus injection of irradiated anti-MBP reactive T cells does not induce EAE, but it nonetheless induces the same regulatory response as EAE does, and the animals become protected from further attempts at disease induction[8,9]. The principle of T cell vaccination is thus the transfer of a lesson learned in antimicrobial immunity many years ago: immunization with the attenuated agent responsible for the disease in question can induce a protective immune response. The agent responsible for autoimmune disease is in most cases the autoreactive CD4-positive T cell. Attenuation can be achieved by various methods in addition to irradiation, such as chemical crosslinking or hydrostatic pressure; the principle of inducing a specific regulatory response remains the same[10,11].

## MECHANISMS OF T CELL VACCINATION

Two components seem to be critical to the success and to the specificity of T cell vaccination: the T cell receptor (TCR) and the state of activation. T cell vaccination is mostly very specific for the T cell clone or line used for vaccination. In the Lewis rat this was beautifully demonstrated with anti-MBP clones responsible for EAE in comparison with T cell clones responsible for adjuvant arthritis (AA) and with specificity for the responsible antigen the 60 kDa heat-shock protein (HSP60) of *Mycobacterium tuberculosis*. Vaccination with anti-MBP T cells protected from EAE but not from AA, while anti-HSP60 T cell clones protected from AA but not from EAE[12,13]. As the critical difference between these two CD4-positive T cell clones is their T cell receptor accounting for their antigen specificity, it was clear that the T cell receptor must be the main target of the regulatory response induced by T cell vaccination. This has since been supported by further data using either peptides from the T cell receptor or DNA vaccination with the TCR-encoding sequence[14–16]. The specificity of T cell vaccination for the vaccinating T cell clone, the idiotype, could also be demonstrated *in vitro* by culturing anti-idiotypic T cells induced by T cell vaccination[12].

However, a second component is essential for the development of an anti-idiotypic response, and this second signal is only poorly understood. In all studies of T cell vaccination it was essential that the vaccinating T cell clone needed to be activated in order to induce a regulatory immune response. After injection of the same or higher numbers of T cells of the same clone as resting cells, i.e. without previous activation with antigen or mitogen *in vitro*, the animals would neither get disease nor mount a regulatory response. These resting autoreactive T cells were simply ignored by the immune system. Teleologically this makes very good sense: only an activated autoreactive T cell can cause tissue damage, and thus only this cell needs to be regulated. Therefore, in order to induce a regulatory response by T cell vaccination, activation of the vaccinating cells is required. The activated T cell, however, provides more than just a 'second signal' for T cell vaccination; it is also an important target of an independent regulatory response. Immunization with activated T cells induces also a population of regulatory T cells that reacts to the activation state of the immunizing clone, but similarly to the activation state of any T cell[17]. We have named these cells anti-ergotypic T cells as they recognize the activation state (the ergotope)[17,18]. These cells are clearly also regulatory cells, as induction of anti-ergotypic cells can also suppress experimental autoimmune disease[18]. It appears that anti-ergotypic cells carry two important functions: one is a direct regulatory role, the other is the provision of help for the development of anti-idiotypic T cells. Anti-ergotypic T cells also develop as part of other ongoing immune responses that lead to the activation of many T cells, and presumably they serve an important regulatory role in physiological immune response[18].

It was mentioned above that T cell receptor peptides can also be used for T cell vaccination, which might appear to contradict the postulate of a second signal provided by the activation state (ergotype) of the vaccinating T cell. However, T cell receptor peptide vaccination always requires application with a suitable adjuvant[14,15], and we have been able to show that adjuvants, by activating many T cells non-specifically, also induced an anti-ergotypic response[18]. Thus these experiments further support the concept of two components as the key to T cell vaccination, the idiotype (T cell receptor) and the ergotype (the activation state).

## T CELL VACCINATION IN THE PREVENTION OF EAH

The murine model of EAH offers the opportunity to study the applicability of T cell vaccination in autoimmune liver disease. EAH is induced in susceptible mouse strains by immunization with the 100 000 g supernatant of crude syngeneic liver homogenate (S-100) in CFA[3]. Immunization intraperitoneally is the most effective mode of immunization inducing histological hepatitis after even a single immunization. Passive transfer of the disease, although not very effective, can be achieved by activated CD4-positive T cells. The exact target antigen recognized by autoreactive T cells in this model is not known; therefore it is not possible to apply T cell vaccination with purified antigen-specific T cell populations or T cell clones. Nonetheless, previous experience in other models had suggested that vaccination with a mixed T cell population that includes the pathogenic cells can be sufficient to induce a protective immune response[10,19]. We thus used splenocytes from animals taken on day 14 after two immunizations (day 0 and day 7) with S-100/CFA activated these cells *in vitro* using the non-specific mitogen concanavalin A (Con A), and after irradiation used these cells for T cell vaccination, again applied twice at weekly intervals[20]. In order to control for the more non-specific effect of T cell vaccination by the anti-ergotypic response against any activated cells, we used as a control Con A activated splenocytes from naive animals as a T cell vaccine. After two vaccinations animals were challenged with the disease-inducing immunization with S-100/CFA twice at weekly intervals, and histology was checked after a further 2 weeks, when maximum activity is expected. It could be clearly shown that only animals vaccinated with cells from diseased animals were protected from EAH, while control vaccinated animals progressed to hepatitis to a similar degree as did control animals[20].

The immunological effect of vaccination could be measured *in vitro* by measuring the proliferative response of splenocytes from vaccinated, control vaccinated and control animals to the various cell populations: while control animals showed no clear response to any of the cell populations used for vaccination, T cell vaccinated animals showed both an anti-idiotypic response to the splenocytes from EAH animals and an anti-ergotypic response to activated control cells, with the maximum response to activated EAH cells[20]. Control vaccinated animals that had been injected with irrelevant activated splenocytes showed an anti-ergotypic response to any activated syngeneic splenocyte population, but no additional response to splenocytes from animals with EAH[20].

## THERAPEUTIC T CELL VACCINATION

In order to apply T cell vaccination in human autoimmune disease it is essential to demonstrate its potential to actually treat ongoing autoimmune disease rather than preventing it by preemptive vaccination. This is likely to be much more difficult, because, as explained earlier, the experimental animal by itself tries to overcome the aberrant autoimmune response and uses mechanism at the basis of T cell vaccination, but it is not clear to what extent these autoregulatory circles are defective in patients with autoimmune disease. All that can be hoped for in T cell vaccination in human autoimmune disease is augmentation of an ongoing beneficial regulatory response. The ability to use therapeutic T cell vaccination in experimental animal models was first demonstrated in adjuvant arthritis (AA) establishing the applicability in principle of therapeutic T cell vaccination[10]. While experimental autoimmune diseases of short duration such as EAE are not suitable for therapeutic T cell vaccination, the relatively long course of EAH makes it suitable for this approach, although this model suffers from the handicap that there is no clinical way of monitoring disease activity on a day-to-day basis as there is in, for example, arthritis models. We applied T cell vaccination as a therapeutic modality in EAH by using the same approach as in preventive T cell vaccination, as explained above, but instead of immunizing with the activated splenocyte population before disease induction, we vaccinated 1 and 2 weeks after disease induction and sacrificed the animals after a further week[20]. Indeed, disease activity as measured by histology was only half in the treated group as compared to the control group[20]. Transaminase levels were also lower, but admittedly transaminase levels are a far less reliable marker than histology in assessing disease activity in this model, which is characterized by more tissue infiltration than hepatocyte damage. Nonetheless, these observations demonstrate the applicability in principle of therapeutic T cell vaccination.

## CLINICAL EXPERIENCE WITH T CELL VACCINATION IN OTHER IMMUNE-MEDIATED DISEASES

Applying T cell vaccination in human autoimmune disease requires the successful transfer of the animal model experience to the clinic. Autoimmune hepatitis as a disease that can usually be treated very successfully by acceptable doses of immunosuppressive drugs is not the disease of choice to apply this experimental immunotherapy. Clinical experience thus far is largely confined to multiple sclerosis (MS)[21–23], with a few pilot studies also in severe rheumatoid arthritis[24,25]. These studies have established the safety and applicability in principle, but many questions are still open. However, studies with anti-MBP specific T cell clones in MS have shown very beautifully that a successful regulatory response can be induced that leads to disappearance of the specific idiotype used for vaccination from the peripheral immune repertoire[22,23]. These studies are enormously work-intensive as they require the culture of individual antigen-specific T cell clones with specificity for the presumed autoantigen. Therefore the approach of using just T cell receptor peptides of TCR rearrangements thought to be used frequently in autoantigen recognition has also been applied in MS, and again induction of an anti-idiotypic response could be established. The clinical effects of these interventions have not been impressive thus far, but are nonetheless encouraging.

## OPEN QUESTIONS AND FUTURE PERSPECTIVES

There are several key questions that need to be answered before T cell vaccination can be considered a realistic approach to immunotherapy for autoimmune diseases. Critical to the concept is the identification of the major target antigen of the autoimmune reaction. While in multiple sclerosis experimental animal models and clinical studies suggest two or three major target antigens, in autoimmune hepatitis we are a long way from identification of the major antigen responsible for the disease. The animal model of EAH has not provided us thus far with a defined antigen, and studies of patients have identified several antigens of autoantibodies, but except for anti-SLA/LP autoantibodies none of these antibodies is disease-specific; therefore the antigens recognized are unlikely to be the disease-specific inducer of the autoimmune response. Whether the newly identified target antigen of SLA/LP autoantibodies might provide such a disease-specific target antigen will need to be studied.

The second key question is one of immunopharmacology: how many cells need to be used for vaccination, what is the best mode of attenuation (irradiation, crosslinking, etc.?), how should the cells be injected, how often should vaccination be repeated, etc.[24,25]? The third and most important question is whether patients with autoimmune disease have the same ability to control autoreactive cells as experimental animals have, or is their disease a consequence of the fact that they cannot regulate these cells effectively. Although this point is important, there are good indications that this pessimistic view is not justified, the most important aspect being the clinical observation that many patients may experience spontaneous fluctuation of their disease activity including spontaneous recoveries, and that others run a very slow course of their disease; both observations strongly suggesting that immunoregulatory circuits are operative in these patients, and that the potential to suppress the aberrant autoimmune response is present, but simply requires augmentation. Understanding these regulatory circuits better will be the basis of a more effective and more specific immunotherapy. T cell vaccination is an important tool in this study, and may lead us to an optimal immunotherapy of autoimmune diseases including autoimmune hepatitis.

## References


1. Arnon R. Experimental allergic encephalomyelitis – susceptibility and suppression. Immuno Rev. 1981;55:5.
2. Ben-Nun A, Wekerle H, Cohen IR. The rapid isolation of clonable antigen-specific T lymphocyte lines capable of mediating autoimmune encephalomyelitis. Eur J Immunol. 1981;11:195–9.
3. Lohse AW, Manns M, Dienes HP, Meyer zum Büschenfelde K-H, Cohen IR. Experimental autoimmune hepatitis: disease induction, time course and T-cell reactivity. Hepatology. 1990;11:24–30.
4. Cohen IR, Young D. Autoimmunity, microbial immunity and the immunological homunculus. Immunol Today. 1991;12:105–10.
5. Lohse AW, Cohen IR. Immunoregulation: studies of physiological and therapeutic autoreactivity by T cell vaccination. Springer Semin Immunopathol. 1992;14:179–86.
6. Cohen IR, Ben-Nun A, Holoshitz J, Maron R, Zerubavel R. Vaccination against experimental disease with lines of autoimmune T lymphocytes. Immunol Today. 1983;4:227–30.
7. Cohen IR. Regulation of autoimmune disease: physiological and therapeutic. Immunol Rev. 1986;94:5–21.
8. Ben-Nun A, Wekerle H, Cohen IR. Vaccination against autoimmune encephalomyelitis with T lymphocyte lines reactive against myelin basic protein. Nature. 1981;292:60–1.
9. Beraud E, Lider O, Baharav E, Reshef T, Cohen IR. Vaccination against experimental autoimmune encephalomyelitis using a subencephalitogenic dose of autoimmune effector cells. I. Characteristics of vaccination. J Autoimmun. 1989;2:75–86.
10. Lider O, Karin N, Shinitzky M, Cohen IR. Therapeutic vaccination against adjuvant arthritis using autoimmune T cells treated with hydrostatic pressure. Proc Natl Acad Sci USA. 1987;84:4577–80.
11. Lohse AW, Cohen IR. Experimental regulation of autoimmune disease. In: Farid NR, editor. The Immunogenetics of Autoimmune Diseases, vol. 1. Boca Raton: CRC Press; 1991:159–65.
12. Lider O, Reshef T, Beraud E, Ben-Nun A, Cohen IR. Anti-idiotypic network induced by T cell vaccination against experimental autoimmune encephalomyelitis. Science. 1988;239:181–3.

13. Lider O, Beraud E, Reshef T, Friedman A, Cohen IR. Vaccination against experimental autoimmune encephalomyelitis using a subencephalitogenic dose of autoimmune effector cells. II. Induction of a protective anti-idiotypic response. J Autoimmun. 1989;2:87–99.
14. Vandenbark AA, Hashim G, Offner H. Immunization with a synthetic T-cell receptor V-region peptide protects against experimental autoimmune encephalomyelitis. Nature. 1989;341:541–4.
15. Offner H, Hashim G, Vandenbark A. T cell receptor peptide therapy triggers autoregulation of experimental encephalomyelitis. Science. 1991;251:430–2.
16. Waisman A, Ruiz PJ, Hirschberg DL *et al.* Suppressive vaccination with DNA encoding a variable region of the T-cell receptor prevents autoimmune encephalomyelitis and activates Th2 immunity. Nat Med. 1996;2:899–905.
17. Lohse AW, Mor F, Karin N, Cohen IR. Control of experimental autoimmune encephalomyelitis by T cells responding to activated T cells. Science. 1989;244:820–2.
18. Lohse AW, Spahn TW, Wölfel T, Herkel J, Cohen IR, Meyer zum Büschenfelde KH. Induction of the anti-ergotypic response. Int Immunol. 1993;5:533–9.
19. Mor F, Lohse AW, Karin N, Cohen IR. Clinical modeling of T cell vaccination against autoimmune disease in rats. Selection of antigen-specific T cells using a mitogen. J Clin Invest. 1990;85:1594–8.
20. Lohse AW, Dienes HP, Meyer zum Büschenfelde KH. Suppression of murine experimental autoimmune hepatitis by T-cell vaccination or immunosuppression. Hepatology. 1998;27:1536–43.
21. Hafler D, Cohen IR, Benjamin DS, Weiner HL. T cell vaccination in multiple sclerosis; a preliminary report. Clin Immunol Immunopathol. 1992;62:307–13.
22. Zhang J, Medaer R, Stinissen P, Hafler D, Raus J. MHC-restricted depletion of human myelin basic protein-reactive T cells by cell vaccination. Science. 1993;261:1451–4.
23. Zhang J, Vanderyver C, Stinissen P, Raus J. *In vivo* clonotypic regulation of human myelin basic protein-reactive T cells by T cell vaccination. J Immunol. 1995;155:5868–76.
24. Lohse AW, Bakker NPM, Hermann E, Poralla T, Jonker M, Meyer zum Büschenfelde KH. Induction of an anti-vaccine response by T cell vaccination in non-human primates and humans. J Autoimmun. 1993;6:121–30.
25. van Laar JM, Miltenburg AM, Verdonk MJ *et al.* Effects of inoculation with attenuated T cells in patients with rheumatoid arthritis. J Autoimmun. 1993;6:159–67.

# 33
# Gene therapy for autoimmune diseases

V. K. TUOHY and P. M. MATHISEN

## INTRODUCTION

Recent investigations have demonstrated efficacy in applying gene therapy strategies for the treatment of autoimmune diseases in animal models[1, 2]. Typically, these strategies involve the use of viral vectors to deliver therapeutic transgene cytokines or cytokine receptors to inflammatory sites[3]. However, it has become increasingly more evident that a considerable refinement of currently used reagents and conditions will be needed before an effective gene therapy strategy can be used in the treatment of human autoimmune diseases. Such refinements will focus on optimizing three basic requirements for effective gene therapy, *viz.*, (1) *targeted delivery* of the therapeutic gene or its gene product in a reliable, efficient manner; (2) *long-term expression* of the therapeutic gene; and (3) *regulated expression* of the therapeutic gene so that it is activated only when needed.

Using an experimental autoimmune encephalomyelitis (EAE) mouse model, we have examined the potential for using the T cell as a gene therapy vector for targeted, long-term, regulated delivery of therapeutic transgene factors to the autoimmune inflammatory milieu. Our data indicate that the autoreactive T cell may serve as a useful endogenous vector for antigen-inducible, site-specific delivery of a variety of therapeutic transgene factors capable of mediating both inhibition of autoimmune inflammation and regeneration and/or protection of damaged tissue.

## PROS AND CONS OF VIRAL VECTORS FOR GENE THERAPY

Modified viruses are the most commonly used vectors for gene therapy[4–6]. Vectors derived from replication-defective retroviruses have the advantage of integrating directly into the host genome. However, transgene delivery by retroviral vectors is restricted to replicating cells expressing appropriate viral receptors. Typically, targeted delivery with retroviral vectors is mediated by transduction of isolated cells *in vitro* before transfer of the modified cells back into the host.

Adenoviral vectors have the advantage over retroviral vectors of being able to transduce nondividing cells *in vivo*. However, targeted delivery is mediated primarily by physical placement of the modified adenovirus into the tissue area of interest. Thus, *in vivo* delivery is not effectively confined to a single cell type. In addition to the difficulties in targeted cell delivery, viral vectors are inherently predisposed to transient gene expression. This may occur as a result of expression of viral regulatory elements that eventually inhibit transgene expression or as a result of inflammation and immune clearance of vector-infected cells. Furthermore, although adenoviral vectors are designed to be replication-defective, reports of low levels of replication-competent adenoviral vectors after infection suggest that vector-induced malignant transformation may occur[6]. Thus, viral vectors may re-acquire pathogenic properties after exposure to the *in vivo* milieu.

Viral vector transgene expression may also be compromised as a result of positional effects following random integration into transcriptionally inactive regions of host DNA, e.g. near centromeres or telomeres[7]. Flanking host chromatin regions may exert *cis*-regulatory effects that inhibit transgene expression. This inhibition may take the form of immediate silencing or gradual temporal extinction of transgene expression. Retroviral vectors appear to be particularly sensitive to positional effects[8, 9]. These positional effects may be overcome to a great extent by genetically modifying viral LTR to remove domains involved in temporal quiescence[10, 11] or by incorporation of chromatin insulators into the design of the vector[12]. Such insulator nucleotide sequences inhibit temporal extinction of transgene expression by serving as domain boundaries, thereby protecting independent domains from the regulatory influences of adjacent domains.

Most viral vector systems use promoters that drive constitutive expression of transgene products. However, recent studies indicate that inducible promoters may provide controlled production of transgene factors. In the doxycycline-inducible gene expression system the addition of doxycycline to the drinking water results in the production of muscle-targeted transgene expression of erythropoietin *in vivo*[13, 14]. In a related application the oral ingestion of rapamycin results in coupling of two complementary fusion transcription factors, one containing a novel DNA binding domain and the other containing only an activation domain. The resultant complex provides regulated expression of transgene erythropoietin by binding to novel sites in the transgene promoter region[15–17].

## THE AUTOREACTIVE T CELLS AS A VECTOR FOR GENE THERAPY

In contrast to the extensive manipulation required for achieving regulated transgene expression with viral vectors, the autoreactive T cell provides regulated, antigen-specific activation as an integral feature of its native design. Thus, we propose that the antigen specificity and migratory properties of autoreactive T cells provide an endogenous system for regulated delivery of therapeutic transgene products to the autoimmune milieu. The autoreactive T cell may be genetically modified to deliver anti-inflammatory factors capable of inhibiting the inflammatory autoreactive Th1 T cell response that mediates target tissue destruction. Moreover, the autoreactive T cell may be genetically modified to produce therapeutic transgene factors capable of regenerating and repairing the damaged target tissue. This view of gene therapy in autoimmunity is depicted in Figure 1, which shows the genetically modified autoreactive T cell in a position to inhibit the autoimmune destruction mediated by the inflammatory Th1 T cell and to regenerate target tissue damaged as a result of the autoimmune attack. The depicted autoimmune target in Figure 1 is the oligodendrocyte believed to be the primary target in multiple sclerosis (MS) and our related EAE animal model.

Our experimental design involved the genetic modification of autoreactive T cells in such a way as to regulate the therapeutic transgene factor, e.g. the anti-inflammatory factor interleukin 10 (IL-10), with an antigen inducible transgene promoter, e.g. an IL-2 promoter region. In this way engagement of the genetically modified T cell with self-antigen would result in the activation of both the native and transgene IL-2 promoters through the same endogenous signalling/transcription factor pathways. This design concept is depicted in Figure 2, which shows the simultaneous antigen-induced activation of both native and transgene T cell promoters that results in the inducible production of the selected therapeutic transgene. The first question we addressed in this study is whether normal autoreactive memory T cells can be genetically modified to produce regulatory transgene cytokines in an antigen-inducible manner. Moreover, we asked whether such modified T cells could inhibit Th1 T cell-mediated autoimmune inflammation and demyelination.

Our initial approach involved the transfection of primed autoreactive T cells with a plasmid construct designed to produce a regulatory cytokine in an antigen-inducible manner[18]. IL-10 was selected as our candidate cytokine because of its well-characterized anti-inflammatory features including down-regulation of MHC class II molecules on antigen-presenting cells (APC), inhibition

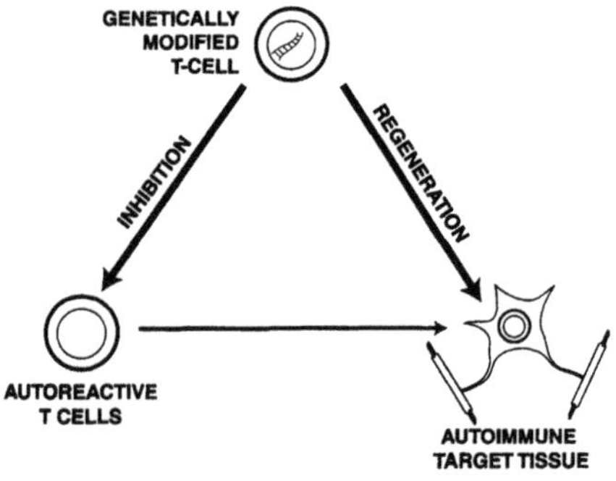


**Fig. 1** Gene therapy in autoimmune disease. The autoreactive memory T cell serves as an endogenous vector for site-specific delivery of therapeutic transgene factors to the autoimmune inflammatory milieu. Autoreactive T cells may be genetically modified to produce immunoregulatory factors capable of inhibiting the Th1 T cell-mediated attack directed against target tissue, e.g. the mature myelinating oligodendrocyte targeted in EAE and MS. In addition, autoreactive T cells may be genetically modified to produce regenerative growth factors capable of mediating repair and regeneration of tissue damaged as a result of autoimmune inflammation

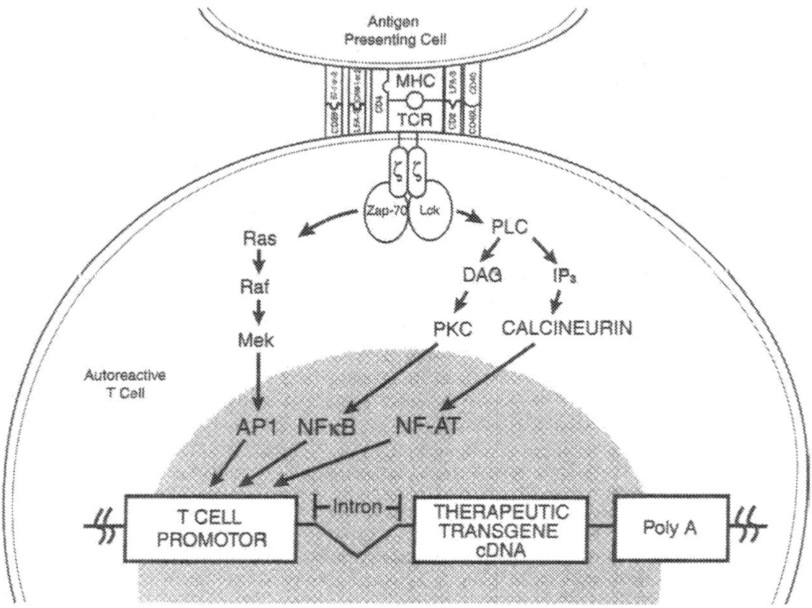


**Fig. 2** Antigen-inducible activation of the therapeutic transgene. Engagement with self-antigen results in the activation of the transfected autoreactive T cell leading to production of transcription factors that regulate transcription of both the native inducible T cell promoters, e.g. IL-2, IL-4, or IL-5 promoters, as well as minimal versions of such promoters incorporated in the design of the transgene plasmid. This design results in the production of the native inducible T cell factor as well as the ectopic therapeutic transgene factor capable of inhibiting inflammation, e.g. IL-10, or regenerating and repairing damaged tissue, e.g. PDGF

of co-stimulatory activity, and inhibition of interferon gamma (IFN-$\gamma$) production by inflammatory Th1 T cells. Our plasmid construct contained a minimal IL-2 promoter region for regulating expression of the IL-10 cDNA (IL-2Prom $\rightarrow$ IL-10cDNA) as well as an intron sequence between the IL-2 promoter region and the IL-10 cDNA and a 3′ SV40 poly A tail to ensure maximum transgene expression. Our design also involved the immunization of SWXJ mice with the immunodominant encephalitogenic determinant PLP 139–151. At 7–10 days after immunization, lymph node cells were removed and activated *in vitro* with PLP 139–151. Three days later the activated T cells were harvested and co-transfected with the IL-2Prom $\rightarrow$ IL-10cDNA plasmid, as well as with a plasmid construct containing the gene for neomycin resistance (pSV2neo plasmid). Transfection was mediated by dimethyl sulphoxide (DMSO) polybrene-assisted gene transfer. Transfected cells were selected by treatment with geneticin, and the surviving cells were expanded by antigen activation and cloned by limiting dilution analysis. Several clones were isolated, and one particular clone called T10.11 was selected for further characterization because of its vigorous growth. Clone T10.11 responded to PLP 139–151 but not to PLP 104–117 by producing high levels of IL-10 and IL-4 but little or no IFN-$\gamma$ and tumour necrosis factor alpha (TNF-$\alpha$). Thus, clone T10.11 showed the characteristic profile of the immunoregulatory Th2 T cell.

Analysis of T10.11 mRNA by an RNase protection assay showed that two distinct IL-10 bands were protected, *viz.* the endogenous IL-10 mRNA and a longer band containing untranslated vector-specific sequences. Clone T10.11 inhibited the development of EAE when transferred into SWXJ mice just prior to EAE onset. Moreover, the transfected line from which the T10.11 clone was derived also inhibited EAE onset, thereby indicating that the therapeutic features of clone T10.11 were shared by other transfected T cells. In addition, the transfected T10.11 clone inhibited progression of EAE when cells were transferred after EAE onset. EAE inhibition was never observed after transfer of cells from an IL-2Prom → IL-10cDNA-transfected KLH-specific T cell line or after transfer of normal splenocytes. From these studies we conclude that autoreactive T cells may be genetically modified to produce immunoregulatory cytokines in a regulated, antigen-inducible manner. Upon adoptive transfer, transfected T cells can inhibit EAE onset and therapeutically alter the course of ongoing disease. Thus, genetically modified T cells may serve as potent vectors for delivering therapeutic transgene factors to the autoimmune inflammatory milieu.

## OPTIMIZING THE THERAPEUTIC POTENTIAL OF THE AUTOREACTIVE T CELL

The experiments described above serve to indicate 'proof of principle' for generating T cells capable of producing therapeutic transgene factors upon engagement with self-antigen. However, as we have indicated previously[19], several challenging considerations remain for optimizing the therapeutic features of genetically modified autoreactive T cells: (1) choosing the therapeutic transgene factor, e.g. does one choose immunoregulatory factors for inhibiting inflammation or regenerative growth factors for repairing damaged target tissue? (2) choosing the regulatory promoter, e.g. does one choose an antigen-inducible promoter? If so, then does one choose a Th1 promoter or a Th2 promoter? Alternatively, does one opt for a constitutive promoter, e.g. the distal *lck* promoter? (3) choosing the antigen specificity, e.g. does one choose to target a determinant capable of eliciting a recall response from an established primed repertoire or does one preemptively target the epitope spreading cascade before endogenous neoautoreactivity has had a chance to develop?

## CHOOSING THE THERAPEUTIC TRANSGENE

Regarding the first consideration, can T cell-mediated gene therapy be used to deliver therapeutic growth factors capable of mediating repair and regeneration of damaged autoimmune target tissue? In the case of EAE and MS, the primary target cell for autoimmune attack is the oligodendrocyte. The mature myelinating oligodendrocyte is derived from progenitor cells that develop through distinct stages of proliferation, migration, and maturation with each sequential stage supported by distinct sets of growth factors. We chose platelet-derived growth factor-A (PDGF) as our initial regenerative transgene growth factor because it plays an important role at several stages of oligodendrocyte development by stimulating progenitor cells to undergo proliferation, migration, differentiation, and survival[20–23]. PDGF induces a limited number of oligodendrocyte progenitor cell divisions and is permissive for oligodendrocyte differentiation. In addition, PDGF is a chemoattractant for oligodendrocyte progenitor cells.

Primed autoreactive T cells were transfected as described above but with the plasmid construct IL-2Prom → PDGFcDNA designed in such a way as to provide expression of PDGF cDNA under the antigen-inducible regulation of a minimal IL-2 promoter region[24]. Twelve PLP 139–151-specific T cell clones were isolated and nine were shown to produce PDGF upon activation with antigen. All nine clones that produce PDGF had a Th2-like cytokine profile producing high levels of IL-5 and IL-10. Two of the three transfected clones that did not produce PDGF were INF-$\gamma$-producing T cells, suggesting perhaps that the Th2 T cell may provide a more favourable milieu for expression of PDGF than the Th1 or Th0 T cell. Alternatively, our conditions may simply provide a bias for selecting Th2 rather than Th1 T cells that produce PDGF.

To show that the PDGF produced by the transfected T cell clones was transgene derived, the mRNAs from activated transfected clones were amplified by reverse transcription polymerase chain reaction (RT-PCR) using a vector-specific 5′ primer and a PDGF-specific 3′ primer. The amplified transgene product was visualized by Southern blot analysis using a PDGF-specific $^{32}$P-labeled nested probe. Our results showed that the PDGF produced by transfected clones was transgene derived.

To show that the secreted transgene-derived PDGF was biologically active, supernatants from transfected clones that produced PDGF, as well as from transfected clones that did not produce PDGF, were added to cultures of PDGF-responsive human gingival fibroblasts (HGF-1)[25], and rat O2A oligodendrocyte progenitor cells[26–29]. Proliferation of both HGF-1 cells and O2A cells occurred only in cultures containing supernatants from PDGF-producing transfected clones.

To determine whether transfected PDGF-producing T cells were capable of migrating to the central nervous system (CNS), three activated clones were labelled with the PKH26 red fluorescent cell linker and transferred into SWXJ mice 3 days after EAE onset. Three days later the mice were perfused, mononuclear cells were isolated from brains by Percoll centrifugation, and the extracted cells were analysed by flow cytometry. Transfected T cells represented a mean of 8.27 ± 1.42% of the total CNS T cell population but only 0.75 ± 0.12% of the total spleen cell population. Moreover, it was evident from the detection of two distinct PKH26-containing T cell populations that the transfected T cells had divided *in vivo* after transfer. The flow cytometry results were corroborated when the PDGF transgene was amplified from CNS-obtained T cells using primers specific for the PDGF transgene. Thus, PDGF-transfected Th2-like T cells are fully capable of migrating to the CNS during autoimmune demyelinating disease and mediating a therapeutic effect on disease outcome.

## CHOOSING THE REGULATORY PROMOTER

Initially, we did not know that we would encounter a strong Th2 T cell bias in selecting for transfected clones. Perhaps we were fortunate that the minimal IL-2 promoter used in our constructs remained active in the selected Th2-like clones. This activity may have been due to the fact that the transgene IL-2 promoter was chosen because it served as the minimal promoter region (1.8 kb) capable of driving high-level recorder gene expression in Jurkat cells[30]. Since the endogenous IL-2 promoter region represents at least 8 kb, it appears likely that several *cis*-regulatory elements may be absent in the transgene promoter region, thereby preventing down-regulation of the transgene IL-2 promoter even in a committed Th2 milieu. Nevertheless, we became convinced that the use of a minimal IL-2 promoter for regulating transgene expression may not be optimal for operating in a Th2 milieu.

We redesigned our plasmid construct so that an antigen-inducible IL-4 promoter region[31] would regulate expression of PDGF (IL-4Prom → PDGFcDNA). We transfected PLP 139–151-specific T cells with the IL-4Prom → PDGFcDNA construct and selected autoreactive neomycin-resistant T cell lines. Expansion of the transfected T cell lines was performed in the presence of antigen and either IL-2 or IL-4. We found that when IL4-Prom → PDGFcDNA-transfected cells were expanded in the presence of IL-4, antigen activation resulted in supernatant levels of PDGF that were equivalent to the concentrations produced for IL-10. Cells selected conventionally in IL-2 produced about 10–12% of the amount of PDGF observed in the IL-4 expanded population. Thus, unlike the results observed with the transgene Th1 IL-2 promoter, the use of the Th2 IL-4 promoter resulted in a level of transgene expression and production that was similar to levels obtained for native genomic cytokines after activation with antigen.

## CHOOSING THE ANTIGEN SPECIFICITY

The choice of antigen specificity is critical. One may target adoptive immunotherapy to a determinant capable of eliciting a recall response at a given selected time during the disease process, i.e. the 'epitope *du jour*' activating the established current autoimmune repertoire[32, 33]. Alternatively, one may target adoptive immunotherapy to a determinant that will inevitably and predictably be involved in the autoimmune response as a consequence of epitope spreading, i.e. the spreading determinants that will ultimately activate the latent autoimmune repertoire[34–37].

We and others have shown that progression of EAE may be inhibited when Th2-like T cells specific for the priming determinant are adoptively transferred into EAE mice after onset of actively induced disease[18, 38]. However, we have also shown that in SWXJ mice primed to PLP 139–151 progression to chronicity is invariably accompanied by the sequential accumulation of Th1 neoautoreactivity as defined by the epitope spreading cascade PLP 139–151 → PLP 249–273 → MBP 87–99 → PLP 173–198[36, 37]. Based on this observation of temporally spaced neoautoreactivity, we examined the therapeutic potential of preemptive targeting of the epitope spreading cascade by adoptive transfer after EAE onset of Th2-like T cells specific for spreading determinants. Our approach involved the generation of stable Th2 T cell lines by transfecting primed lymph node cells with a transgene construct in which a mouse IL-2 promoter region regulated the expression of mouse IL-10 cDNA (IL2-Prom → IL10 cDNA). We found that, after induction of EAE with PLP 139–151, adoptive transfer of Th2 T cells with specificity for components of the epitope spreading cascade resulted in a marked and prolonged inhibition of disease progression accompanied by a significant increase in total spinal cord myelin as measured by quantitative immunocytochemistry. No comparable marked impact on disease progression was observed after transfer of Th2 T cell lines specific for either BSA or PLP 104–117, a determinant not involved in the spreading cascade. The therapeutic effect was accompanied by a profound and prolonged Th1 $\rightarrow$ Th2 immune deviation to the spreading determinant characterized by decreased production of IFN-$\gamma$ and IL-12 and increased production of IL-4 and IL-10 from splenocytes stimulated *ex vivo* with the targeted spreading determinant. Thus, our results indicate that preemptive targeting of the epitope spreading cascade with adoptive Th2 immunotherapy results in a dramatic long-term therapeutic impact on the progression of autoimmune demyelinating disease.

## CONCLUSIONS

Autoreactive T cells may serve as useful vectors for regulated and site-specific delivery of therapeutic transgene factors to the autoimmune inflammatory milieu. Autoreactive T cells may serve to deliver both anti-inflammatory transgene factors as well as regenerative and neuroprotective transgene factors to inflammatory sites. Although this therapeutic approach has not been fully optimized in animal model systems, the authors believe that 'proof of principle' has been established, and that there may be a potential for application of this technology in the future for the treatment of putative human autoimmune diseases such as multiple sclerosis, rheumatoid arthritis, and insulin-dependent diabetes mellitus.

### Acknowledgements

We thanks Dr Min Yu, Dr Ling Yin, Dr Akiko Nishiyama, Justin M. Johnson, and Julie A. Kawczak for their invaluable contribution to the work described in this chapter. We also thank Dr Ellen V. Rothenberg for generously providing the mouse IL-2 promoter region, Dr Richard A. Flavell for generously providing the mouse IL-4 promoter, and Dr Daniel Bowen-Pope for generously providing the mouse PDGF cDNA. This work was supported by grants NS36054 and NS37476 from the National Institutes of Health, USA.

### References

1. Robbins PD, Evans CH. Prospects for treating autoimmune and inflammatory diseases by gene therapy. Gene Ther. 1996;3:187–9.
2. Mathisen PM, Tuohy VK. Gene therapy in the treatment of autoimmune disease. Immunol Today. 1998;19:103–5.
3. Schmidt-Wolf GD, Schmidt-Wolf IGH. Cytokines and gene therapy. Immunol. 1995;16:173–5.
4. Wilson JM. Vectors – shuttle vehicles for gene therapy. Clin Exp Immunol. 1997;107(Suppl. 1):31–2.
5. Morgan RA, Anderson FW. Human gene therapy. Annu Rev Biochem. 1993;62:191–217.
6. Mulligan RC. The basic science of gene therapy. Science. 1993;260:926–32.

7. Karpen GH. Position-effect variegation and the new biology of heterochromatin. Curr Opin Genet Dev. 1994;4:281–91.
8. Neff T, Shotkoski F, Stamatoyannopoulos G. Stem cell gene therapy, position effects and chromatin insulators. Stem Cells. 1997;15(Suppl. 1):265–71.
9. Rivella S, Sadelain M. Genetic treatment of severe hemoglobinopathies: the combat against transgene variegation and transgene silencing. Semin Hematol. 1998;35:112–25.
10. Deng H, Lin Q, Khavari PA. Sustainable cutaneous gene delivery. Nature Biotech. 1997;15:1388–91.
11. Robbins PB, Skelton DC, Yu X-J, Halene S, Leonard EL, Kohn DB. Consistent, persistent expression from modified retroviral vectors in murine hematopoietic stem cells. Proc Natl Acad Sci USA. 1998;95:10182–7.
12. Emery DW, Stamatoyannopoulos G. Stem cell gene therapy for the *b*-chain hemoglobinopathies: problems and progress. Ann NY Acad Sci. 1999;87:94–108.
13. Gossen M. Transcriptional activation by tetracyclines in mammalian cells. Science. 1995;268:1766–9.
14. Bohl D, Naffakh N, Heard JM. Long-term control of erythropoietin secretion by doxycycline in mice transplanted with engineered primary myoblasts. Nature Med. 1997;3:299–305.
15. Burcin MM, Schiedner G, Kochanek S, Tsai SY, O'Malley BW. Adenovirus-mediated regulable target gene expression *in vitro*. Proc Natl Acad Sci USA. 1999;96:355–60.
16. Rivera VM, Clackson T, Natesan S *et al.* A humanized system for pharmacologic control of gene expression. Nature Med. 1996;2:1028–32.
17. Ye X, Rivera VM, Zoltick P *et al.* Regulated delivery of therapeutic proteins after *in vivo* somatic cell gene transfer. Science. 1999;283:88–91.
18. Mathisen PM, Yu M, Johnson JM, Drazba JA, Tuohy VK. Treatment of experimental autoimmune encephalomyelitis with genetically modified memory T cells. J Exp Med. 1997;186:159–64.
19. Tuohy VK, Mathisen PM. T cell design: optimizing the therapeutic potential of autoreactive T cells by genetic modification. Res Immunol. 1998;149:834–42.
20. Raff MC, Abney ER, Fok-Seang J. Reconstruction of a developmental clock *in vitro*: a critical role for astrocytes in the timing of oligodendrocyte differentiation. Cell. 1985;42:61–9.
21. Richardson WD, Pringle N, Mosley MJ, Westermark B, Dubois-Dalq M. A role for platelet-derived growth factor in normal gliogenesis in the central nervous system. Cell. 1988;53:309–19.
22. Pringle N, Collarini EJ, Mosley MJ, Heldin C-H, Westermark B, Richardson WD. PGDF A chain homodimers drive proliferation of bipotential (O2A) glial progenitors cells in the developing rat optic nerve. EMBO J. 1989;8:1049–56.
23. Armstrong RC, Harvath L, Dubois-Dalcq ME. Type-1 astrocytes and oligodendrocytes-type 2 astrocyte glial progenitors migrate toward distinct molecules. J Neurosci Res. 1990;27:400–7.
24. Mathisen PM, Yu M, Yin L, Johnson JM, Kawczak JA, Nishiyama A, Tuohy VK. Th2 T cells expressing transgene PDGF-A serve as vectors for gene therapy in autoimmune demyelinating disease. J Autoimmun. 1999;13:31–8.
25. McAllister BS, Leeb-Lundberg F, Olson MS. Bradykinin inhibition of EGF- and PDGF-induced DNA synthesis in human fibroblasts. Am J Physiol. 1993;265:477–84.
26. Raff MC, Miller RH, Noble M. A glial progenitor cell that develops *in vitro* into an astrocyte or an oligodendrocyte depending on culture medium. Nature. 1983;303:390–6.
27. Barres BA, Hart IK, Coles HSR *et al.* Cell death and control of cell survival in the oligodendrocyte lineage. Cell. 1992;70:31–46.
28. Barres BA, Schmid R, Sendnter M, Raff MC. Multiple extracellular signals are required for long-term oligodendrocyte survival. Development. 1993;118:283–95.
29. Nishiyama A, Lin X-H, Giese N, Heldin C-H, Stallcup WB. Interaction between NG2 proteoglycan and PDGF*a*-receptor on O2A progenitor cells is required for optimal response to PDGF. J Neurosci Res. 1996;43:315–30.
30. Novak TJ, White PM, Rothenberg EV. Regulatory anatomy of the murine interleukin-2 gene. Nuc Acids Res. 1990;18:4523–33.
31. Kamogawa Y, Minasi L, Carding SR, Bottomly K, Flavell RA. The relationship of IL-4- and IFN*g*-producing T cells studied by lineage ablation of IL-4-producing cells. Cell. 1993;75:985–95.

32. Tuohy VK, Yu M, Yin L, Kawczak JA, Kinkel RP. Spontaneous regression of primary autoreactivity during chronic progression of experimental autoimmune encephalomyelitis and multiple sclerosis. J Exp Med. 1999;189:1033–42.
33. Tuohy VK, Yu M, Yin L, Kawczak JA, Kinkel RP. Regression and spreading of self-recognition during the development of autoimmune demyelinating disease. J Autoimmun. 1999;13:11–20.
34. McRae BL, Vanderlugt CL, Dal Canto MC, Miller SD. Functional evidence for epitope spreading in the relapsing pathology of experimental autoimmune encephalomyelitis. J Exp Med. 1995;182:75–85.
35. Vanderlugt CJ, Miller SD. Epitope spreading. Curr Opin Immunol. 1996;8:831–6.
36. Yu M, Johnson JM, Tuohy VK. A predictable sequential determinant spreading cascade invariably accompanies progression of experimental autoimmune encephalomyelitis: a basis for peptide-specific therapy after onset of clinical disease. J Exp Med. 1996;183:1777–88.
37. Tuohy VK, Yu M, Yin L *et al.* The epitope spreading cascade during progression of experimental autoimmune encephalomyelitis and multiple sclerosis. Immunol Rev. 1998;164:93–100.
38. Kuchroo VK, Das MP, Brown JA *et al.* B7-1 and B7-2 costimulatory molecules activate differentially the Th1/Th2 developmental pathways: application to autoimmune disease therapy. Cell. 1995;80:707–18.

# Index

# Falk Symposium Series

43. Reutter W, Popper H, Arias IM, Heinrich PC, Keppler D, Landmann L, eds.: *Modulation of Liver Cell Expression*. Falk Symposium No. 43. 1987 ISBN: 0-85200-677-2*
44. Boyer JL, Bianchi L, eds.: *Liver Cirrhosis*. Falk Symposium No. 44. 1987 ISBN: 0-85200-993-3*
45. Paumgartner G, Stiehl A, Gerok W, eds.: *Bile Acids and the Liver*. Falk Symposium No. 45. 1987 ISBN: 0-85200-675-6*
46. Goebell H, Peskar BM, Malchow H, eds.: *Inflammatory Bowel Diseases – Basic Research & Clinical Implications*. Falk Symposium No. 46. 1988 ISBN: 0-7462-0067-6*
47. Bianchi L, Holt P, James OFW, Butler RN, eds.: *Aging in Liver and Gastrointestinal Tract*. Falk Symposium No. 47. 1988 ISBN: 0-7462-0066-8*
48. Heilmann C, ed.: *Calcium-Dependent Processes in the Liver*. Falk Symposium No. 48. 1988 ISBN: 0-7462-0075-7*
50. Singer MV, Goebell H, eds.: *Nerves and the Gastrointestinal Tract*. Falk Symposium No. 50. 1989 ISBN: 0-7462-0114-1
51. Bannasch P, Keppler D, Weber G, eds.: *Liver Cell Carcinoma*. Falk Symposium No. 51. 1989 ISBN: 0-7462-0111-7
52. Paumgartner G, Stiehl A, Gerok W, eds.: *Trends in Bile Acid Research*. Falk Symposium No. 52. 1989 ISBN: 0-7462-0112-5
53. Paumgartner G, Stiehl A, Barbara L, Roda E, eds.: *Strategies for the Treatment of Hepatobiliary Diseases*. Falk Symposium No. 53. 1990 ISBN: 0-7923-8903-4
54. Bianchi L, Gerok W, Maier K-P, Deinhardt F, eds.: *Infectious Diseases of the Liver*. Falk Symposium No. 54. 1990 ISBN: 0-7923-8902-6
55. Falk Symposium No. 55 not published

55B. Hadziselimovic F, Herzog B, Bürgin-Wolff A, eds.: *Inflammatory Bowel Disease and Coeliac Disease in Children*. International Falk Symposium. 1990 ISBN 0-7462-0125-7

56. Williams CN, eds.: *Trends in Inflammatory Bowel Disease Therapy*. Falk Symposium No. 56. 1990 ISBN: 0-7923-8952-2
57. Bock KW, Gerok W, Matern S, Schmid R, eds.: *Hepatic Metabolism and Disposition of Endo- and Xenobiotics*. Falk Symposium No. 57. 1991 ISBN: 0-7923-8953-0
58. Paumgartner G, Stiehl A, Gerok W, eds.: *Bile Acids as Therapeutic Agents: From Basic Science to Clinical Practice*. Falk Symposium No. 58. 1991 ISBN: 0-7923-8954-9
59. Halter F, Garner A, Tytgat GNJ, eds.: *Mechanisms of Peptic Ulcer Healing*. Falk Symposium No. 59. 1991 ISBN: 0-7923-8955-7
60. Goebell H, Ewe K, Malchow H, Koelbel Ch, eds.: *Inflammatory Bowel Diseases – Progress in Basic Research and Clinical Implications*. Falk Symposium No. 60. 1991 ISBN: 0-7923-8956-5
61. Falk Symposium No. 61 not published
62. Dowling RH, Folsch UR, Löser Ch, eds.: *Polyamines in the Gastrointestinal Tract*. Falk Symposium No. 62. 1992 ISBN: 0-7923-8976-X
63. Lentze MJ, Reichen J, eds.: *Paediatric Cholestasis: Novel Approaches to Treatment*. Falk Symposium No. 63. 1992 ISBN: 0-7923-8977-8
64. Demling L, Frühmorgen P, eds.: *Non-Neoplastic Diseases of the Anorectum*. Falk Symposium No. 64. 1992 ISBN: 0-7923-8979-4

64B. Gressner AM, Ramadori G, eds.: *Molecular and Cell Biology of Liver Fibrogenesis*. International Falk Symposium. 1992 ISBN: 0-7923-8980-8

*These titles were published under the MTP Press imprint.

65. Hadziselimovic F, Herzog B, eds.: *Inflammatory Bowel Diseases and Morbus Hirschprung*. Falk Symposium No. 65. 1992 ISBN: 0-7923-8995-6
66. Martin F, McLeod RS, Sutherland LR, Williams CN, eds.: *Trends in Inflammatory Bowel Disease Therapy*. Falk Symposium No. 66. 1993 ISBN: 0-7923-8827-5
67. Schölmerich J, Kruis W, Goebell H, Hohenberger W, Gross V, eds.: *Inflammatory Bowel Diseases – Pathophysiology as Basis of Treatment*. Falk Symposium No. 67. 1993 ISBN: 0-7923-8996-4
68. Paumgartner G, Stiehl A, Gerok W, eds.: *Bile Acids and The Hepatobiliary System: From Basic Science to Clinical Practice*. Falk Symposium No. 68. 1993 ISBN: 0-7923-8829-1
69. Schmid R, Bianchi L, Gerok W, Maier K-P, eds.: *Extrahepatic Manifestations in Liver Diseases*. Falk Symposium No. 69. 1993 ISBN: 0-7923-8821-6
70. Meyer zum Büschenfelde K-H, Hoofnagle J, Manns M, eds.: *Immunology and Liver*. Falk Symposium No. 70. 1993 ISBN: 0-7923-8830-5
71. Surrenti C, Casini A, Milani S, Pinzani M , eds.: *Fat-Storing Cells and Liver Fibrosis*. Falk Symposium No. 71. 1994 ISBN: 0-7923-8842-9
72. Rachmilewitz D, ed.: *Inflammatory Bowel Diseases – 1994*. Falk Symposium No. 72. 1994 ISBN: 0-7923-8845-3
73. Binder HJ, Cummings J, Soergel KH, eds.: *Short Chain Fatty Acids*. Falk Symposium No. 73. 1994 ISBN: 0-7923-8849-6

73B. Möllmann HW, May B, eds.: *Glucocorticoid Therapy in Chronic Inflammatory Bowel Disease: from basic principles to rational therapy*. International Falk Workshop. 1996 ISBN 0-7923-8708-2

74. Keppler D, Jungermann K, eds.: *Transport in the Liver*. Falk Symposium No. 74. 1994 ISBN: 0-7923-8858-5

74B. Stange EF, ed.: *Chronic Inflammatory Bowel Disease*. Falk Symposium. 1995 ISBN: 0-7923-8876-3

75. van Berge Henegouwen GP, van Hoek B, De Groote J, Matern S, Stockbrügger RW, eds.: *Cholestatic Liver Diseases: New Strategies for Prevention and Treatment of Hepatobiliary and Cholestatic Liver Diseases*. Falk Symposium 75. 1994. ISBN: 0-7923-8867-4
76. Monteiro E, Tavarela Veloso F, eds.: *Inflammatory Bowel Diseases: New Insights into Mechanisms of Inflammation and Challenges in Diagnosis and Treatment*. Falk Symposium 76. 1995. ISBN 0-7923-8884-4
77. Singer MV, Ziegler R, Rohr G, eds.: *Gastrointestinal Tract and Endocrine System*. Falk Symposium 77. 1995. ISBN 0-7923-8877-1
78. Decker K, Gerok W, Andus T, Gross V, eds.: *Cytokines and the Liver*. Falk Symposium 78. 1995. ISBN 0-7923-8878-X
79. Holstege A, Schölmerich J, Hahn EG, eds.: *Portal Hypertension*. Falk Symposium 79. 1995. ISBN 0-7923-8879-8
80. Hofmann AF, Paumgartner G, Stiehl A, eds.: *Bile Acids in Gastroenterology: Basic and Clinical Aspects*. Falk Symposium 80. 1995 ISBN 0-7923-8880-1
81. Riecken EO, Stallmach A, Zeitz M, Heise W, eds.: *Malignancy and Chronic Inflammation in the Gastrointestinal Tract – New Concepts*. Falk Symposium 81. 1995 ISBN 0-7923-8889-5
82. Fleig WE, ed.: *Inflammatory Bowel Diseases: New Developments and Standards*. Falk Symposium 82. 1995 ISBN 0-7923-8890-6

82B. Paumgartner G, Beuers U, eds.: *Bile Acids in Liver Diseases*. International Falk Workshop. 1995 ISBN 0-7923-8891-7
83. Dobrilla G, Felder M, de Pretis G, eds.: *Advances in Hepatobiliary and Pancreatic Diseases: Special Clinical Topics*. Falk Symposium 83. 1995. ISBN 0-7923-8892-5
84. Fromm H, Leuschner U, eds.: *Bile Acids – Cholestasis – Gallstones: Advances in Basic and Clinical Bile Acid Research*. Falk Symposium 84. 1995 ISBN 0-7923-8893-3
85. Tytgat GNJ, Bartelsman JFWM, van Deventer SJH, eds.: *Inflammatory Bowel Diseases*. Falk Symposium 85. 1995 ISBN 0-7923-8894-1
86. Berg PA, Leuschner U, eds.: *Bile Acids and Immunology*. Falk Symposium 86. 1996 ISBN 0-7923-8700-7
87. Schmid R, Bianchi L, Blum HE, Gerok W, Maier KP, Stalder GA, eds.: *Acute and Chronic Liver Diseases: Molecular Biology and Clinics*. Falk Symposium 87. 1996 ISBN 0-7923-8701-5
88. Blum HE, Wu GY, Wu CH, eds.: *Molecular Diagnosis and Gene Therapy*. Falk Symposium 88. 1996 ISBN 0-7923-8702-3
88B. Poupon RE, Reichen J, eds.: *Surrogate Markers to Assess Efficacy of TReatment in Chronic Liver Diseases*. International Falk Workshop. 1996 ISBN 0-7923-8705-8
89. Reyes HB, Leuschner U, Arias IM, eds.: *Pregnancy, Sex Hormones and the Liver*. Falk Symposium 89. 1996 ISBN 0-7923-8704-X
89B. Broelsch CE, Burdelski M, Rogiers X, eds.: *Cholestatic Liver Diseases in Children and Adults*. International Falk Workshop. 1996 ISBN 0-7923-8710-4
90. Lam S-K, Paumgartner P, Wang B, eds.: *Update on Hepatobiliary Diseases 1996*. Falk Symposium 90. 1996 ISBN 0-7923-8715-5
91. Hadziselimovic F, Herzog B, eds.: *Inflammatory Bowel Diseases and Chronic Recurrent Abdominal Pain*. Falk Symposium 91. 1996 ISBN 0-7923-8722-8
91B. Alvaro D, Benedetti A, Strazzabosco M, eds.: *Vanishing Bile Duct Syndrome – Pathophysiology and Treatment*. International Falk Workshop. 1996 ISBN 0-7923-8721-X
92. Gerok W, Loginov AS, Pokrowskij VI, eds.: *New Trends in Hepatology 1996*. Falk Symposium 92. 1997 ISBN 0-7923-8723-6
93. Paumgartner G, Stiehl A, Gerok W, eds.: *Bile Acids in Hepatobiliary Diseases – Basic Research and Clinical Application*. Falk Symposium 93. 1997 ISBN 0-7923-8725-2
94. Halter F, Winton D, Wright NA, eds.: *The Gut as a Model in Cell and Molecular Biology*. Falk Symposium 94. 1997 ISBN 0-7923-8726-0
94B. Kruse-Jarres JD, Schölmerich J, eds.: *Zinc and Diseases of the Digestive Tract*. International Falk Workshop. 1997 ISBN 0-7923-8724-4
95. Ewe K, Eckardt VF, Enck P, eds.: *Constipation and Anorectal Insufficiency*. Falk Symposium 95. 1997 ISBN 0-7923-8727-9
96. Andus T, Goebell H, Layer P, Schölmerich J, eds.: *Inflammatory Bowel Disease – from Bench to Bedside*. Falk Symposium 96. 1997 ISBN 0-7923-8728-7
97. Campieri M, Bianchi-Porro G, Fiocchi C, Schölmerich J, eds. *Clinical Challenges in Inflammatory Bowel Diseases: Diagnosis, Prognosis and Treatment*. Falk Symposium 97. 1998 ISBN 0-7923-8733-3
98. Lembcke B, Kruis W, Sartor RB, eds. *Systemic Manifestations of IBD: The Pending Challenge for Subtle Diagnosis and Treatment*. Falk Symposium 98. 1998 ISBN 0-7923-8734-1

# Falk Symposium Series

99. Goebell H, Holtmann G, Talley NJ, eds. *Functional Dyspepsia and Irritable Bowel Syndrome: Concepts and Controversies.* Falk Symposium 99. 1998 ISBN 0-7923-8735-X
100. Blum HE, Bode Ch, Bode JCh, Sartor RB, eds. *Gut and the Liver.* Falk Symposium 100. 1998 ISBN 0-7923-8736-8
101. Rachmilewitz D, ed. *V International Symposium on Inflammatory Bowel Diseases.* Falk Symposium 101. 1998 ISBN 0-7923-8743-0
102. Manns MP, Boyer JL, Jansen PLM, Reichen J, eds. *Cholestatic Liver Diseases.* Falk Symposium 102. 1998 ISBN 0-7923-8746-5
102B. Manns MP, Chapman RW, Stiehl A, Wiesner R, eds. *Primary Sclerosing Cholangitis.* International Falk Workshop. 1998. ISBN 0-7923-8745-7
103. Häussinger D, Jungermann K, eds. *Liver and Nervous System.* Falk Symposium 102. 1998 ISBN 0-7924-8742-2
103B. Häussinger D, Heinrich PC, eds. *Signalling in the Liver.* International Falk Workshop. 1998 ISBN 0-7923-8744-9
103C. Fleig W, ed. *Normal and Malignant Liver Cell Growth.* International Falk Workshop. 1998 ISBN 0-7923-8748-1
104. Stallmach A, Zeitz M, Strober W, MacDonald TT, Lochs H, eds. *Induction and Modulation of Gastrointestinal Inflammation.* Falk Symposium 104. 1998 ISBN 0-7923-8747-3
105. Emmrich J, Liebe S, Stange EF, eds. *Innovative Concepts in Inflammatory Bowel Diseases.* Falk Symposium 105. 1999 ISBN 0-7923-8749-X
106. Rutgeerts P, Colombel J-F, Hanauer SB, Schölmerich J, Tytgat GNJ, van Gossum A, eds. *Advances in Inflammatory Bowel Diseases.* Falk Symposium 106. 1999 ISBN 0-7923-8750-3
107. Špičák J, Boyer J, Gilat T, Kotrlik K, Mareček Z, Paumgartner G, eds. *Diseases of the Liver and the Bile Ducts – New Aspects and Clinical Implications.* Falk Symposium 107. 1999 ISBN 0-7923-8751-1
108. Paumgartner G, Stiehl A, Gerok W, Keppler D, Leuschner U, eds. *Bile Acids and Cholestasis.* Falk Symposium 108. 1999 ISBN 0-7923-8752-X
109. Schmiegel W, Schölmerich J, eds. *Colorectal Cancer – Molecular Mechanisms, Premalignant State and its Prevention.* Falk Symposium 109. 1999 ISBN 0-7923-8753-8
110. Domschke W, Stoll R, Brasitus TA, Kagnoff MF, eds. *Intestinal Mucosa and its Diseases – Pathophysiology and Clinics.* Falk Symposium 110. 1999 ISBN 0-7923-8754-6
110B. Northfield TC, Ahmed HA, Jazwari RP, Zentler-Munro PL, eds. *Bile Acids in Hepatobiliary Disease.* Falk Workshop. 2000 ISBN 0-7923-8755-4
111. Rogler G, Kullmann F, Rutgeerts P, Sartor RB, Schölmerich J, eds. *IBD at the End of its First Century.* Falk Symposium 111. 2000 ISBN 0-7923-8756-2
112. Krammer HJ, Singer MV, eds. *Neurogastroenterology: From the Basics to the Clinics.* Falk Symposium 112. 2000 ISBN 0-7923-8757-0
113. Andus T, Rogler G, Schlottmann K, Frick E, Adler G, Schmiegel W, Zeitz M, Schölmerich J, eds. *Cytokines and Cell Homeostasis in the Gastrointestinal Tract.* Falk Symposium 113. 2000 ISBN 0-7923-8758-9
114. Manns MP, Paumgartner G, Leuschner U, eds. *Immunology and Liver.* Falk Symposium 114. 2000 ISBN 0-7923-8759-7

www.ingramcontent.com/pod-product-compliance
Ingram Content Group UK Ltd.
Pitfield, Milton Keynes, MK11 3LW, UK
UKHW020134160926
475607UK00003B/36

*9780792387596*